Clinical
Guidelines in
Neonatology

Notice

Medicine is an ever-changing science. As new research and clinical experience broaden our knowledge, changes in treatment and drug therapy are required. The authors and the publisher of this work have checked with sources believed to be reliable in their efforts to provide information that is complete and generally in accord with the standards accepted at the time of publication. However, in view of the possibility of human error or changes in medical sciences, neither the authors nor the publisher nor any other party who has been involved in the preparation or publication of this work warrants that the information contained herein is in every respect accurate or complete, and they disclaim all responsibility for any errors or omissions or for the results obtained from use of the information contained in this work. Readers are encouraged to confirm the information contained herein with other sources. For example and in particular, readers are advised to check the product information sheet included in the package of each drug they plan to administer to be certain that the information contained in this work is accurate and that changes have not been made in the recommended dose or in the contraindications for administration. This recommendation is of particular importance in connection with new or infrequently used drugs.

Clinical Guidelines in Neonatology

Lucky Jain, MD, MBA
George W. Brumley Jr. Professor and
 Chair, Department of Pediatrics
Emory University School of Medicine
Chief Academic Officer,
 Children's Healthcare of Atlanta
Executive Director, Emory and
 Children's Pediatric Institute
Atlanta, Georgia

Gautham K. Suresh, MD, DM, MS, FAAP
Professor of Pediatrics
Baylor College of Medicine
Section Head and Service Chief of Neonatology
Texas Children's Hospital
Houston, Texas

New York   Chicago   San Francisco   Athens   London   Madrid   Mexico City
        Milan   New Delhi   Singapore   Sydney   Toronto

Clinical Guidelines in Neonatology

1 2 3 4 5 6 7 8 9   LCR   24 23 22 21 20 19

ISBN 978-0-07-182025-7
MHID 0-07-182025-6

This book was set in Minion Pro by Cenveo® Publisher Services.
The editor was Andrew Moyer.
The production supervisor was Richard Ruzycka.
Project management was provided by Arushi Chawla, Cenveo Publisher Services.
The cover designer was W2 Design.

Library of Congress Cataloging-in-Publication Data

Names: Jain, Lucky, editor. | Suresh, Gautham K., editor.
Title: Clinical guidelines in neonatology / editors, Lucky Jain, MD, MBA,
  George W. Brumley Jr. Professor and Chair, Department of Pediatrics Emory,
  University School of Medicine, Chief Academic Officer, Children's
  Healthcare of Atlanta, Executive Director, Emory and Children's
  Pediatric Institute, Atlanta, Georgia, Gautham K. Suresh, MD, DM, MS,
  FAAP, Professor of Pediatrics, Baylor College of Medicine, Section Head
  and Service Chief of Neonatology, Texas Children's Hospital, Houston, Texas.
Description: New York : McGraw-Hill Education / Medical, [2019]
Identifiers: LCCN 2019017084 | ISBN 9780071820257 (paperback)
Subjects: LCSH: Neonatology—Handbooks, manuals, etc. |
  Neonatology—Research—Handbooks, manuals, etc. | Pediatrics—Handbooks,
  manuals, etc. | BISAC: MEDICAL / Pediatrics.
Classification: LCC RJ251 .C55 2019 | DDC 618.92/01—dc23

McGraw-Hill Education books are available at special quantity discounts to use as premiums and sales promotions or for use in corporate training programs. To contact a representative, please visit the Contact Us pages at www.mhprofessional.com.

This book is dedicated to neonatologists and pediatricians everywhere who strive to improve the lives of their tiny patients with the highest standards of clinical practice and care delivery.

SECTION EDITORS

Munish Gupta, MD, MMSc
Director, Quality Improvement
Department of Neonatology
Beth Israel Deaconess Medical Center
Assistant Professor of Pediatrics
Harvard Medical School
Boston, Massachusetts

Praveen Kumar, MBBS, DCH, MD, FAAP
Associate Chair
Department of Pediatrics
Visiting Professor of Pediatrics
University of Illinois
Children's Hospital of Illinois
Peoria, Illinois

Ashley Darcy-Mahoney, PhD, NNP, FAAN
Associate Professor
The George Washington University School of Nursing
Director of Infant Research
The George Washington University Autism and Neurodevelopmental
    Disorders Institute
Neonatal Nurse Practitioner, Mednax
Washington, DC

Matthew M. Laughon, MD, MPH
Professor of Pediatrics
Division of Neonatal-Perinatal Medicine
University of North Carolina at Chapel Hill
Chapel Hill, North Carolina

Matthew A. Saxonhouse, MD
Associate Professor
Division of Neonatology
Department of Pediatrics
Levine Children's Hospital at Atrium Healthcare
University of North Carolina Charlotte Campus
Charlotte, North Carolina

Brian Smith, MD, MPH, MHS
Samuel L. Katz Professor of Pediatrics
Division of Neonatal-Perinatal Medicine
Duke University Medical Center
Duke Clinical Research Institute
Durham, North Carolina

Contents

Preface

In the bestselling book, *The Checklist Manifesto*, Atul Gawande laments about the current state of health care in which avoidable failures abound. "We train longer, specialize more, use ever-advancing technologies, and still we fail." Part of the problem, he argues, is that the ever-increasing complexity of medicine makes uniform care delivery impractical or impossible. That is, unless there are guidelines, checklists, or care paths that are readily available to providers.

Standard textbooks, journals, and online resources currently available create excellent repositories of detailed information about the etiology, pathogenesis, clinical picture, diagnosis, and treatment of a condition. However, for a busy clinician looking for the best way to manage a sick patient, a standardized path for effective management of the patient may be impossible to discern. Admittedly, evidence-based practices are simply not available for many maladies, yet for many others, there are conflicting ones. Still, wouldn't it be a lot easier if we all managed simple things in a uniform way using the best available evidence, and tracked easily collated data to make changes? Pediatric oncology groups have done this better than anyone else, and in so doing have transformed their field. Why do we have to wait decades before best practices are made available to every patient?

In neonatology, busy clinicians have all felt the need for a concise, easy-to-use resource at the bedside for evidence-based guidelines, or consensus-driven care paths where high-grade evidence is not available. This book attempts to fill that void and is the product of contributions from numerous authors from all over the world, and the section editors who oversaw the work of individual authors. The book is divided into 11 discrete sections with the chapters in each section having a format different from that of textbooks and manuals. In addition to major recommendations and practice options, chapters also contain suggested quality metrics and descriptions of implementation strategies for the clinical practices. We hope that such an approach will encourage clinicians to apply available evidence to their practice and also track compliance with desired practices. A wide variety of common neonatal problems are addressed in this book. Our goal was not to create an encyclopedic work that included all neonatal topics—we thought that role was best left to the standard, large textbooks of neonatology, of which there are many. We hope that practicing neonatologists, fellows, nurse practitioners, and other NICU personnel will find this book useful in delivering high-quality clinical care to their patients and their families. We remain open to feedback and suggestions about how to improve this resource and how to make it maximally useful to those delivering care at the bedside in the NICU.

Lucky Jain, MD
Gautham K. Suresh, MD
March 2019

Contributors

David H. Adamkin, MD
Professor of Pediatrics
Division of Neonatology
University of Louisville
Louisville, Kentucky

Oluyemisi A. Adeyemi-Fowode, MD, FACOG
Assistant Professor
Department of Obstetrics and Gynecology
Baylor College of Medicine
Division of Pediatric and Adolescent Gynecology
Texas Children's Hospital
Houston, Texas

Saima Aftab, MD
Chief, Section of Neonatology PSA
Medical Director, Perinatal Medicine and
    Fetal Care Program
Nicklaus Children's Hospital
Miami, Florida

Pankaj B. Agrawal, MD, MMSc
Attending Neonatologist
Director
Neonatal Genomics Program
Merton Bernfield Chair in Neonatology
Division of Newborn Medicine
Medical Director
Manton Center Gene Discovery Core
Division of Genetics and Genomics
Boston Children's Hospital
Associate Professor of Pediatrics
Harvard Medical School
Associate Member
Broad Institute of Harvard & MIT
Boston, Massachusetts

Sofia R. Aliaga, MD, MPH, FAAP
Associate Professor of Pediatrics
Neonatal-Perinatal Medicine
University of North Carolina
Chapel Hill, North Carolina

Rajendra Prasad Anne, MBBS, MD, DM
Division of Neonatology
Department of Pediatrics
Postgraduate Institute of Medical Education
    and Research
Chandigarh, India

Wendy A. Araya, DNP, APRN, NNP-BC
Manager
Advance Practice Provider Team
Neonatal Intensive Care Unit
Pediatrics, Department of Neonatology
Monroe Carell Jr. Children's Hospital at
    Vanderbilt
Nashville, Tennessee

Bonnie H. Arzuaga, MD, FAAP
Attending Neonatologist, South Shore Hospital
Instructor of Pediatrics, part-time, Harvard
    Medical School
Course Director for Medical Student Electives in
    Newborn Medicine, Harvard Medical School
Course Director for Observer Education in
    Newborn Medicine, Boston Children's
    Hospital
Division of Newborn Medicine
Boston, Massachusetts

Kamlesh V. Athavale, MD
Assistant Professor
Division of Neonatal Perinatal Medicine
Department of Pediatrics
Duke University
Durham, North Carolina

François Audibert, MD, MSc
Professor
Head, Division of Maternal Fetal Medicine
Department of Obstetrics and Gynecology
CHU Sainte-Justine
Université de Montréal
Montréal, Québec, Canada

Marni Elyse Axelrad, PhD, ABPP
Board Certified in Clinical Child and
    Adolescent Psychology
Psychology Service, Texas Children's Hospital
Professor, Department of Pediatrics
Baylor College of Medicine
Houston, Texas

Eduardo Bancalari, MD
Professor of Pediatrics
University of Miami Miller School of Medicine
Division of Neonatology
Jackson Memorial Holtz Children's Hospital
Miami, Florida

Maria Estefania Barbian, MD
Neonatology Fellow, YR1 PGY4
Emory University
Atlanta, Georgia

Sudeepta K. Basu, MD
Assistant Professor of Pediatrics
Division of Neonatology
Children's National Medical Center
Washington, DC

Beau Batton, MD
Chief of Neonatology and Associate Professor
Department of Pediatrics
Division of Neonatology
Southern Illinois University School of
    Medicine
Springfield, Illinois

David W. Bearl, MD, MA
Assistant Professor
Division of Pediatric Cardiology
Monroe Carell Jr. Children's Hospital at Vanderbilt
Nashville, Tennessee

Daniel K. Benjamin Jr, MD, PhD, MPH
Kiser-Arena Distinguished Professor of
    Pediatrics
Division of Pediatric-Infectious Diseases
Duke University Medical Center
Durham, North Carolina

Vincenzo Berghella, MD
Director of Maternal-Fetal Medicine
Professor of Obstetrics and Gynecology
Thomas Jefferson University
Philadelphia, Pennsylvania

Rupsa C. Boelig, MD
Clinical Instructor
Maternal Fetal Medicine
Thomas Jefferson University Hospital
Philadelphia, Pennsylvania

Isabelle Boucoiran, MD, MSc
Division of Obstetrics and Gynecology
CHU Sainte-Justine
Montreal, Québec, Canada

Andrew C. Bowe, DO, MS, FAAP
Neonatologist
Division of Neonatology
Pediatrix Medical Group of Georgia
Macon, Georgia

Kathleen Brennan, MD
Assistant Professor of Pediatrics
Division of Neonatology
Morgan Stanley Children's Hospital of
    New York Presbyterian
New York, New York

Patrick D. Carroll, MD, MPH
Medical Director, Pediatric and Newborn
Division of Neonatology
Dixie Regional Medical Center
St. George, Utah

Lori Christ, MD
Assistant Professor of Clinical Pediatrics
Division of Neonatology
The Children's Hospital of Philadelphia
Philadelphia, Pennsylvania

Nelson Claure, MSc, PhD
Associate Professor of Pediatrics and
    Biomedical Engineering
Division of Neonatology
Department of Pediatrics
University of Miami Miller School of Medicine
Director
Neonatal Pulmonary Physiology Laboratory
Holtz Children's Hospital
Miami, Florida

Johanna Viau Colindres, MD
Pediatric Endocrinology
Presbyterian Healthcare Services
Albuquerque, New Mexico

C. Michael Cotten, MD, MHS
Chief, Division of Neonatology
Department of Pediatrics
Duke University Medical Center
Durham, North Carolina

Kevin Crezee, BS, RRT-NPS
Clinical Specialist
Division of Medical Affairs
Mallincktodt Pharmaceuticals
Bedminster, New Jersey

Isabelle De Bie, MD, PhD, FRCPC, FCCMG
Medical Geneticist and Clinical Molecular
   Geneticist
Head, Prenatal Diagnosis Program
Clinical Director, Core Molecular Diagnostic
   Laboratory
Division of Medical Genetics, Department of
   Medicine
McGill University Health Centre
Montreal, Québec, Canada

Valérie Désilets, MD
Associate Professor
Department of Pediatrics
Division Medical Genetics
CHU Sherbrooke (Fleurimont)
Sherbrooke, Québec, Canada

Sridevi Devaraj, PhD, DABCC, FAACC, FRSC, CCRP
Medical Director
Clinical Chemistry and Point of
   Care Technology
Texas Children's Hospital and Clearlake
   Health Center
Director of Laboratories
TCH Centers for Women and Children
Professor of Pathology and Immunology
Baylor College of Medicine
Director
Clinical Chemistry Fellowship and Clinical
   Chemistry Resident Rotation
Associate Director
Texas Children's Microbiome Center
Houston, Texas

Robert J. DiGeronimo, MD
University of Washington School of Medicine
Medical Director, NICU
Seattle Children's Hospital
Seattle, Washington

Sourabh Dutta, MBBS, MD, PhD
Division of Neonatology
Department of Pediatrics
Postgraduate Institute of Medical Education
   and Research
Chandigarh, India

Traci Fauerbach, MS, RD, CNSC, LDN
Advanced Practice Clinical Dietitian
Division of Neonatology
Hospital of the University of Pennsylvania
Philadelphia, Pennsylvania

Caraciolo J. Fernandes, MD, MBA, FAAP
Medical Director
Neonatal Transport
Texas Children's Hospital Kangaroo Crew®
Program Director
Congenital Diaphragmatic Hernia/
Pulmonary Hypertension/ECMO Programs
Section of Neonatology
Texas Children's Hospital
Baylor College of Medicine
Associate Professor of Pediatrics
Department of Pediatrics
Houston, Texas

Alejandro Frade Garcia, MD
Pediatric Resident
Nicklaus Children's Hospital
Miami, Florida

Paraskevi Georgiadis, MD, FAAP
Assistant Professor
Department of Pediatrics
Baylor College of Medicine
Division of Neonatology Texas Children's
   Hospital
Houston, Texas

Susan E. Gerber, MD, MPH
Associate Professor, Obstetrics and Gynecology
Division of Maternal-Fetal Medicine
Northwestern Memorial Hospital
Chicago, Illinois

Vani V. Gopalareddy, MD
Director, Hepatology and Liver
   Transplant Program
Division of Gastroenterology
Levine Children's Hospital
Carolinas Medical Center
Charlotte, North Carolina

Phillip V. Gordon, MD, PhD
Director of Neonatology
Mobile Infirmary
Mobile, Alabama

Vinayak Govande, MD, MS, MBA
Neonatologist
Medical Director, NICU
Division of Neonatology
McLane Children's Hospital
Temple, Texas

Sheila K. Gunn, MD
Section of Diabetes and Endocrinology
Department of Pediatrics
Baylor College of Medicine
Houston, Texas

Aaron Hamvas, MD
Raymond and Hazel Speck Barry Professor of
   Neonatology
Head, Division of Neonatology
Ann and Robert H. Lurie Children's Hospital
   of Chicago
Northwestern University Feinberg School of
   Medicine
Chicago, Illinois

Paula Harmon, MD
Director of Hearing Loss
Children's Healthcare of Atlanta
Adjunct Professor, Department of Medicine
   and Pediatrics
Morehouse School of Medicine
Division of Otolaryngology
Children's Healthcare of Atlanta/Pediatric
   ENT of Atlanta
Atlanta, Georgia

Andrew Z. Heling, MD
Neonatologist
Division of Neonatology
Atrium Health, NorthEast Hospital
Vice Chief of Pediatrics
University Hospital
Adjunct Assistant Professor, UNC Department
   of Pediatrics
Concord, North Carolina

Kevin Hill, MD, MS
Associate Professor of Pediatrics
Division of Pediatric Cardiology
Duke University Medical Center
Durham, North Carolina

Catherine Huskins, MSN, APRN, NNP-BC
Team Lead, NICU Advanced Practice Providers
Division of Neonatalogy
The Monroe Carell Jr Children's Hospital at
   Vanderbilt
Nashville, Tennessee

Saleem Islam, MD, MPH
Professor and Division Chief
Division of Pediatric Surgery
University of Florida, College of Medicine
Gainesville, Florida

Kendall R. Johnson, MD
Assistant Professor
Division of Neonatology
Connecticut Children's Medical Center
Hartford, Connecticut

Usama Kanaan, MD
Assistant Professor
Emory University School of Medicine
Division of Pediatric Cardiology
Director, Pulmonary Hypertension Program
Children's Healthcare of Atlanta
Atlanta, Georgia

Lefkothea Karaviti, MD, PhD
Section of Diabetes and Endocrinology
Department of Pediatrics
Baylor College of Medicine
Houston, Texas

Lakshmi Katakam, MD, MPH, FAAP
Medical Director, NICU
Texas Children's Hospital
Associate Professor of Pediatrics
Baylor College of Medicine
Houston, Texas

Sarah D. Keene, MD, FAAP
Assistant Professor
Division of Neonatal-Perinatal Medicine
Emory University School of Medicine
Atlanta, Georgia

Matthew S. Kelly, MD, MPH
Assistant Professor of Pediatrics
Division of Pediatric Infectious Diseases
Duke University
Durham, North Carolina

Martin Keszler, MD
Professor of Pediatrics
Alpert Medical School of Brown University
Division of Neonatology
Women and Infants Hospital of Rhode Island
Providence, Rhode Island

Megan Lagoski, MD
Assistant Professor of Pediatrics
Division of Pediatrics, Neonatology
Ann & Robert H. Lurie Children's Hospital
Northwestern University Feinberg School of
    Medicine
Chicago, Illinois

Satyan Lakshminrusimha, MD
Dennis and Nancy Marks Chair
Professor of Pediatrics
Division Pediatrician-in-Chief
UC Davis Children's Hospital
Sacramento, California

Kiersten LeBar, DNP, MMHC, CPNP-AC
Director Advanced Practice
Vanderbilt University Medical Center
Nashville, Tennessee

Heena K. Lee, MD, MPH
Pediatrics Instructor
Department of Pediatrics
Harvard Medical School
Attending Pediatrician
Department of Neonatology
Beth Israel Deaconess Medical Center
Boston, Massachusetts

Stephanie Si-Tang Lee, MD
Division of Newborn Medicine
St. Louis Children's Hospital/Washington
    University School of Medicine
St. Louis, Missouri

Shannon N. Liang, MD
Assistant Clinical Professor
Division of Child Neurology
University of California Davis Medical Center
Sacramento, California

Ashley M. Lucke, MD, FAAP
Instructor
Fetal Medicine Fellow
Division of Neonatology
Children's National Medical Center
Washington, DC

Renee M. Madden, MS, MD
Assistant Medical Director
The Bleeding and Clotting Disorders Institute
Peoria, Illinois

Sarah Mapp, MD
Staff Physician
Division of Neonatology
Mednax
San Antonio, Texas

Bobby Mathew, MBBS
Assistant Professor of Pediatrics
University of Buffalo
Division of Neonatology
Oishei Children's Hospital
Buffalo, New York

Amit M. Mathur, MBBS, MD, MRCP(UK)
Professor of Pediatrics
Newborn Medicine
Washington University School of Medicine
    and St. Louis Children's Hospital
St. Louis, Missouri

Ross McKinney Jr, MD
Professor Emeritus
Pediatric Infectious Diseases
Duke University Medical Center
Durham, North Carolina

Amy R. Mehollin-Ray, MD
Associate Professor, Department of Radiology
Baylor College of Medicine
Staff Radiologist
E.B. Singleton Department of Pediatric
    Radiology
Texas Children's Hospital
Houston, Texas

James E. Moore, MD, PhD
Division Chief Neonatology
Division of Neonatal-Perinatal Medicine
Connecticut Children's Medical Center
Hartford, Connecticut

Hallie Morris, MD
Division of Neonatology
Washington University School of Medicine
St. Louis, Missouri

Sarah U. Morton, MD, PhD
Physician-in-Medicine
Division of Newborn Medicine
Boston Children's Hospital
Boston, Massachusetts
Instructor, Department of Pediatrics
Harvard Medical School
Boston, Massachusetts

Colleen Moss, MSN, APRN, NNP-BC
Neonatal Nurse Practitioner
Neonatal Advanced Practice Providers
Division of Neonatology
Monroe Carell Jr. Children's Hospital at
 Vanderbilt
Nashville, Tennessee

Sagori Mukhopadhyay, MD, MMSc
Assistant Professor of Pediatrics
Perelman School of Medicine
University of Pennsylvania
Division of Neonatology
Children's Hospital of Philadelphia
Philadelphia, Pennsylvania

**Helen L. Nation, MSN, APRN, NNP-BC,
 C-NPT**
Division of Neonatology
Vanderbilt University School of Nursing
Nashville, Tennessee

Elizabeth K. Oh, MD
Instructor, Department of Pediatrics
Harvard Medical School
Attending Pediatrician
Department of Neonatology
Beth Israel Deaconess Medical Center
Boston, Massachusetts

Mitali Pakvasa, MD
Assistant Professor of Pediatrics
Division of Neonatology
Emory University
Atlanta, Georgia

Ravi M. Patel, MD, MSc
Associate Professor of Pediatrics
Division of Neonatology
Emory University School of Medicine and
 Children's Healthcare of Atlanta
Atlanta, Georgia

Roberta Pineda, PhD, OTR/L
Assistant Professor
Washington University School of Medicine
Program in Occupational Therapy, Pediatrics
St. Louis, Missouri

Richard A. Polin, MD, FAAP
William T Speck Professor of Pediatrics
Columbia University
Executive Vice-Chair, Department of Pediatrics
Division of Neonatology
Columbia University Medical Center
New York, New York

Michael A. Posencheg, MD
Associate Chief Medical Officer
Value Improvement
Penn Medicine
Medical Director, Intensive Care Nursery
Hospital of the University of Pennsylvania
Professor of Clinical Pediatrics
Perelman School of Medicine
University of Pennsylvania
Attending Neonatologist
Division of Neonatology
Children's Hospital of Philadelphia
Philadelphia, Pennsylvania

Wayne A. Price, MD
Professor, Pediatrics
Division of Neonatal-Perinatal Medicine
North Carolina Children's Hospital
University of North Carolina at Chapel Hill
Chapel Hill, North Carolina

Karen M. Puopolo, MD, PhD
Associate Professor of Pediatrics
University of Pennsylvania Perelman School of
 Medicine
Division of Neonatology
Children's Hospital of Philadelphia
Philadelphia, Pennsylvania

Roy Rajan, MD
Pediatric Otolaryngologist
Pediatric Surgical Specialties
Lehigh Valley Health Network
Allentown, Pennsylvania

Charlotte Ramieh, DNP, APRN, NNP-BC
Neonatal Nurse Practitioner
Pediatrix Medical Group of Tennessee
Nashville, Tennessee

Mary R. Raney, MSN, NNP-BC, WCC
Neonatal Nurse Practitioner
Neonatal Intensive Care Unit
St. Louis Children's Hospital
St. Louis, Missouri

Cynthia E. Rogers, MD
Associate Professor
Departments of Psychiatry and Pediatrics
Division of Child and Adolescent Psychiatry
Washington University School of Medicine
St. Louis, Missouri

Robert W. Rothstein, MD
Interim Chief, Newborn Medicine
Assistant Professor Pediatrics
University of Massachusetts Medical School
Worcester, Massachusetts
Adjunct Assistant Professor of Pediatrics
Tufts University School of Medicine
Boston, Massachusetts
Division of Newborn Medicine
Baystate Children's Hospital
Springfield, Massachusetts

Grant J. Shafer, MD, MA, FAAP
Neonatal-Perinatal Medicine Fellow
Department of Pediatrics, Division of
    Neonatology
Baylor College of Medicine/Texas Children's
    Hospital
Houston, Texas

Yunru Shao, MMSc, LCGC
Invitae Corporation
San Francisco, California

Prem S. Shekhawat, MD
Associate Professor
Department of Pediatrics
Division of Neonatal-Perinatal Medicine
Vice Chair of Research
MetroHealth Medical Center
Case Western Reserve University
MetroHealth Medical Center
Cleveland, Ohio

Jeffrey S. Shenberger, MD
Professor of Pediatrics
Division of Neonatology
Brenner Children's Hospital
Winston-Salem, North Carolina

Dawn Simon, MD
Associate Professor of Pediatrics
Division of Pulmonary Medicine
Emory University School of Medicine
Atlanta, Georgia

Rachana Singh, MD, MS
Medical Director, NICU
Associate Professor of Pediatrics
University of Massachusetts Medical
    School–Baystate
Division of Newborn Medicine
Baystate Children's Hospital
Springfield, Massachusetts

Joan R. Smith, PhD, RN, NNP-BC
Director Quality, Safety & Practice Excellence
Division of Nursing
St. Louis Children's Hospital
St. Louis, Missouri

Christopher D. Smyser, MD, MSCI
Associate Professor of Neurology, Pediatrics,
    and Radiology
Division of Pediatric and Developmental
    Neurology
Washington University in St. Louis/St. Louis
    Children's Hospital
St. Louis, Missouri

Moeun Son, MD, MSCI
Assistant Professor
Division of Maternal Fetal Medicine
Department of Obstetrics and Gynecology
Northwestern University
Feinberg School of Medicine
Chicago, Illinois

Diane L. Spatz, PhD, RN-BC, FAAN
Professor of Perinatal Nursing
Helen M. Shearer Professor of Nutrition
University of Pennsylvania School of Nursing
Nurse Researcher
Manager of Lactation Program
The Children's Hospital of Philadelphia (CHOP)
Clinical Coordinator of the CHOP's Mothers'
    Milk Bank
Philadelphia, Pennsylvania

Poyyapakkam R. Srivaths, MD, MS, FAAP
Associate Professor
Division Renal Section
Department of Pediatrics
Hospital Baylor College of Medicine
Houston, Texas

Nathan C. Sundgren, MD, PhD
Assistant Professor of Pediatrics
Division of Neonatology
Texas Children's Hospital
Houston, Texas

Gautham K. Suresh, MD, DM, MS, FAAP
Professor of Pediatrics
Baylor College of Medicine
Section Head and Service Chief of
    Neonatology
Texas Children's Hospital
Houston, Texas

Vernon R. Sutton, MD
Department of Molecular and Human
    Genetics
Baylor College of Medicine
Houston, Texas

Jonathan R. Swanson, MD, MSc
Associate Professor of Pediatrics
Medical Director, NICU
Department of Pediatrics
Division of Neonatology
University of Virginia Children's Hospital
Charlottesville, Virginia

Michael D. Tarantino, MD
Medical Director and President
The Bleeding and Clotting Disorders Institute
Professor of Pediatrics and Medicine
University of Illinois College of
    Medicine-Peoria
Peoria, Illinois

Sarah N. Taylor, MD, MSCR
Associate Professor of Pediatrics
Yale School of Medicine
New Haven, Connecticut

Wendy L. Timpson, MD, MEd
Instructor of Pediatrics
Division of Newborn Medicine
Harvard Medical School
Boston, Massachusetts

Jennifer M. Trzaski, MD
Assistant Professor of Pediatrics
Division of Neonatology
Connecticut Children's Medical Center
University of Connecticut School of
    Medicine
Hartford, Connecticut

Duong D. Tu, MD
Assistant Professor
Department of Urology
Texas Children's Hospital
Baylor College of Medicine
Houston, Texas

Kelly C. Wade, MD, PhD, MSCE
Associate Professor of Clinical Pediatrics
Perelman School of Medicine
Division Neonatology
Children's Hospital of Philadelphia
CHOP Newborn Care at Pennsylvania
    Hospital
Philadelphia, Pennsylvania

Ari J. Wassner, MD
Director, Thyroid Program
Boston Children's Hospital
Fellowship Program Director
Division of Endocrinology
Boston Children's Hospital
Assistant Professor of Pediatrics
Harvard Medical School
Boston, Massachusetts

Monica Hsiung Wojcik, MD
Fellow
Divisions of Newborn Medicine and Genetics
    and Genomics
Boston Children's Hospital
Boston, Massachusetts

Bradley A. Yoder, MD
Professor of Pediatrics
Division Chief, Division of Neonatology
Hospital University of Utah
Salt Lake City, Utah

Kanecia Zimmerman, MD, MPH
Assistant Professor
Division of Pediatric Critical Care Medicine
Duke Children's Hospital
Durham, North Carolina

Antenatal and Perinatal Management

Preterm Labor

Rupsa C. Boelig, MD • Vincenzo Berghella, MD

SCOPE

DISEASE/CONDITION(S)

Preterm labor (PTL) and preterm premature rupture of membranes (PPROM)

GUIDELINE OBJECTIVE(S)

Define PTL and PPROM; outline diagnosis and initial assessment of PTL and PPROM; review evidence-based management practices in PTL and PPROM including the appropriate initiation and selection of tocolytics, antibiotics, corticosteroids, and magnesium sulfate.

BRIEF BACKGROUND

Preterm birth (PTB) is one of the leading causes of neonatal morbidity and mortality. In the United States in 2013, 11.39% of all births were preterm. Neonatal complications of PTB include respiratory, gastrointestinal, and neurological difficulties as well as long-term neurodevelopmental deficits. The annual cost of PTB in the United States was estimated to be $26.2 billion in 2005. While approximately 35% of PTBs are iatrogenic for maternal or fetal indications, the majority are spontaneous preterm births (sPTB), of which 40–45% are related to preterm labor (PTL) and 25–30% are due to preterm premature rupture of membranes (PPROM). Both PTL and PPROM are considered to be part of a syndrome with multiple inciting mechanisms including inflammation, infection, uterine overdistension, uteroplacental ischemia/hemorrhage, and other immune-mediated processes that ultimately lead to PTB. In most cases, a precise mechanism or cause cannot be identified.

TABLE 1.1. Risk Factors for Preterm Birth

Maternal Demographic and Social History
- Race (African American at higher risk compared to Asian, Caucasian, and Hispanic)
- Age ≥35 or <17
- BMI >35 or <19
- Tobacco use
- Substance use disorder (opiate or cocaine)
- Low socioeconomic status

Obstetric/Gynecologic History
- Prior preterm birth (>20 weeks) or late second trimester loss (>16 weeks)
- Multiple dilation and evacuations
- History of sexually transmitted infections
- Prior cervical surgery
- Uterine anomaly

Current Pregnancy Characteristics
- Short-interval pregnancy (<6 months)
- Fetal disease: growth restriction, poly or oligohydramnios, major congenital or chromosomal anomaly
- Assisted reproductive technologies
- Abnormal placentation
- Bacterial vaginosis this pregnancy
- Vaginal bleeding
- Maternal infection: urinary tract, sexually transmitted
- Depression/anxiety/significant psychosocial stressors
- Maternal medical comorbidities: hypertension, diabetes, asthma, thyroid disease
- Abdominal surgery
- Multiple gestations
- Cervical length ≤25 mm between 16 and 24 weeks

Risk factors for sPTB are outlined in Table 1.1; although there are a number of demographic, medical, social, and antepartum factors associated with PTB, the most significant historical risk factor is a history of a prior sPTB.

DIAGNOSIS OF PRETERM LABOR

PTL has been traditionally defined by the clinical criteria of regular uterine contractions with a change in cervical dilation and/or effacement, or by the presentation of regular uterine contractions and a cervical dilation of at least 2 cm in pregnant women between 20 and 36 6/7 weeks' gestation. Unfortunately, this clinical criteria alone has a limited positive predictive value, with >70% of women presenting in this manner ultimately delivering at term. A more accurate definition may be regular uterine contractions with a transvaginal ultrasound cervical length (TVU CL) <20 mm or TVU CL 20–29 mm, with a positive fetal fibronectin (FFN) between about 22 and 36 weeks. The sensitivity of this approach in predicting sPTB within 7 days is >70%, and the negative predictive value is >98%, with a positive predictive value of ~45%. The sensitivity and positive likelihood for this screening approach is highest for predicting PTB risk within 7 days at earlier gestational ages, <28 weeks. Knowledge of the CL and FFN has been shown to

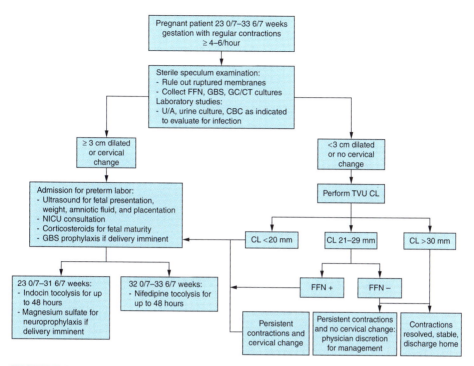

FIGURE 1.1 • Diagnosis and management of preterm labor. (Adapted from Berghella V. Preterm labor. In: Berghella V, ed. *Obstetric Evidence-Based Guidelines*. 2nd ed. London, UK: Informa Healthcare;2012:164-76.)

improve the ability of the physician to decrease evaluation time and prevent unnecessary hospital admissions among women with CL ≥30 mm with no increased rate of sPTB or failure to appropriately administer steroids in those who delivered before 34 weeks. Figure 1.1 outlines the diagnosis of PTL and basic management strategy.

INITIAL ASSESSMENT OF PRETERM LABOR

The evaluation of women with possible PTL includes a thorough history, physical examination including sterile speculum and vaginal examination, laboratory studies, and ultrasound.

HISTORY

The history should include a review of symptoms of PTL such as cramping, abdominal pain, back pain, pelvic pressure, and vaginal bleeding. It should also evaluate for risk factors of PTB (Table 1.1).

PHYSICAL EXAMINATION

- Sterile speculum examination and evaluation for any genital tract infection, evaluate for ruptured membranes (nitrazine, ferning, pooling), collect group B streptococcal (GBS) culture, and FFN
- Sterile vaginal examination to evaluate for dilation

- Uterine tone, tenderness
- Evaluation for signs of chorioamnionitis—two or more of the following: uterine tenderness, fever ≥100.4, maternal tachycardia, fetal tachycardia, in the absence of other sources of infection

LABORATORY STUDIES

- Urine analysis and urine culture
- CBC if indicated to evaluate for infection
- Gonorrhea and chlamydia cultures
- GBS culture

ULTRASOUND

- Confirmation of gestational age
- Estimated fetal weight and amniotic fluid index
- Transvaginal cervical length

RECOMMENDATIONS FOR PRETERM LABOR

MAJOR RECOMMENDATIONS

Following the diagnosis of PTL, the following steps should be taken to maximize neonatal outcome: for pregnancies between 24 0/7 and 33 6/7 weeks, a course of corticosteroids for fetal maturity; for pregnancies between 24 0/7 and 31 6/7 weeks, magnesium sulfate for neuroprotection if delivery is anticipated; for pregnancies between 24 0/7 and 36 6/7 weeks, antibiotic prophylaxis for GBS should be initiated if GBS status is positive or unknown and delivery is anticipated. Magnesium sulfate and GBS prophylaxis may be discontinued after 12 hours if delivery is no longer considered imminent. Once stable, transfer to a center with the appropriate neonatal capabilities should be strongly considered.

In the event of PTL in pregnancies between 24 0/7 and 33 6/7 weeks, in the absence of contraindications, tocolytics should be given with the intention of delaying delivery at least 48 hours to allow for the administration of corticosteroids and transfer if necessary. Between gestational ages 24 0/7 and 31 6/7, the tocolytics of choice are indomethacin or nifedipine; between 32 0/7 and 33 6/7, the tocolytic of choice is nifedipine. Tocolytics are not indicated ≥34 0/7 weeks.

PRACTICE OPTIONS

Practice Option #1: Counseling

The patient should be appropriately counseled regarding the morbidity and mortality for neonates at her gestational age using the most up-to-date, institution-specific if possible, outcome data. Patients at risk for a periviable delivery (22–25 weeks' gestation) are particularly challenging to counsel. The morbidity and mortality along with options for intervention at this gestational age are often institution dependent. For more details on the management of periviable gestations see Chapter 2.

Practice Option #2: Transfer

Once a patient has been diagnosed with PTL or PPROM, the first step in management is to assess the available resources. If appropriate care is not available for the gestational age of the neonate, transfer to a tertiary care center with appropriate neonatal support is recommended. Transport of the mother prior to delivery has been shown to improve outcomes compared to neonatal transport after delivery, including decreased rates of respiratory distress syndrome (RDS), grade III or IV intraventricular hemorrhage, and neonatal mortality.

Practice Option #3: Interventions for Neonatal Benefit

During the initial management of a patient diagnosed with PTL or PPROM, it is often difficult to predict whether labor will be able to be arrested or delayed. As such, the following interventions should be considered to maximize the neonatal outcome should the patient deliver preterm.

Corticosteroids. Betamethasone and dexamethasone are the only two corticosteroids that cross the placenta, and are used for fetal benefit for gestational ages 24 0/7–33 6/7.

Dose. Betamethasone 12 mg IM q24h × 2 doses or dexamethasone 6 mg IM q6h × 4 doses.

Contraindications. None

Effectiveness. Antenatal corticosteroids are effective in reducing the risk of RDS, intraventricular hemorrhage (IVH), and neonatal mortality. The benefit of corticosteroids applies to gestational ages 24 0/7–33 6/7 weeks and is most marked at 48 hours to 7 days from the first dose. Some studies have demonstrated benefit in reducing neonatal death at 23 0/7–23 6/7 weeks. Dexamethasone is associated with a reduced risk of IVH compared to betamethasone, and one trial found an association with decreased neonatal intensive care unit (NICU) stay. When compiling data to calculate indirect comparisons of dexamethasone and betamethasone, betamethasone was associated with a decreased risk of RDS and chorioamnionitis. A rescue course of steroids received before 33 weeks may have additional benefit if the initial treatment was given at least 7–14 days prior; beyond this, multiple courses (>2) are not recommended due to an association with reduced birth weight and smaller infant head size.

Conclusion. Women at risk for PTB within 7 days at gestational ages 23 0/7–33 6/7 should receive a course of antenatal corticosteroids to improve neonatal outcomes. An additional rescue dose may be given if the patient presents again at less than 33 weeks and the initial course was over 2 weeks ago. Multiple courses of steroids (>2) are not recommended due to an association with reduced birth weight and head circumference.

Magnesium Sulfate for Neuroprotection

Dose. Magnesium sulfate 6 g loading dose IV over 20–30 minutes followed by maintenance infusion 2 g/hour until delivery.

Contraindications. Myasthenia gravis is the only absolute contraindication. Caution should be used with cardiac disease, conduction defects, and significant renal impairment.

Effectiveness. The administration of magnesium sulfate significantly reduces the rate of cerebral palsy and gross motor dysfunction when administered prior to 32 weeks.

Conclusion. Magnesium sulfate should be administered for neuroprotection between gestational ages 24 0/7 and 31 6/7. If delivery has not occurred within 12 hours and is not considered imminent, it may be discontinued.

Antibiotics for Group B Streptococcal Sepsis Prophylaxis. Any patient at risk of imminent delivery <37 weeks who are either GBS unknown or GBS positive should receive antibiotic GBS prophylaxis according to Centers for Disease Control and Prevention (CDC) guidelines to prevent neonatal GBS sepsis. Antibiotics may be discontinued if delivery is no longer considered imminent.

Practice Option #4: Tocolysis for Preterm Labor

The goals of tocolysis are to prolong pregnancy for 48 hours to allow for the administration of steroids for fetal lung maturity and to allow for safe maternal transfer to an appropriate institution if needed. Tocolysis should be limited to those women who have met diagnostic criteria for PTL with intact membranes (Figure 1.1) and is generally not indicated after 34 weeks' gestation. Tocolysis is contraindicated in certain scenarios. Maternal contraindications include chorioamnionitis, heavy vaginal bleeding concerning for abruption, or other antepartum conditions such as severe preeclampsia that warrant delivery. Fetal contraindications include demise, major congenital or chromosomal abnormality, especially one that is not compatible with life. There are several classes of tocolytics: betamimetics, calcium channel blockers (CCBs), cyclooxygenase (COX) inhibitors, oxytocin receptor antagonist (ORA), nitric oxide donors (NODs), and magnesium sulfate. See Table 1.2 for a summary of the different classes of tocolytics.

Betamimetics. The most commonly used betamimetic is terbutaline, although ritodrine is also an option.

Dose. Ritodrine: 50–100 µg/min IV initial dose, may increase 50 µg/min q10min (max dose 350 µg/min) 1–2 mg PO q2–4h. Terbutaline: 0.25 mg SQ q20–30min initially up to four doses, then q2–4h; 2.5–5 µg/min IV, increase every 20–30 minutes by 2.5–5 µg/min (max 30 µg/min); 2.5–5 mg PO q2–4h for 24 hours. Hold for heart rate ≥120 bpm.

Contraindications. Significant cardiac disease, arrhythmia, poorly controlled diabetes, poorly controlled thyroid disease (for ritodrine specifically).

Effectiveness. A Cochrane review in 2014 of 12 trials found that betamimetics decreased the number of women in PTL giving birth within 48 hours, and within 7 days, but there was no evidence of reduction in PTB (<37 weeks). There was also no significant reduction in neonatal outcomes. There was a significant association with withdrawal from treatment due to adverse effects, and a significantly greater number of adverse effects compared to placebo. There were insufficient data to support the use of one betamimetic over another.

Conclusion. Betamimetics are effective at reducing the rate of delivery within 48 hours and 7 days, thus allowing for the administration of corticosteroids for fetal lung maturity and transfer to a tertiary care institution; however they should be used with caution, given multiple frequent adverse effects.

Calcium Channel Blockers. The main CCB used for tocolysis is nifedipine, although nicardipine may also be used.

Dose. Initial dose of nifedipine is 20–30 mg PO, then 10–20 mg PO q4–8h (max 90 mg/day).

Contraindications. Left ventricular dysfunction or congestive heart failure, hypotension (<90/50). Due to a theoretical concern for synergistic suppression of muscle contractility, use with magnesium sulfate is not recommended.

TABLE 1.2. Summary of Tocolytic Therapies

Tocolytic Class	Dose	Contraindication	Major Adverse Effects	Summary of Efficacy
Betamimetics				
Ritodrine	50–100 μg/min IV initial dose, may increase 50 μg/min q10min (max dose 350 μg/min); 1–2 mg PO q2–4h	Significant cardiac disease, arrhythmia, poorly controlled diabetes, poorly controlled thyroid disease (for ritodrine)	Maternal: Hypokalemia, hyperglycemia, tachycardia, chest pain, shortness of breath, arrhythmia, EKG changes, pulmonary edema, rare myocardial ischemia	Effective in delaying preterm birth to allow for administration of corticosteroids and transfer if necessary; however should be used with caution given multiple, frequent adverse effects
Terbutaline	0.25 mg SQ q20–30min initially up to four doses, then q2–4h; 2.5–5 μg/min IV, increase every 20–30 minutes by 2.5–5 μg/min (max 30 μg/min); 2.5–5 mg PO q2–4h for 24 hours; hold for heart rate ≥120 bpm		Fetal: Tachycardia, hyperinsulinemia, hypoglycemia, hypocalcemia, hypobilirubinemia, hypotension, rare myocardial ischemia	
Calcium Channel Blockers				
Nifedipine	20–30 mg PO, then 10–20 mg PO q4–8h (max 90 mg/day)	Left ventricular dysfunction or congestive heart failure, hypotension (<90/50) Due to a theoretical concern for synergistic suppression of muscle contractility, use with magnesium sulfate is not recommended	Maternal: Hypotension, tachycardia Fetal: None	Effective in delaying birth to allow for administration of corticosteroids with fewer adverse effects compared with other tocolytics

(Continued)

TABLE 1.2. Summary of Tocolytic Therapies (Continued)

Tocolytic Class	Dose	Contraindication	Major Adverse Effects	Summary of Efficacy
Cyclooxygenase Inhibitors				
Indomethacin	50–100 mg vaginal, rectal, or oral followed by 25 mg q6h for 48 hours	Renal or hepatic disease, active peptic ulcers, poorly controlled hypertension, NSAID-sensitive asthma, platelet or coagulative dysfunction Gestational age ≥32 weeks	Maternal: GERD, gastritis Fetal/neonatal: Short-term use not associated with significant adverse effects Prolonged use >48 hours associated with oligohydramnios and renal insufficiency Use after 32 weeks associated with constriction of ductus arteriosus, hydrops, pulmonary hypertension, and death	Effective in delaying birth and reducing preterm birth with few maternal and fetal effects when used for a short course up to 48 hours prior to 32 weeks' gestation.
Magnesium Sulfate	4–6 g IV bolus over 20 minutes, then continuous infusion 2 g/hour	Myasthenia gravis, cardiac disease, cardiac conduction defects; significant renal impairment	Maternal: Rare pulmonary edema and cardiac arrest Fetal: Lethargy, hypotonia, hypocalcemia, respiratory depression	Current evidence does not demonstrate significant benefit in the use of magnesium sulfate for the purpose of tocolysis

Agent	Dosing		Adverse Effects	Comments
Oxytocin Receptor Antagonist Atosiban	6.75 ng bolus then 300 μg/min IV× 3 hours, then 100 μg/min up to 45 hours	None	Maternal: No serious adverse effects Fetal: None	Studies with mixed results Currently there is insufficient evidence to support use of oxytocin receptor antagonists as a tocolytic for the delay or prevention of preterm birth
Nitric Oxide Donors Nitroglycerine	0.4 mg/hour transdermal patch			Current evidence does not support the benefit of nitroglycerine as a tocolytic to delay or prevent preterm birth
Progestational Agents	Variable dosing for oral, vaginal, intramuscular	None	Maternal: No serious adverse effects Fetal: None	Current evidence does not support the benefit of progesterone as a tocolytic, although vaginal progesterone and 17-alpha-hydroxyprogesterone may be beneficial for maintenance tocolysis once preterm labor has been arrested

Effectiveness. A Cochrane review of 26 trials found that CCBs compared to no treatment or placebo were effective at decreasing birth within 48 hours with an increase in adverse maternal effects. CCBs were superior to betamimetics in that they had fewer maternal adverse effects, less discontinuation of treatment, decreased rate of preterm and very preterm birth, and improved neonatal outcomes. Compared with ORAs, one study found an increase in gestational age at birth (1.2 weeks) and a reduction in PTB, admission to NICU, and duration of stay in NICU, but also a higher rate of adverse maternal effects. Compared with magnesium sulfate, CCBs were associated with reduced maternal adverse effects, reduced pulmonary edema, and reduced duration of NICU stay. There is no significant difference in gestational age at delivery or delay of birth for 48 hours or 7 days between nifedipine and magnesium sulfate. No differences were found in comparisons with NOs or NSAIDs, although the numbers were small.

Conclusion. CCBs have been demonstrated to be beneficial over placebo in delaying birth to allow for the administration of corticosteroids and possible transfer; they are also associated with few, not severe, maternal side effects and no adverse fetal or neonatal effects, making them a favorable tocolytic to use in practice.

Cyclooxygenase Inhibitors. The main COX inhibitor used is indomethacin, although others used include ketorolac and sulindac.

Dose. Indomethacin 50–100 mg vaginal, rectal, or oral followed by 25 mg q6h for 48 hours prior to 32 weeks.

Contraindications. Renal or hepatic disease, active peptic ulcers, poorly controlled hypertension, NSAID-sensitive asthma, platelet or coagulative dysfunction. Gestational age ≥32 weeks.

Effectiveness. A Cochrane review in 2005 found that indomethacin compared with placebo resulted in a reduction in PTB (<37 weeks), an increase in gestational age (weighted MD 3.53 weeks) and birthweight. There was also found to be a trend toward reduction in delivery within 48 hours. Two reviews found no difference in perinatal outcomes including mortality, RDS, premature closure of ductus arteriosus, and persistent pulmonary hypertension of the newborn, IVH, and necrotizing enterocolitis (NEC). A more recent review did find that antenatal exposure to indomethacin was associated with an increased risk of grade II–IV IVH, NEC, and periventricular leukomalacia. Compared to other tocolytics, COX inhibitors resulted in a reduction in PTB (<37 weeks) and reduced maternal adverse reaction requiring cessation in treatment. There was a trend toward a reduction in the number of women delivering within 48 hours for COX inhibitors, but no difference in the number of women delivering within 7 days. There was also a trend toward increased oligohydramnios associated with COX inhibitors, although this has been shown to be reversible on discontinuation of therapy. There was no difference found between nonselective COX inhibitors versus selective COX-2 inhibitors in maternal or neonatal outcomes.

Conclusion. Given few maternal adverse effects and few fetal/neonatal effects with short-term use as well as the favorable outcomes compared to both placebo and other tocolytics, indomethacin is a relatively safe and effective option for tocolysis for up to 48 hours at gestational ages <32 weeks.

Magnesium Sulfate

Dose. 4–6 g IV bolus over 20 minutes, then continuous infusion at 2 g/hour. In the setting of renal impairment, the continuous infusion may be reduced to 1 g/hour.

Contraindications. Myasthenia gravis, cardiac disease, cardiac conduction defects, significant renal impairment.

Effectiveness. A Cochrane review of 37 trials found no benefit for magnesium sulfate in reducing birth within 48 hours or PTB compared to placebo or alternative tocolytics. There was also no difference found in gestational age at birth, or serious adverse neonatal outcomes, except there was borderline increased risk of total death when compared with placebo (RR 4.56, 95% CI 1.00 to 20.86). Multiple other prior reviews have found similar lack of efficacy in magnesium as a tocolytic agent. That being said, there was one meta-analysis that found that magnesium sulfate compared to placebo significantly reduced birth within 48 hours.

Conclusion. Current evidence does not demonstrate significant benefit in the use of magnesium sulfate for the purpose of tocolysis in PTL.

Oxytocin Receptor Antagonists

Dose. Atosiban 6.75-mg bolus, then 300 µg/min IV × 3 hours, then 100 µg/min up to 45 hours.

Contraindications. None.

Effectiveness. A Cochrane review of four studies found that compared to placebo there was no difference in birth within 48 hours, PTB <38 weeks perinatal mortality, or major neonatal morbidity. Another review found that women receiving atosiban were less likely to deliver within 48 hours if randomized ≥25.5 weeks and less likely to deliver within 7 days if randomized ≥26.4 weeks, based on one randomized trial. Compared to betamimetics there was no significant difference in birth within 48 hours, PTB, perinatal mortality, or major neonatal morbidity. ORAs were associated with fewer maternal adverse effects requiring cessation of treatment. In two studies that compared ORA to CCBs there was no difference in birth within 48 hours or in extremely PTB. One trial demonstrated an increase in PTB <37 weeks, a lower gestational age at birth, and an increase admission to the NICU with ORA. ORA did have fewer maternal adverse effects.

Conclusion. Although ORAs may have fewer maternal side effects compared with other tocolytics, given the mixed results on efficacy there is insufficient evidence to suggest a benefit compared to placebo or other tocolytics in delaying or preventing PTB.

Nitric Oxide Donors

Dose. Nitroglycerine transdermal patch 0.4 mg/hour.

Effectiveness. Compared to placebo, there was no evidence that NOD delayed delivery >48 hours or reduced PTB <37 weeks or reduced neonatal morbidity or mortality. Compared to other tocolytics, there was no significant evidence that NODs were more effective at prolonging pregnancy, although they did tend to be associated with fewer adverse effects.

Conclusion. There is insufficient evidence to support the use of NODs for the purpose of tocolysis in delaying or preventing PTB.

Progesterone

Dose. Various dosage forms of vaginal, oral, and intramuscular progesterone of a variety of formulations.

Effectiveness. A Cochrane review of eight trials found no difference in PTB <34 weeks or birthweight <2.5 kg when compared with placebo or in combination with other tocolytic agents. There was also no significant difference in RDS, NICU admission, IVH, NEC, or mortality. When used in combination with other tocolytics, there was a significant reduction in PTB <37 weeks and increase in birth weight.

Conclusion. Given the small studies and limited evidence we do not recommend the use of progestational agents as a tocolytic for the delay or prevention of PTB.

Practice Option #5: Combination Tocolytic Therapy for Preterm Labor

Few studies exist on combinations of tocolytic therapies for PTL, and current evidence does not support the use of combination therapy for tocolysis. A Cochrane review examined eleven studies with seven different comparisons and found insufficient evidence to support the use of combination tocolytic regimens. Another recent prospective study found that combination of salbutamol and nifedipine compared to nifedipine alone was associated with increased adverse effects and decreased delivery interval.

Practice Option #6: Refractory Tocolysis

There are insufficient data to support the use of additional tocolytic agents when the primary agent fails. One small trial compared the use of indomethacin and sulindac in women who had failed initial therapy with magnesium and found similar results in both groups; there was no placebo arm.

Practice Option #7: Maintenance Tocolysis

Although there are some promising data on the use of progesterone, at this time there is insufficient evidence to support the use of any medication for the purpose of maintenance tocolysis in PTL.

Betamimetics. Reviews on both oral and subcutaneous pump betamimetic therapy for maintenance tocolysis similarly found no benefit compared to placebo in PTB, prolonging pregnancy 48 hours or 1 week, or in neonatal outcomes.

Calcium Channel Blockers. A review on maintenance therapy with CCB similarly found no reduction in PTB or birth within 48 hours or neonatal mortality when compared with placebo or no treatment.

COX Inhibitors. Given the fetal side effects, COX inhibitors should not be used for prolonged maintenance therapy.

Magnesium Sulfate. A review on the use of magnesium maintenance therapy found no significant difference in the incidence of PTB of perinatal mortality when compared with placebo, no treatment, or alternative therapies.

Oxytocin Receptor Antagonists. One review on ORA for maintenance therapy also found no benefit.

Progesterone. There is some evidence that progesterone may prolong pregnancy. A randomized controlled trial of oral micronized progesterone compared to placebo found a significant prolongation in pregnancy, decreased PTB, and higher birth weight with similar adverse effects and perinatal outcomes when using progesterone. A review of 17-alpha-hydroxyprogesterone for maintenance tocolysis found that it significantly prolonged pregnancy by 8 days with significantly higher birth weights. Two other studies of vaginal progesterone compared to placebo or no treatment similarly found increased latency period to delivery, although no decrease in PTB <37 weeks with progesterone. A meta-analysis of vaginal progesterone also found a significantly longer latency, mean 13 days, decreased recurrent PTL, and lower rates of neonatal sepsis. These studies are small but warrant further investigation.

Practice Option #8: Non-Tocolytic Interventions

Antibiotics. There is no benefit to prophylactic antibiotic treatment in women with PTL with intact membranes for the purpose of delaying or preventing PTB. A Cochrane review in 2013 found no difference in reduction of PTB or perinatal or infant mortality for women receiving prophylactic antibiotics compared with placebo. There was also an indication that cerebral palsy was significantly increased in women allocated to macrolide and beta-lactam antibiotics, compared to placebo.

Hydration. There is no evidence to support the use of hydration to prevent or delay PTB. Two studies comparing IV hydration with bedrest alone found no decrease in the risk of preterm delivery before 37 or 34 weeks, or in NICU admission.

Bed Rest. Current evidence does not support the use of bed rest in the prevention or delay of PTB in the setting of PTL. There are few randomized studies on bed rest in the prevention of PTB. A recent trial found no benefit to bed rest for women treated for PTL, including no difference in the incidence of preterm delivery or interval to delivery. Recent reviews on bed rest in pregnancy have come to similar conclusions.

Practice Option #9: Intrapartum Interventions

Mode of Delivery. There is insufficient evidence to support planned cesarean delivery for PTB at any gestational age except for fetal indications—there are few studies on this, and more research needs to be done in this area.

Delayed Cord Clamping. Delayed cord clamping for 30–120 seconds in women between 24 0/7 and 35 6/7 weeks' gestation is associated with fewer transfusions, less IVH, and decreased risk of NEC compared to immediate cord clamping; however, it was also associated with higher peak bilirubin.

DIAGNOSIS OF PRETERM PREMATURE RUPTURE OF MEMBRANES

PPROM is defined as ruptured membranes prior to 37 weeks' gestation before the onset of labor. It may be diagnosed by the direct visualization of pooling of fluid during the speculum examination. Confirmatory testing includes nitrazine test on a cervicovaginal swab of the fluid, and the presence of ferning when the fluid sample is examined under the microscope. If the diagnosis is uncertain, 1 mL indigo carmine in 9 mL normal saline may be injected in the amniotic cavity under ultrasound guidance. If blue-dyed fluid is found on a perineal pad, rupture is confirmed.

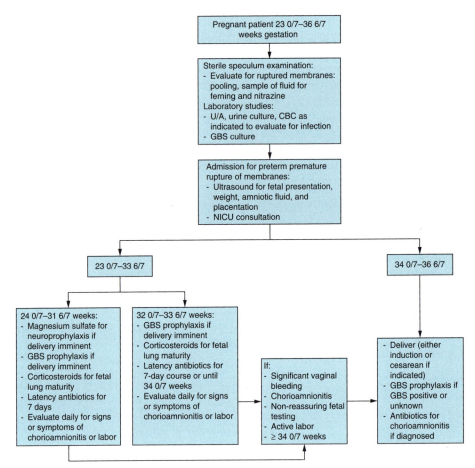

FIGURE 1.2 • Diagnosis and management of preterm premature rupture of membranes.

INITIAL ASSESSMENT OF PRETERM PREMATURE RUPTURE OF MEMBRANES

The evaluation of women with PPROM is similar to that of PTL and includes a thorough history, physical examination including sterile speculum examination, laboratory studies, and ultrasound. The only notable exceptions are that a sterile speculum, rather than vaginal, examination should be done to evaluate for dilation, and there is no utility of a TVU CL in this setting. See Figure 1.2 for outline of diagnosis and management of PPROM.

RECOMMENDATIONS FOR PRETERM PREMATURE RUPTURE OF MEMBRANES

MAJOR RECOMMENDATIONS

In the event of PPROM in pregnancies between 23 0/7 and 33 6/7, antibiotics to prolong latency should be initiated for a total 7-day course or until 34 0/7 weeks. For pregnancies between 34 0/7 and 36 6/7 diagnosed with PPROM, delivery should be initiated.

Regardless of gestational age, delivery is indicated in the setting of chorioamnionitis, non-reassuring fetal testing, significant active bleeding, active labor, or gestational age ≥34 weeks. See Figure 1.2 for an outline of diagnosis and management of PPROM. Similar to PTL, following steps should be taken to maximize neonatal outcome: for pregnancies between 23 0/7 and 33 6/7 weeks, a course of corticosteroids for fetal maturity; for pregnancies between 23 0/7 and 31 6/7 weeks, magnesium sulfate for neuroprotection if delivery is anticipated; for pregnancies between 23 0/7 and 36 6/7 weeks, antibiotic prophylaxis for GBS should be initiated if GBS status is positive or unknown and delivery is anticipated. Magnesium sulfate and GBS prophylaxis may be discontinued after 12 hours if delivery is no longer considered imminent. Once stable, transfer to a center with the appropriate neonatal capabilities should be strongly considered (see Practice Options #1–3 for PTL).

PRACTICE OPTIONS
Practice Option #1: Antibiotics

Preferred Regimen. Ampicillin 2 g IV q6h and erythromycin 250 mg IV q6h × 48 hours followed by amoxicillin 250 mg PO q8h and erythromycin 333 mg PO q8h × 5 days. Azithromycin may be substituted for erythromycin.

Alternative Regimens. Erythromycin 250 mg PO q8h × 10 days. Azithromycin may be substituted for erythromycin.

Contraindications. None.

Effectiveness. Compared to placebo, antibiotics for women with PPROM are associated with a significant reduction in chorioamnionitis, PTB within 48 hours and within 7 days, neonatal infection, RDS, NEC, need for respiratory therapy. Of note, amoxicillin/clavulanate was associated with an increased risk of NEC and should be avoided. A single dose of azithromycin may be substituted for erythromycin, although this has not been studied in a randomized manner.

Recommendation. Antibiotics, preferably a 7-day course of amoxicillin/erythromycin, should be administered prior to 34 weeks in PPROM for maternal and neonatal benefit.

Practice Option #2: Tocolysis

Effectiveness. Tocolytic therapy compared to no therapy was associated with an increased latency and reduced risk of birth within 48 hours but was also associated with higher incidence of neonatal ventilation. In the subgroup of women <34 weeks, there was no benefit and an increased risk chorioamnionitis. However, the studies were small and limited in the use of corticosteroid and latency antibiotic use, which significantly affects neonatal outcomes. Maintenance tocolysis is associated with an increased risk of chorioamnionitis and postpartum endometritis with no decrease in neonatal complications.

Recommendation. Given the limited benefit and the potential for neonatal harm, tocolysis in the setting of PPROM is not recommended.

Practice Option #3: Amnioinfusion

Effectiveness. A Cochrane review found that transabdominal amnioinfusion was associated with a reduction in neonatal death, sepsis, and pulmonary hypoplasia as well as decreased rate of delivery within 7 days; however, the trials were small and unblinded.

Recommendations. Although initial studies on the benefit of transabdominal amnioinfusion in the setting of PPROM are promising, currently there is insufficient evidence to recommend it as standard practice.

IMPLEMENTATION OF GUIDELINE

DESCRIPTION OF IMPLEMENTATION STRATEGY

Recommend following Figure 1.1 for diagnosis and management of PTL and Figure 1.2 for diagnosis and management of PPROM. Provide written guidelines for appropriate interventions by gestational age.

QUALITY METRICS

Monitor rates of admission for PTL and subsequent preterm delivery. Monitor rates of admission for PPROM, administration of latency antibiotics, and time from admission to delivery. Monitor timing and rate of administration of corticosteroids, magnesium sulfate, and GBS prophylaxis in preterm deliveries prior to 34 weeks, 32 weeks, and 37 weeks, respectively.

SUMMARY

In the setting of PTL or PPROM, there are certain interventions for neonatal benefit that when given at the appropriate gestational age have been shown to improve outcomes, including corticosteroids for fetal lung maturity, magnesium sulfate for neuroprotection, and GBS prophylaxis for neonatal sepsis prophylaxis.

In the setting of PTL <34 weeks in the absence of ruptured membranes, single-agent tocolysis may be effective in delaying delivery for the purpose of corticosteroid administration and transfer if necessary. The two tocolytics of choice are nifedipine and indomethacin, depending on gestational age. Additional studies are needed to evaluate the efficacy of progesterone for maintenance tocolysis to prolong latency following arrested PTL. Delivery is indicated for non-reassuring fetal testing, significant vaginal bleeding, chorioamnionitis.

In the setting of PPROM, antibiotics have been demonstrated to improve maternal and neonatal outcomes, including prolonging latency, and should be administered prior to 34 weeks. Short-term tocolysis for the administration of corticosteroids may be considered in the absence of other contraindications, but maintenance tocolysis is not indicated. Delivery is indicated in the setting of chorioamnionitis, non-reassuring fetal testing, significant vaginal bleeding, active labor, or gestational age ≥34 weeks.

BIBLIOGRAPHIC SOURCE(S)

Alfirevic Z, Milan SJ, Livio S. Caesarean section versus vaginal delivery for preterm birth in singletons. *Cochrane Database Syst Rev.* 2013;9:CD000078.

American College of Obstetricians and Gynecologists, Committee on Practice Bulletins-Obstetrics. ACOG practice bulletin no. 127: management of preterm labor. *Obstet Gynecol.* 2012; 119(6):1308-17.

Arikan I, Barut A, Harma M, Harma IM. Effect of progesterone as a tocolytic and in maintenance therapy during preterm labor. *Gynecol Obstet Invest.* 2011;72(4):269-73.

Berghella V. Preterm labor. In: Berghella V, ed. *Obstetric Evidence-Based Guidelines*. 2nd ed. London (UK): Informa Healthcare;2012:164-76.

Borna S, Sahabi N. Progesterone for maintenance tocolytic therapy after threatened preterm labour: a randomised controlled trial. *Aust N Z J Obstet Gynaecol*. 2008;48(1):58-63.

Brownfoot FC, Gagliardi DI, Bain E, Middleton P, Crowther CA. Different corticosteroids and regimens for accelerating fetal lung maturation for women at risk of preterm birth. *Cochrane Database Syst Rev*. 2013;8:CD006764.

Carlan SJ, O'Brien WF, O'Leary TD, Mastrogiannis D. Randomized comparative trial of indomethacin and sulindac for the treatment of refractory preterm labor. *Obstet Gynecol*. 1992;79(2):223-8.

Chawanpaiboon S, Laopaiboon M, Lumbiganon P, Sangkomkamhang US, Dowswell T. Terbutaline pump maintenance therapy after threatened preterm labour for reducing adverse neonatal outcomes. *Cochrane Database Syst Rev*. 2014;3:CD010800.

Choudhary M, Suneja A, Vaid NB, Guleria K, Faridi MM. Maintenance tocolysis with oral micronized progesterone for prevention of preterm birth after arrested preterm labor. *Int J Gynaecol Obstet*. 2014;126(1):60-3.

Crowther CA, Brown J, McKinlay CJ, Middleton P. Magnesium sulphate for preventing preterm birth in threatened preterm labour. *Cochrane Database Syst Rev*. 2014;8:CD001060.

Decavalas G, Mastrogiannis D, Papadopoulos V, Tzingounis V. Short-term versus long-term prophylactic tocolysis in patients with preterm premature rupture of membranes. *Eur J Obstet Gynecol Reprod Biol*. 1995;59(2):143-7.

DeFranco EA, Lewis DF, Odibo AO. Improving the screening accuracy for preterm labor: is the combination of fetal fibronectin and cervical length in symptomatic patients a useful predictor of preterm birth? A systematic review. *Am J Obstet Gynecol*. 2013;208(3):233.e1-e6.

Dodd JM, Crowther CA, Middleton P. Oral betamimetics for maintenance therapy after threatened preterm labour. *Cochrane Database Syst Rev*. 2012;12:CD003927.

Doyle LW, Crowther CA, Middleton P, Marret S, Rouse D. Magnesium sulphate for women at risk of preterm birth for neuroprotection of the fetus. *Cochrane Database Syst Rev*. 2009;(1):CD004661.

Duckitt K, Thornton S, O'Donovan OP, Dowswell T. Nitric oxide donors for treating preterm labour. *Cochrane Database Syst Rev*. 2014;5:CD002860.

Elliott JP, Miller HS, Coleman S, et al. A randomized multicenter study to determine the efficacy of activity restriction for preterm labor management in patients testing negative for fetal fibronectin. *J Perinatol*. 2005;25(10):626-30.

Flenady V, Hawley G, Stock OM, Kenyon S, Badawi N. Prophylactic antibiotics for inhibiting preterm labour with intact membranes. *Cochrane Database Syst Rev*. 2013;12:CD000246.

Flenady V, Reinebrant HE, Liley HG, Tambimuttu EG, Papatsonis DN. Oxytocin receptor antagonists for inhibiting preterm labour. *Cochrane Database Syst Rev*. 2014;6:CD004452.

Flenady V, Wojcieszek AM, Papatsonis DN, et al. Calcium channel blockers for inhibiting preterm labour and birth. *Cochrane Database Syst Rev*. 2014;6:CD002255.

Goldenberg RL, Culhane JF, Iams JD, Romero R. Epidemiology and causes of preterm birth. *Lancet*. 2008;371(9606):75-84.

Goldenberg RL, McClure EM. Epidemiology of Preterm Birth. In: Berghella V, ed. *Preterm Birth: Prevention and Management*. Hoboken, NJ: Wiley-Blackwell;2010:22-38.

Haas DM, Caldwell DM, Kirkpatrick P, McIntosh JJ, Welton NJ. Tocolytic therapy for preterm delivery: systematic review and network meta-analysis. *BMJ*. 2012;345:e6226.

Hammers AL, Sanchez-Ramos L, Kaunitz AM. Antenatal exposure to indomethacin increases the risk of severe intraventricular hemorrhage, necrotizing enterocolitis, and periventricular leukomalacia: a systematic review with metaanalysis. *Am J Obstet Gynecol*. 2015;212(4)505.e1-13.

Han S, Crowther CA, Moore V. Magnesium maintenance therapy for preventing preterm birth after threatened preterm labour. *Cochrane Database Syst Rev*. 2013;5:CD000940.

Haram K, Mortensen JH, Morrison JC. Tocolysis for acute preterm labor: does anything work. *J Matern Fetal Neonatal Med*. 2015;28(4):371-8.

Hayes EJ, Paul DA, Stahl GE, et al. Effect of antenatal corticosteroids on survival for neonates born at 23 weeks of gestation. *Obstet Gynecol*. 2008;111(4):921-6.

Hofmeyr GJ, Eke AC, Lawrie TA. Amnioinfusion for third trimester preterm premature rupture of membranes. *Cochrane Database Syst Rev*. 2014;3:CD000942.

Institute of Medicine (US) Committee on Understanding Premature Birth and Assuring Healthy Outcomes. 2007.

Kenyon S, Boulvain M, Neilson JP. Antibiotics for preterm rupture of membranes. *Cochrane Database Syst Rev*. 2013;12:CD001058.

King J, Flenady V, Cole S, Thornton S. Cyclo-oxygenase (COX) inhibitors for treating preterm labour. *Cochrane Database Syst Rev*. 2005;(2)(2):CD001992.

Klauser CK, Briery CM, Martin RW, Langston L, Magann EF, Morrison JC. A comparison of three tocolytics for preterm labor: a randomized clinical trial. *J Matern Fetal Neonatal Med*. 2014;27(8):801-6.

Loe SM, Sanchez-Ramos L, Kaunitz AM. Assessing the neonatal safety of indomethacin tocolysis: a systematic review with meta-analysis. *Obstet Gynecol*. 2005;106(1):173-9.

Mackeen AD, Seibel-Seamon J, Muhammad J, Baxter JK, Berghella V. Tocolytics for preterm premature rupture of membranes. *Cochrane Database Syst Rev*. 2014;2:CD007062.

Martin JA, Hamilton BE, Osterman MJ, Curtin SC, Matthews TJ. Births: final data for 2013. *Natl Vital Stat Rep*. 2015;64(1):1-65.

Mittendorf R, Pryde PG. A review of the role for magnesium sulphate in preterm labour. *BJOG*. 2005;112(Suppl 1):84-8.

Naik Gaunekar N, Raman P, Bain E, Crowther CA. Maintenance therapy with calcium channel blockers for preventing preterm birth after threatened preterm labour. *Cochrane Database Syst Rev*. 2013;10:CD004071.

Neilson JP, West HM, Dowswell T. Betamimetics for inhibiting preterm labour. *Cochrane Database Syst Rev*. 2014;2:CD004352.

Ness A, Visintine J, Ricci E, Berghella V. Does knowledge of cervical length and fetal fibronectin affect management of women with threatened preterm labor? A randomized trial. *Am J Obstet Gynecol*. 2007;197(4):426.e1-e7.

Nikbakht R, Taheri Moghadam M, Ghane'ee H. Nifedipine compared to magnesium sulfate for treating preterm labor: a randomized clinical trial. *Iran J Reprod Med*. 2014;12(2):145-50.

Ng QJ, Abdul Rahman MF, Lim ML, Chee JJ, Tan KH. Single versus combination tocolytic regimen in the prevention of preterm births in women: a prospective cohort study. *J Perinat Med*. 2015;43(4):423-8.

Padovani TR, Guyatt G, Lopes LC. Nifedipine versus terbutaline, tocolytic effectiveness and maternal and neonatal adverse effects: A randomized, controlled pilot trial. *Basic Clin Pharmacol Toxicol*. 2015;116(3):244-50.

Papatsonis DN, Flenady V, Liley HG. Maintenance therapy with oxytocin antagonists for inhibiting preterm birth after threatened preterm labour. *Cochrane Database Syst Rev*. 2013;10: CD005938.

Peaceman AM, Bajaj K, Kumar P, Grobman WA. The interval between a single course of antenatal steroids and delivery and its association with neonatal outcomes. *Am J Obstet Gynecol*. 2005;193(3 Pt 2):1165-9.

Pierson RC, Gordon SS, Haas DM. A retrospective comparison of antibiotic regimens for preterm premature rupture of membranes. *Obstet Gynecol*. 2014;124(3):515-9.

Practice bulletins no. 139: Premature rupture of membranes. *Obstet Gynecol*. 2013;122(4):918-30.

Rabe H, Diaz-Rossello JL, Duley L, Dowswell T. Effect of timing of umbilical cord clamping and other strategies to influence placental transfusion at preterm birth on maternal and infant outcomes. *Cochrane Database Syst Rev*. 2012;8:CD003248.

Raju TN, Mercer BM, Burchfield DJ, Joseph GF Jr. Periviable birth: executive summary of a joint workshop by the Eunice Kennedy Shriver National Institute of Child Health and Human Development, Society for Maternal-Fetal Medicine, American Academy of Pediatrics, and American College of Obstetricians and Gynecologists. *Am J Obstet Gynecol.* 2014;210(5):406-17.

Roberts D, Dalziel S. Antenatal corticosteroids for accelerating fetal lung maturation for women at risk of preterm birth. *Cochrane Database Syst Rev.* 2006;(3)(3):CD004454.

Saccone G, Suhag A, Berghella V. 17-alpha-hydroxyprogesterone caproate for maintenance tocolysis: A systematic review and metaanalysis of randomized trials. *Am J Obstet Gynecol.* 2015;213(1):16-22.

Sciscione AC. Maternal activity restriction and the prevention of preterm birth. *Am J Obstet Gynecol.* 2010;202(3):232.e1-5.

Shlossman PA, Manley JS, Sciscione AC, Colmorgen GH. An analysis of neonatal morbidity and mortality in maternal (in utero) and neonatal transports at 24-34 weeks' gestation. *Am J Perinatol.* 1997;14(8):449-56.

Sosa C, Althabe F, Belizan J, Bergel E. Bed rest in singleton pregnancies for preventing preterm birth. *Cochrane Database Syst Rev.* 2004;(1):CD003581.

Stan CM, Boulvain M, Pfister R, Hirsbrunner-Almagbaly P. Hydration for treatment of preterm labour. *Cochrane Database Syst Rev.* 2013;11:CD003096.

Su LL, Samuel M, Chong YS. Progestational agents for treating threatened or established preterm labour. *Cochrane Database Syst Rev.* 2014;1:CD006770.

Suhag A, Saccone G, Berghella V. Vaginal progesterone for maintenance tocolysis: a systematic review and meta-analysis of randomized trials. *Am J Obstet Gynecol.* 2015;213(4):479-87.

Usta IM, Khalil A, Nassar AH. Oxytocin antagonists for the management of preterm birth: a review. *Am J Perinatol.* 2011;28(6):449-60.

Verani JR, McGee L, Schrag SJ, Division of Bacterial Diseases, National Center for Immunization and Respiratory Diseases, Centers for Disease Control and Prevention (CDC). Prevention of perinatal group B streptococcal disease--revised guidelines from CDC, 2010. *MMWR Recomm Rep.* 2010;59(RR-10):1-36.

Vogel JP, Nardin JM, Dowswell T, West HM, Oladapo OT. Combination of tocolytic agents for inhibiting preterm labour. *Cochrane Database Syst Rev.* 2014;7:CD006169.

Xiao C, Gangal M, Abenhaim HA. Effect of magnesium sulfate and nifedipine on the risk of developing pulmonary edema in preterm births. *J Perinat Med.* 2014;42(5):585-9.

Fetal Management at the Limit of Viability

Bonnie H. Arzuaga, MD, FAAP

SCOPE

DISEASE/CONDITION(S)

Anticipated delivery and/or birth within the margin of viability, generally considered to be between 22 weeks 0 days and 25 weeks 6 days estimated gestational age.

GUIDELINE OBJECTIVE(S)

To address the following aspects of management of the fetus at the limits of viability. 1) Decrease variation in practice among individual clinicians providing antenatal counseling and/or delivery room care of infants born between 22 weeks 0 days and 25 weeks 6 days estimated gestational age. 2) Promote utilization of a shared decision-making strategy with the infant's parents when providing antenatal counseling. 3) Describe how to appropriately use the ethical standard of "best interests" for an infant when making care plan decisions. 4) Define a "trial of therapy" and understand some of the limitations associated with this practice. 5) Understand how the law may influence decision-making about delivery room management of a periviable infant.

BRIEF BACKGROUND

Definition of Viability

Human viability is most commonly defined as the time in fetal development when there is a reasonable likelihood of sustained survival of the fetus outside the womb, with or without artificial aid. Despite the relative simplicity of this definition, the practical concept of viability is actually quite complex. In reality, the point in time when viability occurs varies between individual pregnancies and is dependent on differences in fetal maturation rates as well as a multitude of other biologic and environmental factors (i.e., intrauterine growth restriction, presence of chorioamnionitis, and availability of antenatal steroid treatment). Furthermore, as medical innovation and technology have advanced over the past century, the definition of viability has evolved with it. Infants who would have not survived 50 years ago because of complications related to their prematurity are now not only surviving, but also thriving. This rapidly changing environment coupled with a "periviable" gray zone in which infants can be delivered has led to complex scientific, social, and ethical considerations.

Survival of Periviable Infants

In 2001, the National Institute for Child Health and Human Development (NICHD) Neonatal Research Network, which comprises 20 large academic centers across the United States, collected and published survival data for premature infants born weighing at least 500 g during the years 1995 and 1996. At that time, overall mortality was 100% for infants born at 21 weeks' gestation, 79% for those at 22 weeks, 70% for those at 23 weeks, and 50% for those at 24 weeks. A decade later this data was reported again; however, due to shifts in resuscitation practices, the new report included all babies born with birth weights greater than 401 g. Despite the addition of smaller infants, the results were similar. The mortality rate for infants born at 22 weeks' gestation was 94% with a reported range of 50% to 100% depending on the particular institution in which the data was taken; 74% (range 47–98%) at 23 weeks; and 45% (range 0–80%) at 24 weeks. The report was unable to examine the etiology of the wide inter-institutional variation in survival due to inadequate data; however, it suggested a lack of standardization in decision-making and clinical practices across the country.

Despite the modest to good survival rates of infants born between 22 and 24 weeks' gestation, these babies are at high risk of suffering from eventual mortality or serious long-term morbidities such as chronic lung disease, growth failure, and neurodevelopmental or cognitive delays. It has been found that clinicians are frequently inaccurate when attempting to predict future morbidities, and that during the early part of the hospitalization course of these infants, there is not much objective data that can improve this prognostication.

Current Resuscitation Practices

Due to the uncertainty of the eventual outcome for any individual extremely premature infant, the appropriate management of a baby born within the margins of viability is a topic that continues to be debated within both national and international forums. No scientific society recommends actively treating a woman in labor for the benefit of her fetus at less than 22 weeks' gestation, beyond offering compassionate or comfort-focused care. A general agreement also exists that active interventions, such as the use of antenatal steroids, prenatal transport, and cesarean section if needed for fetal indications, be pursued for fetuses of at least 25 weeks' gestational age. For all those anticipated births that fall within these two extremes, the long-term outcomes have been found to be too variable to accurately or ethically promote one all-encompassing recommendation.

In 2010, the International Liaison Committee on Resuscitation for neonates at the margins of viability demonstrated that beliefs and practices pertaining to perinatal management and delivery room resuscitation vary widely according to region and availability of resources. An extensive array of available literature has shown that a variety of specific factors, such as geographic location of practice, provider belief of likely neurodevelopmental outcomes, race of the infant, and even belief regarding the moral worth of a premature infant, play important roles in individual physician decision-making regarding delivery room resuscitation of periviable infants.

Variation in beliefs about what constitutes appropriate clinical care for periviable infants also exists between medical specialists. Neonatal and obstetric providers have frequently been found to disagree about the management of a mother-fetus dyad, depending on the estimated gestational age of the fetus. These disagreements have detrimental effects and have even been shown to increase the odds of infant death in the first day of life. Consequently, it is imperative that providers not only understand the complex interplay of factors that occurs with the anticipated birth of a periviable infant, but they must also be able to reconcile the medical and ethical conflicts that can arise in order to provide optimal care to both the mother and her extremely premature infant.

RECOMMENDATIONS

MAJOR RECOMMENDATIONS

Professional specialty societies provide the individual clinician with some guidance on how to care for a mother anticipating a periviable delivery or for an infant born at a periviable gestation. The American College of Obstetricians and Gynecologists (ACOG) and the American Academy of Pediatrics (AAP) both have written guidelines on the topic but stress the importance of individualizing each particular clinical case.

Obstetrical Management

Women and/or families faced with an imminent periviable delivery should be provided with local or regional outcomes data specific to the gestational age and weight of their fetus. If those data are unavailable, clinicians may alternatively opt to utilize the NICHD Neonatal Research Network: Extremely Preterm Birth Outcome Data calculator to provide general outcomes information. Information should include both short-term and long-term expectations, including information on possible morbidities if the infant were to survive until hospital discharge. If an accurate gestational age has not been well established, the clinician should present a wide range of prognoses while emphasizing that the infant's actual gestational age and overall condition can be assessed more accurately following delivery. In this particular circumstance, ACOG recommends that if a discrepancy exists between available ultrasound and menstrual dating of greater than 2 weeks, the clinician should utilize fetal measurements obtained by ultrasound to aid in management decisions. This is particularly true if ultrasound findings suggest a fetus is older than what menstrual dating predicts. However, caution should be used if ultrasound measurements are consistent with a significantly younger fetus compared to menstrual dating, as this may indicate the possibility of growth restriction.

Gestational Age–Specific Recommendations. A joint workshop of the NICHD, the Society for Maternal-Fetal Medicine, AAP, and ACOG produced an executive summary addressing clinical management and counseling issues of women anticipated to deliver at a periviable gestation. The summary included clinical guidance for both obstetricians and neonatologists and had detailed recommendations for active medical intervention for fetuses of younger gestational ages than previously published guidelines, thus representing general practice shift toward more active management of younger infants.

The summary recommendations for obstetric interventions for threatened and imminent periviable birth are summarized in Table 2.1. If parents of a periviable fetus request active medical management, most interventions are either recommended or encouraged at 23 weeks or more, while provision of comfort-focused care is the only recommendation for fetuses less than 22 weeks. Based on the outcomes listed in the summary, infants born at 23 weeks' gestation should be treated as potentially viable.

TABLE 2.1. General Guidance Regarding Obstetric Interventions for Threatened and Imminent Periviable Birth

	Weeks of Gestation		
	<22 0/7 Weeks	*22 0/7 to 22 6/7 Weeks*	*23 0/7 Weeks or More*
Antenatal corticosteroids	Not recommended	Consider if delivery at or later than 23 0/7 weeks is anticipated	Recommended
Tocolytics to enhance latency for potential steroid benefit	Not recommended	Not recommended unless concurrent with antenatal steroids	Consider
Magnesium sulfate for neuroprotection	Not recommended	Not recommended	Recommended
Antibiotics for premature rupture of membranes to enhance latency	Consider if delivery is not imminent	Consider if delivery is not imminent	Recommended if delivery is not imminent
Intrapartum antibiotics for GBS prophylaxis	Not recommended	Not recommended	Recommended
Continuous intrapartum electronic fetal monitoring	Not recommended	Not recommended	Recommended
Cesarean delivery for fetal indication	Not recommended	Not recommended	Recommended
Aggressive newborn resuscitation	Not recommended; comfort care only	Not recommended unless considered potentially viable based on individual circumstances	Recommended unless considered nonviable based on individual circumstances

Reprinted by permission from Macmillan Publishers Ltd: *Journal of Perinatology*. Raju TNK, Mercer BM, Burchfield DJ, Joseph GF. Periviable birth: executive summary of a Joint Workshop by the Eunice Kennedy Shriver National Institute of Child Health and Human Development, Society for Maternal-Fetal Medicine, American Academy of Pediatrics, and American College of Obstetricians and Gynecologists. *J Perinatol*. 2014;34:333-42, copyright 2014.

Infants born at 22–23 weeks' gestation may be potentially viable based on individual factors, and in many institutions, are provided with a trial of intensive care if the parents desire resuscitation. If at all feasible, these deliveries should be undertaken at a facility with the resources to care for such extremely premature infants.

Transportation Considerations. In cases that may require maternal transfer to a center that can provide a higher level of care, the family should be encouraged to actively participate in decisions regarding transport. Physicians should be able to provide patients with information regarding available modes of transportation (i.e., ground vs air transport) and regional resources as well as the benefits and risks of maternal versus infant transport. In general, periviable infants born at a center that can provide an appropriate level of care suffer less complications and have greater rates of survival when compared to those who require transport from one hospital to another immediately following birth. In addition, it is best that mothers not be separated from their newborn infants, so for these reasons, maternal transport prior to delivery should always be preferred over infant transport. More detailed counseling and local data information will invariably be available at the institution providing the higher level of care, and this should be clearly conveyed to the patient and her family.

Maternal or infant transfer should only be considered if the tertiary center would be able to provide care not available at the local hospital. Generally speaking, infants born at less than 32 weeks require Level III or higher NICU care. Mothers anticipated to deliver at a gestational age below this threshold should be cared for at an institution with an available NICU whenever possible. Transport is expensive and can be traumatic, so should be avoided if the newborn's condition is believed to be incompatible with prolonged life. Local protocols regarding appropriate transfers between the tertiary center and community hospitals should be developed to help individual providers in their decision-making.

Neonatal Management

Neonatal care decisions should be made with an emphasis on individualization of decision-making in each case using parental preferences, known facts about the particular fetus, and any confounding influences (e.g., locally available resources). Coordination of obstetric and pediatric services is instrumental in providing optimal care to an extremely premature infant. Care plans based on the best available evidence for both the mother and infant should complement each other using a risk-benefit assessment.

All current clinical guidelines emphasize the importance of re-evaluation of any decisions made as new information becomes available to the medical team. Care plans should be continuously tailored depending on the neonate's condition at birth, the postnatal gestational age assessment, and the infant's response to resuscitative measures. Similarly, frequent re-evaluation of the appropriateness of ongoing intensive care support should be done with parental input and should be based on the infant's evolving condition and prognosis.

Development of Local Guidelines. Some institutions have developed standardized medical staff guidelines to aid in antenatal counseling and subsequent decision-making regarding resuscitation of periviable infants. The most successful of these guidelines tend to be those that were developed using pooled local outcomes data as well as clinician preferences. After implementation of such consensus-based guidelines, it has been found that pregnant women at these institutions view the information provided during antenatal counseling as highly understandable, useful, consistent, and respectful. Guidelines should not replace individualized decision-making based on parental preferences but are effective in standardizing the overall approach to cases of anticipated periviable birth and can minimize inter-provider variability in practice.

Withholding Care. Decisions to withhold resuscitation, discontinue resuscitation, or forgo other life-supporting interventions should be made with an emphasis on maintaining patient dignity and supporting the needs of the infant's family. Practices that promote these concepts include emphasis on careful handling of the infant, maintaining warmth, and avoidance of invasive or painful procedures and intrusive monitoring. Families should be allowed time to interact and hold their infant during the dying process and also for an extended period of time after death occurs. Clergy, palliative care specialists, and other support personnel should be made available and families should be encouraged to request this type of support if desired. Memory making with personalized information, such as recording of anthropometric measurements at birth, completion of a crib card, and obtaining photographs and footprints are important modalities of family bereavement.

Ongoing emotional support for clinicians and hospital staff working in situations of either continued intensive care for a periviable infant or of infant death should be made available due to the inherently complex nature of the decision-making process regarding delivery room management of a periviable infant.

Summary of Recommendations

Using the most recent executive summary recommendations, Figure 2.1 provides a comprehensive algorithm for appropriate coordination of obstetric and neonatal care as well as basic guidelines for treatment pathways based on the gestational age of a periviable fetus.

Many clinicians rely on gestational age more heavily than parental preference for infant resuscitation when making delivery room management decisions. However, as the shift in practice continues to favor resuscitation of younger infants at parental request and more information becomes available regarding long-term outcomes of *survivors*, clinicians should continue to encourage active parental input during decision-making discussions and use this information to help standardize management strategies between obstetric and neonatal providers.

PRACTICE OPTIONS

Practice Option #1: Antenatal Counseling

Antenatal counseling has traditionally focused on providing as much information as possible to parents anticipating a periviable delivery and using this information to make a decision about the amount of intervention the infant should receive at birth. In current practice, this information and the way it is provided to families varies widely between institutions, providers of varying specialties, and providers within the same specialty. Pregnant women most often do not receive any counseling regarding prematurity until they present in preterm labor, so they must therefore hear, comprehend, and attempt to understand the implications of complicated medical information in a compromised and inherently stressful physical and mental state. As a consequence, clinicians should strive to provide counseling about periviable birth in a sensitive, efficient, and effective way.

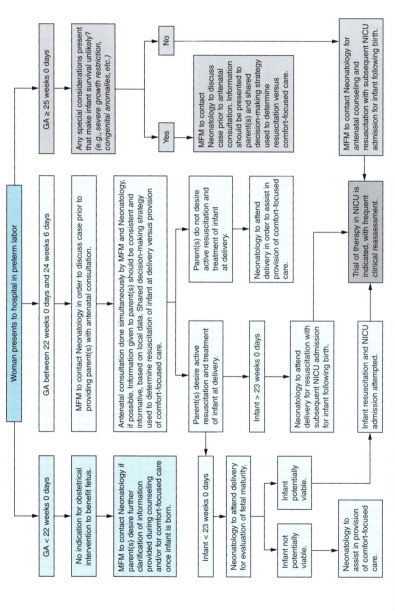

FIGURE 2.1 • Counseling and resuscitation algorithm for fetuses at limit of viability.

Parents should be provided with the most accurate prognostic data available in order to help them make decisions. This is most often local institutional data; however, it can also be regional or national if hospital-specific data is unavailable. The best data uses gestational age in concert with other individual factors, such as estimated fetal weight, gender, and use of prenatal steroids and magnesium as a basis for estimating risks and providing parents with recommendations. The NICHD NRN: Extremely Preterm Birth Outcome Data online calculator can provide clinicians with the best estimate of expected survival and survival without morbidity if local data is not available at the time of the consultation. Traditional models of counseling advocate conveying such information to parents in a nondirective manner and leaving them to decide whether they want their infant resuscitated. However, it has been argued that this pure "parental autonomy" approach can lead to feelings of guilt or regret by parents who may later question their decisions. Instead, a "shared decision-making" model should be employed during any periviable consultation. Information should be presented as clearly and informatively as possible. If the involved clinician feels that there is no chance of survival, (s)he should advocate for comfort-focused care over resuscitation. In instances where survival is unlikely and the chance of morbidity is high, the clinician should describe the possible outcomes in as much detail as possible and make his or her clinical recommendations, but respect whatever decision the parents come to. Written material on potential complications can help the parents process and understand the complex information being discussed. Importantly, the clinician should emphasize that the decision to resuscitate a periviable infant is not the end of the decision-making algorithm. Parents and clinicians alike gain more information throughout the first hours to days of an infant's hospitalization, and this data can aid in more accurate prognostication following initial delivery room management.

In order to decrease interspecialty variation in counseling techniques, the AAP advocates that antenatal consultations be done simultaneously by neonatal and obstetric providers whenever possible. Toolkits and/or written materials can also help accomplish this goal. Translator services should be used if a family is not proficient in English; utilizing other family members and/or friends to interpret consultation discussions for a patient should be avoided whenever possible.

Importantly, if parents are undecided about their preference for infant resuscitation, initiation of resuscitative efforts is appropriate pending further discussions. Clinicians should emphasize that decisions made during an antenatal consultation are not firm and may require modification after an appropriate physical evaluation of the infant immediately following birth.

Practice Option #2: Infant Resuscitation

The ethical standards that direct medical decision-making in pediatrics emphasize consideration of the "best interests" of the child for whom the decision is being made. By invoking a "best-interests standard," decision-makers can justify one course of action over another. This practice becomes complicated, however, when clinicians attempt to determine what is in the best interests of a newborn baby who may not yet experience self-awareness in a way akin to that of older children and adults. In these cases, if one were to consider withholding resuscitation on an infant based on the assumption that it would not be preferable to continue to live, one would have to have a high degree of certainty that the state of pain and suffering experienced by that infant would be indeed intolerable, and that the known risks of aggressive intervention drastically outweigh any foreseeable benefit.

Rather than using this narrow definition of best interests, clinicians anticipating a periviable delivery should consider the infant's interests to be a "primary consideration," while also taking into account competing interests from affected parties, namely the parent(s), sibling(s), or other intimately involved family members.

Thorough yet sensitive antenatal counseling techniques, as previously discussed, should be to able to support a shared decision-making strategy between the clinician(s) and parent(s) by using the infant's best interests as the primary consideration, supported by parental interests.

If it is decided that comfort-focused care should be pursued at birth, obstetrics and neonatology providers should determine which team members will be most successful in providing that care. Many hospitals have protocols and order sets particularly for this purpose. A major dictum of these protocols is to treat the newly born infant in a respectful manner by ensuring 1) that he/she stays warm either under a radiant warmer or in parents' arms, 2) that the infant is wrapped in a blanket, and 3) that if there is any concern of discomfort or pain during the dying process, the appropriate measures are taken to relieve these symptoms.

Alternatively, if it is agreed upon that the infant should have resuscitation attempted at delivery, a "trial of therapy" in the neonatal intensive care unit (NICU) would then be appropriate. During the first hours to days of a periviable infant's NICU stay, some information may be available to aid in ultimate survival predictions. Unfortunately, providers' intuitions regarding survival of any particular infant are also imprecise. As new diagnostic information becomes available during an infant's hospitalization, parents must be counseled on an ongoing basis as to the implications of this information and about any uncertainty of the eventual outcome for their infant.

Practice Option #3: Legal Considerations

Discourse regarding human viability in the legal realm has traditionally fallen within cases regarding terminations of pregnancy. The landmark Supreme Court case of *Planned Parenthood of Southeastern PA v Casey* (1992) provided one of the most specific legal definitions of viability in case law and emphasized that viability marks the earliest "point" at which the State has a significant interest in fetal life.

Interestingly, this keen interest in promoting State interest in the life of periviable fetus in relation to abortions has not extended to situations of unanticipated birth of a periviable infant. Instead, the law most often presumes that parents act in the best interests of their children and therefore grants them rights to make difficult medical decisions, including decisions regarding withdrawal of care, for their infants.

Cases that have directly touched upon medical decision-making within the periviable period are exceedingly rare and generally reflect situations in which intractable conflicts have occurred between families and physicians. In these cases, the courts have generally ruled under the presumption that "continued life is in the best interests of the patient." Despite the existence of these rulings, in reality their influence on clinical practice remains minimal. In general, the law does not dictate what the treatment obligations are for obstetric and neonatal patients within the periviable period, and as a consequence, institutional variation has become customary in the United States.

CLINICAL ALGORITHM(S)

While each anticipated periviable delivery should be approached by taking into account case-specific clinical factors and patient values, Figure 2.1 provides an algorithm to be used as a general guide to navigate this complex decision-making scenario. Separate pathways are outlined for anticipated births of infants less than 22 weeks' gestation, 22 0/7–24 6/7 weeks' gestation, and greater than or equal to 25 weeks' gestation.

IMPLEMENTATION OF GUIDELINE

DESCRIPTION OF IMPLEMENTATION STRATEGY

Educate clinicians and staff on aspects of the Counseling and Resuscitation Algorithm for Fetuses at Limit of Viability; provide clinicians with general guidelines to improve consistency of information given to parents during antenatal consultation for anticipated periviable delivery; track institutional-specific outcomes of infants resuscitated and admitted to the NICU; track gestational ages of infants in which resuscitation was initiated but not successful in the delivery room.

QUALITY METRICS

Survey parent comprehension of information provided during antenatal consultation; track cases of periviable delivery and pursue efforts to minimize individual provider variability in decision-making regarding delivery room resuscitation of infants between 22 0/7 and 25 6/7 weeks' gestational age.

SUMMARY

When faced with an anticipated periviable delivery, decisions about infant resuscitation in the delivery room should be individualized and based on a combination of likelihood of survival coupled with consideration of parental wishes and the infant's best interests. Prognostic information should be based on local data whenever possible. Decisions made prior to an infant's birth should never be firm, and parents should be made aware that care plans may change based on postnatal evaluation of the periviable infant.

BIBLIOGRAPHIC SOURCE(S)

American Congress of Obstetricians and Gynecologists. ACOG Practice Bulletin No. 38: perinatal care at the threshold of viability. *Int J Gynaecol Obstet.* 2002;79:181-8.

Arzuaga BH, Lee BH. Limits of human viability in the united states: a medicolegal review. *Pediatrics.* 2011;128(6):1047-52.

Arzuaga BH, Meadow W. National variability in neonatal resuscitation practices at the limit of viability. *Am J Perinatol.* 2014;31(6):521-8.

Assembly, UN General. Convention on the Rights of the Child. *United Nations, Treaty Series.* 1989;1577(3):Part I, Article 3.

Batton DG; American Academy of Pediatrics, Committee on Fetus and Newborn. Antenatal counseling regarding resuscitation at an extremely low gestational age. *Pediatrics.* 2009;124: 422-7.

Catlin A, Carter B. Creation of a neonatal end-of-life palliative care protocol. *J Perinatol* 2002;22:184-95.

Chervenak FE, McCullough LB, Levene MI. An ethically justified, clinically comprehensive approach to peri-viability: gynaecological, obstetric, perinatal and neonatal dimensions. *J Obstet Gynaecol.* 2007;27(1):3-7.

deLeeuw R, Cuttini M, Nadai M, et al. Treatment choices for extremely premature infants: an international perspective. *J Pediatr.* 2000;137:608-15.

Guinsburg R, Branco de Almeida MF, dos Santos Rodrigues Sadeck L, et al. Proactive management of extreme prematurity: disagreement between obstetricians and neonatologists. *J Perinatol.* 2012;32:913-9.

https://neonatal.rti.org/about/map.cfm. Accessed January 23, 2015.

International Liaison Committee on Resuscitation. The International Liaison Committee on Resuscitation (ILCOR) consensus on science with treatment recommendations for pediatric and neonatal patients: neonatal resuscitation. *Pediatrics.* 2006;117(5):e978.

Janvier A, Barrington KJ, Deschenes M, et al. Relationship between site of training and attitudes about neonatal resuscitation. *Arch Pediatr Adolesc Med.* 2008;162(6):532-7.

Janvier A, Leblanc I, Barrington KJ. The best-interest standard is not applied for neonatal resuscitation decisions. *Pediatrics.* 2008;121:963-9.

Lantos J, Meadow W. *Neonatal Bioethics: The Moral Challenges of Medical Innovation.* Baltimore, MD: Johns Hopkins University Press; 2006.

Lemons JA, Bauer CR, Oh W, et al. Very low birth weight outcomes of the National Institute of Child Health and Human Development Neonatal Research Network, January 1995 through December 1996. *Pediatrics.* 2001;107(1):e1-8.

Kaempf JW, Tomlinson MW, Campbell B, Ferguson L, Stewart VT. Counseling pregnant women who may deliver extremely premature infants: medical care guidelines, family choices, and neonatal outcomes. *Pediatrics.* 2009;123;1509.

Kakkilaya V, Groome LJ, Platt D, et al. Use of a visual aid to improve counseling at the threshold of viability. *Pediatrics.* 2011;128(6):e1511-9.

Meadow W. Ethics at the margins of viability. *NeoReviews.* 2013;14(12):e588-91.

Meadow W, Lagatta J, Andrews B, et al. Just, in time: ethical implications of serial predictions of death and morbidity for ventilated premature infants. *Pediatrics.* 2008;121(4):732-40.

Mehrota A, Lagatta J, Simpson P, et al. Variations among US hospitals in counseling practices regarding prematurely born infants. *J Perinatol.* 2013;33:509-13.

Mercurio MR. Parental authority, patient's best interest and refusal of resuscitation at borderline gestational age. *J Perinatol.* 2006;26:452-7.

Miller v HCA, 118 S.W. 3d 758 (2003).

Montalvo v Borkovec. 647 N.W. 2d 413 (Wis. App. 2002).

Nuffield Council on Bioethics. *Critical Care Decisions in Fetal and Neonatal Medicine: Ethical Issues.* London: Clyvedon Press; 2006.

Pignotti MS. The definition of human viability: a historical perspective. *Acta Paediatr.* 2010;99(1):33-6.

Raju TNK, Mercer BM, Burchfield, DJ, et al. Periviable birth: executive summary of a Joint Workshop by the Eunice Kennedy Shriver National Institute of Child Health and Human Development, Society for Maternal-Fetal Medicine, American Academy of Pediatrics, and American College of Obstetricians and Gynecologists. *J Perinatol.* 2014;34:333-42.

Sayeed S. The marginally viable newborn: legal challenges, conceptual inadequacies, and reasonableness. *J Law Med Ethics.* 2006;34(3):600-10.

Sayeed S. Peri-viable birth: legal considerations. *Seminars Perinatol.* 2014;38:52-5.

Singh J, Fanaroff J, Andrews B, et al. Resuscitation in the "gray zone" of viability: determining physician preferences and predicting infant outcomes. *Pediatrics.* 2007;120(3):519-26.

Stoll BJ, Hansen NI, Bell EF, et al. Neonatal outcomes of extremely preterm infants from the NICHD Neonatal Research Network. *Pediatrics.* 2010;126(3):443-56.

Truog RD, Sayeed SA. Neonatal decision-making: beyond the standard of best interests. *Am J Bioethics.* 2011;11(2):44-5.

Tucker-Edmonds B, Fager C, Srinivas S, Lorch S. Racial and ethnic differences in use of intubation for periviable neonates. *Pediatrics.* 2011;127:e1120-7.

Tucker Edmonds B, McKenzie F, Farrow V, Raglan G, Schulkin J. A national survey of obstetricians' attitudes toward and practice of periviable intervention. *J Perinatol.* 2014;doi:10.1038/jp.2014.201.

Tyson JE, Parikh NA, Langer J, Green C, Higgins RD; National Institute of Child Health and Human Development Neonatal Research Network. Intensive care for extreme prematurity: moving beyond gestational age. *N Engl J Med.* 2008;358(16):1672-81.

Weiss AR, Binns HJ, Collins JW, deRegnier R-A. Decision-making in the delivery room: a survey of neonatologists. *J Perinatol.* 2007;27:754-60.

Nonimmune Hydrops

Isabelle Boucoiran, MD, MSc • Isabelle De Bie, MD, PhD, FRCPC, FCCMG • Valérie Désilets, MD • François Audibert, MD, MSc

SCOPE

DISEASE/CONDITION(S)

Counseling and management of prenatally diagnosed nonimmune hydrops.

GUIDELINE OBJECTIVE(S)

Describe the current investigations and management of nonimmune fetal hydrops with a focus on treatable or recurring etiologies.

BRIEF BACKGROUND

Hydrops fetalis is defined as an abnormal accumulation of fluid in at least two different fetal compartments. Generally it carries a poor prognosis; however, several etiologies can be treated in utero with potential good results. The growing number of recognized etiologies requires a comprehensive and systematic search for causes, in particular, for treatable or recurrent conditions.

RECOMMENDATIONS

1. All pregnant women with fetal hydrops should be referred promptly to a maternal-fetal medicine unit for evaluation. Some conditions amenable to prenatal treatment represent a therapeutic emergency after 18 weeks.
2. Fetal chromosome analysis through comparative genomic hybridization microarray molecular testing should be offered in all cases of nonimmune fetal hydrops.

3. Imaging studies should include comprehensive obstetrical ultrasound (including arterial and venous fetal Doppler) and fetal echocardiography.
4. To evaluate the risk of fetal anemia, Doppler measurement of the middle cerebral artery peak systolic velocity should be performed in all hydropic fetuses after 16 weeks of gestation. In cases of suspected fetal anemia, fetal blood sampling and intrauterine transfusion should be offered rapidly.
5. Investigation for maternal-fetal infections, and alpha-thalassemia in women at risk based on ethnicity, should be performed in all cases of unexplained fetal hydrops.
6. All cases of unexplained fetal hydrops should be referred to a medical genetics service where available. Detailed postnatal evaluation by a medical geneticist should be performed on all cases of newborns with unexplained nonimmune hydrops.
7. Autopsy should be recommended in all cases of fetal or neonatal death or pregnancy termination. Amniotic fluid and/or fetal cells should be stored for future genetic and/or metabolic testing.

DEFINITIONS

Hydrops fetalis is defined as an abnormal accumulation of fluid in at least two different fetal compartments. It implies an extracellular accumulation of fluid in tissues and serous cavities. It generally presents as subcutaneous edema, accompanied by effusions in two or more serous cavities, including pericardial or pleural effusions and ascites. Polyhydramnios or placental thickening (>6 cm) is often associated. The primary mechanisms associated with hydrops fetalis are anemia, heart failure, increase of central venous pressure/compromised venous return, and hypoproteinemia.

IMMUNE HYDROPS

Maternal red cell alloimmunization occurs when a pregnant woman presents an immunological response to a paternally-derived antigen that is foreign to the mother and inherited by the fetus. Maternal antibodies may cross the placenta, bind to antigens present on the fetal erythrocytes, and cause hemolysis, hydrops fetalis, and fetal death. The complete description and management of this condition is beyond the scope of this chapter.

NONIMMUNE HYDROPS

Nonimmune hydrops fetalis (NIHF) refers to hydrops in the absence of maternal circulating red cell antibodies. With the introduction of widespread immunoprophylaxis for red cell alloimmunization and the use of in utero transfusions for immune hydrops therapy, nonimmune causes have become responsible for at least 85% of all cases of fetal hydrops. The incidence is around 3/10,000 births but is much higher at the time of the first- and second-trimester ultrasounds, due to higher fetal death rates.

NIHF occurring in one or both twins of a monochorionic pregnancy suggests twin-to-twin transfusion syndrome (TTTS). Review articles discussing assessment and management of TTTS and other complications specific to twin pregnancies are available to the reader.

ETIOLOGIES

A growing number of conditions can result in NIHF (Table 3.1). Despite thorough investigations, 9–28% of cases remain unexplained.

TABLE 3.1. Conditions Associated with Nonimmune Fetal Hydrops

	Cardiovascular	Hemato-logic	Chromo-somal	Infections	Thoracic	Syndromic	Placental (TTTS)	Lymphatic Dysplasia	Idio-pathic	Various[*]
Number of cases	1181	564	727	366	327	237	304	310	966	455
%	**21.7**	**10.4**	**13.4**	**6.7**	**6.0**	**4.4**	**5.6**	**5.7**	**17.8**	**8.4**
Potential fetal therapy	Yes[+] (antiarrythmic drugs)	Yes (IUT)	No	Yes (IUT for parvo)	Yes (thoraco-amniotic shunting)	No	Yes (placental laser therapy)	No	No	

Based on a total number of 5437 cases of NIHF.

[*]Including inborn storage diseases, urinary tract malformations, extrathoracic tumors, gastrointestinal, miscellaneous.

[+]For fetal tachyarrythmias only.

IUT, intrauterine transfusion; TTTS, twin-to-twin transfusion syndrome.

Adapted from Braun T, Brauer M, Fuchs I, et al. Mirror syndrome: a systematic review of fetal associated conditions, maternal presentation and perinatal outcome. *Fetal Diagn Ther.* 2010;27:191-203 and Bellini C, Hennekam RC, Bonioli E. A diagnostic flow chart for non-immune hydrops fetalis. *Am J Med Genet A.* 2009;149A:852-3.

CARDIAC ETIOLOGIES

Cardiac etiologies account for 10–20% of cases of NIHF. These include structural abnormalities, especially right heart defects, cardiac arrhythmias, tumors, and physiological dysfunction due to infection, inflammation, infarction, and arterial calcification.

Cardiac arrhythmia may be primary or may occur secondary to a systemic etiology, such as hyperthyroidism, or in mothers with autoimmune conditions associated with high titers of circulating anti-SS-A or anti-SS-B antibodies. The most common clinically significant fetal arrhythmias are 1) supraventricular tachyarrhythmia, the cardiac etiology of hydrops fetalis most amenable to treatment and 2) severe bradyarrhythmias, associated with complete heart block, which can cause NIHF if the fetal heart rate is persistently below 50 beats per minute.

Congestive heart failure may be secondary to other systemic causes that need to be evaluated. When identifying a cardiac component in the context of NIFH, this important finding should not be considered as a final diagnosis in itself. A careful search for maternal underlying illness, chromosomal anomaly, or single-gene disorder is still indicated.

HEMATOLOGICAL DISORDERS

Hematological disorders can be identified in 7% of NIFH. The incidence may be higher in certain ethnic groups with higher carrier frequencies of alpha-thalassemia. For example, homozygous alpha-thalassemia is an autosomal recessive condition that occurs at higher frequency in some ethnic groups such as Mediterranean, African, and Southeast Asian populations. Carriers are suspected on the basis of the presence of low red blood cell volume (microcytosis) with normal ferritin.

CHROMOSOME ABNORMALIES

Chromosome anomalies are the cause of NIFH in 25–70% of cases. The risk of fetal aneuploidy is higher when hydrops is identified earlier in gestation or if fetal structural anomalies are detected. Fetal chromosome analysis is indicated in all cases of hydrops. Microarray comparative genomic hybridization molecular testing should be considered in all NIFH cases, where available, as the National Institute of Child Health and Human Development (NICHD) microarray study has shown additional genetic chromosomal anomalies in 7% of fetuses with congenital anomalies and normal karyotype.

INFECTIOUS DISEASES

Intrauterine infections are a common cause of fetal hydrops (4–15%) with parvovirus B19 infection and secondary anemia being the most frequent. Fetal toxoplasmosis, syphilis, cytomegalovirus (CMV), and varicella infection can also present as fetal hydrops, with commonly associated findings such as hepatomegaly, splenomegaly, or calcifications (Tables 3.1 and 3.2). For more information on congenital infectious disease diagnosis and management, consult specific guidelines.

STRUCTURAL CONGENITAL ANOMALIES

Structural congenital anomalies should be evaluated, as they represent a large group of disorders that can be identified through detailed fetal imaging, some of which being amenable to treatment. A list of congenital anomalies associated with fetal hydrops is presented in Table 3.1. Primary chylothorax, congenital cystic adenomatoid malformation, and various fetal tumors have been also described as underlying etiologies of hydrops.

TABLE 3.2. Ultrasound Findings in Fetal Infections Causing Fetal Hydrops

Infection	CNS	Cardiac	Abdominal	Placental/AF	IUGR
Toxoplasmosis	+		+	+	Rare
Syphilis			+	+	Rare
Rubella	+	+	+		+
Parvovirus		+	+	+	
Cytomegalovirus	+	+	+	+	+
Varicella	+		+	+	+

AF, amniotic fluid; CNS, central nervous system; IUGR, intrauterine growth retardation.

Adapted from Klein JO, Baker CJ, Remington JS, Wilsonn CB. Current concepts of infections of the fetus and newborn infant. In: Remington JS, Klein JO, eds. *Infectious Diseases of the Fetus and Newborn Infant*. 6th ed. Philadelphia, PA: Elsevier Saunders; 2006:3-25.

SINGLE-GENE DISORDERS

Known single-gene disorders associated with metabolic pathways, hematological conditions, skeletal dysplasias, neurologic disorders, cardiomyopathies, congenital nephrosis, congenital lymphedema, and mitochondrial dysfunctions have been reported as causes of potentially recurring fetal hydrops. The identification of a single gene disorder not only helps in predicting the outcome of the current pregnancy but also has an impact on the management or screening of future pregnancies in the family, as it may carry a 3–50% recurrence risk, depending on the gene involved. Thus, prenatal testing for Noonan syndrome should be considered in fetuses with normal caryotype.

Lysosomal storage disorders, such as mucopolysaccharidosis (MPS) type VII, infantile galactosialidosis, type 2 Gaucher disease, and infantile free sialic acid storage disease, are the group of metabolic disorders most commonly involved in NIHF. At least 15 other inborn errors of metabolism may cause NIHF. Specific enzyme assays are available to test for these disorders on cultured amniocytes or specific metabolite measurement in amniotic fluid supernatant.

INVESTIGATIONS

Multiple mechanisms of hydrops may coexist, and the primary cause is often not obvious. We propose a standardized approach to the investigation and management of NIFH with focus on the treatable or potentially recurring causes (Table 3.3). One should not wait for complete results before initiating referral to a maternal-fetal medicine unit, invasive diagnostic procedures, or treatments.

DOPPLER ULTRASOUND

- **Middle cerebral artery (MCA) peak systolic velocity:** Its measurement to assess fetal anemia is essential to the management of fetuses with hydrops. After 16 weeks of gestation, there is a significant association between delta-MCA peak flow and delta-Hb concentration, especially when the fetal hemoglobin concentration is very low. A peak systolic above 1.5 MoM has a 100% (CI 86–100%) sensitivity for detecting fetal anemia from various causes.

TABLE 3.3. Step-Wise Investigation of Nonimmune Fetal Hydrops

Step 1: Urgent

Clinical Evaluation
- Parental past medical history, ethnic background, and consanguinity
- Three-generation pedigree, including specific questions on fetal losses, death in infancy, developmental delay, congenital malformation, genetic syndrome, skeletal dysplasia, chronic infantile illness, inherited cardiomyopathies, and neurodegenerative disorders
- Reproductive history, including previous fetal, neonatal, or infantile deaths
- History of viral exposure/illness, sexually transmitted diseases, traveling
- Bleeding
- Medication or drug during the pregnancy
- Physical examination

Fetal Imaging
- Detailed morphology obstetrical ultrasound in a tertiary care center and the assessment of the fetal venous and arterial circulation
- Doppler (MCA, venous, arterial)
- Fetal echocardiogram

Maternal Blood
- CBC and hemoglobin electrophoresis
- Kleihauer-Betke
- ABO type and antigen status
- Indirect Coombs (antibody screen)
- Syphilis enzyme immunoassay
- Serologies +/– avidity for parvovirus, toxoplasmosis, cytomegalovirus, rubella, and other infection according to history and clinical presentation (also on archived serum from routine first-trimester baseline tests if available)
- Liver function tests, uric acid, coagulation tests (suspected mirror syndrome)
- SS-A, SS-B antibodies (fetal bradyarrhythmia)
- TSH, TSH receptor antibodies (Graves disease, fetal tachycardia)
- Depending on ethnic origin: hemoglobin electrophoresis, G6PD deficiency screen

Step 2: Invasive Procedures

Amniocentesis
- Rapid aneuploidy testing through FISH or QF-PCR on uncultured amniocytes followed by chromosome analysis through microarray (comparative genomic hybridization) if rapid aneuploidy testing reported as normal
- PCR for CMV
- PCR for parvovirus B19/toxoplasmosis and other viral infections according to clinical presentation and serologies
- Molecular analysis of fetal DNA from amniocytes if alpha-thalassemia is suspected
- Keep amniotic cells and supernatant for potential future studies (metabolite measurement)

Fetal Blood Sampling (MFM specialist)
- CBC, WBC differential, platelets
- Direct Coombs test
- Blood group and type
- TORCH/viral serologies (IgM)
- Protein/albumin/liver function tests (not on all cases)

(Continued)

TABLE 3.3. Step-Wise Investigation of Nonimmune Fetal Hydrops (Continued)

Cavity Aspiration (may be done at the time of amniocentesis)
- Lymphocyte count (pleural effusion, cystic hygroma)
- Protein/albumin
- Creatinine/ionogram (ascites)
- PCR for CMV parvovirus B19 toxoplasmosis
- Cytology

Step 3: Post-delivery
Examination of the placenta
Neonatal Survival
- Detailed physical examination
- Cardiac monitoring
- Cranial ultrasound
- Abdominal ultrasound
- Cardiac monitoring
- Echocardiography
- CBC, liver function tests, creatinine kinase, albumin, protein
- TORCH, viral culture
- Specialized testing guided by results of prenatal workup

Neonatal/Fetal Demise
- Clinical pictures
- Skeletal survey
- Fetal cells culture (skin, others)
- Freeze fetal tissues and amniotic fluid supernatant
- Bank fetal DNA
- Placental pathology
- Autopsy

- **Ductus venosus (DV):** Abnormal DV waveform helps identify fetuses at risk for cardiac anomalies as well as predicting prognosis.
- **Umbilical venous pulsation:** Its presence is the best predictor of perinatal death because the most common pathway of perinatal demise is fetal congestive heart failure.
- **Umbilical artery (UA):** Changes in UA Doppler appear later than the venous Doppler and cardiac function alterations. Absent or reverse diastolic flow, reflecting elevated placental resistance, is common in non-survivors and often associated with increased cardiac afterload.

INVESTIGATIONS FOR FETAL INFECTIONS

Most congenital infections which lead to fetal hydrops are asymptomatic in the pregnant women. Toxoplasmosis, syphilis, CMV, and parvovirus B19 serologies should be ordered. Additional serologies such as herpes simpex or rubella should be ordered on a case-by-case basis depending on clinical and serological history and recent exposure. Two samples separated by a significant time period are required for determination of seroconversion or a substantial rise in titer. Serology performed by using ELISA assays is very sensitive but often cannot conclusively determine the time of primary infection and the occurrence of a reactivation or a reinfection (CMV), which may be critical for risk assessment. IgM identification is more in favor of a recent infection; however, IgM may persist for several months or even years, and false positive results are common. IgM can also be negative at the time of fetal hydrops if the seroconversion has occurred several weeks earlier or if congenital infection is due to CMV reactivation or reinfection. Avidity test can help to discriminate recent versus old (>4 month) infections. Testing for other infectious diseases may be considered in particular clinical situations (ultrasound findings, HIV-positive pregnant women, clinical symptoms).

Direct detection of infectious agent is possible in amniotic fluid and other fetal samples by polymerase chain reaction (PCR). For CMV detection, timing is critical: amniotic fluid should be collected after 21 gestational weeks and at least 6 weeks post maternal infection.

FETAL BLOOD SAMPLING

Fetal blood sampling should be performed under the following circumstances: MCA Doppler results suggestive of fetal anemia, documented parvovirus B19 seroconversion, parental microcytic anemia from at-risk ethnicity, and documented fetal bleeding. Baseline studies to consider on fetal blood sampling are presented in Table 3.3. If fetal anemia is strongly suspected, O-negative CMV-negative maternally crossmatched blood should be ready for transfusion. The fetal loss rate after cordocentesis was 11% in a group of hydropic fetuses, probably due in part to the high loss rate associated with hydrops itself.

METABOLIC INVESTIGATIONS

The recommended metabolic investigations for unexplained fetal hydrops are listed in Table 3.4. The laboratory should be instructed to keep frozen supernatant and amniotic cells for future studies.

PROGNOSIS

NIHF, all causes together, has a high mortality rate. Fetal chromosomal anomaly, gestational age <24 weeks, and fetal structural anomalies other than chylothorax are indicators of a poor prognosis. However, fetal treatment has significantly improved the survival in selected cases.

PERINATAL MANAGEMENT

Fetal hydrops is a medical emergency and mandates urgent referral to a maternal-fetal medicine specialist and medical geneticist for rapid evaluation. The hydropic fetus is usually in a precarious state, and even minimal delays may prevent access to life-saving procedures.

TABLE 3.4. Lysosomal Enzymatic Assays Used for Nonimmune Fetal Hydrops

Beta galactosidase (GM1)
Beta-glucuronidase (MPS VII)
Beta-glucosidase (Gaucher)
Neuraminidase (sialidosis)
Beta galactosidase and neuraminidase (galactosialidosis)
Sphingomyelin lipidosis or sphingomyelinase deficiency (Niemann-Pick A and B)
Mucolipidosis type II

TABLE 3.5. Fetal Therapies for Nonimmune Hydrops

1. **Intrauterine transfusion**
   Maternal acquired pure red cell aplasia
   Maternal fetal hemorrhage
   Fetal hemolysis (G6PD)
   Fetal parvovirus infection
2. **Repeated centesis or shunt insertion**
   Pleural effusion
   Ascites
   Thoracic cystic lesions
   Congenital cystic adenomatoid malformation (CCAM)
   Pulmonary sequestration
   Pulmonary lymphangiectasia
3. **Intravascular or maternal treatment with anti-arrhythmic drugs**
   Fetal tachyarrhythmia
   Atrioventricular block (anti-SSA/SSB)
4. **Fetal procedures: open fetal surgery or laser vessel ablation/ radiofrequency ablation**
   CCAM
   Sequestration
   Sacrococcygeal teratoma
   Twin-to-twin transfusion syndrome (stage IV)
5. **Others**
   Antithyroid drugs (fetal thyrotoxicosis)

Fetal treatment options for NIHF depend on the underlying etiology(ies) and the gestational age at diagnosis. A maternal-fetal specialist should undertake this evaluation. Clinically available treatment options a are presented in Table 3.5.

When a pregnancy is continued with a known fetal hydrops, the occurrence of a maternal "mirror" syndrome should be carefully monitored. This is defined as the development of maternal edema secondary to fetal hydrops and is usually associated with severe preeclampsia. Because the maternal prognosis can be poor, the option of continuing a pregnancy with a fetal hydrops should be carefully discussed.

Women with pregnancies presenting with fetal hydrops should deliver in a tertiary care center with prenatal consultation with appropriate subspecialties including maternal fetal medicine specialists, medical geneticists, neonatologists, and pediatric surgeons. Antenatal consultation with neonatology allows for parental counseling, adequate preparation of the resuscitation team, and planning of specialized equipment required in the delivery room. Pre-delivery cavity aspiration (pleural effusions, severe ascites, severe polyhydramnios) may facilitate neonatal management and reduce maternal complications. Postnatal therapy begins with vigorous resuscitation, including thoracocentesis and/or paracentesis, in order to establish adequate lung expansion, followed by efforts to determine the cause and correct the condition responsible for the hydrops. Once the neonate is stabilized, a detailed physical examination, cardiac monitoring, and chest radiograph along with ultrasound examinations (head, cardiac, and abdominal) are performed. Additional testing is guided by the investigations initiated antenatally.

It is mandatory to pursue diagnostic investigations after the death of the fetus or newborn with NIHF. Referral to a genetic service should be made to plan for additional analyses.

SUMMARY

The prognosis of NIHF differs markedly between different etiological groups. Recent progress in prenatal genetics and maternal-fetal medicine provides us with newer tools to identify potential underlying etiologies. Prompt access to maternal-fetal medicine units for fetal evaluation and treatment has improved outcome. It is essential to attempt to identify the etiology to better predict prognosis, offer treatment when appropriate, and assess recurrence risk to plan for the management of future pregnancies.

BIBLIOGRAPHIC SOURCE(S)

Abrams ME, Meredith KS, Kinnard P, Clark RH. Hydrops fetalis: a retrospective review of cases reported to a large national database and identification of risk factors associated with death. *Pediatrics.* 2007;120:84-9.

Acar A, Balci O, Gezginc K, et al. Evaluation of the results of cordocentesis. *Taiwan J Obstet Gynecol.* 2007;46:405-9.

Ayida GA, Soothill PW, Rodeck CH. Survival in non-immune hydrops fetalis without malformation or chromosomal abnormalities after invasive treatment. *Fetal Diagn Ther.* 1995;10:101-5.

Bellini C, Hennekam RC, Bonioli E. A diagnostic flow chart for non-immune hydrops fetalis. *Am J Med Genet A.* 2009;149A:852-3.

Berg C, Geipel A, Kohl T, et al. Atrioventricular block detected in fetal life: associated anomalies and potential prognostic markers. *Ultrasound Obstet Gynecol.* 2005;26:4-15.

Braun T, Brauer M, Fuchs I, et al. Mirror syndrome: a systematic review of fetal associated conditions, maternal presentation and perinatal outcome. *Fetal Diagn Ther.* 2010;27:191-203.

Burin MG, Scholz AP, Gus R, et al. Investigation of lysosomal storage diseases in nonimmune hydrops fetalis. *Prenat Diagn.* 2004;24:653-7.

Carvalho S, Martins M, Fortuna A, Ramos U, Ramos C, Rodrigues MC. Galactosialidosis presenting as nonimmune fetal hydrops: a case report. *Prenat Diagn.* 2009;29:895-6.

Chalouhi GE, Stirnemann JJ, Salomon LJ, Essaoui M, Quibel T, Ville Y. Specific complications of monochorionic twin pregnancies: twin-twin transfusion syndrome and twin reversed arterial perfusion sequence. *Semin Fetal Neonatal Med.* 2010;15:349-56.

Cosmi E, Dessole S, Uras L, et al. Middle cerebral artery peak systolic and ductus venosus velocity waveforms in the hydropic fetus. *J Ultrasound Med.* 2005;24:209-13.

Crane J, Mundle W, Boucoiran I, et al. Parvovirus B19 infection in pregnancy. *J Obstet Gynaecol Can.* 2014;36:1107-16.

Crino JP. Ultrasound and fetal diagnosis of perinatal infection. *Clin Obstet Gynecol.* 1999;42:71-80; quiz 174-5.

Croonen EA, Nillesen WM, Stuurman KE, et al. Prenatal diagnostic testing of the Noonan syndrome genes in fetuses with abnormal ultrasound findings. *Eur J Hum Genet.* 2013;21:936-42.

Désilets V, De Bie I, Audibert F. Investigation and management of non-immune fetal hydrops. *J Obstet Gynaecol Can.* 2018;40(8):1077-90.

Dwinnell SJ, Coad S, Butler B, et al. In utero diagnosis and management of a fetus with homozygous alpha-thalassemia in the second trimester: a case report and literature review. *J Pediatr Hematol Oncol.* 2011;33:e358-60.

Enders M, Weidner A, Zoellner I, Searle K, Enders G. Fetal morbidity and mortality after acute human parvovirus B19 infection in pregnancy: prospective evaluation of 1018 cases. *Prenat Diagn.* 2004;24:513-8.

Fallet-Bianco C, De Bie I, Désilets V, Oligny LL. No. 365-Fetal and perinatal autopsy in prenatally diagnosed fetal abnormalities with normal chromosome analysis. *J Obstet Gynaecol Can.* 2018;40:1358-66.

Fouron JC. Fetal arrhythmias: the Saint-Justine hospital experience. *Prenat Diagn.* 2004;24:1068-80.

Fung Kee Fung K, Eason E, Crane J, et al. Prevention of Rh alloimmunization. *J Obstet Gynaecol Can.* 2003;25:765-73.

Gedikbasi A, Oztarhan K, Gunenc Z, et al. Preeclampsia due to fetal non-immune hydrops: mirror syndrome and review of literature. *Hypertens Pregnancy.* 2011;30:322-30.

Hansen T. Non immune hydrops fetalis. In: Rudolph A, Kamei R, Overby K, eds. *Rudolph's Pediatrics.* 21st ed. New York: McGraw-Hill; 2003.

Has R. Non-immune hydrops fetalis in the first trimester: a review of 30 cases. *Clin Exper Obstet Gynecol.* 2001;28:187-90.

Hernandez-Andrade E, Scheier M, Dezerega V, Carmo A, Nicolaides KH. Fetal middle cerebral artery peak systolic velocity in the investigation of non-immune hydrops. *Ultrasound Obstet Gynecol.* 2004;23:442-5.

Hofstaetter C, Hansmann M, Eik-Nes SH, Huhta JC, Luther SL. A cardiovascular profile score in the surveillance of fetal hydrops. *J Matern Fetal Neonatal Med.* 2006;19:407-13.

Huang HR, Tsay PK, Chiang MC, Lien R, Chou YH. Prognostic factors and clinical features in liveborn neonates with hydrops fetalis. *Am J Perinatol.* 2007;24:33-8.

Huhta JC. Guidelines for the evaluation of heart failure in the fetus with or without hydrops. *Pediatr Cardiol.* 2004;25:274-86.

Isaacs H Jr. Fetal hydrops associated with tumors. *Am J Perinatol.* 2008;25:43-68.

Jauniaux E, Van Maldergem L, De Munter C, Moscoso G, Gillerot Y. Nonimmune hydrops fetalis associated with genetic abnormalities. *Obstet Gynecol.* 1990;75:568-72.

Klein JO, Baker CJ, Remington JS, Wilsonn CB. Current concepts of infections of the fetus and newborn infant. In: Remington JS, Klein JO, eds. *Infectious Diseases of the Fetus and Newborn Infant.* 6th ed. Philadelphia, PA: Elsevier Saunders; 2006:3-25.

Knilans TK. Cardiac abnormalities associated with hydrops fetalis. *Semin Perinatol.* 1995;19:483-92.

Knisely AS. The pathologist and the hydropic placenta, fetus, or infant. *Semin Perinatol.* 1995;19(6):525-31.

Kooper AJ, Janssens PM, de Groot AN, et al. Lysosomal storage diseases in non-immune hydrops fetalis pregnancies. *Clin Chim Acta.* 2006;371:176-82.

Langlois S, Ford JC, Chitayat D, et al. Carrier screening for thalassemia and hemoglobinopathies in Canada. *J Obstet Gynaecol Can.* 2008;30:950-71.

Lee FL, Said N, Grikscheit TC, Shin CE, Llanes A, Chmait RH. Treatment of congenital pulmonary airway malformation induced hydrops fetalis via percutaneous sclerotherapy. *Fetal Diagn Ther.* 2012;31(4):264-8.

L'Hermine-Coulomb A, Beuzen F, Bouvier R, et al. Fetal type IV glycogen storage disease: clinical, enzymatic, and genetic data of a pure muscular form with variable and early antenatal manifestations in the same family. *Am J Med Genet A.* 2005;139A:118-22.

Liao C, Wei J, Li Q, Li J, Li L, Li D. Nonimmune hydrops fetalis diagnosed during the second half of pregnancy in Southern China. *Fetal Diagn Ther.* 2007;22:302-5.

Mari G. Middle cerebral artery peak systolic velocity for the diagnosis of fetal anemia: the untold story. *Ultrasound Obstet Gynecol.* 2005;25:323-30.

Mari G, Deter RL, Carpenter RL, et al. Noninvasive diagnosis by Doppler ultrasonography of fetal anemia due to maternal red-cell alloimmunization. Collaborative Group for Doppler Assessment of the Blood Velocity in Anemic Fetuses. *N Engl J Med.* 2000;342:9-14.

McCoy MC, Katz VL, Gould N, Kuller JA. Non-immune hydrops after 20 weeks' gestation: review of 10 years' experience with suggestions for management. *Obstet Gynecol.* 1995;85:578-82.

Mendelson E, Aboudy Y, Smetana Z, Tepperberg M, Grossman Z. Laboratory assessment and diagnosis of congenital viral infections: rubella, cytomegalovirus (CMV), varicella-zoster virus (VZV), herpes simplex virus (HSV), parvovirus B19 and human immunodeficiency virus (HIV). *Reprod Toxicol.* 2006;21:350-82.

Milunsky A. *Genetic Disorders of the Fetus: Diagnosis, Prevention and Treatment.* 5th ed. Baltimore, MD: The Johns Hopkins University Press; 2004.

Morin L, Lim K. Ultrasound in twin pregnancies. *J Obstet Gynaecol Can.* 2011;33:643-56.

Negishi H, Yamada H, Okuyama K, Sagawa T, Makinoda S, Fujimoto S. Outcome of non-immune hydrops fetalis and a fetus with hydrothorax and/or ascites: with some trials of intrauterine treatment. *J Perinat Med.* 1997;25:71-7.

Pajkrt E, Weisz B, Firth HV, Chitty LS. Fetal cardiac anomalies and genetic syndromes. *Prenat Diagn.* 2004;24:1104-15.

Picone O, Benachi A, Mandelbrot L, Ruano R, Dumez Y, Dommergues M. Thoracoamniotic shunting for fetal pleural effusions with hydrops. *Am J Obstet Gynecol.* 2004;191:2047-50.

Ramsay SL, Maire I, Bindloss C, et al. Determination of oligosaccharides and glycolipids in amniotic fluid by electrospray ionisation tandem mass spectrometry: in utero indicators of lysosomal storage diseases. *Molec Genet Metab.* 2004;83:231-8.

Randenberg AL. Nonimmune hydrops fetalis part I: etiology and pathophysiology. *Neonatal Netw.* 2010;29:281-95.

Rodriguez MM, Bruce JH, Jimenez XF, et al. Nonimmune hydrops fetalis in the liveborn: series of 32 autopsies. *Pediatr Devel Pathol.* 2005;8:369-78.

Saudubray J, Van der Berghe G, Walter J. *Inborn Metabolic Diseases: Diagnosis and Treatment.* Berlin: Springer-Verlag; 2007.

Senat MV, Deprest J, Boulvain M, Paupe A, Winer N, Ville Y. Endoscopic laser surgery versus serial amnioreduction for severe twin-to-twin transfusion syndrome. *N Engl J Med.* 2004;351:136-44.

Shah A, Moon-Grady A, Bhogal N, et al. Effectiveness of sotalol as first-line therapy for fetal supraventricular tachyarrhythmias. *Am J Cardiol.* 2012;109(11):1614-8.

Stone DL, Sidransky E. Hydrops fetalis: lysosomal storage disorders in extremis. *Adv Pediatr.* 1999;46:409-40.

Turgal M, Ozyuncu O, Boyraz G, Yazicioglu A, Sinan Beksac M. Non-immune hydrops fetalis as a diagnostic and survival problems: what do we tell the parents? *J Perinat Med.* 2015;43(3):353-8.

Venkat-Raman N, Sebire NJ, Murphy KW. Recurrent fetal hydrops due to mucopolysaccharidoses type VII. *Fetal Diagn Ther.* 2006;21:250-4.

Wapner RJ, Driscoll DA, Simpson JL. Integration of microarray technology into prenatal diagnosis: counselling issues generated during the NICHD clinical trial. *Prenat Diagn.* 2012;32:396-400.

Yamamoto M, Ville Y. Twin-to-twin transfusion syndrome: management options and outcomes. *Clin Obstet Gynecol.* 2005;48:973-80.

Yinon Y, Farine D, Yudin MH, et al. Cytomegalovirus infection in pregnancy. *J Obstet Gynaecol Can.* 2010;32:348-54.

Yong PJ, Von Dadelszen P, Carpara D, et al. Prediction of pediatric outcome after prenatal diagnosis and expectant antenatal management of congenital cystic adenomatoid malformation. *Fetal Diagn Ther.* 2012;31:94-102.

Fetal Anemia

Moeun Son, MD, MSCI • Susan E. Gerber, MD, MPH

SCOPE

DISEASE/CONDITION(S)

An insufficient number or quality of red blood cells in the fetal circulatory system to adequately carry oxygen to the cells and organs of the fetus.

GUIDELINE OBJECTIVE(S)

Review important etiologies of fetal anemia; examine different clinical approaches to identifying at-risk or already affected fetuses; compile recommendations for antenatal surveillance, fetal diagnostic and therapeutic interventions, delivery planning, and immediate postnatal management.

BRIEF BACKGROUND

Fetal anemia is defined as a hematocrit or hemoglobin concentration more than two standard deviations below the mean for a given gestational age. It can develop as the result of three general causes: increased fetal red blood cell (RBC) destruction, decreased fetal RBC production, or fetal blood loss. There are several different scenarios in which fetal anemia may be detected in the antenatal period (Table 4.1). Anemia leads to decreased oxygen delivery to tissue, but mild to moderate anemia is generally well tolerated by the fetus and can resolve without sequelae. However, if the anemia becomes more severe, it can lead to fetal compensatory responses, resulting in the development of fetal hydrops and/or death. Unfortunately, in the antenatal period, most clinical signs of fetal anemia only become apparent at this severe stage. Thus most diagnostic efforts have focused on the surveillance of pregnant women identified as carrying fetuses at particular risk of developing anemia.

TABLE 4.1. Conditions Associated with Fetal Anemia

Identifying the at-risk mother
  Red cell alloimmunization
  Thalassemia
  Parvovirus infection
  Twin anemia-polycythemia sequence
Fetal hydrops on ultrasound
Fetomaternal hemorrhage

RECOMMENDATIONS

MAJOR RECOMMENDATIONS

Management of the At-Risk Mother

Positive Maternal Antibody Screen The presence of maternal red blood cell (RBC) antibodies, also known as alloimmunization, may lead to fetal hemolysis with subsequent anemia depending on the degree of antigenicity and the amount and type of antibodies involved. Therefore, a maternal antibody screen should be performed on all women at their first prenatal visit. If the antibody screen is positive, the detected antibody should be identified and characterized for its potential to cause fetal hemolytic disease (Figure 4.1). If the identified antibody has never been associated with fetal hemolysis, no further evaluation is necessary. However, if the identified antibody is clinically significant, the next step is to determine paternal antigen carrier status. If paternal testing is not possible or if it is positive, serial antibody titers (indirect Coombs test) should be followed, with further testing only if a critical threshold is reached. Titer values are conventionally reported as the integer of the greatest tube dilution with a positive agglutination reaction. A *critical* titer is defined as the titer associated with a significant risk for fetal hydrops, and thus is used as the threshold for further evaluation. Critical titer thresholds vary depending upon the antigen given different degrees of risk. For example, anti-Kell antibodies cause fetal anemia both by suppression of erythropoiesis and cell-mediated hemolysis. As such, there is risk of fetal anemia even at low titers, and for this antibody there is no threshold to accurately predict the absence of severe fetal anemia. If paternal blood typing is negative for the involved red cell antigen and correct paternity is ensured, further maternal and fetal testing is not indicated. In the case of heterozygous or unknown paternal genotype for the involved red cell antigen, amniocentesis may be performed after 15 weeks of gestation to determine fetal antigen status. The use of cell-free DNA (cfDNA) testing may be used to determine the fetal RhD status, but this is not yet widely implemented in the United States. A homozygous paternal genotype signifies an antigen-positive fetus, and further testing with cfDNA or amniocentesis is unnecessary.

Until recently, the standard test to evaluate the need for fetal transfusion was serial amniocentesis for the determination of bilirubin levels in amniotic fluid. The bilirubin level is quantified by spectrophotometry and expressed as the change in optical density at a wavelength of 450 nm (ΔOD_{450}). Since fetal hemolysis leads to accumulation of bilirubin in amniotic fluid, the ΔOD_{450} values were plotted on a chart devised by Liley to estimate the severity of anemia. However, this invasive approach has been largely replaced by Doppler ultrasonography after seminal work showed that Doppler measurement of the peak velocity of systolic blood flow in the fetal middle cerebral artery

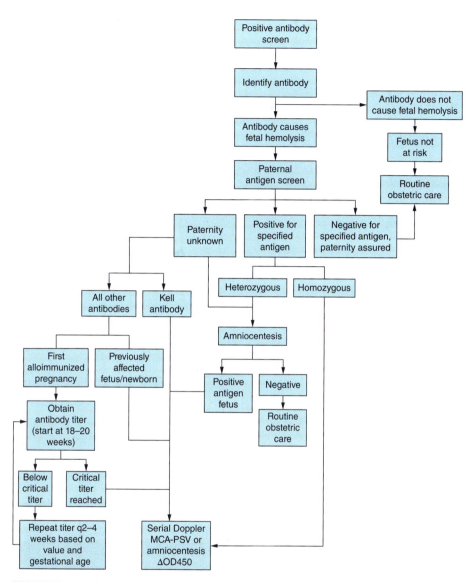

FIGURE 4.1 • Algorithm for the management of the pregnant patient with red cell alloimmunization.

(MCA-PSV) more accurately detected moderate and severe fetal anemia. This method is based on the principle that the anemic fetus preserves oxygen delivery to the brain by increasing cerebral flow of low viscosity blood. MCA-PSV can be measured as early as 16 weeks of gestation if there is a prior history of early severe fetal anemia, but Doppler evaluation is generally initiated later since intrauterine fetal transfusions are technically challenging before 20 weeks of gestation.

Infectious Exposure. Parvovirus B19 is the most common infectious cause of fetal anemia, as the virus has a predilection for erythroid progenitor cells, leading to inhibition of erythropoiesis in the bone marrow. Parvovirus leads to a common childhood illness, but about half of all reproductive-aged women have no immunity to this virus and are therefore susceptible to infection during pregnancy. Most infected adults will be asymptomatic or have vague nonspecific symptoms. As such, cases are more often discovered when a known exposure prompts serologic testing for IgG and IgM antibodies. The risk of vertical transmission to the fetus from an infected mother is about 33%, and the fetal death rate is highest if infection occurs before 20 weeks' gestation. Even if fetal death does not occur, significant fetal anemia can ensue. Thus when a diagnosis of maternal parvovirus infection is made, the fetus should be examined weekly by ultrasound to assess MCA-PSV and look for signs of hydrops. If the MCA-PSV values remain <1.5 multiples of the median (MoM), weekly ultrasound scans should be continued for 12 weeks after the exposure. If severe anemia is suspected because of elevated MCA-PSV or signs of hydrops (Figure 4.2), assessment of fetal hematocrit by fetal blood sampling is warranted with intrauterine transfusion, if severe anemia is confirmed. In most cases, the anemia is transient, and fetal intrauterine transfusion (IUT) can support a fetus through this aplastic crisis.

Maternal Microcytic Anemia. Hereditary RBC disorders such as hemoglobin-opathies can cause increased fetal RBC destruction leading to anemia. Among the hemoglobinopathies, the most common cause of fetal anemia and subsequent hydrops is alpha-thalassemia. As such, all pregnant women should have a complete blood count (CBC) with RBC indices performed at their first prenatal visit to screen for thalassemia. A mean corpuscular volume (MCV) less than 80 fL in the absence of iron deficiency suggests thalassemia, and further testing with hemoglobin analysis is indicated. Hemoglobin electrophoresis identifies women with sickle cell and beta-thalassemia, but DNA-based testing for alpha globin gene deletions is needed to assess for alpha-thalassemia. Alpha-thalassemia is an autosomal recessive disorder most commonly affecting women of Southeast Asian descent, and results in the reduced production of alpha globin chains of hemoglobin. If a woman is found to be a carrier for alpha-thalassemia, paternal testing is recommended; if both parents are determined to be carriers, fetal diagnostic testing should be offered with DNA-based testing using chorionic villi obtained by chorionic villus sample (CVS) at 10 to 12 weeks of gestation or using cultured amniotic fluid cells obtained by amniocentesis after 15 weeks of gestation. Hemoglobin (Hb) H disease, which is caused by the deletion of three alpha-globin chain genes, is usually associated with mild to moderate hemolytic anemia prenatally since only one alpha globin chain gene is functional. As such, affected fetuses should be monitored with ultrasounds to monitor MCA-PSV and assess for signs of hydrops. Most will be symptomatic at birth, often presenting with neonatal jaundice and anemia since alpha globin synthesis is required in utero for the production of hemoglobin F, the major hemoglobin found during late gestation. Alpha-thalassemia major (Hb Bart) is caused by the absence of all four alpha-globin genes. Without any production of alpha globin, fetal hemoglobin cannot be formed, and affected fetuses will universally become hydropic. This condition is typically incompatible with extrauterine life, and infants usually die within a few hours after birth unless supported with massive total exchange transfusions.

Monochorionic Diamniotic Twin Gestation. Twin anemia-polycythemia sequence (TAPS) is an atypical chronic form of twin-twin transfusion syndrome (TTTS) that presents as a large inter-twin hemoglobin difference, without

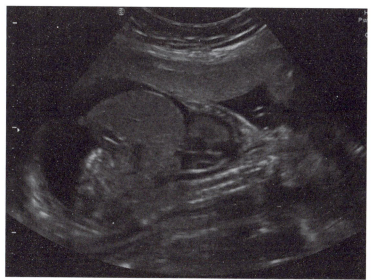

A.

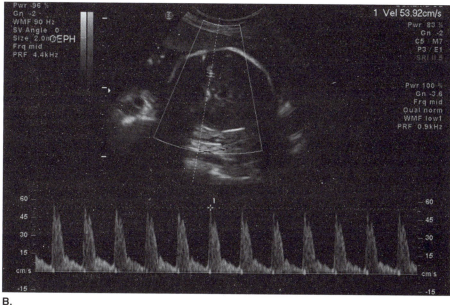

B.

FIGURE 4.2 • Prenatal ultrasound images of a fetus at 21 weeks of gestation with severe anemia and nonimmune hydrops as a result of parvovirus infection. **A.** Sagittal view demonstrates extensive ascites and pericardial effusions. **B.** Doppler assessment of MCA-PSV reveals elevated value of >2 MoM based on gestational age. (Courtesy of the Division of Maternal Fetal Medicine, Department of Obstetrics and Gynecology, Northwestern University Feinberg School of Medicine.)

oligohydramnios-polyhydramnios sequence. While it can spontaneously occur, it is more likely to develop after a pregnancy complicated by TTTS is treated with laser ablation; the small residual anastomoses remaining post ablation lead to the gradual development of anemia in one twin and polycythemia in the other. Prenatal diagnosis is made when the MCA-PSV is greater than 1.5 MoM in the donor twin and less than 0.8 MoM (or less than 1.0 MoM in some studies) in the recipient twin. Postnatal diagnosis is made with an inter-twin hemoglobin difference of more than or equal to 8.0 g/dL, an inter-twin reticulocyte ratio of greater than 1.7 (reticulocyte count of the donor twin divided by the reticulocyte count of the recipient twin), and/or a placental injection examination showing a small number of miniscule (<1 mm) vascular anastomoses.

Management of the Ultrasonographic Detection of Fetal Hydrops

Fetal hydrops is typically defined as the presence of extracellular fluid in at least two fetal body compartments. These fluid body collections include scalp and body wall edema, pleural effusions, pericardial effusions, and ascites. Fetal anemia is identified in 10–27% of hydropic fetuses and generally associated with fetal high output cardiac failure. Once hydrops is identified, a detailed maternal medical history, including ethnic background, should be obtained to determine the etiology. Targeted ultrasound with Doppler assessment of the fetal MCA-PSV should be performed. Laboratory evaluation of CBC with RBC indices, blood type and antibody screen, and infectious serologies (IgM and IgG for cytomegalovirus, toxoplasmosis, rubella, and parvovirus B19; nontreponemal test for syphilis) should also be performed. A Kleihauer-Betke acid elution stain should be used to exclude the possibility of fetomaternal hemorrhage. Definitive fetal testing for infectious diseases with amniocentesis, CVS, or cordocentesis may also be considered.

Management of Fetomaternal Hemorrhage

Fetomaternal hemorrhage (FMH) leading to significant fetal anemia may occur as either an isolated acute event or as a chronic ongoing hemorrhage. There is no universally accepted threshold, but a definition of ≥20% of the fetoplacental blood volume is often utilized because this threshold has been associated with significant fetal and neonatal morbidity and mortality. The rosette test, a qualitative yet sensitive test for FMH, can first be performed if there is an index of suspicion. If the rosette test is positive, a Kleihauer-Betke test can then be performed to assess for the presence of fetal cells in the maternal peripheral blood, or flow cytometry can also be used to estimate the volume of fetal bleeding into the maternal circulation (both based on identification of hemoglobin F). Fetal findings associated with massive FMH include absent or persistently decreased movement, fetal heart rate abnormality (e.g., sinusoidal fetal heart rate pattern, recurrent late decelerations, tachycardia), low biophysical profile score, fetal hydrops, and death. Fetal compromise from FMH is usually an indication for delivery. However, fetal anemia from FMH may be treated with IUT. Still, if the pregnancy is at an advanced gestational age and risks associated with delivery are considered to be less than those associated with the IUT procedure, delivery should be considered.

PRACTICE OPTIONS

Practice Option #1: Antepartum Fetal Surveillance

Various ultrasound parameters have been studied that allow for noninvasive antenatal detection of fetal anemia. Unfortunately, parameters such as amniotic fluid index, diameter of the umbilical vein, and placental thickness have failed to accurately predict fetal anemia. Fetal hydrops can be easily identified by ultrasound, but this is a late sign of fetal anemia. Doppler assessment of the MCA-PSV has proved to be a reliable method for detecting fetal anemia. This test has a sensitivity of 88%, specificity of 82%, and accuracy of 85% in a large prospective, international, multicenter study. It outperformed amniocentesis with ΔOD_{450} analysis, with a 9% improvement in accuracy. Measurements of the MCA-PSV are usually initiated at 18 weeks of gestation and should be repeated at 1- to 2-week intervals. Because the normal MCA-PSV increases with advancing gestational age, data should be adjusted for gestational age using the MoM. Using receiver operating characteristic curve (ROC) analysis, a threshold of 1.5 MoM was used to predict moderate to severe anemia (<0.65 MoM for fetal hemoglobin). An MCA-PSV >1.5 MoM is an indication for fetal blood sampling for fetal hematocrit determination and transfusion as needed.

Practice Option #2: Antenatal Diagnostic Testing and Fetal Therapy

Ultrasound-directed fetal blood sampling (also called percutaneous umbilical blood sampling or cordocentesis) allows direct access to the fetal circulation by puncturing the umbilical vein in the portion of the cord near its insertion into the placenta or as it enters the fetal liver. This allows for measurement of fetal hematocrit, reticulocyte count, direct Coombs, fetal blood type, and total bilirubin. Because fetal blood sampling is associated with a 1–2% rate of fetal death, this procedure is generally reserved for the detection of fetal anemia once the peak MCA Doppler has exceeded 1.5 MoM. Furthermore, the procedure may not be possible prior to 20 weeks' gestation due to the narrow caliber of the fetal vessels. Red blood cells are prepared for intravascular IUT, and are typically from a blood type O, RhD-negative, cytomegalovirus-negative, irradiated unit collected in the previous 72 hours, and are packed to a hematocrit of 75–85% to prevent volume overload in the fetus. The total amount of red cells to transfuse is based on the initial fetal hematocrit, fetoplacental blood volume (estimated from fetal weight), and hematocrit of donor blood unit. Subsequent transfusions are scheduled to support continued fetal growth in the setting of ongoing hemolysis.

Practice Option #3: Timing of Delivery

The appropriate timing of delivery should be individualized for each case, as there are many factors to consider. Recommendations will vary based on the suspected etiology for fetal anemia and its acuity, the gestational age and risks of iatrogenic prematurity, the severity of fetal anemia with the presence or absence of fetal hydrops, the conditions of additional antenatal surveillance (e.g., non-stress test or biophysical profile), and the expected utility of fetal therapy with IUT with its associated risks. For women who are at risk of delivering prior to 32 weeks of gestation, we suggest antenatal administration of magnesium sulfate for neonatal neuroprotection as well as a course of corticosteroids to improve neonatal outcomes.

Practice Option #4: Mode of Delivery

Cesarean delivery should be reserved for usual obstetric indications. There is no evidence of improved neonatal outcome with cesarean delivery in an otherwise uncomplicated gestation. Thus when timing of delivery is determined, induction of labor should be utilized for women who are candidates for vaginal delivery. Operative vaginal delivery is not contraindicated in fetuses with anemia, but caution should be taken given the associated small risks of neonatal intracranial hemorrhage, subgaleal hematomas, and neonatal lacerations.

Practice Option #5: Delivery Room and Postnatal Management

The peripartum care of a woman with a hydropic fetus should be undertaken in a tertiary care center whenever possible, as coordinated efforts by the obstetrician, perinatologist, and neonatal team is needed to optimize neonatal outcome. Resuscitation of hydropic neonates can be difficult, as the majority of these neonates will require respiratory assistance and mechanical ventilation. Ventilation may be compromised by pulmonary hypoplasia, pulmonary edema, air leaks, or with the accumulation of pleural or peritoneal fluid. Abdominal paracentesis of fetal ascites and/or thoracentesis of fetal pleural effusions may be needed prior to delivery or immediately after to facilitate resuscitation. Neonates with severe anemia and cardiovascular instability may benefit from isovolumetric or partial exchange transfusion with packed RBCs. Management of neonatal anemia is further discussed in Chapter 34. Passively acquired antibodies from alloimmunized mothers remain in the neonatal circulation for weeks. This results in a postnatal period of 1 to 3 months in which weekly neonatal hematocrit and reticulocyte counts should be monitored, as infants require several subsequent red cell transfusions. In one series, more than three-quarters of fetuses who received IUT subsequently needed neonatal transfusions. It is also important to note that after birth, a neonate's immature liver may be unable to metabolize the bilirubin that has accumulated in its blood, and the level of bilirubin may rise dramatically, resulting in kernicterus if the bilirubin enters the neonatal brain. Furthermore, severe anemia may prompt the liver, spleen, and other organs to increase their production of RBCs to compensate, resulting in hepatosplenomegaly. Therefore, a neonate affected by significant anemia must be monitored closely in the postpartum period.

IMPLEMENTATION OF GUIDELINE

QUALIFYING STATEMENTS

1. There is variation in the critical titer thresholds at which antenatal surveillance for fetal anemia should be initiated in pregnancies affected by red cell alloimmunization.
2. There are limited data regarding the optimal time intervals of fetal testing and therapy for fetal anemia.
3. There are limited data regarding the optimal timing of delivery for an anemic fetus.

DESCRIPTION OF IMPLEMENTATION STRATEGY

Recommend written guidelines for the management of pregnancies identified to be at risk for the development of fetal anemia; provide written guidelines for the management of ultrasonographic detection of fetal hydrops and pregnancies affected by fetomaternal hemorrhage; provide written guidelines for the initiation and continuation of fetal testing and therapy for fetal anemia; recognize that Doppler assessment of the MCA-PSV is the standard method for the detection of fetal anemia and needs to be calculated based on gestational age.

BIBLIOGRAPHIC SOURCE(S)

ACOG Committee on Obstetrics. ACOG Practice Bulletin no. 78: hemoglobinopathies in pregnancy. *Obstet Gynecol.* 2007;109(1):229-37.

Cosmi E, Mari G, Delle Chiaie L, et al. Noninvasive diagnosis by Doppler ultrasonography of fetal anemia resulting from parvovirus infection. *Am J Obstet Gynecol.* 2002;187(5):1290-3.

Davies SC, Cronin E, Gill M, Greengross P, Hickman M, Normand C. Screening for sickle cell disease and thalassaemia: a systematic review with supplementary research. *Health Technol Assess.* 2000;4(3):i-v, 1-99.

De Boer IP, Zeestraten EC, Lopriore E, van Kamp IL, Kanhai HH, Walther FJ. Pediatric outcome in Rhesus hemolytic disease treated with and without intrauterine transfusion. *Am J Obstet Gynecol.* 2008;198(1):54.e51-4.

Forouzan I. Hydrops fetalis: recent advances. *Obstet Gynecol Surv.* 1997;52(2):130-8.

Harman CR, Bowman JM, Manning FA, Menticoglou SM. Intrauterine transfusion—intraperitoneal versus intravascular approach: a case-control comparison. *Am J Obstet Gynecol.* 1990;162(4): 1053-9.

Lee SY, Chow CB, Li CK, Chiu MC. Outcome of intensive care of homozygous alpha-thalassaemia without prior intra-uterine therapy. *J Paediatr Child Health.* 2007;43(7-8):546-50.

Liley AW. Liquor amnil analysis in the management of the pregnancy complicated by resus sensitization. *Am J Obstet Gynecol.* 1961;82:1359-70.

Lopriore E, Slaghekke F, Middeldorp JM, Klumper FJ, Oepkes D, Vandenbussche FP. Residual anastomoses in twin-to-twin transfusion syndrome treated with selective fetoscopic laser surgery: localization, size, and consequences. *Am J Obstet Gynecol.* 2009;201(1): 66.e1-4.

Lopriore E, Slaghekke F, Oepkes D, Middeldorp JM, Vandenbussche FP, Walther FJ. Hematological characteristics in neonates with twin anemia-polycythemia sequence (TAPS). *Prenat Diagn.* 2010;30(3):251-5.

Lorey F, Charoenkwan P, Witkowska HE, et al. Hb H hydrops foetalis syndrome: a case report and review of literature. *Br J Haematol.* 2001;115(1):72-8.

Mari G, Deter RL, Carpenter RL, et al. Noninvasive diagnosis by Doppler ultrasonography of fetal anemia due to maternal red-cell alloimmunization. Collaborative Group for Doppler Assessment of the Blood Velocity in Anemic Fetuses. *N Engl J Med.* 2000;342(1):9-14.

Moise KJ Jr. Management of rhesus alloimmunization in pregnancy. *Obstet Gynecol.* 2008;112(1):164-76.

Oepkes D, Seaward PG, Vandenbussche FP, et al. Doppler ultrasonography versus amniocentesis to predict fetal anemia. *N Engl J Med.* 2006;355(2):156-64.

Prospective study of human parvovirus (B19) infection in pregnancy. Public Health Laboratory Service Working Party on Fifth Disease. *BMJ.* 1990;300(6733):1166-70.

Remington JS. *Infectious Diseases of the Fetus and Newborn Infant.* 7th ed. Philadelphia: Saunders/Elsevier; 2011.

Rubod C, Deruelle P, Le Goueff F, Tunez V, Fournier M, Subtil D. Long-term prognosis for infants after massive fetomaternal hemorrhage. *Obstet Gynecol.* 2007;110(2 Pt 1):256-60.

Slaghekke F, Kist WJ, Oepkes D, et al. Twin anemia-polycythemia sequence: diagnostic criteria, classification, perinatal management and outcome. *Fetal Diagn Ther.* 2010;27(4):181-90.

Van Kamp IL, Klumper FJ, Oepkes D, et al. Complications of intrauterine intravascular transfusion for fetal anemia due to maternal red-cell alloimmunization. *Am J Obstet Gynecol.* 2005;192(1):171-7.

van Wamelen DJ, Klumper FJ, de Haas M, Meerman RH, van Kamp IL, Oepkes D. Obstetric history and antibody titer in estimating severity of Kell alloimmunization in pregnancy. *Obstet Gynecol.* 2007;109(5):1093-8.

Neonatal Transition

Neonatal Resuscitation

Nathan C. Sundgren, MD, PhD

SCOPE

DISEASE/CONDITION(S)

Respiratory distress syndrome, respiratory failure, prematurity, cardiopulmonary resuscitation.

GUIDELINE OBJECTIVE(S)

Review best practice of stabilization for premature infants at birth. Review best practice of resuscitation when positive pressure and/or cardiac compressions are required.

BRIEF BACKGROUND

Newborn babies, and especially premature newborns, are at risk for requiring resuscitation. This risk is highest on the day of birth when the newborn makes the cardiorespiratory transition to extrauterine life. Some have called the day a preterm baby is born the most dangerous of its life. In the delivery room, 4–10% of all term and late preterm newborns will receive positive-pressure ventilation (PPV), but only 1 to 3 per 1000 will receive chest compressions or emergency medications. Of those who are sick and require admission to the neonatal intensive care unit (NICU), resuscitation outside of the delivery room may still be needed. The incidence of infants who receive cardiopulmonary resuscitation (CPR) in the NICU is 1–6% of all admissions.

The great majority of neonates who require resuscitation require this because of respiratory failure or decompensation, whether at delivery or later during NICU admission.

Therefore, the American Heart Association and American Academy of Pediatrics, through the Neonatal Resuscitation Program (NRP), have long emphasized that ventilation of the lungs is the single most important step in neonatal resuscitation. Stabilization of the respiratory system must be the primary focus for intervention in nearly every baby at birth and during periods of decompensation later in the initial hospitalization. Stabilization of the respiratory system of premature babies has shifted in recent years from primarily intubation and subsequent surfactant administration to stabilizing with continuous positive airway pressure (CPAP). CPAP with selective surfactant use is superior to routine intubation and surfactant administration with continued ventilation by the endotracheal tube (ETT) for prevention of bronchopulmonary dysplasia (BPD) and death. Preterm infants treated with early CPAP alone are not at increased risk of adverse outcomes. Several trials have demonstrated that babies as preterm as 24 weeks can be stabilized on CPAP without intubation, PPV, or surfactant. Thus the spontaneously breathing preterm newborn should always be stabilized on CPAP if possible.

If the baby is not breathing (apnea), is gasping, or has a heart rate below 100 beats per minute, then PPV is required for these signs of ineffective ventilation. Knowing how to provide effective ventilation of the lungs is the foundation for resuscitation skills in the delivery room and NICU. The purpose of ventilation is to aerate the lungs and displace fetal lung fluid and then to maintain functional residual capacity. It should be appreciated that giving an adequate tidal volume with each PPV breath is needed to accomplish this. However, devices used in the delivery room for PPV do not measure tidal volumes. Rather the resuscitation team uses heart rate response and level of chest rise to judge if PPV breaths are adequate. Conversely, tidal volume breaths that are too large are injurious to premature lungs. Data suggests as few as five large tidal volume breaths delivered at birth can cause lung and cerebral injury. Therefore, attention should be paid to limiting pressures and tidal volumes when providing PPV, particularly in preterm infants.

There are cases where ventilatory resuscitation alone will not be adequate. In these cases, the circulation must be supported by chest compressions and medications (primarily epinephrine). However, the team must ensure that effective ventilation has already been established before beginning chest compressions. Current guidelines emphasize, in the absence of a rising heart rate, 30 seconds of PPV through an alternative airway (laryngeal mask airway [LMA] or ETT) that is moving the chest is the best sign of adequate ventilation. Once this has been done, chest compressions are coordinated in a 3:1 ratio with ventilation breaths. Limited studies have tested uncoordinated chest compressions with PPV and various ratios, but so far none have been superior to a coordinated 3:1 ratio. If the need for CPR is felt to be primarily cardiac in origin, for example, for older infants in the NICU, then a 15:2 ratio of chest compressions to PPV breaths can be considered.

RECOMMENDATIONS

MAJOR RECOMMENDATIONS

Guidelines from the NRP should be the foundation for resuscitation of newborn infants. All facilities caring for newborn infants should ensure clinical staff are appropriately trained and certified in NRP protocols.

For preterm infants, a "CPAP first" strategy should be employed for stabilizing spontaneously breathing premature babies in the delivery room. PPV is indicated when the baby is not breathing, is gasping, or has a heart rate of <100. Starting PPV does not preclude a team from transitioning back to CPAP when the baby establishes a consistent breathing pattern and a heart rate is maintained >100; many preterm infants who require PPV can be successfully transitioned to CPAP.

RESPIRATORY SUPPORT PRACTICE OPTIONS

Practice Option #1: CPAP Stabilization

A CPAP-first strategy requires a team effort focused on a successful transition without intubation. Patient providers must be willing to give the newborn time to transition to a consistent breathing effort, establish lung volume, and stabilize oxygen requirement. We recommend that all babies ≤30 weeks gestational age (GA) at time of birth be placed on CPAP immediately on arrival to the warmer. Babies 31–34 weeks GA can be considered for this "prophylactic" approach or be given CPAP in early response if signs of respiratory distress develop. The initial steps of providing warmth and gentle stimulation and assessment of respiratory effort and heart rate can be performed while the baby is receiving CPAP. PPV is indicated before 60 seconds of life if the baby is not breathing or is gasping, or if the heart rate is <100 beats per minute. Neonates may require several periods of time alternating between PPV and CPAP until a consistent spontaneous breathing pattern is established. PPV is the delivery of a volume of air in and out of the lungs using a device such as a flow inflating (anesthesia) bag, t-piece resuscitator, or self-inflating bag. In the delivery room, starting pressures are targeted to avoid large injurious tidal volumes. A starting peak inspiratory pressure (PIP) of 20–25 cm H_2O is recommended and a positive end expiratory pressure (PEEP) of 5 to maintain lung volumes between breaths. The need for limiting PIP may make the t-piece resuscitator the ideal device in the delivery room, but there is little evidence comparing flow-inflating bags to t-piece resuscitators. In the NICU, ventilation pressures used in resuscitation should take into consideration previous support the infant was on and disease process. Assessment of effective ventilation relies on heart rate and chest rise. The most important indicator of effective ventilation is a rising heart rate. The secondary assessment of chest rise in the absence of a rising heart rate can guide further interventions to establish effective ventilation. Strategies to maintain CPAP must continue after stabilization and NICU admission. CPAP failure occurs in ~50% of babies stabilized with a CPAP-first strategy. Early caffeine administration and nasal noninvasive PPV (NIPPV) may be strategies employed to prevent CPAP failure. A rising or persistent FiO_2 >40–60% will likely additionally benefit from surfactant administration. Surfactant administration strategies that minimize the ventilation time used to deliver surfactant should be used when feasible.

Practice Option #2: Intubation

The longtime standard for treating respiratory distress syndrome (RDS) in very preterm infants has been intubation and early surfactant administration. Extremely preterm babies, especially those who did not receive antenatal steroids, are at very high risk for CPAP failure even if a CPAP-first strategy is attempted. Therefore, some practitioners may choose to intubate at the beginning of resuscitation in those preterm babies at the highest risk for CPAP failure and/or need for surfactant administration. Otherwise, initial attempts at resuscitation will start with mask PPV as described in Practice Option #1 above. However, if PPV by face mask is not able to provide effective ventilation, then an ETT should be placed quickly to establish effective ventilation. An alternative airway to an ETT is an LMA. The LMA usually only fits babies that are >1500 g.

In this population, randomized trials have shown the LMA to be superior to face mask ventilation in newborns who require resuscitation, and has been used for surfactant administration. In very preterm infants <1500 g, it is currently not practical to use an LMA for resuscitation.

OXYGEN THERAPY PRACTICE OPTIONS

Practice

Oximeters should be used in the delivery room (and in the NICU) to guide resuscitation when oxygen or positive pressure support are needed. As per NRP guidelines, the FiO_2 used for resuscitation should begin at 0.21 for term infants and 0.21–0.30 for preterm infants, and should then be titrated to achieve oxygen saturation targets. Oxygen saturation targets vary by postnatal age, beginning at 60–65% at 1 minute of life and increasing gradually to 85–95% by 10 minutes of life. Minute-specific oxygen saturation targets are provided in NRP. Of note, it is common for newly born preterm infants to require higher FiO_2 to achieve target saturations until the lungs are optimally recruited. Allow higher FiO_2 temporarily in the delivery room to give time for the lungs to open and FiO_2 to decrease.

CARDIAC RESUSCITATION PRACTICE OPTIONS

Practice

If attempts at ventilatory resuscitation as in options 1 and 2 have failed and the heart rate is <60 beats per minute despite effective ventilation, then chest compressions are begun and continued for at least 1 minute and until the heart rate is >60 bpm. The ratio of coordinated chest compression to breaths is 3:1. If the need for resuscitation is thought to be primarily of cardiac origin, then a higher ratio of 15:2 may be used. If chest compressions do not bring the heart rate >60 bpm, epinephrine should be given. Epinephrine should be given IV or IO (0.1–0.3 mL/kg of 1 mg/10 mL concentration); it can be given via endotracheal tube once (0.5–1.0 mL/kg of 1 mg/10 mL concentration) while access is being obtained. For resuscitations in the NICU beyond the immediate post-delivery period, patient diagnosis and cause for decompensation may make other medications and interventions life-saving that should be tailored for each patient's diagnoses.

CLINICAL ALGORITHM(S)

The clinical algorithm and guidelines for neonatal resuscitation are based on recommendations from the International Liaison Committee on Resuscitation (ILCOR). New guidelines are published every 5 years (http://www.ilcor.org/home/). These recommendations are then put into guidelines by several national organizations. In the United States, the resuscitation guidelines and training recommendations are created by the NRP (https://www.aap.org/en-us/continuing-medical-education/life-support/NRP/Pages/NRP.aspx).

IMPLEMENTATION OF GUIDELINE

DESCRIPTION OF IMPLEMENTATION STRATEGY

All providers involved in resuscitation of newborns should be trained in NRP. Institutions can then develop and agree on clinical guidelines and how to best adopt and use these guidelines in their population. Simulation and frequent practice of resuscitation helps providers be prepared for "high acuity, low occurrence" (HALO) events.

QUALITY METRICS

Although there are no nationally recommended quality measures for neonatal resuscitation, centers should develop local quality indicators. These could include measures around clinical care, teamwork, communication, and more. As an example, the number of babies receiving chest compressions or epinephrine in the delivery room could be a valuable quality metric. The need for these interventions should be uncommon, and higher rates of chest compression or epinephrine use may signal a need to improve team performance on establishing effective ventilation. Potential quality indicators related to neonatal resuscitation have been described in the literature by Lapcharoensap and Lee.

SUMMARY

The need for resuscitation in very preterm babies is a common occurrence. Ventilation of the newborn lungs is the single most important step in resuscitation. Most preterm babies can be stabilized with a combination of PPV and CPAP. Some babies will further require intubation to establish effective ventilation. The need for cardiac compressions should be rare if effective ventilation is established quickly.

BIBLIOGRAPHIC SOURCE(S)

American Academy of Pediatrics. *Textbook of Neonatal Resuscitation*. 7th ed. American Academy of Pediatrics; American Heart Association; 2016.

Lapcharoensap W, Lee HC. Tackling quality improvement in the delivery room. *Clin Perinatol*. 2017;44(3):663-81.

Perlman JM, Wyllie J, Kattwinkel J, et al. Part 7: Neonatal Resuscitation: 2015 International Consensus on Cardiopulmonary Resuscitation and Emergency Cardiovascular Care Science With Treatment Recommendations. *Circulation*. 2015;132(16 Suppl 1):S204-S41.

Qureshi MJ, Kumar M. Laryngeal mask airway versus bag-mask ventilation or endotracheal intubation for neonatal resuscitation. *Cochrane Database Sys Rev*. 2018;3:CD003314.

Subramaniam P, Ho JJ, Davis PG. Prophylactic nasal continuous positive airway pressure for preventing morbidity and mortality in very preterm infants. *Cochrane Database Sys Rev*. 2016;14(6):CD001243.

Wyckoff MH, Aziz K, Escobedo MB, et al. Part 13: Neonatal Resuscitation: 2015 American Heart Association Guidelines Update for Cardiopulmonary Resuscitation and Emergency Cardiovascular Care. *Circulation*. 2015;132(18 Suppl 2): S543-60.

The Well Newborn

Elizabeth K. Oh, MD • Heena K. Lee, MD, MPH

SCOPE

DISEASE/CONDITION(S)

Well newborn.

GUIDELINE/OBJECTIVE(S)

Review best practices in caring for the infants in the well newborn nursery.

BRIEF BACKGROUND

Newborns admitted to the well nursery often include term, late preterm, and stable infants with special diagnoses. Healthy infants may room-in with their parent(s) while they remain in the hospital. The hospital stay of the parent and the newborn allows identification of early problems, ensures that the family is prepared to care for the infant at home, and reduces the risk of readmission.

RECOMMENDATIONS

MAJOR RECOMMENDATIONS

Thorough history and physical examination should be completed within 24 hours of birth to determine if there are any risk factors or findings that may require further evaluation and management. Routine care of the well newborn also includes important screening and prevention measures. This chapter reviews practice recommendations for term infants, late preterm infants, and infants with Trisomy 21.

PRACTICE OPTIONS

Practice Option #1: Term Infant

History

Maternal History. Age, gravida, parity, medical or psychological issues, medications.

Pregnancy History. Prenatal labs (blood type, blood group sensitizations, hepatitis B, group B strep, rubella, gonorrhea, chlamydia, syphilis, HIV); fertility issues; ultrasound results or other screening results; prenatal consultations with specialists; tobacco, alcohol, or drug use; other complications (gestational diabetes, gestational thrombocytopenia, gestational hypertension, pre-eclampsia, thyroid abnormalities such as Graves disease).

Family History. Inherited diseases (genetic disorders, bleeding disorders, metabolic diseases); disorders that require follow up (congenital heart disease, developmental hip dysplasia, early hearing loss, sibling with jaundice).

Intrapartum History. Gestational age; mode of delivery (with or without assistance, such as vacuum); Apgar score and resuscitation needed; sepsis risk factors (fever, duration of rupture of membranes, intrapartum antibiotics, chorioamnionitis); appearance of amniotic fluid; multiple gestation; complications (shoulder dystocia).

Social History. Involvement of father, partner, or other support person; history of domestic violence; custody of other children; drug or alcohol use; cultural background of family; family stressors.

Physical Examination

General Examination
- Infants should be examined whenever possible in the presence of their parents.
- Infants should be fully undressed with proper lighting.

Vital Signs
- Temperature: Should be initially screened in the axilla. Normal axillary temperature is 97.7–99.3°F. If axillary temperature is outside of this range, temperature can be confirmed via rectal temperature. Normal rectal temperature is 98.1–99.9°F.
- Respiratory rate: Normal respiratory rate is 30–60 breaths per minute.
- Heart rate: Normal heart rate is 100–160 beats per minute (bpm). If resting heart rate is 80–100 bpm, heart rate should increase to the normal range with stimulation.

Measurements
- Weight, length, and head circumference: Plot measurements on standard growth chart.
- Assess weight for appropriate for gestational age (AGA), small for gestational age (SGA) or large for gestational age (LGA). In general, SGA is defined as less than 10% and LGA is greater than 90% for gestational age.

Head and Neck
- Scalp
  - Inspect the scalp for abrasions, cuts, or bruises.
  - Anterior and posterior fontanelles should be open, soft, and flat. Bulging fontanelle can be a sign of increased intracranial pressure.
  - Palpate the sutures and assess for mobility. If the sutures are immobile, evaluate for craniosynostosis.

- Molding can be common and resolves spontaneously.
- Swelling of the scalp is commonly due to caput succedaneum or cephalohematoma. Subgaleal hemorrhage is rare, urgent, and associated with vacuum-assisted deliveries. It is characterized by a diffuse, fluctuant swelling that shifts with movement. Significant blood loss is possible and should be followed with serial occipital-frontal head circumference, hematocrit, and vital signs.
- Craniotabes can be palpated over the parietal region and resolves spontaneously.
- Face
  - Evaluate for symmetry and dysmorphic features (see Chapter 8).
- Eyes
  - Red reflex should be assessed to rule out congenital cataracts.
  - Evaluate for scleral/conjunctival hemorrhage, scleral icterus, extra ocular eye movements, shape and reactivity of the pupils.
- Ears
  - Evaluate for shape, position, size, and presence of pits and skin tags.
- Nose
  - Evaluate for patency of nares. Nasal congestion can be common. If obstruction is suspected, feeding tube or suction catheter can be inserted to evaluate patency.
- Mouth
  - Inspect for cleft palate (soft and hard palate) or cleft lip.
  - Evaluate for Epstein pearls, mucoceles, natal teeth, and ankyloglossia.
- Neck
  - Extend neck to evaluate for masses, including cystic hygroma, goiter, thyroglossal duct cysts, or branchial cleft cysts.

Thorax

- Check for shape and symmetry.
- Note presence of supernumerary nipples. Breast buds are due to maternal hormones and will resolve spontaneously.
- Palpate the clavicles for crepitus or step-off, which may indicate a clavicular fracture.

Cardiorespiratory System

- Color
  - Newborns are generally reddish-pink. Acrocyanosis is common.
- Respiratory
  - Observe for any retractions or flaring of the nares.
  - Listen for audible grunting or stridor.
  - Periodic breathing can be normal.
  - Auscultation with stethoscope should note symmetry of breath sounds.
- Heart
  - Auscultation can determine the rate, rhythm, and presence of any murmurs.
  - Murmur: Persistent heart murmurs can be evaluated for specific congenital heart diseases. Evaluation may include measurement of pre- and postductal oxygen saturations, measurement of four extremity blood pressures, EKG, CXR, and echocardiogram (ECHO).
  - Arrhythmias: Irregular rhythm can be confirmed with EKG.
  - Femoral pulses: The presence of bilateral femoral pulses should be confirmed.

Abdomen

- Observation of the abdomen should note masses, asymmetry, general abdominal girth, and abdominal wall defects.
- Palpation of the abdomen should start from the lower quadrant and progress to the upper quadrant. Liver edge may be felt 1–2 cm below right costal margin. Kidneys may be felt with deep palpation.
- Examine the umbilical stump for signs of infection (odor, erythema, discharge).
- Umbilical hernias are common and generally resolve spontaneously.

Genitourinary

- Male: External male genitalia should be inspected.
  - Penis: Phimosis is normal at birth. Length of the penis should be ≥2.5 cm for term infants. Confirm placement of the meatus. If hypospadias or other penile anomalies are present, consult with urologist prior to circumcision.
  - Scrotum: Evaluate for presence of the testicles in the scrotal sac. Palpable undescended testicles can be followed for descent within 6–12 months in the outpatient setting. Bilateral nonpalpable testicles require prompt evaluation for ambiguous genitalia. Hydroceles are common and can be evaluated by transillumination of the scrotal sac.
  - Testicular torsion: Prenatal testicular torsion presents with firm, nontender testicle and discolored hemiscrotum. Postnatal testicular torsion presents with acute tenderness and swelling of the testicle and requires prompt surgical evaluation.
- Female
  - Labia minora and majora are often enlarged in the newborn period due to maternal hormones. Withdrawal of maternal hormones can cause creamy white vaginal discharge, which may be blood-tinged (pseudomenses).
  - Vagina: Vaginal skin tags are common and normal. The hymen should be evaluated for a small opening. Presence of a bulge can indicate an imperforate hymen.
  - Clitoris: Clitoral enlargement, labial fusion, and formation of a urogenital sinus can be signs of androgen excess, which require evaluation for congenital adrenal hyperplasia (see Chapter 49).
- Anus: Evaluate for patency and position.

Extremities

- Hips: Developmental dysplasia of the hip should be evaluated with Barlow and Ortolani maneuvers. Hip clicks are common and can be followed for the first month in the outpatient setting. Hip clunks (dislocation) require ultrasound and orthopedic evaluation.
- Abnormalities of the digits: Note polydactyly, syndactyly, clinodactyly.
- Metatarsus adductus: Forefoot adduction is most likely due to positioning in utero. As long as the foot has full range of motion, this generally resolves over days to weeks.
- Talipes equinovarus (clubfoot): Excessive plantar flexion and may be associated with other genetic syndromes. Further management can be referred to orthopedic surgery.
- Spine: Infant should be observed for straight spine. Sacral dimples require further radiographic evaluation if presence of multiple dimples, dimple diameter larger than 5 mm, location greater than 2.5 cm above the anal verge, and association of the dimple with other cutaneous markers (hypertrichosis, capillary hemangioma, atretic meningocele, subcutaneous mass, or a caudal appendage).

Neurologic Examination

- Behavior: Evaluate the infant's level of alertness and response to stimuli.
- Motor: Evaluate symmetric movements of all extremities and muscular tone.
- Autonomic: Disturbances of the autonomic system can include excessive jitteriness, sneezing, frequent yawning, and mottling. Consider evaluation for neonatal abstinence syndrome if relevant maternal prenatal history.
- Developmental reflexes: Assess for the suck, Moro, palmar and plantar grasp, stepping, Galant and asymmetrical tonic neck reflexes.
- Disturbances of the neurologic examination require further evaluation.

Skin

- Normal newborn rashes
  - Milia: White papules typically found on nose and cheeks caused by retention of keratin and sebaceous material.
  - Transient pustular melanosis neonatorum: Pustules that may transform to hyper-pigmented macules. This is more common in darker-pigmented infants and resolves in weeks to months.
  - Erythema toxicum neonatorum: White papules with an erythematous base. Resolves spontaneously within 2 weeks.
  - Nevus simplex/salmon patch/angel kiss/stork bite: Erythematous patches due to capillary malformations which appear generally over forehead, eyelid, nose, upper lip, and nape of the neck.
  - Congenital dermal melanocytosis/slate grey patch/Mongolian spots: Blue-gray patch, typically over the buttocks. More common in darker-pigmented and Asian infants.
- Jaundice: Presence of jaundice within the first 24 hours of life requires evaluation.
- Other skin findings: It is important to note other findings such as nevus flammeus (port wine stain), café au lait spots, large nevi, or other congenital dermatologic findings.

Management of the Well Newborn

Transitional Care. The first 4 to 6 hours after an infant is born is considered the transitional period during which circulatory and respiratory changes occur. Decrease in pulmonary vascular resistance, increase in pulmonary blood flow, constriction or closure of the ductus arteriosus, and lung inflation help facilitate uptake of fetal lung fluid.

Complications during labor and delivery can interrupt normal transition and cause signs of distress in the newborn, such as respiratory distress, cyanosis, and/or poor perfusion. Infants with delayed transition should be monitored more closely and may require transfer to a higher level of care.

Transient tachypnea of the newborn (TTN) is a delayed reabsorption of fetal lung fluid. TTN is a self-limited condition that can last 48–72 hours after birth.

Routine Care

- Healthy newborns may room-in with their mothers while they remain in the hospital. Research has shown that rooming-in can lead to many benefits for the parent and newborn dyad.
- If the gestational age of the infant is uncertain, assess the infant's gestational age using the expanded Ballard score.

- Record the infant's measurements (weight, length, head circumference). Classify the infant as AGA, SGA, or LGA.
- Record and follow the infant's vital signs frequently in the first hours after birth until stable, and then at least every 8 hours.
- Stabilize temperature, ideally by skin-to-skin contact with the mother, or by servo-controlled open warmer.
- Follow universal precautions.
- Bathe infant once temperature is stable.
- Ensure proper umbilical cord care. Dry cord care is generally sufficient and has not shown to increase infection rates in developed countries. However, antiseptics, such as alcohol or triple dye, or topical antibiotics can be considered if there is concern for omphalitis.
- Perform physical examination by a physician within 24 hours of birth.
- Record urine and stool output. Delayed urination (beyond 30 hours of life) and delayed first meconium (beyond 48 hours of life) should be investigated.
- Document weights in the infant's chart. Weight loss over 10–12% of birth weight, although common, should be monitored closely.

Routine Medications
- Administer 0.5% erythromycin ointment within 1 to 2 hours of birth, as a single ribbon placed in the conjunctiva bilaterally for prophylaxis against gonococcal ophthalmia neonatorum.
- Administer single dose of vitamin K (phytonadione) 0.5–1 mg to all newborns, as an intramuscular injection within 6 hours of birth to prevent vitamin K deficiency bleeding (VKDB). Current oral vitamin K preparations are not recommended as they have not been shown to prevent late VKDB (2–12 weeks of age).
- Administer first dose of hepatitis B immunization, 0.5 mL, as an intramuscular injection after parental consent. Hepatitis B vaccine should be administered within the first 24 hours. Updated vaccine information statements are available at: www.cdc.gov/vaccines/hcp/vis. If mother is hepatitis B surface antigen–positive or unknown, hepatitis B immunoglobulin may be indicated in addition to hepatitis B vaccine (see AAP Red Book for current recommendations).

Screenings
Screening for neonatal sepsis risk: Group B streptococcus (GBS) is the leading cause of early-onset neonatal sepsis. Upon admission to the newborn nursery, all newborns should be screened for the risk of perinatally acquired GBS disease, as outlined by the Centers for Disease Control and the American Academy of Pediatrics (AAP).

Risk factors for GBS disease include maternal GBS colonization, chorioamnionitis, gestational age <37 weeks, and prolonged rupture of membranes.

Cord blood screening: Cord blood may be saved up to 30 days, depending on the institution's blood bank policy. Obtain infant's blood type and direct Coombs test (also known as direct antiglobulin test [DAT]) if 1) jaundice is present within the first 24 hours of age, 2) the mother is Rh-negative or has a positive antibody screen, or 3) sibling had Coombs-positive hemolytic anemia.

Glucose screening: Well-appearing infants should be screened for hypoglycemia if risk factors are present, including: 1) infant of a diabetic mother, 2) SGA status, 3) LGA status, and 4) preterm birth. Guidelines for hypoglycemia screening are available from the AAP and the Pediatric Endocrine Society.

Newborn metabolic screening: Universal newborn screening is recommended for specific disorders for which there are demonstrated benefits of early detection and efficacious treatment. Newborn screening programs are state-based, and an updated list of screened conditions in each state can be found at http://www.babysfirsttest.org.

Bilirubin screening: Prior to discharge, all newborns should be screened with a serum or transcutaneous bilirubin to assess the risk of developing significant hyperbilirubinemia. In many centers, a total serum bilirubin measurement is obtained at the time of the newborn metabolic screen.

Risk factors for developing severe hyperbilirubinemia include hemolytic disease, exclusive breastfeeding with excessive weight loss, prematurity, certain ethnicities including East Asian, cephalohematoma or significant bruising, and history of a sibling requiring phototherapy treatment.

Jaundice prior to 24 hours of age is pathologic and requires evaluation with a serum bilirubin level.

Bilirubin results should be interpreted on an hour-specific nomogram to determine the need for treatment.

Critical congenital heart disease screening: In 2011, the U.S. Secretary of Health and Human Services recommended that screening for critical congenital heart disease (CCHD) using pulse oximetry be added to the uniform newborn screening panel. This has been endorsed by the AAP, American Heart Association, and the American College of Cardiology Foundation.

Congenital heart disease is the most common type of birth defect in the United States, affecting approximately 8 per 1000 live births and accounting for almost 30% of infant deaths due to birth defects. Although some forms of congenital heart disease cause minimal problems for infants and adults, *critical* congenital heart diseases are congenital heart defects requiring surgery or catheter intervention within the first year of life. CCHDs account for one-quarter of all cases of congenital heart disease and are associated with increased risk of morbidity and mortality if detection is delayed.

In combination with a physical examination, pulse oximetry has been demonstrated to increase the ability to identify certain CCHDs in newborns prior to discharge from the hospital, and in some newborns before audible murmurs or other symptoms/signs appear. Of note, pulse oximetry screening may not detect all types of CCHD.

Suggested protocols for CCHD screening are provided by the AAP. Abnormal pulse oximetry screening requires evaluation; of note, infants with abnormal screening may have a respiratory etiology such as retained fetal lung fluid rather than congenital heart disease.

Hearing screening: One to three/1000 newborns are diagnosed with hearing loss. Routine screening for hearing loss is mandated in most states as outlined by the AAP and The Joint Commission on Infant Hearing. Automated auditory brainstem response (AABR) and otoacoustic emissions (OAE) can be used to screen newborns. Abnormal hearing screens require follow-up with diagnostic audiologic evaluation.

As up to one-third of congenital hearing loss is associated with congenital cytomegalovirus (CMV) infection, consideration should be given to test for CMV in newborns with failed hearing screen.

Feeding. Exclusive breastmilk feeding for the first 6 months of a newborn's life has long been the goal of the World Health Organization (WHO), U.S. Department of Health and Human Services, AAP, and American College of Obstetrics and Gynecologists. In 1992, the WHO and the United Nations Children's Fund (UNICEF) launched the Baby-Friendly Hospital Initiative to strengthen maternity practices in hospitals and improve exclusive breastfeeding.

To establish and sustain exclusive breastfeeding:

- Every effort should be made to avoid separation of mother and infant, especially during the first hour of life (the "golden hour") in order to promote immediate initiation of breastfeeding and early bonding through skin-to-skin contact.
- Delaying birth weight measurements is acceptable to allow the opportunity to breastfeed.
- Family-centered maternity care, in which the nurse cares for the mother and baby together in the mother's room (couplet care), facilitates teaching.
- Infants breastfeed on demand, approximately 8–12 times/day.
- Infants receive breastmilk without any additional food or drink unless medically indicated.
- Delay the use of artificial nipples or pacifiers until breastfeeding is well established, usually about 3–4 weeks after birth.
- Consultation with a lactation specialist is recommended, whenever available, during the postpartum hospitalization.

Breastfeeding may be contraindicated with certain maternal infections, medications, and substance use. If breastmilk feeding is contraindicated or if formula feeding is requested by the mother, standard 19- or 20-cal/oz, iron-containing formula is recommended. Infants who are SGA and/or preterm may require different types of formula (e.g., 22 cal/oz or premature formula).

Circumcision. The AAP policy statement, last updated in 2012, states, "Evaluation of current evidence indicates that the health benefits of newborn male circumcision outweigh the risks, and the benefits of newborn male circumcision justify access to this procedure for those families who choose it." However, the evidence is not sufficient to recommend routine circumcision. Parents of newborn males should be made aware of the health benefits and risks while taking into consideration their cultural, religious, and personal preferences.

Potential health benefits include reduced risks of urinary tract infections and some sexually transmitted infections, and reduced risk of penile cancer.

The overall complication rate for newborn circumcision is approximately 0.5%. The most common complication is bleeding (~0.1%), followed by infection.

Contraindications to circumcision in the immediate newborn period that may require further consultation include the following:

- Sick or unstable clinical status.
- Family history of bleeding disorder, such as hemophilia or von Willebrand disease, need to be explored prior to circumcision.
- Disorders of the penis, such as hypospadias, ambiguity, chordee, or micropenis.
- Inconspicuous or "buried" penis.
- Inadequate size—circumcision should be delayed until infant is of adequate size to perform the procedure safely.
- Bilateral cryptorchidism—circumcision should be delayed until cleared by a pediatric urologist.

Adequate analgesia should be provided for neonatal circumcision. If used, topical analgesia creams may cause a higher incidence of skin irritation in low birth weight infants compared with infants of normal weight. Therefore, penile nerve block techniques should be used in this group of newborns.

In addition to analgesia, other methods of comfort are provided to the infant during circumcision such as sucrose and swaddling.

Circumcision in the newborn can be performed using Gomco clamp, Mogen clamp, or Plastibell device.

Oral or written instructions explaining post-circumcision care should be given to all parents.

Discharge Preparation. Parent education should be reviewed:
- Feeding: A minimum of eight feeds per day, adequate wet diapers (one wet diaper per day of age, constant at the sixth day of life), at least one stool a day
- Umbilical cord care
- Signs of illness (fever, irritability, lethargy, bilious emesis, poor feeding)
- Observation for neonatal jaundice
- Routine post-circumcision care (when indicated)
- Safe sleep environment, including supine flat position, tight fitting crib sheet, no loose blankets, pillows, or bumpers, no stuffed animals, swaddling at or below the level of the shoulders, and no bed sharing
- Proper use of a car seat
- Other infant safety matters, such as maintaining a smoke-free environment, checking smoke detectors, lowering the hot water temperature at home, and hand hygiene

The AAP offers comprehensive minimum criteria for term newborns being discharged from the hospital.

Practice Option #2: Late Preterm Infant

Late preterm infants who are 35 0/7 to 36 6/7 weeks' gestation may be eligible for admission to the well newborn nursery or couplet care. At some centers, infants 35 0/7 to 35 6/7 weeks are monitored for a period of time in the newborn intensive care unit prior to admission to the well newborn nursery.

Late preterm infants are at higher risk for morbidity and readmission than term infants.

Risks of Late Preterm Infants
- Temperature instability
  - Baby should be kept skin-to-skin or swaddled. Vital signs should be monitored more closely than term infant for the first 48 hours.
- Hypoglycemia
  - Screening for hypoglycemia should be initiated within the first hour of birth and continued for at least 24 hours.
- Breastfeeding difficulties
  - Early lactation consultation should be arranged.
  - Baby should be offered frequent feedings, at least every 3 hours.
  - Supplementation with expressed breastmilk (or formula, if necessary) can be considered if infant is feeding poorly or if weight loss is excessive.

- Jaundice
  - Bilirubin screening should be completed prior to discharge and plotted on a nomogram based on age in hours. Late preterm infants are at high risk for developing severe hyperbilirubinemia and require closer monitoring and follow-up.

Car Seat Safety. Car seat testing should be performed for all preterm infants to observe for apnea, bradycardia, or oxygen desaturation.

- Car seat should fit the infant appropriately prior to testing:
  - Shoulder straps are at or below the shoulders.
  - Chest clip and buckle do not occlude the airway.
  - Restraint straps can be tightened securely.
  - Crotch strap does not allow legs to cross.
- Car seat should be less than 6 years old.
- Infant should be placed on a cardiopulmonary monitor and observed in the car seat for 1–2 hours.
- Infant should be able to maintain heart rate, respirations, and oxygen saturations.
- If the infant does not pass the car seat test, the infant should be retested in a car bed.

Follow-Up. Early follow-up with the infant's primary care provider should be within 48 hours of discharge.

Practice Option #3: Infant with Down Syndrome (Trisomy 21)

A physical examination is the most sensitive test in the first 24 hours of life to diagnose trisomy 21 in an infant. Confirmation of diagnosis should be done by blood sample for chromosome evaluation, including karyotype and fluorescent in situ hybridization (FISH) testing. Result from FISH testing which should be available within 24 to 48 hours.

Typical physical examination findings include hypotonia, small brachycephalic head, epicanthic folds, flat nasal bridge, upward slanting palpebral fissures, Brushfield spots, small mouth, small ears, excessive skin at the nape of the neck, single transverse palmar crease, short fifth finger with clinodactyly, and a wide space between the first and second toes, often with a deep plantar groove.

Obstetricians and pediatricians should inform parents of their suspicion immediately and offer support and guidance for families while waiting for confirmation of the diagnosis.

In the newborn period, an infant with Down syndrome may have increased risk of certain medical problems, such as:

- Congenital heart defects (40–50%)—perform an echocardiogram to be read by a pediatric cardiologist.
- Feeding problems—infants can usually breastfeed successfully. Occasionally, some will need early supplementation and need to be awakened to feed.
- Cataracts (15%)—document red reflex and any eye abnormalities.
- Congenital hearing loss (75%)—perform hearing screening by AABR or OAE; arrange for follow-up audiological diagnostic evaluation by 3 months of age.
- Gastrointestinal disorders
  - Duodenal atresia (12%) and anorectal atresia/stenosis—perform physical examination and monitor for bilious emesis.

- Hirschsprung disease (<1%)—ensure spontaneous meconium passage within the first 48 hours, and subsequent regular stooling pattern.
- Constipation and gastroesophageal reflux are common and require close outpatient monitoring.
- Apnea, bradycardia, or oxygen desaturation in an infant car seat is possible due to cardiac disease or hypotonia—perform car seat testing prior to hospital discharge.
- Stridor, wheezing, or noisy breathing—if severe or causing feeding difficulty, refer to pediatric pulmonologist to assess for airway anomalies.
- Hematologic problems (3–10%)—obtain CBC to look for transient myeloproliferative disorder (10%) or polycythemia (18–64%).
- Congenital hypothyroidism (1%)—evaluation can be done through the state metabolic screening if TSH and free T4 concentrations are both measured.

The infant, as well as the parents, will require support upon discharge. Therefore, it is important to provide thorough anticipatory guidance, referral to early intervention services, and information for parental support groups.

CLINICAL ALGORITHM(S)

Hypoglycemia

Committee on Fetus and Newborn, Adamkin DH. Postnatal glucose homeostasis in late-preterm and term infants. *Pediatrics.* 2011;127:575-9.

Thornton PS, Stanley CA, De Leon DD, et al. Recommendations from the Pediatric Endocrine Society for evaluation and management of persistent hypoglycemia in neonates, infants, and children. *J Pediatr.* 2015;167:238-45.

Hyperbilirubinemia

Maisels MJ, Bhutani VK, Bogen D, Newman TB, Stark AR, Watchko JF. Hyperbilirubinemia in the newborn infant ≥35 weeks' gestation: an update with clarifications. *Pediatrics.* 2009;124:1193-8.

CCHD

Kemper AR, Mahle WT, Martin GR, et al. Strategies for implementing screening for critical congenital heart disease. *Pediatrics.* 2011;128:e1259-67.

Hearing Screening

U.S. Preventive Services Task Force. Universal screening for hearing loss in newborns: U.S. Preventive Services Task Force Recommendation Statement. *Pediatrics.* 2008;122:143-8.

Safe Sleep

Task Force on Sudden Infant Death Syndrome. SIDS and other sleep-related infant deaths: updated 2016 recommendations for a safe infant sleeping environment. *Pediatrics.* 2016;138:1-12.

Discharge Criteria

Benitz WE; Committee on Fetus and Newborn, American Academy of Pediatrics. Hospital stay for healthy term newborn infants. *Pediatrics.* 2015; 135:948-53.

IMPLEMENTATION OF GUIDELINE

DESCRIPTION OF IMPLEMENTATION STRATEGY

Essential elements of newborn care include thorough maternal history, including pre-natal course; standardized physical examination; written guidelines for recommended screenings, including neonatal sepsis, cord blood, glucose, metabolic, bilirubin, critical congenital heart disease, and hearing; breastfeeding support; and discharge preparation.

Following the guidelines in the Baby-Friendly Initiative, ideal practice should encourage rooming-in all or nearly all of the time to improve exclusive breastmilk feeding rates.

QUALITY METRICS

The Joint Commission Perinatal Care quality measure set includes a neonatal measure: exclusive breastmilk feeding rates for term infants (PC-05 and PC-05a).

Centers should develop additional local quality metrics related to normal newborn care. Potential measures include CCHD screening compliance, timely completion of metabolic screening, identification of infants at risk for hypoglycemia and neonatal sepsis, and readmission rates for hyperbilirubinemia.

SUMMARY

Family-centered postpartum care helps promote the initiation of breastfeeding and early bonding. In conjunction with a thorough history and physical examination of the infant, the hospital stay of the parent and the newborn allows screening and identification of early problems, ensures that the family is prepared to care for the infant at home, and reduces the risk of readmission.

BIBLIOGRAPHIC SOURCE(S)

American Academy of Pediatrics Subcommittee on Hyperbilirubinemia. Management of hyperbilirubinemia in the newborn infant 35 or more weeks of gestation. *Pediatrics*. 2004;114(1):297-316.

American Academy of Pediatrics Task Force on Circumcision. Circumcision policy statement. *Pediatrics*. 2012;130(3):585-6.

Barbi M, Binda S, Caroppo S, Primache V. Neonatal screening for congenital cytomegalovirus infection and hearing loss. *J Clin Virol*. 2006;35(2):206-9.

Benitz WE; Committee on Fetus and Newborn, American Academy of Pediatrics. Hospital stay for healthy term newborns. *Pediatrics*. 2015;135(5):948-53.

Britton J. The transition to extrauterine life and disorders of transition. *Clin Perinatol*. 1998;25(2):271-94.

Bull MJ; Committee on Genetics. Health supervision for children with Down syndrome. *Pediatrics*. 2011;128(2):393-406.

Flaherman VJ, Schaefer EW, Kuzniewicz MW, Li SX, Walsh EM, Paul IM. Early weight loss nomograms for exclusively breastfed newborns. *Pediatrics*. 2015;135(1):e16-23.

Kemper AR, Mahle WT, Martin GR, et al. Strategies for implementing screening for critical congenital heart disease. *Pediatrics*. 2011;128:e1259-67.

Lee HK, Oh E. Care of the well newborn. In: Eichenwald EC, Hansen AR, Martin CR, Stark AR, eds. *Cloherty and Stark's Manual of Neonatal Care*. 8th ed. Philadelphia: Wolters Kluwer; 2017:106-16.

Pass RF. Congenital cytomegalovirus infection and hearing loss. *Herpes*. 2005;12(2):50-5.

Task Force on Sudden Infant Death Syndrome. SIDS and other sleep-related infant deaths: updated 2016 recommendations for a safe infant sleeping environment. *Pediatrics*. 2016;138:1-12.

U.S. Preventive Services Task Force. Universal screening for hearing loss in newborns: U.S. Preventive Services Task Force Recommendation Statement. *Pediatrics*. 2008;122:143-8.

Zywicke HA, Rozzelle CJ. Sacral dimples. *Pediatr Rev*. 2011;32:109-14.

Birth Injuries

Wendy L. Timpson, MD, MEd

SCOPE

DISEASE/CONDITION(S)

Newborn care.

GUIDELINE OBJECTIVE(S)

All newborns are at risk for birth-related injuries. Pediatricians and neonatologists involved in newborn care should be familiar with the presentation and management of common birth injuries.

BRIEF BACKGROUND

Birth injuries are a common reason for neonatology consultation. The overall incidence is decreasing with early identification of risk factors and improving obstetrical techniques. The most common risk factors are fetal macrosomia, maternal obesity, abnormal fetal presentation, and operative deliveries (forceps or vacuum-assisted).

RECOMMENDATIONS

MAJOR RECOMMENDATIONS

Routine newborn care should include assessment for, and management of, common birth injuries. Review of the pregnancy and delivery can reveal important risk factors for injury, and physical examination can detect important signs and symptoms.

PRACTICE OPTIONS

Risk factors, presentation, and management of common birth injuries are presented next by injury type.

Practice Option #1: Musculoskeletal and Soft Tissue Injuries

Fracture

Introduction. Several risk factors for birth-related fractures have been identified. In addition to those known to be associated with increased risk for all birth injuries, prematurity in particular is an important risk factor for fracture. Of note, premature infants are also at increased risk for multiple fractures, with ribs being the most common site.

Clavicular Fracture

Background

- Most common birth-related fractures, with a 0.4–4.4% incidence overall
- Risk increases with instrumented delivery, birth weight >4 kg, shoulder dystocia

Presentation

- Displaced fractures are more likely to be observed in the immediate postpartum period and be accompanied by other physical examination findings (swelling, crepitus, decreased spontaneous arm movement, asymmetrical bone contour, pain with passive motion, asymmetric Moro reflex).
- Nondisplaced fractures are often asymptomatic and may not present for weeks when visible or palpable callus forms, or as an incidental finding on chest radiograph.

Evaluation and management recommendations

- Differential diagnosis includes humeral fracture, shoulder dislocation, and brachial plexus injury.
- Diagnosed by plain radiograph: include chest and upper extremities to evaluate for other associated fractures.
- Most nondisplaced fractures heal spontaneously within 2–3 weeks without sequelae; provide parental reassurance.
- Careful handling to decrease pain; pinning sleeve at 90-degree angle may help with comfort, but is not necessary for healing.
- Repeat radiograph at 2 weeks will delineate proper healing, but callus formation and resolution of tenderness are usually predictive of appropriate healing.
- Significantly displaced fractures should prompt orthopedic consultation.

Humeral Fracture

Background

- Rare, occurring in 0.002–0.005% of births.
- Most are located in the medial 1/3 of the humerus and are transverse and complete.
- Risk increases with shoulder dystocia, macrosomia, breech extraction, cesarean delivery, and weight <2500 or >4500 g.

Presentation

- Infants typically have decreased arm movement, an asymmetric Moro reflex, local swelling or crepitus, or pain with palpation and passive motion.
- Occasionally the obstetrician will feel the break or hear an audible sound at delivery.

Evaluation and management recommendations

- Diagnosis by plain radiograph of the upper extremity; in the rare case the epiphysis has yet to ossify (e.g., premature infants), MRI or ultrasound can be utilized.
- Infants should also be evaluated for accompanying brachial plexus injury.
- Orthopedic consultation is recommended.

- Requires flexed immobilization at 90-degree angle to prevent rotational deformities.
- Reassure parents; spontaneous movement returns with healing and angulation remodels as infant grows.
- Most humeral fractures heal completely; repeat radiograph at 3–4 weeks to confirm callus formation and proper healing.

Femoral Fracture
Background
- Rare, occurring in 0.013–0.017% of births.
- Spiral fracture is most common, typically involving the proximal femur.
- Risk increases with multiples, breech presentation, prematurity, and osteopenia.

Presentation
- Obstetrical team may report an audible sound during delivery.
- Infant may be asymptomatic or have pain on passive motion or local swelling.

Evaluation and management recommendations
- Diagnosis by plain radiograph.
- Orthopedic consultation is recommended.
- Requires reduction, typically with Pavlik harness (less commonly with Spica casting), for proper healing.
- Inadequate reduction can lead to femoral nerve palsy and avascular necrosis of the hip.
- Full recovery is common; reassure parents that angulation will remodel with infant growth.
- Radiographs to confirm callus formation and proper healing should be done at 3–4 weeks.

Skull Fracture
Background
- Depressed skull fractures are rare, occurring in 0.004% of births; most are associated with forceps-assisted deliveries.
- Incidence of linear skull fractures is undefined, as it is often clinically silent.

Presentation
- Depressed skull fractures are noted as a visible or palpable indentation in the head, described as the "ping-pong ball" type due to inward buckling of calvarial bones.
- Linear fractures are not clinically significant and do not require treatment.

Evaluation and management recommendations
- Diagnosis can be made by plain radiograph of the head.
- Neurosurgical consultation is recommended.
- Fractures <2 cm can be managed conservatively; >2 cm often require surgical intervention.
- Use of vacuum extractor to elevate depressed fractures has not been proven to be a safe practice and is therefore not recommended.
- Most heal without intervention; management is conservative.
- While some suggest that basilar skull fractures should be prophylaxed with antibiotics due to risk for developing bacterial meningitis, a 2011 Cochrane review does not support this practice.
- Due to increased risk of intracranial bleeding in depressed fractures that are associated with forceps deliveries, head CT is recommended to evaluate for this complication.

Dislocation

Overview. Dislocations related to birth trauma are rare. Many dislocations noted at birth are congenital, secondary to in utero positioning, rather than birth trauma. Note that epiphyseal plate separation from the metaphysis (Salter Harris type I fracture) can occur in the shoulder, elbow, or hip and is often misdiagnosed as dislocation. Plain radiography is limited in diagnosis of neonatal dislocations, especially in premature infants, due to lack of ossification. Ultrasound or MRI can aid diagnosis.

Nasal Septal Dislocation

Background

- Incidence ranges widely from 1% to as high as 20% in a recent study, likely indicative of variation in definition and underdiagnosis.
- Secondary to in utero positioning or caused by compression from the maternal pubic symphysis or sacral promontory.

Presentation

- Nasal deviation with asymmetric nares and flattening of dislocated side
- Symptoms consistent with airway obstruction

Evaluation and management recommendations

- Diagnosed by rhinoscopy
- Requires manual reduction by an otolaryngologist within 72 hours of life to avoid permanent deformity

Bruising and Petechiae

Background

- Epidemiology is not elucidated in the literature.
- Usually self-limited and evident on the presenting fetal part.

Presentation

- Birth-related bruising presents immediately after birth (as opposed to bleeding diathesis, which typically presents later).
- Breech infants may have genital bruising or edema due to in utero positioning.
- Vertex- or face-presenting infants may have facial petechiae.

Evaluation and management recommendations

- Most cases do not progress; if progression or other bleeding occurs, check platelet count and coagulation studies; consider further hematologic evaluation if abnormal.
- Obtain family history of bleeding diathesis in cases of extensive petechiae or ecchymosis.
- Consider viral etiology (congenital cytomegalovirus, rubella, human immunodeficiency virus).
- Increased risk for hyperbilirubinemia in cases of significant bruising; the AAP Subcommittee of Hyperbilirubinemia recommends follow-up within 2 days of discharge for all infants with significant bruising.

Subcutaneous Fat Necrosis

Background

- Incidence has not been described in the literature, though it is thought to be rare as a result of birth injury alone.
- Significantly increased risk in population undergoing therapeutic hypothermia.

Presentation

- Firm, indurated nodules or plaques on adipose tissue of the back, buttocks, trunk, thighs, forearms, or cheeks; color ranges from flesh to erythematous or blue
- Typically develops within weeks of birth secondary to peripartum ischemia, local trauma, or hypothermia
- Also associated with maternal factors: gestational diabetes, preeclampsia, and maternal exposure to cocaine or calcium antagonists

Evaluation and management recommendations

- Typically self-limited with resolution by 6–8 weeks of age.
- Case series review indicates that roughly half (51%) develop hypercalcemia.
  - Most cases of hypercalcemia occur within 30 days of identification of fat necrosis and only 4% occur at greater than 70 days.
  - 76% of cases had resolution of hypercalcemia within 4 weeks of detection of elevated calcium level.
  - Higher birth weight associated with increased risk of development of hypercalcemia.
  - Baseline and repeat calcium levels should be obtained weekly for 3–4 months.
- Infants with significant bruising should be followed for jaundice.

Laceration
Background

- Most common birth injury related to cesarean delivery
- Incidence ranges from 0.7% to 3% with increased occurrence in emergent cesarean sections

Presentation

Typically occur on the presenting fetal part, most commonly the scalp and face.

Evaluation and management recommendations

- Majority are mild, requiring minimal intervention, such as sterile adhesive strips.
- A small percentage require plastic surgery for repair, including those that involve the eyelid or nasolabial fold, or extend to the subcutaneous tissue.

Ocular Injury
Minor Eye Injury
Background
Minor eye injuries are relatively common, including retinal and subconjunctival hemorrhages and eyelid edema.

Evaluation and management recommendations

- Retinal hemorrhages typically resolve spontaneously in 1–5 days without long-term sequelae.
- Subconjunctival hemorrhages also usually resolve spontaneously, but over a slightly longer period of time, taking 1–2 weeks until complete resolution.

Serious Eye Injury
Background

- Serious eye injuries are rare, estimated at 0.2% of deliveries, with a higher incidence in forceps-assisted deliveries.

- Most common include hyphema (blood in anterior chamber), vitreous hemorrhage, orbital fracture, lacrimal duct or gland injury, and disruption of Descemet's membrane of the cornea.

Evaluation and management recommendations

These injuries pose a potential threat to vision and should prompt immediate ophthalmologic consultation.

Practice Option #2: Neurological Injuries

Brachial Plexus Injury

Background

- Multiple mechanisms can lead to injury, including stretching, downward lateral traction, compression, and hypoxia.
- Most classically associated with shoulder dystocia and birth weight >4000 g, though only 46% of cases occur in presence of one or more risk factor, some following uncomplicated deliveries.
- A recent ACOG systematic review estimates the overall incidence at 0.15%.

Presentation

- Most cases are unilateral, with bilateral involvement in only about 5% of cases.
- Five patterns of involvement can occur:
  - Erb palsy (50% of cases): C5 and C6 injury, upper arm adducted and internally rotated, forearm extended, while hand and wrist are spared
  - Erb palsy plus (35% of cases): C5, C6, and C7 injury (waiter's tip posture)
  - C5 to T1 injury (uncommon): arm paralysis with some sparing of finger flexion
  - C5 to T1 severe nerve root damage (uncommon): flail arm and Horner syndrome (miosis, ptosis, enophthalmos with or without anhidrosis on the ipsilateral side caused by damage to sympathetic outflow via T1)
  - C8 and T1 injury (rarest form): isolated hand and forearm paralysis (Klumpke palsy), and Horner syndrome
- Decreased passive range of motion suggests either in utero injury or other etiology, as it takes time for contractures and joint subluxation to develop.

Evaluation and management recommendations

- Diagnosis is clinical, often presenting with arm posturing in one of the distributions described above or asymmetric Moro reflex.
- There is not sufficient evidence to support early electrodiagnostic studies or neuroimaging of lesions that appear to be related to birth; however, these evaluations and neurology consultation are indicated if there is concern that the injury may be secondary to a spinal cord lesion.
- Infant should be evaluated for clavicular and humeral fractures as well, given their common association.
- Initial management involves physical therapy to maintain range of motion and prevent contractures.
- Supportive splints may be indicated, depending on resting position.
- Referral to a multidisciplinary center with input from neurology and physical therapy within 1 month may improve outcomes.
- Surgical intervention is recommended only in select cases of severe and persistent injury and remains controversial.
- If symptoms persist at 2–3 months, infant should be referred to a specialized center.

- Recovery rate varies widely in published series; though most agree that the outcome is generally favorable, rates of residual functional impairment range from 18% to 50% of patients.
- Degree of recovery depends on the distribution and extent of the injury; one prospective population-based study demonstrated the highest recovery rate in C5/C6 palsy (95%), less in C5/C6/C7 palsy (64%), and lowest in C5 to T1 palsy (21%).
- Birth weight greater than 4 kg and younger maternal age are independently associated with disability lasting greater than 1 year of age.

Facial Nerve Injury
Background

Occurs in 0.06–0.7% of births; most commonly occurs in forceps-assisted deliveries, though risk is also increased with weight >3.5 kg and prematurity.

Presentation
- Typically only the mandibular branch is affected, and symptoms usually present immediately after birth.
- Diminished movement on the affected side, loss of nasolabial fold, partial closing of the eye, and drooping mouth.
- The mouth is drawn toward the unaffected side with crying.

Evaluation and management recommendations
- Must be differentiated from syndromic or developmental etiologies (e.g., Moebius, Goldenhar's, Poland's, DiGeorge, and trisomies) and congenital hypoplasia of the depressor anguli oris muscle.
- Traumatic facial nerve palsy has an excellent prognosis: greater than 90% spontaneously resolve in the first 2 weeks of life.
- Management focuses on protecting involved eye (artificial tears and taping) to prevent corneal injury.

Phrenic Nerve Injury
Background
- Caused by extreme lateral traction on the shoulder with delivery of the shoulder during cephalic extraction or with delivery of the head during breech extraction.
- Involvement of the third to fifth cervical nerve root can result in diaphragmatic paralysis.
- Considered rare, though exact incidence is not described in the literature.
- Associated with macrosomia, shoulder dystocia, breech delivery, and malposition of forceps.
- Strongly associated with brachial plexus injury (80–90% of cases).

Presentation
- Presents on first day of life with respiratory distress, decreased movement, and diminished aeration of affected side.
- Maintain a high index of suspicion following traumatic or breech delivery.
- Some infants present with Kienböck's sign: paradoxical diaphragmatic movement (rising with inspiration and falling with expiration) that results in seesaw movement of abdomen.
- The belly dancer's sign is rarely observed: umbilicus moves toward affected side during inspiration.

- Rarely, abdominal percussion or palpation reveals caudal liver displacement in right-sided lesions.
- Some infants with left diaphragmatic paralysis have frequent regurgitation due to displacement of the lower esophagus or stomach.
- Should be considered when other etiologies (cardiac, pulmonary) have been ruled out and the infant is unable to wean from respiratory support.

Evaluation and management recommendations
- Evaluate for diaphragmatic hernia, pulmonary and cardiac disease.
- Obtain chest radiograph and blood gas, consider hyperoxia test and echocardiogram.
- AP chest film typically reveals elevation of the affected diaphragm with mediastinal shift toward the contralateral side.
- Affected right hemidiaphragm is typically two intercostal spaces above the left.
- Affected left hemidiaphragm is typically one intercostal space higher than the right.
- Traditionally diagnosed by fluoroscopy, though there is some evidence to suggest that ultrasound may be more sensitive with the additional benefit of bedside application and avoidance of radiation exposure.
- Pediatric surgery consultation is recommended.
- Roughly one-third have spontaneous recovery of phrenic nerve function within a month.
- For infants with protracted mechanical ventilation requirement, surgical plication should be considered.
- Appropriate timing of diaphragmatic plication is unclear, as most cases will resolve spontaneously in the first 6 months of life.
- Due to the untoward effects of long-term ventilation, earlier surgery is usually recommended, typically after 1 month without spontaneous recovery.
- Post-plication recovery is generally good, with rapid improvement in uncomplicated cases: most infants are weaned from mechanical ventilation within 1 week of surgery.

Recurrent Laryngeal Nerve Injury
Background
- Caused by stretching or compression of the neck during delivery, increased risk with breech extraction, may result in vocal cord paralysis.
- Incidence of nerve injury is unknown, though it is estimated that 5–26% of all congenital vocal cord paralysis is due to birth trauma.

Presentation
Presents with stridor, respiratory distress, hoarse/absent/weak cry, dysphagia, and coughing with feeds (aspiration).

Evaluation and management recommendations
- Otolaryngology consultation is recommended.
- Diagnosis by flexible nasolaryngoscopy in the awake child or direct laryngoscopy under anesthesia.
- Treatment depends on severity of injury (unilateral vs bilateral cord paralysis and presence of aspiration or respiratory distress).
- Paralysis due to birth injury resolves over time in most cases.
- Treatment is supportive.

Spinal Cord Injury

Background

- Rare, roughly 0.001% of births, with upper cord lesions being more common than lower.
- High cervical lesions most often associated with forceps-assisted rotation from vertex position.
- Low cervical and thoracic lesions typically occur during vaginal breech delivery due to hyperextension of the head or head entrapment due to cephalopelvic disproportion.

Presentation

- Injury occurs secondary to stretching during longitudinal traction or rotation of the cord.
- Infants present immediately after birth with decreased spontaneous movement and reflexes, periodic breathing, and decreased sensation below the level of the cord lesion.
- Lesions above C4 are almost always associated with apnea, whereas those between C4 and T4 may result in respiratory compromise due to phrenic and intercostal nerve involvement.
- Can occur in the setting of neonatal depression and encephalopathy, which may obscure the symptoms.

Evaluation and management recommendations

- Differential includes intracranial injury, neuromuscular diseases, and congenital spinal anomalies.
- If spinal cord injury is suspected in the delivery room, infant should be immobilized immediately and neurosurgery consulted.
- Ultrasound can be performed at the bedside, though MRI is more likely to be diagnostic.
- Therapy is supportive, and prognosis is generally poor, especially in those remaining ventilator dependent after 24 hours of life.

Practice Option #3: Extracranial Injuries of the Head

Caput Succedaneum

Background

- Caused by prolonged engagement of the fetal head in the birth canal or following vacuum extraction
- Common, though exact incidence is not delineated in the literature

Presentation

- Presents immediately after birth with edema and a serosanguinous fluid collection above the periosteum that extends across suture lines
- Typically presents with ecchymosis and/or purpura over the presenting portion of the scalp

Evaluation and management recommendations

- Benign; usually resolves in a few days without intervention
- Sporadic reports of necrotic lesions causing scarring, alopecia, or infection

Cephalohematoma
Background

- Less common than caput succedaneum, occurring in 1–2.5% of births, though risk increases to 6% and 11% of forceps and vacuum-assisted deliveries, respectively
- Caused by ruptured blood vessels beneath the periosteum, typically over parietal or occipital bones

Presentation

- Swelling typically over parietal or occipital bones that does not cross suture lines, often without discoloration of the overlying scalp.
- Subperiosteal bleeding is slow and therefore may not present immediately after birth.

Evaluation and management recommendations

- Majority resolve over a few weeks without intervention.
- Rare complications can occur:
  - Large hemorrhages may result in significant intravascular blood loss causing anemia and hypotension.
  - Skull fractures may present in up to 5% of cases; most are linear, non-depressed, and do not require intervention.
  - Calcification: bony swelling for months that can potentially lead to skull deformities.
  - Infection or sepsis: consider if cephalohematoma rapidly enlarges, becomes erythematous or fluctuant, or the infant is otherwise unwell.
    - *Escherichia coli* is the most common pathogen.
    - Needle aspiration for culture is diagnostic.
    - MRI or CT will delineate extent.
    - Treatment includes incision and drainage with debridement of skull and IV antibiotics.

Subgaleal Hemorrhage
Background

- Occurs in 0.04% of spontaneous deliveries, risk increases to 0.6–3.8% of vacuum-assisted deliveries
- Caused by sheering or laceration of the large emissary veins between the scalp veins and the dural sinuses, as a result of traction during delivery

Presentation

- Bleeding in the loose areolar tissue in the space between the periosteum and the galea aponeurotica
- Presents as diffuse, indurated, fluctuant swelling of the posterior head that straddles cranial sutures and shifts with repositioning
- Typically noted in the first 4 hours after birth and may progress over the following 12–72 hours

Evaluation and management recommendations

- High mortality rate (14–22%) due to risk of massive blood loss into this large potential space that extends from the superior orbital ridges anteriorly, to nape of neck posteriorly, to edge of ears laterally, that can contain up to 40% of infant's entire blood volume (50–100 mL).
- Early recognition of injury and close monitoring are crucial to survival.
- Monitor for tachycardia, pallor, or evidence of shock with frequent vital signs (minimum q1h), serial hematocrits (33% require transfusions); consider coagulation studies.

- Obtain frequent head circumference measurements: increases by an estimated 1 cm with each 40 mL of subgaleal blood.
- Follow jaundice closely; up to 56% can develop hyperbilirubinemia.
- CT or MRI can be helpful to delineate extent and identify other accompanying injuries.
- Treatment is generally supportive; prevention of shock with aggressive fluid resuscitation and volume expansion (normal saline, fresh frozen plasma, packed red blood cells).
- Early neurosurgical consultation is recommended; transfer to facility with appropriate services is recommended for evidence of lesion expansion.
- Rare cases of brain compression require surgical evacuation of hematoma.

Practice Option #4: Intracranial Hemorrhage

Overview. Birth-related intracranial hemorrhage is not uncommon. One retrospective MRI study of 97 asymptomatic neonates born by spontaneous unassisted vaginal delivery described an incidence of 26% in this healthy population. Other studies describe lower incidence that increases with forceps and vacuum-assisted delivery.

Epidural Hemorrhage
Background
- Very rare in neonates
- Typically caused by middle meningeal artery injury that accompanies a linear skull fracture in the parietotemporal area; risk increases in operative vaginal deliveries

Presentation
- Can coexist with cephalohematoma with communication through a skull fracture
- Presents with nonspecific neurological symptoms: seizures, hypotonia, lethargy

Evaluation and management recommendations
- Diagnosis by head CT or MRI.
- Neurosurgical consultation is recommended.
- Potential for rapid deterioration due to arterial bleeding.
- Monitor for evidence of increased intracranial pressure (ICP) with bulging fontanel, vital sign instability, altered consciousness.
- Infants with very small lesions and a stable course can be managed with supportive therapy.
- Evidence of increased ICP or large hemorrhage prompts surgical evacuation.
- When an epidural hemorrhage is accompanied by a cephalohematoma, in the setting of either an overt or suspected cranial fracture, aspiration of the latter may result in resolution of the epidural hemorrhage, though this should only be prefromed in consultation with neurosurgery.

Subdural Hemorrhage
Background
Most common type of intracranial hemorrhage, though still low overall incidence of 0.03%, 0.08%, 0.1%, and 0.2% of deliveries for spontaneous, vacuum, forceps-assisted, and combined vacuum/forceps deliveries, respectively.

Presentation
- Most infants are asymptomatic and likely never diagnosed.
- Symptomatic infants present at 24–48 hours with apnea, seizure, irritability, altered tone or consciousness.
- Rarely present with evidence of increased ICP: expanding head circumference, tense fontanel, bradycardia, altered mental status.

Evaluation and management recommendations
- Diagnosed by head CT or MRI.
- Neurosurgical consultation is recommended; management depends on size and location of hematoma, and most cases managed conservatively due to plasticity of neonatal skull.
- Surgical evacuation indicated when there is evidence of increased ICP (more likely for posterior fossa hemorrhages).

Subarachnoid Hemorrhage
Background
- Reported incidence of 0.01%, 0.02%, 0.03%, and 0.11% for spontaneous, vacuum, forceps, and combined vacuum/forceps-assisted deliveries, respectively
- Caused by rupture of bridging veins in the subarachnoid space or small leptomeningeal blood vessels

Presentation
Typically presents at 24–48 hours of life with apnea, respiratory depression, seizures.

Evaluation and management recommendations
- Diagnosed by head CT or MRI.
- Neurosurgical consultation is recommended.
- Treatment is usually conservative; rarely post-hemorrhagic hydrocephalus can develop.

Intraventricular Hemorrhage
Background
- Usually associated with prematurity but can rarely occur in term infants.
- Incidence in healthy, asymptomatic term infants ranges from 0.01% to 4% with increased incidence in operative deliveries.
- In a large prospective study of term infants, all were subependymal (grade I).
- Incidence in premature infants varies depending on gestational age.

Presentation
Generally asymptomatic, though in setting of severe birth trauma symptoms may develop if hemorrhage extends.

Evaluation and management recommendations
- In setting of severe birth trauma, observation is recommended due to potential for extension into surrounding parenchyma and complication of post-hemorrhagic hydrocephalus.
- Preterm neonates require surveillance cranial ultrasound at regular intervals due to increased risk.
- Most cases resolve spontaneously without long-term sequelae.

Practice Option #5: Intra-Abdominal Injuries
Background
- Uncommon, tend to occur in association with overtly traumatic birth
- Include rupture or subcapsular hemorrhage of the liver (most common), spleen, or adrenal gland

Presentation

- Varies according to degree of blood loss: infants with solid organ rupture may present with pallor, abdominal distension and discoloration and hemorrhagic shock.
- Infants with subcapsular organ hemorrhage have a more insidious onset of anemia with symptoms of poor feeding, tachycardia, tachypnea.
- Unilateral adrenal hemorrhage may present as a palpable mass.

Evaluation and management recommendations

- Diagnosis by abdominal ultrasonography.
- Follow serial hematocrit and coagulation studies.
- Pediatric surgery consultation is recommended.
- Treatment is supportive with fluid resuscitation, treatment of coagulopathy.
- Laparotomy may be required to control bleeding in cases of solid organ rupture.

IMPLEMENTATION OF GUIDELINE

QUALITY METRICS

Several national organizations include birth injury rates as core perinatal quality measures. The Agency for Healthcare Research and Quality (AHRQ) includes "Birth Trauma Rate – Injury to Neonate" as one of its Patient Safety Indicators (www.qualityindicators. ahrq.gov). The Joint Commission includes "Unexpected Complications in Term Newborns" as one of its Perinatal Care core measures; this measure includes birth trauma in addition to other unexpected complications. Both these measures are based on ICD coding.

It is likely that most hospitals will report the AHRQ or Joint Commission measures externally. In addition, hospitals are encouraged to define local measures through joint collaboration of their obstetric and newborn providers to help monitor incidence of common and important birth injuries.

SUMMARY

Birth injuries are common in newborns. Many can be managed without subspecialty consultation and should resolve without sequalae; some are more severe and require significant intervention and follow-up. Pediatricians caring for newborns should evaluate for injury as part of their routine history and physical examination, and centers should have collaborative programs between obstetrics and pediatrics to monitor rates of birth injuries and identify practices to limit their risk.

BIBLIOGRAPHIC SOURCE(S)

Ahn ES, Jung MS, Lee YK, Ko SY, Shin SM, Hahn MH. Neonatal clavicular fracture: recent 10 year study. *Pediatr Int.* 2015;57(1):60-3.

Alexander JM, Leveno KJ, Hauth J, et al. Fetal injury associated with cesarean delivery. *Obstet Gynecol.* 2006;108(4):885-90.

Amar AP, Aryan HE, Meltzer HS, Levy ML. Neonatal subgaleal hematoma causing brain compression: report of two cases and review of the literature. *Neurosurgery.* 2003;52(6):1470-4; discussion 4.

American Academy of Pediatrics Subcommittee on Hyperbilirubinemia. Management of hyperbil-irubinemia in the newborn infant 35 or more weeks of gestation. *Pediatrics*. 2004;114(1):297-316.

Anglen JO, Choi L. Treatment options in pediatric femoral shaft fractures. *J Orthop Trauma*. 2005;19(10):724-33.

Basha A, Amarin Z, Abu-Hassan F. Birth-associated long-bone fractures. *Int J Gynaecol Obstet*. 2013;123(2):127-30.

Bishop HC, Koop CE. Acquired eventration of the diaphragm in infancy. *Pediatrics*. 1958;22(6):1088-96.

Broker FH, Burbach T. Ultrasonic diagnosis of separation of the proximal humeral epiphysis in the newborn. *J Bone Joint Surg Am*. 1990;72(2):187-91.

Burden AD, Krafchik BR. Subcutaneous fat necrosis of the newborn: a review of 11 cases. *Pediatr Dermatol*. 1999;16(5):384-7.

Caviglia H, Garrido CP, Palazzi FF, Meana NV. Pediatric fractures of the humerus. *Clin Orthop Relat Res*. 2005(432):49-56.

Coroneos CJ, Voineskos SH, Christakis MK, et al. Obstetrical brachial plexus injury (OBPI): Canada's national clinical practice guideline. *BMJ Open*. 2017;7(1):e014141.

Daya H, Hosni A, Bejar-Solar I, Evans JN, Bailey CM. Pediatric vocal fold paralysis: a long-term retrospective study. *Arch Otolaryngol Head Neck Surg*. 2000;126(1):21-5.

Demissie K, Rhoads GG, Smulian JC, et al. Operative vaginal delivery and neonatal and infant adverse outcomes: population based retrospective analysis. *BMJ*. 2004;329(7456):24-9.

Dessole S, Cosmi E, Balata A, et al. Accidental fetal lacerations during cesarean delivery: experience in an Italian level III university hospital. *Am J Obstet Gynecol*. 2004;191(5):1673-7.

de Vries TS, Koens BL, Vos A. Surgical treatment of diaphragmatic eventration caused by phrenic nerve injury in the newborn. *J Pediatr Surg*. 1998;33(4):602-5.

Dupuis O, Silveira R, Dupont C, et al. Comparison of "instrument-associated" and "sponta-neous" obstetric depressed skull fractures in a cohort of 68 neonates. *Am J Obstet Gynecol*. 2005;192(1):165-70.

Eiff MP. Management of clavicle fractures. *Am Fam Physician*. 1997;55(1):121-8.

Executive summary: neonatal brachial plexus palsy. Report of the American College of Obste-tricians and Gynecologists' Task Force on Neonatal Brachial Plexus Palsy. *Obstet Gynecol*. 2014;123(4):902-4.

Foad SL, Mehlman CT, Ying J. The epidemiology of neonatal brachial plexus palsy in the United States. *J Bone Joint Surg Am*. 2008;90(6):1258-64.

Grossman JA. Early operative intervention for selected cases of brachial plexus birth injury. *Arch Neurol*. 2006;63(7):1031-2.

Harugop AS, Mudhol RS, Hajare PS, Nargund AI, Metgudmath VV, Chakrabarti S. Prevalence of nasal septal deviation in new-borns and its precipitating factors: a cross-sectional study. *Indian J Otolaryngol Head Neck Surg*. 2012;64(3):248-51.

Hayden CK Jr, Shattuck KE, Richardson CJ, Ahrendt DK, House R, Swischuk LE. Subependymal germinal matrix hemorrhage in full-term neonates. *Pediatrics*. 1985;75(4):714-8.

Heyman R, Heckly A, Magagi J, Pladys P, Hamlat A. Intracranial epidural hematoma in newborn infants: clinical study of 15 cases. *Neurosurgery*. 2005;57(5):924-9; discussion 9.

Holden R, Morsman DG, Davidek GM, O'Connor GM, Coles EC, Dawson AJ. External ocular trauma in instrumental and normal deliveries. *Br J Obstet Gynaecol*. 1992;99(2):132-4.

Hsu TY, Hung FC, Lu YJ, et al. Neonatal clavicular fracture: clinical analysis of incidence, predis-posing factors, diagnosis, and outcome. *Am J Perinatol*. 2002;19(1):17-21.

Jones GP, Seguin J, Shiels WE 2nd. Salter-Harris II fracture of the proximal humerus in a preterm infant. *Am J Perinatol*. 2003;20(5):249-53.

Lagerkvist AL, Johansson U, Johansson A, Bager B, Uvebrant P. Obstetric brachial plexus palsy: a prospective, population-based study of incidence, recovery, and residual impairment at 18 months of age. *Devel Med Child Neurol*. 2010;52(6):529-34.

Looney CB, Smith JK, Merck LH, et al. Intracranial hemorrhage in asymptomatic neonates: prevalence on MR images and relationship to obstetric and neonatal risk factors. *Radiology.* 2007;242(2):535-41.

Miller SG, Brook MM, Tacy TA. Reliability of two-dimensional echocardiography in the assessment of clinically significant abnormal hemidiaphragm motion in pediatric cardiothoracic patients: comparison with fluoroscopy. *Pediatr Crit Care Med.* 2006;7(5):441-4.

Morris S, Cassidy N, Stephens M, McCormack D, McManus F. Birth-associated femoral fractures: incidence and outcome. *J Pediatr Orthop.* 2002;22(1):27-30.

Nichols MM. Shifting umbilicus in neonatal phrenic palsy (the belly dancer's sign). *Clin Pediatr.* 1976;15(4):342-3.

Podoshin L, Gertner R, Fradis M, Berger A. Incidence and treatment of deviation of nasal septum in newborns. *Ear Nose Throat J.* 1991;70(8):485-7.

Ratilal BO, Costa J, Sampaio C, Pappamikail L. Antibiotic prophylaxis for preventing meningitis in patients with basilar skull fractures. *Cochrane Database Syst Rev.* 2011(8):CD004884.

Smith BT. Isolated phrenic nerve palsy in the newborn. *Pediatrics.* 1972;49(3):449-51.

Stefanko NS, Drolet BA. Subcutaneous fat necrosis of the newborn and associated hypercalcemia: a systematic review of the literature. *Pediatr Dermatol.* 2019;36(1):24-30.

Towner D, Castro MA, Eby-Wilkens E, Gilbert WM. Effect of mode of delivery in nulliparous women on neonatal intracranial injury. *New Engl J Med.* 1999;341(23):1709-14.

Tsugawa C, Kimura K, Nishijima E, Muraji T, Yamaguchi M. Diaphragmatic eventration in infants and children: is conservative treatment justified? *J Pediatr Surg.* 1997;32(11):1643-4.

Uchil D, Arulkumaran S. Neonatal subgaleal hemorrhage and its relationship to delivery by vacuum extraction. *Obstet Gynecolog Surv.* 2003;58(10):687-93.

Uhing MR. Management of birth injuries. *Pediatr Clin North Am.* 2004;51(4):1169-86, xii.

van Dijk JG, Pondaag W, Malessy MJ. Obstetric lesions of the brachial plexus. *Muscle Nerve.* 2001;24(11):1451-61.

Volpe J. *Neurology of the Newborn.* 4th ed. Philadelphia: WB Saunders; 2001.

Zuarez-Easton S, Zafran N, Garmi G, Hasanein J, Edelstein S, Salim R. Risk factors for persistent disability in children with obstetric brachial plexus palsy. *J Perinatol.* 2017;37(2):168-71.

Congenital Anomalies

Monica Hsiung Wojcik, MD • Pankaj B. Agrawal, MD, MMSc

SCOPE

DISEASE/CONDITION(S)

Major congenital anomalies, common genetic syndromes.

GUIDELINE OBJECTIVE(S)

To review the approach to the evaluation and management of major congenital anomalies that often present to the neonatal intensive care unit.

BRIEF BACKGROUND

Congenital anomalies, also referred to as birth defects, are present in 2–3% of liveborn births. *Major congenital anomalies* are those that have a substantial impact on health or cosmetic appearance (such as critical congenital cardiac defects, cleft lip and palate, or absence of a limb) and are not on the spectrum of normal variation within a population, while *minor congenital anomalies* are relatively common and do not affect the health of the individual (such as an ear tag, a supernumerary nipple, or a single palmar crease). The neonatal intensive care unit (NICU) is enriched for infants with these conditions due to the potential that many have to impact survival after birth. Indeed, prior literature has shown that congenital anomalies are responsible for 25–50% of mortality in the NICU setting, and birth defects, along with chromosomal anomalies, are the most common cause of infant deaths in the United States.

The underlying etiology of congenital anomalies may be environmental or genetic, with environmental causes including teratogenic exposures such as to thalidomide or excessive alcohol consumption in addition to exposures to maternal conditions, as seen in diabetic embryopathy. Genetic causes of congenital anomalies are quite diverse and may include chromosomal aneuploidy syndromes, such as trisomies 13, 18, and 21, chromosomal microdeletion or duplication syndromes, such as 22q11 deletion syndrome or Cri-du-Chat (5p deletion) syndrome, in addition to monogenic disorders such as CHARGE (coloboma, heart defects, atresia choanae, retarded growth, genitourinary anomalies, ear abnormalities) syndrome, caused by pathogenic variants in single genes. It is important to recognize which infants are at higher risk for genetic syndromes, as testing may be available for these conditions. Multiple developmental mechanisms can be responsible for congenital anomalies, including malformation, deformation, and disruption. A *malformation* is the abnormal development of an embryonic tissue due to intrinsic factors, such as a congenital heart defect. A *deformation* is an abnormally formed structure due to mechanical forces (without which the structure would appear normal), such as the flattened face seen in Potter sequence. *Disruptions* are defects occurring when normal tissue is damaged or interrupted, as in amniotic band sequence. It is helpful to distinguish between these types of congenital anomalies, as deformations and disruptions are less likely to be related to genetic causes than malformations.

Furthermore, while the majority (75%) of major anomalies are isolated, they can occur together in an association, a sequence, or as a syndrome. An *association* is a group of anomalies that tend to occur together (more often than would be expected by chance) such as VACTERL (vertebral, anal, cardiac, tracheoesophageal fistula, renal, and limb defects) association. Occasionally, greater understanding of the underlying genetic contributions to congenital anomalies leads to a shift in classification, as occurred with CHARGE syndrome, which was known as an association prior to the discovery that it was caused by variants in the gene *CHD7*. A *sequence* is a group of anomalies that occur together due to a single cause (such as a malformation, disruption, or deformation), such as Robin sequence (micrognathia leading to posterior tongue positioning resulting in cleft palate). A *syndrome* is a group of congenital anomalies that are thought to be related to each other with a unifying underlying cause that can be genetic, environmental, or a combination of both, such as trisomy 21 (Down syndrome) or fetal alcohol syndrome. Again, it is helpful to categorize congenital anomalies in this way as those that are "syndromic" in nature are more likely to have an identifiable genetic cause.

It is important for the neonatologist to recognize congenital anomalies in neonates and infants under their care, and to investigate the underlying cause of the congenital anomalies in addition to providing appropriate clinical management.

RECOMMENDATIONS

MAJOR RECOMMENDATIONS

The broad treatment goals for managing infants with congenital anomalies are as follows:

1. Initial stabilization: For major anomalies impacting the airway or lung parenchyma, intubation may be required (i.e., an infant with severe microretrognathia or an infant with giant omphalocele and corresponding pulmonary hypoplasia with an inability to adequately oxygenate and ventilate). Certain anomalies require particular attention when establishing an airway, and continuous positive airway pressure (CPAP)

applied noninvasively may be relatively contraindicated in certain circumstances. In some cases, the presence of a pediatric surgeon either at birth or shortly thereafter may be recommended; these infants are ideally identified prenatally in order to co-ordinate delivery at a tertiary or quaternary care center with the appropriate specialists available. For any anomaly impacting the ability to tolerate enteral feedings, central access may be recommended for nutritional support.

2. Characterization of the number and type of congenital anomalies and identify those warranting a medical genetics evaluation: Guidelines toward categorizing and describing congenital anomalies are presented, as are clinical features that warrant consultation with a clinical geneticist and consideration of genetic testing.

3. Targeted history, genetic testing, and ancillary studies: Ideally, this should take place under the guidance of a clinical geneticist, although general guidelines that could be followed by any provider are discussed.

PRACTICE OPTIONS

Practice Option #1

Initial Stabilization. As with any neonatal admission, the first priority is ensuring respiratory and circulatory stabilization. Depending on the severity of the malformation, intubation may be required for respiratory stability. If a critical congenital cardiac defect is suspected that is dependent on the patent ductus arteriosus to support circulation postnatally, a prostaglandin infusion may be warranted. Certain skeletal dysplasias, such as achondroplasia, require special attention to neck positioning during intubation or other procedures to avoid spinal injuries at the craniocervical junction. Many infants with gastrointestinal malformations or other major anomalies requiring surgery will require central access for long-term nutritional support. The particulars of management of any single disorder are outside the scope of this review, but an excellent resource for the neonatologist regarding the surgical management of critically ill neonates is the *Manual of Neonatal Surgical Intensive Care* by Hansen and Puder.

Once the infant has been stabilized, the remainder of the evaluation can be performed. Of note, as many of these infants will receive blood transfusions either due to critical illness or in the setting of surgery, it may be helpful to draw a 3–5 mL blood sample in a purple top (EDTA) tube for future DNA extraction and 3–5 mL in a green top (sodium heparin) tube for cytogenetic studies such as karyotype prior to transfusion to save for potential genetic testing, particularly for life-threatening anomalies where the opportunity to do so may be later lost. These blood samples are stable refrigerated (4°C) for several days, and the purple top tube can be frozen (–20° to –70°C) for future use.

Practice Option #2

Characterize Number and Type of Congenital Anomalies. While at least one minor anomaly may be seen in about 20% of newborns, less than 1% will have two minor anomalies and these newborns have a 10% risk of also having a major congenital anomaly. The presence of three minor anomalies is associated with a 20% risk of having a concurrent major congenital anomaly. It is important to be aware of these risks when evaluating a healthy-appearing newborn with multiple minor anomalies, as screening for a major congenital anomaly, such as with a cardiac or renal ultrasound, may be warranted. Infants with more than one (unrelated) major anomaly are said to have *multiple congenital anomalies*.

Certain congenital anomalies, even minor ones, may be suggestive of other specific anomalies. For example, asymmetric crying facies are often associated with congenital cardiac anomalies and an echocardiogram may be helpful for these infants. Preauricular tags and pits are associated with hearing loss, and a hearing evaluation should be undertaken in these patients, but a renal ultrasound (to evaluate for anomalies as can be seen in branchio-oto-renal syndrome) may not be necessary unless the infant also has dysmorphic features or other anomalies, or in the presence of a positive family history of ear anomalies or hearing loss, or a maternal history of exposure to teratogenic drugs or gestational diabetes. Infants with components of the VACTERL association, such as esophageal atresia, should have an evaluation for the other components, such as an echocardiogram, renal ultrasound, and a spinal ultrasound due to the association with or a tethered cord. Further recommendations can be found in a recent review by Jones and Adam.

Identify Infants in Need of a Medical Genetics Evaluation. Certain types of congenital anomalies, such as malformations and those present in conjunction with other clinical features, such as dysmorphic facial features or growth retardation suggestive of a syndrome, are more likely to have an identifiable genetic cause using available clinical diagnostic techniques. Other anomalies, such as those occurring in the setting of environmental factors (i.e., oligohydramnios in the setting of preterm prolonged rupture of membranes leading to Potter sequence of pulmonary hypoplasia and flattened facial features) may not be as suggestive. However, the attribution of congenital anomalies to environmental factors alone should be considered a diagnosis of exclusion in the absence of overwhelming evidence to the contrary. It has been suggested that infants with more than one major and one minor malformation (including dysmorphic features) should be evaluated by a clinical geneticist; however, certain anomalies that are more frequently associated with genetic syndromes (i.e., tetralogy of Fallot) may also warrant referral even if observed in isolation. Indeed, a retrospective analysis of infants admitted to the cardiac intensive care unit with congenital structural cardiac defects by Ahrens-Nicklas et al. demonstrated that 25% were identified to have a genetic disorder confirmed by testing, although certain cardiac defects, such as a complete atrioventricular canal defect, were more likely to be associated with a genetic diagnosis, whereas no genetic diagnoses were made for infants with D-transposition of the great arteries. As another example, asymmetric crying facies can be seen in 22q11 deletion syndrome, attributed to hypoplasia or absence of the depressor anguli oris muscle. Asymmetric crying facies can also be seen in CHARGE syndrome when attributed to cranial nerve abnormalities. An overview of the genetic syndromes associated with commonly seen congenital anomalies is presented in Table 8.1.

Other constellations of anomalies are more likely attributable to environmental causes, particularly in the setting of a positive family history or maternal history. Diabetic embryopathy, caused by maternal diabetes mellitus, can present with neural tube defects, holoprosencephaly, congenital heart defects, microcolon, caudal regression syndrome (including sacral agenesis), vertebral anomalies, and limb deformities such as preaxial polydactyly and tibial hemimelia.

Practice Option #3

Targeted History. For infants presenting with congenital anomalies, a detailed maternal, prenatal, and family history is important. For pregnancies conceived using in vitro fertilization (IVF), particularly intracytoplasmic sperm injection (ICSI), the risk of

TABLE 8.1. **Selected Major Anomalies Commonly Seen in the NICU and Associated Genetic Syndromes**

Organ System	Anomaly	Genetic Syndrome	Gene(s)
Craniofacial			
	Aplasia cutis congenita	Patau syndrome	Trisomy 13
		Adams-Oliver syndrome	*ARHGAP31, DLL4, DOCK6, EOGT, RBPJ, NOTCH1*
	Craniosynostosis	Apert syndrome	*FGFR2*
		Crouzon syndrome	*FGFR2*
		Muenke syndrome	*FGFR3*
		Pfeiffer syndrome	*FGFR1, FGFR2*
		Saethre-Chotzen syndrome	*TWIST1, FGFR2*
	Cleft lip and palate	Patau syndrome	Trisomy 13
		Van der Woude	*IRF6*
	Cleft palate	22q11 deletion syndrome	Deletion on chromosome 22
		Smith-Lemli-Opitz syndrome	*DHCR7*
		CHARGE syndrome	*CHD7*
		Stickler syndrome	*COL2A1, COL9A1, COL9A2, COL11A1,* and *COL11A2*
	Asymmetric crying facies	22q11 deletion syndrome	Deletion on chromosome 22
		CHARGE syndrome	*CHD7*
Respiratory			
	Congenital diaphragmatic hernia	Fryns syndrome	*NIPBL, SMC1A, HDAC8, SMC3, RAD21*
		Cornelia de Lange syndrome	
		Pallister-Killian syndrome	Tetrasomy 12p
		Donnai-Barrow syndrome	*LRP2*
Cardiac			
	Tetralogy of Fallot	22q11 deletion syndrome	Deletion on chromosome 22
	Interrupted aortic arch	22q11 deletion syndrome	Deletion on chromosome 22
	Coarctation of the aorta	Turner syndrome	Monosomy X
		Kabuki syndrome	*KMT2D, KDM6A*
	Atrioventricular canal defect	Down syndrome	Trisomy 21
	Pulmonary valve stenosis	Noonan syndrome	*PTPN11* or other RASopathy genes

(Continued)

TABLE 8.1. Selected Major Anomalies Commonly Seen in the NICU and Associated Genetic Syndromes (Continued)

Organ System	Anomaly	Genetic Syndrome	Gene(s)
	Peripheral pulmonary artery stenosis	Alagille syndrome	*JAG1*
	Supravalvular aortic stenosis (SVAS)	Williams syndrome	Deletion on chromosome 7
		Isolated SVAS	*ELN*
Gastrointestinal			
	Duodenal atresia	Down syndrome	Trisomy 21
	Esophageal atresia	Down syndrome	Trisomy 21
		Edward syndrome	Trisomy 18
		CHARGE syndrome	*CHD7*
		Fanconi anemia	Chromosomal breakage studies, gene panel
	Anal atresia or imperforate anus		
	Omphalocele	Beckwith-Wiedemann syndrome	Methylation analysis
	Hirschsprung disease	Smith-Lemli-Opitz syndrome	*DHCR7*
		Mowat-Wilson syndrome	*ZEB2*
		Down syndrome	Trisomy 21
		Waardenburg-Shah syndrome	*EDNRB, EDN3, SOX10*
Urogenital			
	Polycystic kidneys	Autosomal recessive polycystic kidney disease	*PKHD1*
	Nephronophthisis	Multiple genes	Gene panel
	Ambiguous genitalia	Disorders of sexual differentiation	
Skeletal			
	Shortened long bones	Skeletal dysplasia	Gene panel
Central Nervous System			
	Brain malformations	Multiple genes	Gene panel
	Perinodular heterotopia		*FLNA*
	Holoprosencephaly	Nonsyndromic	*SHH*, others
		Syndromic	Trisomy 13, trisomy 18
			DHCR7

congenital anomalies and of imprinting defects is higher. Certain maternal infections, such as rubella, are also associated with congenital anomalies, as are teratogenic drugs such as warfarin and thalidomide, though with many drugs the risk of congenital malformations depends substantially on the dose and timing of exposure. However, in the absence of overwhelming evidence suggesting an environmental cause of the anomalies, environmental factors should be considered a diagnosis of exclusion.

A history of prenatal genetic testing should also be obtained, with the caveat that "negative" prenatal genetic testing does not eliminate the possibility of a genetic disorder in the neonate, even one that had been theoretically screened for. For pregnancies achieved using IVF, preimplantation genetic screening (PGS) may have been performed. This is a limited screening evaluation for chromosomal disorders and is likely to miss smaller chromosomal abnormalities; it will also fail to detect abnormalities at the level of the single gene. Many women are now pursuing noninvasive prenatal screening (NIPS) using cell-free fetal DNA testing, which is a maternal blood test that is able to detect chromosomal imbalances in the fetal DNA. While this test is highly sensitive, it is typically used to detect common trisomies such as 21, 18, and 13 and sex chromosome aneuploidies (such as Turner and Klinefelter syndromes) and generally is not commonly used for chromosomal microdeletion syndromes. At this time, it is also not being used for the detection of single-gene disorders. In addition, as the test evaluates fetal DNA from the placenta, either false negatives or false positives are possible in the setting of chromosomal disorders that are present either only in the placenta or only in the fetus. A diagnostic test, such as karyotype performed via chorionic villus sampling or amniocentesis, is recommended in the setting of a positive NIPS. In addition to NIPS, traditional serum screening is also standardly performed, as is a fetal anatomy survey during which many congenital anomalies are detected.

Ancillary Studies. Additional evaluations may be suggested by a clinical geneticist to aid in delineating the patient's phenotype either prior to or in the process of obtaining genetic test results. These include consultations for specialized examinations, such as a dilated eye examination by a pediatric ophthalmologist to assess for features such as cataracts, coloboma, or posterior embryotoxon that may be suggestive of certain genetic disorders, or bedside laryngoscopy by an otorhinolaryngologist to evaluate for laryngeal clefts or other anomalies not otherwise visible. Radiologic evaluations are often helpful to fully understand a patient's anatomy, such as echocardiography, an abdominal or renal ultrasound, a skeletal survey, or head imaging such as computed tomography (helpful in the evaluation of craniosynostosis or for the evaluation of other bony structures) or magnetic resonance imaging (MRI). Finally, electrographic studies such as electroencephalography (EEG) or electromyography (EMG) may be useful in identifying neurologic features of suspected genetic syndromes that may present with congenital anomalies.

Genetic Laboratory Testing. A substantial proportion of congenital anomalies are attributed to identifiable genetic disorders, and this proportion is likely to increase as the frequency of genetic testing in the NICU increases. Currently, single gene changes are thought to cause about 17% of congenital anomalies, while 10% have been attributed to chromosomal changes and 4–10% to identifiable maternal or environmental causes.

Many options now exist for genetic testing in the neonatal period. A traditional karyotype can be performed on a blood sample to evaluate for chromosomal abnormalities of number and/or structure, such as trisomies 21, 18, and 13, and chromosomal rearrangements, deletions, or duplications that are visible under a microscope. A chromosomal microarray is able to detect submicroscopic deletions or duplications in addition to detecting runs of homozygosity (depending on the technology) as can be seen in consanguinity. However, chromosomal microarrays will generally not detect balanced chromosomal rearrangements and, depending on the technology used, a chromosomal microarray may miss cases of triploidy (in which three copies of every chromosome are present). The American College of Medical Genetics recommends chromosomal microarray testing as the first line for infants with multiple congenital anomalies that are not suggestive of a specific genetic disorder (i.e., CHARGE syndrome, trisomy 21) that would warrant targeted testing. It has also been suggested that a chromosomal microarray should be considered for all cases of fetal growth restriction or macrosomia.

A normal karyotype and chromosomal microarray does not indicate that a disorder is not genetic, as these tests lack resolution at the level of single gene or nucleotide changes. Sequencing studies, which can be performed on single genes or multiple genes at once (in a gene panel test), look for single nucleotide variants (SNVs) or small insertions or deletions (indels) that may be disease causing. Exome sequencing (ES) involves sequencing all of the coding regions of the genome and has greatly augmented the capacity for neonatal genetic diagnosis, particularly among infants with multiple congenital anomalies. Additional studies, such as triplet repeat or methylation studies, look for other types of changes that can occur at the level of the gene and cause disorders such as fragile X syndrome (a triplet repeat disorder) or Prader-Willi syndrome (an imprinting disorder). Importantly, while ES is now being used more frequently in the NICU, this test will generally not detect disorders such as fragile X or Prader-Willi that occur via these other mechanisms.

IMPLEMENTATION OF GUIDELINE

DESCRIPTION OF IMPLEMENTATION STRATEGY

In order to implement the practice strategies outlined above, continuing education of the neonatal team regarding the identification and management of particular congenital anomalies is recommended. In addition, coordination between the prenatal providers and postnatal care team is paramount in order to deliver the best possible care.

SUMMARY

Congenital anomalies are encountered frequently in the NICU, and a basic understanding of the approach to evaluation and management is important for the neonatologist. These anomalies range from life threatening to primarily cosmetic in nature, and some may be suggestive of an underlying genetic disorder. Where possible, a genetic diagnosis should be pursued, as management changes may be indicated depending on the underlying genetic etiology. Furthermore, accurate recurrence risks for parents cannot be estimated without the knowledge of the underlying genetic disorder.

BIBLIOGRAPHIC SOURCE(S)

Ahrens-Nicklas RC, Khan S, Garbarini J, et al. Utility of genetic evaluation in infants with congenital heart defects admitted to the cardiac intensive care unit. *Am J Med Genet A*. 2016; 170(12):3090-7.

Brent RL. Environmental causes of human congenital malformations: the pediatrician's role in dealing with these complex clinical problems caused by a multiplicity of environmental and genetic factors. *Pediatrics.* 2004;113:957-68.

Centers for Disease Control and Prevention. Appendix C: Causes of congenital anomalies and classification according to developmental mechanism and clinical presentation. 2015. Retrieved from https://www.cdc.gov/ncbddd/birthdefects/surveillancemanual/appendices/appendix-c.html.

Centers for Disease Control and Prevention. Congenital Anomalies – Definitions. 2015. Retrieved from https://www.cdc.gov/ncbddd/birthdefects/surveillancemanual/chapters/chapter-1/chapter1-4.html.

Hansen A, Puder M. *Manual of Neonatal Surgical Intensive Care.* 3rd ed. Shelton, CT: People's Medical Publishing House; 2016.

Jones KL, Adam MP. Evaluation and diagnosis of the dysmorphic infant. *Clin Perinatol.* 2015;42(2):243-viii.

Mathews TJ, Driscoll AK. Trends in Infant Mortality in the United States, 2005–2014. NCHS data brief, no 279. Hyattsville, MD: National Center for Health Statistics; 2017.

Miller DT, Adam MP, Aradhya S, et al. Consensus statement: chromosomal microarray is a first-tier clinical diagnostic test for individuals with developmental disabilities or congenital anomalies. *Am J Hum Genet.* 2010;86:749-64.

Nelson K, Holmes LB. Malformations due to presumed spontaneous mutations in newborn infants. *N Engl J Med.* 1989;320:19-23.

O'Neill BR, Yu AK, Tyler-Kabara EC. Prevalence of tethered spinal cord in infants with VACTERL. *J Neurosurg Pediatr.* 2010;6(2):177-82.

Parisi MA. Hirschsprung disease overview. 2002 [Updated 2015]. In: Adam MP, Ardinger HH, Pagon RA, et al, eds. GeneReviews® [Internet]. Seattle, WA: University of Washington, Seattle; 1993-2018. Available from https://www.ncbi.nlm.nih.gov/books/NBK1439/.

Pober BR, Russell MK, Ackerman KG. Congenital diaphragmatic hernia overview. 2006 [Updated 2010]. In: Adam MP, Ardinger HH, Pagon RA, et al, eds. GeneReviews® [Internet]. Seattle, WA: University of Washington, Seattle; 1993-2018. Available from https://www.ncbi.nlm.nih.gov/books/NBK1359/.

Simpson CD, Ye XY, Hellmann J, Tomlinson C. Trends in cause-specific mortality at a Canadian outborn NICU. *Pediatrics.* 2010;126(6):1538.

Solomon BD, Gropman A, Muenke M. Holoprosencephaly overview. 2000 [Updated 2013]. In: Adam MP, Ardinger HH, Pagon RA, et al, eds. GeneReviews® [Internet]. Seattle, WA: University of Washington, Seattle; 1993-2018. Available from https://www.ncbi.nlm.nih.gov/books/NBK1530/.

Stark Z, Tan TY, Chong B, et al. A prospective evaluation of whole-exome sequencing as a first-tier molecular test in infants with suspected monogenic disorders. *Genet Med.* 2016;18:1090-6.

Weiner J, Sharma J, Lantos J, Kilbride H. How infants die in the neonatal intensive care unit: trends from 1999 through 2008. *Arch Pediatr Adolesc Med.* 2011;165(7):630-4.

Wenger T, Bhoj E. Contemporary evaluation of the neonate with congenital anomalies. *NeoReviews.* 2017;18;e522.

Temperature Management

Patrick D. Carroll, MD, MPH

SCOPE

DISEASE/CONDITION(S)

Maintaining normothermia in the immediate postpartum period and beyond.

GUIDELINE OBJECTIVE(S)

Review definition and classification of temperature ranges; risks of hypothermia; clinical management options for prevention of hypothermia.

BRIEF BACKGROUND

Normothermia has been defined by the World Health Organization (WHO) as a neonatal temperature of 36.5–37.5°C (97.7–99.5°F). Any neonatal temperatures above this are considered hyperthermia and those below this range are considered hypothermia. Hypothermia is further separated into mild hypothermia (36–36.5°C; also referred to as "cold stress"), moderate hypothermia (32–35.9°C), and severe hypothermia (<32°C). Hypothermia is frequent in preterm infants. A California-based cohort of 8782 very low birth weight (VLBW) neonates born in 2006–2007 reported a 56.2% rate of hypothermia. A report from 18 hospitals included in the National Institute of Child Health and Human Development (NICHD) Neonatal Research Network reported 38.6% of moderately preterm infants (29–33 weeks) and 40.9% of extremely preterm infants (<29 weeks) had admission temperatures <36.5 °C. A Canadian cohort of 9833 neonates born at <33 gestational age in 2010–2012 reported a 35.8% rate of hypothermia.

The incidence of hypothermia in term infants is not well defined. A single-institution study from a resource-poor setting in Zambia reported 73% of term infants experienced hypothermia. It is likely that resource-rich settings also experience a non-trivial rate of hypothermia in term infants.

Hypothermia has been associated with increased morbidity and mortality. In a population-based study, admission temperature less than 35°C was an independent predictor of death and bronchopulmonary dysplasia (BPD) among neonates born less than 26 weeks. A separate study which included 8782 neonates born between 23 and 32 weeks' gestation also found strong associations between moderate to severe hypothermia and stage 3–4 retinopathy of prematurity (ROP), late onset sepsis, BPD, intraventricular hemorrhage (IVH), and death.

On the basis of these findings, both obstetric and neonatal organizations have issued guidelines addressing prevention of hypothermia as part of the delivery and resuscitation process. Organizations with such statements or recommendations include the American Academy of Pediatrics (AAP), American College of Obstetrics and Gynecology, American Heart Association, International Liaison Committee on Resuscitation, Neonatal Resuscitation Program, and European Resuscitation Council.

Although the pathophysiology is beyond the scope of this chapter, it should be recognized that the general mechanisms for heat loss are evaporation, conduction, convection, and radiation. Interventions to prevent hypothermia target one or more of these mechanisms. Interventions that are discussed below include delivery room temperature standards, use of a radiant warmer, attention to thermoregulation during transport of preterm infants to the neonatal intensive care unit (NICU), use of occlusive wrap or bag including plastic cap, use of an exothermic mattress, use of heated-humidified gas, and skin-to-skin (kangaroo) care.

RECOMMENDATIONS

MAJOR RECOMMENDATIONS

Adopt strategies to prevent hypothermia during resuscitation and thereafter. While preterm infants are at greater risk of hypothermia, particularly moderate/severe hypothermia, term infants are not immune from developing hypothermia.

PRACTICE OPTIONS

Practice Option #1: Regulate the Delivery Room Temperature

The WHO has recommended maintaining delivery room temperature at 25°C. The International Liaison Committee on Resuscitation, European Resuscitation Council, and American Heart Association have recommended a delivery room temperature of 23–25°C for all neonates and >25°C for all babies less than 28 weeks gestational age at birth. AAP Guidelines for Perinatal Care recommends a delivery room temperature of 26°C. This intervention has been demonstrated to be effective in both term and preterm infants. This strategy decreases evaporative and radiation heat loss. (Class I evidence)

Practice Option #2: Resuscitate Neonates in a Prewarmed Radiant Warmer

Any infant requiring resuscitation should be placed under a radiant warmer during resuscitation regardless of gestational age. The International Liaison Committee on

Resuscitation has recommended "if the baby needs support in transition or resuscitation then place the baby on a warm surface under a preheated radiant warmer." Preheating the radiant warmer decreases conductive heat loss while the overhead warmer provides radiant heat. Especially in smaller neonates the sidewalls of the radiant warmer may be raised. This will decrease air flow over the neonate and reduce convective heat loss while still allowing resuscitation measures to continue. Hyperthermia may be prevented by using the servo-control mode with a temperature probe on the neonate. (Class III evidence)

Practice Option #3: Maintain Attention to Thermoregulation During Neonatal Transfer

The transfer of a neonate from the delivery room or resuscitation room to the NICU should be considered an extension of resuscitation. Use of a prewarmed incubator or radiant warmer along with occlusive wrap have both been shown to be equally effective in maintaining normothermia during transfer to the NICU. Use of polyethylene bags reduces the occurrence of hypothermia during hospital to hospital transport of very low birth weight infants. (Class I evidence)

Practice Option #4: Use of Occlusive Plastic Bag or Wrap Immediately After Delivery

Infants less than 29 weeks' gestation benefit from the use of occlusive plastic bag or wrap without drying first. This strategy is recommended by multiple organizations. Infants should be placed in a plastic bag or wrap from the neck down throughout the resuscitation. This practice option reduces evaporative and convective heat loss. (Class I evidence)

Practice Option #5: Covering the Head with Occlusive Wrap

Covering the head with occlusive wrap in addition to the body did not further decrease frequency of hypothermia or increase hyperthermia in one study but demonstrated additional benefit in another. Benefits of occlusive plastic bag or wrap for infants 29 weeks or above has been demonstrated in resource-limited settings which may not have radiant warmers or ability to control delivery room temperatures. This practice option reduces evaporative and convective heat loss. (Class II evidence)

Practice Option #6: Use of an Exothermic Mattress During Resuscitation

The International Liaison Committee on Resuscitation includes the use of an exothermic mattress among possible interventions to prevent hypothermia among infants <32 weeks' gestation. Infants can be placed on an exothermic mattress to prevent heat loss. Chemical reaction (sodium acetate mattress)–mediated and paraffin-based phase change material have been effective in preventing hypothermia in preterm infants immediately after delivery. This intervention has been described both in place of and in addition to use of plastic bag/wrap. Increased risk of hyperthermia has been reported and must be monitored. (Class II evidence)

Practice Option #7: Use Heated-Humidified Gas

The International Liaison Committee on Resuscitation includes the use of heated humidified gas at delivery in the bundle of interventions to prevent hypothermia. This practice,

TABLE 9.1. Guidelines for Term Newborns: "The Warm Chain"

1. Warm delivery room
2. Immediate drying
3. Skin-to-skin contact
4. Breastfeeding
5. Bathing and weighing postponed
6. Appropriate clothing/bedding
7. Mother and baby together
8. Warm transportation
9. Warm resuscitation
10. Training and awareness raising

Guidelines for all newborns including term and resource limited settings. (World Health Organization. *Thermal Protection of the Newborn: A Practical Guide*. Geneva, World Health Organization; 1997.)

where heated humidified gas is used from the time of birth including during resuscitation, is effective in decreasing hypothermia when done in addition to heated delivery rooms, the use of radiant warmers, body wrap, and head covering. (Class I evidence)

Practice Option #8: Encourage Skin-to-Skin Contact (Kangaroo Mother Care)

Infants not requiring active resuscitation can be placed in direct skin-to-skin contact (kangaroo mother care) with the mother. This intervention is particularly important in resource-limited settings where radiant warmers are not available. It has been demonstrated to be effective in decreasing hypothermia among infants born at 34–40 weeks' gestation and among low birth weight infants. (Class I evidence)

CLINICAL ALGORITHM(S)

Two guidelines exist for thermoregulation immediately after birth. The first (Table 9.1) is "The Warm Chain" developed for term newborns. This guideline was developed by the World Health Organization and can be used in resource-rich and resource-poor countries. The second guideline (Table 9.2) is for preterm newborns, published by the International Liaison Committee on Resuscitation.

TABLE 9.2. Guidelines for Preterm Newborns

Radiant warmer
Environmental temperature 23–25°C
Warm blankets
Plastic wrapping without drying
Plastic cap
Thermal mattress

International Liaison Committee on Resuscitation guidelines for neonates <32 weeks gestational age at birth. These interventions may be used individually or in various combinations. (Perlman JM, Wyllie J, Kattwinkel J, Wyckoff MH, Aziz K, Guinsburg R, Kim HS, Liley HG, Mildenhall L, Simon WM, Szyld E, Tamura M, Velaphi S. Part 7: Neonatal Resuscitation: 2015 International Consensus on Cardiopulmonary Resuscitation and Emergency Cardiovascular Care Science with Treatment Recommendations. *Circulation*. 2015;132(16 Suppl 1): S204-241.)

IMPLEMENTATION OF GUIDELINE

QUALIFYING STATEMENTS

- Not all interventions have been studied independently or in combination with all other interventions. Therefore, institutions may be successful in preventing hypothermia through implementation of various combinations of practice options.
- Care to prevent hyperthermia must be exercised. Hyperthermia also increases mortality.
- Delayed cord clamping has *not* been shown to cause hypothermia and is *not* a contraindication to thermal regulation strategies.

DESCRIPTION OF IMPLEMENTATION STRATEGY

- Create institutional thermoregulation guidelines based on consensus standards and existing reliable published literature.
- Ensure that multidisciplinary teams including obstetrics and neonatology, and key stakeholders including physicians, nurse practitioners, nurses, respiratory therapists, and facilities management are involved in the development of institutional guidelines.
- Monitor and report compliance to guidelines and neonatal temperature outcomes.
- Provide ongoing education and promote future research.

QUALITY METRICS

- Institutions should measure the frequency of hypothermia in neonates. This can be further measured by population (i.e., gestational age, birth weight, type of delivery) and hypothermia subgroups (mild/cold stress, 36.0–36.4; moderate, 35.0–35.9; and severe <35.0).
- Institutions should measure the frequency of hyperthermia (>37.5) and severe hyperthermia (>38.0).
- Consideration may be given to reporting aggregate data as well as physician-specific data as determined by the institution.

SUMMARY

Thermoregulation is a critical aspect of neonatal care that begins in the first minutes of life. Hypothermia has been shown in multiple studies to increase mortality. A number of strategies have been shown to reduce the odds of hypothermia including regulation of delivery room temperature, resuscitation on prewarmed radiant warmers, ongoing attention to thermoregulation during transfer from the delivery room to the neonatal intensive care unit, use of occlusive plastic bag or wrap for the body and head, use of an exothermic mattress, heated-humidified gas, and skin-to-skin contact. These strategies have been used in various combinations to decrease hypothermia in neonates, particularly among preterm neonates.

BIBLIOGRAPHIC SOURCE(S)

American Academy of Pediatrics and American College of Obstetricians and Gynecologists. *Guidelines for Perinatal Care*. Elk Grove Village, IL, American Academy of Pediatrics; 2012.
Belsches TC, Tilly AE, Miller TR, et al. Randomized trial of plastic bags to prevent term neonatal hypothermia in a resource-poor setting. *Pediatrics*. 2013;132(3):e656-61.

Bhat SR, Meng NF, Kumar K, Nagesh KN, Kawale A, Bhutani VK. Keeping babies warm: a non-inferiority trial of a conductive thermal mattress. *Arch Dis Child Fetal Neonatal Ed.* 2015;100(4):F309-12.

Carroll PD, Nankervis CA, Giannone PJ, Cordero L. Use of polyethylene bags in extremely low birth weight infant resuscitation for the prevention of hypothermia. *J Reprod Med.* 2010;55(1-2): 9-13.

Conde-Agudelo A, Diaz-Rossello JL. Kangaroo mother care to reduce morbidity and mortality in low birthweight infants. *Cochrane Database Sys Rev.* 2016;(8):CD002771.

Costeloe K, Hennessy E, Gibson AT, Marlow N, Wilkinson AR. The EPICure study: outcomes to discharge from hospital for infants born at the threshold of viability. *Pediatrics.* 2000;106(4):659-71.

Costeloe KL, Hennessy EM, Haider S, Stacey F, Marlow N, Draper ES. Short term outcomes after extreme preterm birth in England: comparison of two birth cohorts in 1995 and 2006 (the EPICure studies). *BMJ.* 2012;345:e7976.

Doglioni N, Cavallin F, Mardegan V, et al. Total body polyethylene wraps for preventing hypothermia in preterm infants: a randomized trial. *J Pediatr.* 2014;165(2):261-6, e261.

Hu XJ, Wang L, Zheng RY, et al. Using polyethylene plastic bag to prevent moderate hypothermia during transport in very low birth weight infants: a randomized trial. *J Perinatol.* 2018;38(4):332-6.

Kent AL, Williams J. Increasing ambient operating theatre temperature and wrapping in polyethylene improves admission temperature in premature infants. *J Paediatr Child Health.* 2008;44(6):325-31.

Knobel RB, Wimmer JE Jr, Holbert D. Heat loss prevention for preterm infants in the delivery room. *J Perinatol.* 2005;25(5):304-8.

Laptook AR, Bell EF, Shankaran S, et al. Admission temperature and associated mortality and morbidity among moderately and extremely preterm infants. *J Pediatr.* 2018;192:53-9; e52.

Lyu Y, Shah PS, Ye XY, et al. Association between admission temperature and mortality and major morbidity in preterm infants born at fewer than 33 weeks' gestation. *JAMA Pediatr.* 2015;169(4):e150277.

Mathew B, Lakshminrusimha S, Sengupta S, Carrion V. Randomized controlled trial of vinyl bags versus thermal mattress to prevent hypothermia in extremely low-gestational-age infants. *Am J Perinatol.* 2013;30(4):317-22.

McCarthy LK, Molloy EJ, Twomey AR, Murphy JF, O'Donnell CP. A randomized trial of exothermic mattresses for preterm newborns in polyethylene bags. *Pediatrics.* 2013;132(1):e135-41.

Meyer MP, Bold GT. Admission temperatures following radiant warmer or incubator transport for preterm infants <28 weeks: a randomised study. *Arch Dis Child Fetal Neonatal.* 2007;92(4):F295-7.

Meyer MP, Hou D, Ishrar NN, Dito I, te Pas AB. Initial respiratory support with cold, dry gas versus heated humidified gas and admission temperature of preterm infants. *J Pediatr.* 2015;166(2):245-50; e241.

Miller SS, Lee HC, Gould JB. Hypothermia in very low birth weight infants: distribution, risk factors and outcomes. *J Perinatol.* 2011;31(Suppl 1):S49-56.

Nimbalkar SM, Patel VK, Patel DV, Nimbalkar AS, Sethi A, Phatak A. Effect of early skin-to-skin contact following normal delivery on incidence of hypothermia in neonates more than 1800 g: randomized control trial. *J Perinatol.* 2014;34(5):364-8.

Perlman JM, Wyllie J, Kattwinkel J, et al. Part 7: neonatal resuscitation: 2015 international consensus on cardiopulmonary resuscitation and emergency cardiovascular care science with treatment recommendations. *Circulation.* 2015;132(16 Suppl 1): S204-241.

Pinheiro JM, Boynton S, Furdon SA, Dugan R, Reu-Donlon C. Use of chemical warming packs during delivery room resuscitation is associated with decreased rates of hypothermia in very low-birth-weight neonates. *Adv Neonatal Care.* 2011;11(5):357-62.

Singh A, Duckett J, Newton T, Watkinson M. Improving neonatal unit admission temperatures in preterm babies: exothermic mattresses, polythene bags or a traditional approach? *J Perinatol.* 2010;30(1):45-9.

Talakoub S, Shahbazifard Z, Armanian AM, Ghazavi Z. Effect of two polyethylene covers in prevention of hypothermia among premature neonates. *Iran J Nurs Midwifery Res.* 2015;20(3):322-6.

Vohra S, Frent G, Campbell V, Abbott M, Whyte R. Effect of polyethylene occlusive skin wrapping on heat loss in very low birth weight infants at delivery: a randomized trial. *J Pediatr.* 1999;134(5): 547-51.

Vohra S, Roberts RS, Zhang B, Janes M, Schmidt B. Heat loss prevention (HeLP) in the delivery room: a randomized controlled trial of polyethylene occlusive skin wrapping in very preterm infants. *J Pediatr.* 2004;145(6):750-3.

World Health Organization. *Thermal Protection of the Newborn: A Practial Guide.* Geneva, World Health Organization; 1997.

Wyllie J, Bruinenberg J, Roehr CC, Rudiger M, Trevisanuto D, Urlesberger B. European Resuscitation Council Guidelines for Resuscitation 2015: Section 7. Resuscitation and support of transition of babies at birth. *Resuscitation.* 2015;95:249-63.

Neonatal Sepsis

Sagori Mukhopadhyay, MD, MMSc • Karen M. Puopolo, MD, PhD

SCOPE

DISEASE/CONDITION(S)

Neonatal early-onset sepsis (EOS).

GUIDELINE OBJECTIVE(S)

Review EOS epidemiology and microbiology; approach for prevention of group B *Streptococcus* (GBS)-specific EOS; identification and management of infants at increased risk for EOS.

BRIEF BACKGROUND

Definition

Neonatal EOS is defined as blood and/or cerebrospinal fluid (CSF) culture-proven infection occurring in the newborn at less than 7 days of age. Among preterm infants, time frame is limited to infection occurring <72 hours of age.

Incidence

Current EOS incidence is ~0.8 cases per 1000 live births in United States. Incidence and case fatality rate are strongly influenced by preterm birth. Among preterm, very-low birth weight (VLBW) infants (birth weight <1500 g) EOS incidence is ~11 cases per 1000 live births; for infants born 22–24 weeks' gestation, the incidence is as high as 30–35 cases per 1000 live births. Case-fatality rates also track with prematurity; 1–2% among term infants but ~50% among those born ≤24 weeks' gestation.

Microbiology

GBS is the leading cause of EOS in the term population, accounting for ~40% of EOS cases. *Escherichia coli* accounts for ~15% of term cases. In contrast, among infants born

<34 weeks' gestation, *E. coli* accounts for ~50% of EOS cases among preterm infants and GBS ~20%. Enterococcus, viridans streptococcus, and gram-negative organisms account for most other cases. Fungal species, staphylococcus, and *Listeria* are all uncommon causes of EOS, each accounting for <1–3% of reported cases. Centers where anaerobic cultures are obtained have reported ~15% of EOS cases occurring among VLBW infants to be caused by strict anaerobic bacteria, primarily *Bacteroides* species.

Pathogenesis and Prevention

EOS pathogenesis predominantly occurs by ascending colonization and infection of the uterine compartment and fetus with microbial species from the maternal genitourinary flora during labor and/or during vaginal delivery. Clinical risk factors for EOS include those factors that provide opportunity for this pathogenesis (such as preterm and/or prolonged rupture of membranes [ROM]) or reflect progressive maternal inflammation and infection (such as maternal fever). Although the pathogenesis of EOS primarily occurs during labor and delivery for term infants, rarely intraamniotic infection may occur prior to the onset of labor and may even cause stillbirth. In contrast, onset of infection is often uncertain among preterm infants. Intraamniotic infection may precede and cause preterm labor or premature ROM (PROM) and prolonged periods of premature cervical dilatation and/or PROM may facilitate ascending infection. Occasionally, preterm EOS may be caused by bloodborne spread of infection across the placenta, as is the case with *Listeria monocytogenes* infection. Primary prevention of GBS-specific EOS can be achieved via the administration of intrapartum antibiotic prophylaxis (IAP) to mothers colonized with GBS, to reduce the burden of maternal and fetal colonization with this organism. Although IAP has reduced incidence, EOS-associated mortality and morbidity remain substantial. Thus assessing a newborn infant for risk of EOS, appropriate determination of infection and timely institution of treatment constitute critical parts of early newborn care.

RECOMMENDATIONS

MAJOR RECOMMENDATIONS

Primary Prevention of EOS

Multiple obstetric management strategies aim to protect both mother and fetus from infection and are not within the scope of this chapter. Current national recommendations from the American Academy of Pediatrics (AAP), American College of Obstetricians and Gynecologists (ACOG), and Centers for Disease Control (CDC) address prevention of GBS-specific EOS and are summarized here:

- All pregnant women should be screened for rectovaginal GBS colonization at 35–37 weeks' gestation, as well as at any point in gestation where there is concern for premature ROM and/or preterm labor.
  - If GBS colonization has been documented by urine culture prior to 35–37 weeks, third trimester screening is not needed.
  - Some centers use GBS nucleic acid–based point-of-care testing at the time of presentation for delivery.
- IAP should be administered if any of the following are present:
  - Mother is GBS-positive (by rectovaginal culture, urine culture, or intrapartum nucleic acid testing).

- Mother has previously delivered an infant with GBS disease.
- Mother is GBS unknown and any of the following occur:
  - Delivery at <37 0/7 weeks gestation
  - Intrapartum maternal temperature ≥38.0°C (≥100.4°C)
  - ROM ≥18 hours

GBS IAP should consist of penicillin G, ampicillin, or cefazolin. Alternatives for women with serious penicillin allergy are clindamycin or vancomycin, but neither of these antibiotics will provide adequate newborn prophylaxis.

Secondary Prevention of EOS

The goal of clinical risk assessment in EOS is to identify newborns at highest risk of EOS and subsequently attempt to prevent the progression of the disease by instituting appropriate antibiotic therapy. Optimized EOS screening aims to identify newborns for which early treatment may prevent severe disease while reducing unnecessary medical intervention among uninfected infants. Due to differences in epidemiology and microbiology of infection between term and preterm infants, risk assessment strategies also differ. Information used to estimate the risk of infection includes the following:

- **Perinatal risk factors:** Gestational age, maternal GBS colonization, evidence of maternal intraamniotic infection (such as maternal intrapartum fever), duration of ROM, onset of preterm labor, administration of intrapartum antibiotic prophylaxis.
- **Clinical status of the newborn:** Most cases of EOS present within the first 24–36 hours after birth, and a well-appearing condition is associated with decreased risk.
- **Laboratory tests:** Markers of host response to infection such as complete blood count and C-reactive protein (CRP) can provide surrogate evidence for infection. However, in the immediate postnatal period these tests lack sensitivity and specificity for predicting EOS, and among term infants their value is impacted by the very low rate of disease.
- **Microbiology tests:** Definitive diagnosis is made by blood and/or CSF culture.

PRACTICE OPTIONS: TERM AND LATE PRETERM INFANTS

Among *term and late preterm infants* (born ≥35 weeks' gestation), there are three general approaches to EOS risk assessment.

Practice Option #1: Categorical Use of Risk Factors

Such strategies dichotomize infants in categories of "at risk" or "not at risk" based on the presence or absence of specific risk factors such as maternal chorioamnionitis, often defined as maternal intrapartum temperature ≥38.0°C (≥100.4°C). The secondary prevention of EOS algorithm contained within the CDC 2010 perinatal GBS prevention guidelines is an example of this approach. The CDC 2010 algorithm recommended that newborns

- Have laboratory testing, blood culture, and empiric antibiotics administered if they have clinical illness consistent with EOS.
- Have laboratory testing, blood culture, and empiric antibiotics administered if born to a mother with a diagnosis of chorioamnionitis, regardless of infant clinical condition.
- Born to mothers with inadequate indicated GBS IAP and no additional risk factors be observed in hospital for a minimum 48 hours.
- Born to mothers with inadequate indicated GBS IAP and the additional risk factor of with ROM ≥18 hours or gestational age <37 weeks have laboratory testing and blood culture.

The CDC algorithm approach requires that clinicians define both the clinical obstetric diagnosis of "chorioamnionitis" and delineate the timing and content of newborn "clinical illness." Local algorithms based on specific cutoffs for maternal fever or ROM can be developed but will lack external validation.

Practice Option #2: Multivariate Use of Risk Factors

Multivariate modeling can optimize the use of clinical risk factors to increase the accuracy of risk assessment for individual infants. The Neonatal Early-Onset Sepsis Calculator is based on two multivariate models that account multiple clinical risk factors for EOS as well as for newborn clinical condition and provide quantitative risk estimates for the individual newborn. This is available at: https://neonatalsepsiscalculator.kaiserpermanente.org. The approach takes a Bayesian perspective and begins with the baseline incidence of EOS in the population. Empiric antibiotic administration and laboratory testing are based on the estimated risk of infection at birth and the evolving newborn clinical condition. Threshold values for such decisions have been validated in prospective studies, but the quantitative risk output of these models allows centers to determine local thresholds for such actions if desired.

Practice Option #3: Clinical Observation

The approaches in both Practice Options #1 and #2 can be used to assess newborn risk of EOS with the goal of administering empiric antibiotics only to infants who appear to manifest signs of illness. Under this approach, all newborns who are symptomatic at birth are administered empiric antibiotics and subject to laboratory testing. Well-appearing newborns deemed at risk by Practice Option #1 or #2 are placed in a specific setting (such as the neonatal intensive care unit) and/or on a specific clinical pathway for enhanced medical observation. Initially well-appearing infants are treated and/or tested only if they develop signs of illness. Centers choosing this option must define the content and timing of newborn "signs of illness" and establish safety audits in place to monitor time to antibiotics in confirmed cases.

PRACTICE OPTION: PRETERM INFANTS

Among *preterm infants* (born ≤34 weeks' gestation), the frequency of EOS risk factors and clinical instability make it difficult to apply the approaches described above. Consequently, in most centers, 70–90% of preterm infants are administered empiric antibiotics and subject to laboratory testing.

Practice Option #1: Identify Preterm Infants at Differential Risk of EOS

Infants born by cesarean section without labor, any attempt to induce labor, and without ROM prior to delivery have not been exposed to factors associated with risk of ascending bacterial colonization and infection. As long as such infants are born for maternal non-infectious reasons (e.g., preeclampsia), then such infants are at low risk of EOS regardless of their clinical condition at birth. Single-center and multicenter studies suggest that such infants are at 5- to 12-fold lower risk compared to infants that do not meet such criteria. Because the need for respiratory support is common among preterm infants, those that meet these low-risk criteria could be spared empiric antibiotic therapy unless they manifest significant cardiovascular instability. In contrast, infants born in the setting of preterm labor or cervical dilatation, premature rupture of membranes, concern for maternal intraamniotic infection (chorioamnionitis), or acute onset of unexplained non-reassuring fetal status are at the highest risk of EOS. Such preterm infants should undergo EOS evaluation with blood culture, CSF culture if appropriate, and empiric antibiotics should be administered pending culture results.

TESTING AND TREATMENT

Testing and Treatment Practice

White blood cell count and its components, platelet counts, and CRP levels have all been studied for use in predicting EOS. None are sensitive or specific enough to be used alone to determine the need for empiric antibiotic therapy. When blood cultures are indicated, at least one blood culture bottle should be incubated with 1 mL of blood. Both infecting organism recovery and opportunity to distinguish contaminant species may be optimized if two blood culture bottles are incubated, each with 1 mL blood. Anaerobic culture may be considered, particularly for preterm infants. Blood may be obtained via peripheral venous or arterial phlebotomy, or from central catheters using sterile technique. Empiric antibiotics most commonly include ampicillin (100 mg/kg/dose every 12 hours) and gentamicin (5 mg/kg/dose every 48 hours for gestation <29 weeks, 4.5 mg/kg/dose every 36 hours for gestation 30–34 weeks, and 4 mg/kg/dose every 24 hours for gestation >34 weeks). Approximately 60–70% of *E. coli* EOS isolates are now resistant to ampicillin; therefore, for severely ill infants at highest risk of EOS the addition of a cephalosporin or other extended-spectrum beta-lactam antibiotic may be warranted until culture results are known. Duration of empiric therapy is based on time for most confirmed infections to be identified. For centers using automated blood culture growth detection methods, a duration of 36–48 hours is sufficient prior to discontinuation of therapy.

IMPLEMENTATION OF GUIDELINE

DESCRIPTION OF IMPLEMENTATION STRATEGY

For all described approach(s) used, the following principles can be useful in establishing successful implementation.

1. **Multidisciplinary approach:** EOS approach spans multiple specialties (obstetrics, neonatology, general pediatricians, hospitalists, and occasionally infectious disease) and care providers (nurses in labor floor, intensive care units, well baby units, physician assistants, trainees, lactation consultants, and physicians). Identifying the local participants and involving them in the planning and implementation of the EOS approach can ensure compliance.
2. **Standardizing local care:** Every birth center and neonatal care unit should consider a written protocol that clarifies the institute's approach to identifying high-risk infants, details the use and interpretation of diagnostic testing, prescribes methods for optimal blood culture collection, and identifies choice for first-line empiric therapy.
3. **Baby-friendly practices:** In the care of well-appearing newborns identified as at risk for EOS, timing and location of intervention should consider minimizing maternal/infant separation when feasible.
4. **Antibiotic stewardship:** Nonspecific elevations of acute-phase markers used in diagnostics must be considered before mandating prolonged duration of antibiotics and/or further testing such as lumbar puncture in well-appearing infants. Optimizing blood culture collection practices can increase confidence in negative results.

Clear documentation of indication for diagnosis of culture-negative sepsis can provide information for ongoing stewardship efforts.

5. **Auditing practice:** Monitoring of implementation for practice drift and noncompliance can prevent unanticipated consequences and can inform future changes.

QUALITY METRICS

- **Obstetrics:** Monitor compliance with GBS screening guidelines and IAP administration.
- **Newborn care:** Monitor compliance with written protocol, incidence of antibiotic exposure, and incidence of culture confirmed EOS.

SUMMARY

Early-onset neonatal sepsis is a low-frequency, high-morbidity disease occurring more commonly in preterm infants. Different approaches exist based on perinatal risk factors, clinical condition of the infant, and laboratory testing that can inform the management of these infants. In the absence of a prediction model or laboratory test that is accurate at 100%, clinicians must balance minimizing unnecessary intervention while maximizing safety. Standardized approaches modified to local disease incidence and practice are recommended to improve consistency of care.

BIBLIOGRAPHIC SOURCE(S)

Benitz WE. Adjunct laboratory tests in the diagnosis of early-onset neonatal sepsis. *Clin Perinatol.* 2010;37(2):421-38.

Escobar GJ, Puopolo KM, Wi S, et al. Stratification of risk of early-onset sepsis in newborns >=34 weeks' gestation. *Pediatrics.* 2014;133(1):30-6.

Joshi NS, Gupta A, Allan JM, et al. Clinical monitoring of well-appearing infants born to mothers with chorioamnionitis. *Pediatrics.* 2018;141(4):e20172056.

Puopolo KM, Draper D, Wi S, et al. Estimating the probability of neonatal early-onset infection on the basis of maternal risk factors. *Pediatrics.* 2011;128(5):e1155-63.9.

Puopolo K, Mukhopadhyay S, Hansen N, et al. Identification of extremely premature infants at low risk for early-onset sepsis. *Pediatrics.* 2017;140(5). pii: e20170925.

Stoll BJ, Hansen NI, Sanchez PJ, et al. Early onset neonatal sepsis: the burden of group B Streptococcal and E. coli disease continues. *Pediatrics.* 2011;127(5):817-26.

Verani JR, McGee L, Schrag SJ, Division of Bacterial Diseases, National Center for Immunization and Respiratory Diseases, Centers for Disease Control and Prevention (CDC). Prevention of perinatal group B streptococcal disease--revised guidelines from CDC, 2010. *MMWR Recomm Rep.* 2010;59(RR-10):1-36.

Weston EJ, Pondo T, Lewis MM, et al. The burden of invasive early-onset neonatal sepsis in the United States, 2005-2008. *Pediatr Infect Dis J.* 2011;30(11):937-41.

Neonatal Abstinence Syndrome

Rachana Singh, MD, MS • Jeffrey S. Shenberger, MD
• Robert W. Rothstein, MD

SCOPE

DISEASE/CONDITION(S)

In utero exposure to maternal illicit drugs and/or medication assisted treatment (MAT) with potential for neonatal abstinence syndrome.

GUIDELINE OBJECTIVE(S)

Review best practices for antenatal and postnatal care plans for both the substance exposed newborns and their families to assist in successful transition home.

BRIEF BACKGROUND

The well-documented epidemic of opioid use in the United States and internationally has resulted in a rising incidence of births by mothers with opioid use disorder (OUD). It is estimated that in the United States, one child is born each hour requiring treatment for neonatal abstinence syndrome (NAS). Complications of OUD in pregnancy include miscarriage, preterm labor, preterm premature rupture of membranes, intrauterine growth restriction, preeclampsia, and stillbirth. Accordingly, substance-exposed newborns (SENs) born to mothers with OUD are at increased risk of adverse health and social outcomes both short term (e.g., NAS) and long term (e.g., foster care placement, neurodevelopmental impairment). In the United States, the current incidence of NAS is 3–4 infants/1000 live births, though a significant variation is noted geographically. Mirroring this are increases in resources utilized, with an average NAS admission costing $53,400. The outcomes of substance-exposed pregnancies and infants depend on multiple factors including, but not limited to, socioeconomic factors/influences, co-occurring psychiatric disorders, family infrastructure, community support, the types of substances used, genetic and metabolic factors, treatment medications, feeding type and mode (breastfeeding vs breastmilk vs formula), parental education, and the degree of parental involvement in infant care. Efforts to improve neonatal outcomes must address multiple factors such as maternal sobriety, breastfeeding and bonding, and best practices for NAS treatment. To improve care of the SENs, the requisite interventions need to be implemented ideally in the preconception and antenatal period. Well thought out clinical care plans are also needed in the early neonatal period as well as in the long-term post-discharge follow-up care aimed at monitoring growth and neurodevelopmental outcomes.

RECOMMENDATIONS

RECOMMENDATION 1

Establishing a consistent preconception and antenatal care and counseling program for families affected by OUD is paramount. It is well known that women with chronic medical conditions will have greater success at conceiving and carrying a healthy pregnancy to term if there is good control of their preexisting conditions, such as obesity, diabetes, and hypertension. Therefore, it stands to reason that a mother enrolled in a structured rehabilitative program utilizing a MAT program prior to conception and during pregnancy will have a greater potential for achieving a healthy term pregnancy.

Practice Option #1

Females in childbearing age of 15–44 years who are in stable MAT programs should discuss pregnancy plans and contraception options with their primary care and obstetric providers. These discussions should be incorporated into routine annual as well as post conception visits. Attention should focus on standard pregnancy counseling as per American College of Obstetricians and Gynecologists guidelines, smoking cessation (tobacco, cannabinoids), mental health counseling if warranted, breastfeeding, and the potential for their infants to develop NAS. A multidisciplinary prenatal consulting team, including neonatology/pediatrics, anesthesiology, and social service is critical in preparing families for potential immediate and long-term outcomes (Figure 11.1). The inclusion of anesthesiology to the prenatal consulting team is valuable, as opioid-dependent women fear their labor pain may be inadequately treated (tolerance or hyperalgesia). These fears have been associated with self-medication prior to admission. In addition, community resources should be made readily available to the families to help provide the much needed, and often lacking, peer and family support crucial to successful transitioning to home.

Practice Option #2

Females in childbearing age of 15–44 years who are actively abusing substances and not in stable MAT programs should be identified as early as possible (emergency department visit, first prenatal visit, primary care visit) and enrolled in a stable MAT program. Two models of MAT programs, methadone clinics or buprenorphine individual

```
NEONATAL CONSULT MATERNAL DRUG USE
Neonatology consulted to discuss NAS.                     Requested by (Referring MD): _____
Consult to speak with mom about pregnancy complicated by:       Pt. name: _____
Neonatal/fetal drug exposure to                                 Date:_____
_____Methadone            _____Opiates
_____Buprenorphine        _____Cannabinoids
_____Heroin               _____Other
_____Cocaine

Maternal history and chart reviewed.

_____The following anticipated problems were discussed and reviewed with

Mother and                    _____FOB                    _____Family support members

This includes but is not limited to the following:
_____Illicit and treatment medications use in pregnancy
_____Illicit and treatment medication dosing in pregnancy
_____Toxicology testing during pregnancy
_____Support systems during pregnancy
_____Breastfeeding
_____Post-delivery newborn observation
_____Nonpharmacologic treatment for NAS
_____Pharmacologic treatment for NAS (meds, escalating and weaning protocol)
_____Need for NICU admission
_____Social Service consult
_____Filing 51A and DSS
_____Discharge and length of stay
_____NICU visitation policy
_____Newborn follow-up (EI, VNA)

Mother received:
_____Parent information sheet
_____Tips for parents
_____Tour of NICU (Social Service)
_____CDC Hep B and C infections (only for moms testing +)

Comments:

Provider signature                                Date
```

FIGURE 11.1 • Prototype of antenatal neonatal consultation for pregnancy complicated by substance use disorder.

prescribers, currently exist. Methadone clinics are closely regulated and provide consistent behavioral and mental health counseling, require daily or weekly visits, enhance adherence, and lessen the risk of diversion. However, methadone can be associated with a greater severity of NAS. Buprenorphine prescribers/clinics are currently less regulated, provide ease of prescription, have minimal to no mandate for behavioral and/or mental health counseling, and require less frequent (monthly) clinic visits. An additional advantage of buprenorphine is that it is associated with less severe NAS symptoms, requires less morphine, and had shorter duration of NAS treatment and hospital length of stay (LOS). Despite these advantages, concerns exist for higher maternal relapse rates and ease of medication diversion. The choice of MAT (methadone vs buprenorphine) should therefore be based on the parturient preference and tailored to the response achieved. While transitioning them to a MAT program, all of Practice Option #1 should be concurrently incorporated in care. In addition, pathways, including psychosocial support, should be put in place to help the parents secure stable housing and employment, which will assist in making the transition to home seamless. Community resources as well as social service teams should be identified and be actively involved prenatally (Figure 11.2).

Western Massachusetts Substance Abuse Treatment and Prevention Services Directory	Western Massachusetts Substance Abuse Treatment and Prevention Services Directory
Programs Funded and/or Licensed by: The Department of Public Health Bureau of Substance Abuse Services Ruth Jacobson-Hardy, Western Massachusetts Regional Manager X3128 Erica Piedade, Director of Licensing X3182 Jennifer Babich, Licensing Inspector Western Region X3132 Ben Cluff, Veterans Services Coordinator X3126 Department of Public Health 23 Service Center Road Northampton, MA 01060 Voice: (413) 586-7525 Fax: (413) 784-1037 TTY: (800) 769 -9991 Boston Office: (617) 624-5175 www.mass.gov/dph/bsas/bsas.htm Statewide HELPLINE: 1-800-327-5050 www.helpline-online.com For services for pregnant women and family residential treatment call the Institute for Health and Recovery at 617-661-3991 Or 866-705-2807	**Table of Contents**
March, 2015	

FIGURE 11.2 • Prototype of the listings of local community resources available to providers and families.

Practice Option #3

Females in child bearing age of 15–44 years of age who actively take illicit drugs and present at the time of birth with absent prenatal care, not enrolled in a MAT program and with lack of support systems are commonly encountered. Multiple issues need to be addressed in such cases, including acute withdrawal in the mother, pain management in the intra- and postpartum periods, legal custody issues, as well as infant care plans. Institutional protocols in such situations may provide consistent care plans and relay educational information to both family members and the staff caring for them. Though the protocols may vary between institutions based on available resources and geographical variations, having a protocol in place is a good clinical care practice. Protocols have been shown to improve NAS outcomes, including a shorter duration of opioid treatment, as well as decreasing length of hospital stay and need for adjunctive medication therapy.

RECOMMENDATION 2

Establish guidelines for the management of SENs, detailing the monitoring as well as the treatment of the infant with NAS. As mentioned earlier (Recommendation 1), having well-established protocols in place generally improves outcome. These should provide consistent guidelines to the practitioner while allowing flexibility to tailor them to the individual patient's needs, and should be reassessed regularly to incorporate new emerging evidence-based practices.

Practice Option #1

Create a single scoring system for SENs and train clinical staff to perform the scoring objectively and consistently. Of the available scoring systems, the modified Finnegan scoring is the most commonly used and has the advantage of being easily taught and validated. A novel scoring system "Eat, Sleep, Console" tool is currently being developed, piloted, and tested, with some initial promising results. The nursing staff taking care of infants in well-baby nurseries as well as neonatal intensive care units (NICUs) should be trained and periodically validated to perform the scoring and document results in the infant's medical record. Since the choice of initiating and weaning pharmacotherapy is dependent on the scores, validating the staff in scoring is a best practice that should be universally embraced. In efforts to assure interobserver reliability, an educational manual for those using the Finnegan neonatal abstinence score is available. Parents should be educated about the scoring system, and when feasible, be invited to score the infant along with the medical staff. This improves communication between the parents and the medical team, while engaging the parents to play a more active role in the treatment plan for their infant.

Practice Option #2

Foster the mother-infant dyad while monitoring the infant for NAS by providing well-developed nonpharmacological treatment protocols. Current AAP guidelines recommend inpatient observation of SENs for 7 days prior to discharge home. The first week of life is critical for parent-infant bonding and breastfeeding success, making it vital to keep this dyad intact. In addition, promoting and succeeding with nonpharmacological treatment interventions, such as breastfeeding, skin-to-skin care, environmental modifications, and soothing techniques helps reduce the need for pharmacotherapy, further reinforcing the importance of an intact dyad. These treatment strategies should be shared with parents and families, and enable them to provide the first line of care. This practice creates an opportunity to provide good parenting education to families who frequently feel overwhelmed by their overall complex medical and social situation (Figure 11.3).

Practice Option #3

Create a NAS treatment protocol tailored to the infant's in utero drug exposure. Opioid abuse in the general population and the incidence of NAS are increasing at a steady rate. Polydrug use combined with tobacco and multiple psychoactive agents (anxiolytics, antidepressants), superimposed upon comorbid psychiatric conditions, have complicated the course of NAS. These confounders impart a significant clinical variability in the NAS severity, even when excluding infant's genotype and phenotype for individual neonate. In addition, variability in the time to initiate pharmacotherapy, the medications used, and locations of treatment (inpatient vs outpatient) all exist without any strong evidence supporting that one strategy is superior to another. Commonly used medications that are the mainstay for therapy include opioids (neonatal morphine sulfate, methadone) as the first line and non-opioids as adjunctive therapies (phenobarbital, clonidine, diazepam). These medications are used either as a single agent, combination therapy at initiation, or added later as an adjunct therapy if monotherapy fails. Evidence

What To Do IF?
Tips for Parents

What do I do if my baby can't sleep? Difficulty sleeping is a common problem during withdrawal. It is best not to wake your sleeping baby.	What do I do if my baby won't stop crying?	What do I do if my baby won't eat?	What do I do if my baby won't stop eating? Tummy cramps, gas, and loose stools are frequent symptoms of withdrawal.	What do I do if my baby doesn't look at me? Is the baby restless, fussy, or turning away from you?
Here are some tips: • *To soothe your baby (after feeding), offer a pacifier.* • *Wrap snugly in a blanket.* • *Gently rock.* • *Sing softly.* • *Gently pat on the back.* • *Make sure that the baby's bedside is dim and quiet—no lights, no loud voices.*	*Here are some tips:* • *Again, try soft voices, dim lights, gentle handling.* • *Skin-to-skin (also called kangaroo care) (Dads and Moms can both do this!)* • *Soft music.* • *If sweating or trembling, a warm bath or massage may soothe the baby.*	*Here are some tips:* • *Try a different nipple when feeding your baby.* • *Try laying the baby in your lap with their face away from you.* • *With no distractions, your baby may be able to focus better on eating.*	*Here are some tips:* • *Talk to your baby's nurse about feedings.* • *Together, you can decide when your baby needs to eat, and when the baby needs to be soothed in other ways.* • *Remember: breastfeeding is best for you and your baby. Talk to your baby's doctor. Sometimes there is a reason not to breastfeed. If that is the case, you can keep your baby safe and comfortable with formula.*	*Here are some tips:* • *The baby may be overstimulated and ready for quiet time.*

FIGURE 11.3 • Prototype of nonpharmacological treatment options to be shared with caregivers of SENs and utilized during inpatient treatment.

suggests that having a consistent protocol in place can be more important than the actual medications used. Accordingly, each unit should have a single evidence-based protocol in place that is then adhered to by multiple providers (Figure 11.4).

RECOMMENDATION 3

Establish well-defined post-discharge medical and follow-up plans for the SENs. Since family support is critical for success, post-discharge community support programs should not only be readily available, but families should be connected to them prior to discharge.

Practice Option #1

Define post-discharge medical and neurodevelopmental follow-up plans for the SENs. If the infant is being discharged home on medications, such as methadone and/or phenobarbital, then parents/caregivers should be given clear, precise written instructions about administration and storage of medications, along with a weaning protocol. There should be provision for regular post-discharge follow-up visits with the primary care providers in order to ensure monitoring of medication weaning as well as growth. All SENs should have an Early Intervention (or its equivalent) referral made prior to discharge, and routine neurodevelopmental screenings. Opiate-exposed infants are significantly more likely to have neurodevelopmental impairments at 18 months and 3 years old. A significant number of NAS infants have long-term neuromotor, cognitive, and/or behavioral morbidities, including insecure and disorganized attachment, impaired speech and language development, aggressive behavior, peer conflicts, hyperactivity, inattention, anxiety, depression, and substance abuse. Early identification and intervention have been shown to improve outcome.

	NAS MEDICATION CALCULATION WORKSHEET		
Tier	**Neonatal morphine sulfate (NMS)'**	**Clonidine**	**Phenobarbital**
	(0.4 mg/mL)	(10 µg/mL)	(20 mg/5 mL)
1 (FS 8-10)	0.32 mg/kg/day divided q3h	6 µg/kg/day divided q6h	1. Loading: Phenobarbital 10 mg/kg po every 12 hours for 2 doses total
2 (FS 11-13)	0.48 mg/kg/day divided q3h	8 µg/kg/day divided q6h	
3 (FS 14-16)	0.64 mg/kg/day divided q3h	10 µg/kg/day divided q6h	2. Maintenance: Phenobarbital 5 mg/kg po every 24 hours, started
4 (FS ≥17)	0.80 mg/kg/day divided q3h	12 µg/kg/day divided q6h	12 h after 2nd loading dose
	When needing more than 0.80 mg/kg/day NMS, then increase dose in increments of 0.16 mg/kg/day until neonatal abstinence score is less than 8		Check Phenobarbital level 72 hours after starting Phenobarbital and then repeat again in 72 hours, unless otherwise indicated.

*Infants <35 weeks are treated with NMS alone.
Neonatal morphine sulfate dosage escalation:
After initiation of medications, during the first 48 hours: if 2 or more NAS scores are >8: increase dosage to the next tier up.

Standard neonatal morphine sulfate (NMS) weaning:
- NMS is weaned by 10% of the highest dose. For example, if the infant is getting 0.2 mg q3h then wean will be by 0.02 mg per dose, the weans can be q12h or 24 h.
- Hold the weaning if 2 or more consecutive scores >8.
- In the first 48 hours increase to the next Tier up if needed for early capture. Any time after initial 48 hours, if NAS scores ≥10 give a NMS rescue dose of 0.05 mg/kg.
- Up to two (2) NMS rescue doses may be given in a 24-hour period, before reverting to last effective dose.
- If scores continue to be ≥10 despite 2 rescue doses; increase scheduled NMS and clonidine to next dosing range.
- NMS to be discontinued once daily dose is at 0.12 mg/kg/day.

Standard clonidine weaning:
- Once infant is off NMS for 12–24 hours with scores primarily <8 then clonidine weaning can be initiated
- The weaning is a two-step process—first wean to $\frac{1}{2}$, dose and then discontinue it. If starting with 6 µg/kg/day then wean to 3 µg/kg/day and then 12–24 hours later discontinue if scores permit.
- Infant ready for discharge home after 24 hours off all medications with scores primarily <8.

Standard phenobarbital weaning:
- Phenobarbital weaning should begin 48 hours after NMS has been stopped.
- Phenobarbital can be weaned by 20% of the maximum maintenance total daily dose every 3 days.
- An infant may be discharged home 24-48 hours after the first phenobarbital wean.
- The remaining phenobarbital wean will be outlined in the discharge prescription and followed by the primary care pediatrician.
- With weaning every 3 days, the infant should be weaned off phenobarbital within a 2-week period to minimize any adverse long-term effects.
- If the infant starts to exhibits signs of phenobarbital withdrawal (hyperactivity, tremors, hyperreflexia), the dose should be increased to the last effective dose.
- Once stabilized, the wean can be resumed as described above.

FIGURE 11.4 • Prototype of a pharmacotherapy protocol with specific guidelines for type, dose, route of medications to be used along with the inpatient/outpatient weaning instructions.

Practice Option #2

Define postpartum follow-up plans for mothers of SENs and identify community support groups for the mothers to connect with. For families affected with substance use disorders (SUDs), behavioral health comorbidities are frequently seen, and social support systems are often tenuous. In one study, almost 65% of opioid-dependent pregnant women screened positive for one or more psychiatric diagnoses, such as a mood (48.6%), anxiety (40%), or depressive (33%) disorders. In addition, a significant history of trauma and posttraumatic stress disorder is often observed in women with substance abuse. Accordingly, mothers of SENs should have closer follow-up to monitor for postpartum depression and anxiety, with readily available referrals and management protocols in place. In addition to programs aimed at minimizing recurrence of substance abuse, it is equally important that interventions are put in place to improve frequently associated problematic parenting. A review of such interventions, examining 21 outcomes studies, provides insight into identifying barriers and targeting strategies to improve outcomes. The authors suggest that concurrent dual treatment of both substance abuse and parenting difficulties synergistically improves both areas, with the treatment of one enhancing the outcome of the other. For the developing infant, the importance of a good relationship with their primary provider of care, most often their mother, and avoiding severe stress and enhancing attachment, are important for optimal brain development and lessening mental health issues later in life. Given the burden and complexities of community resources needed, the Department of Health in most states has federally funded resources available. Identification and providing mechanisms to connect families to these resources is vital not only for successful transition home, but also for future treatment retention and success.

CLINICAL ALGORITHM(S)

To achieve successful outcome for maternal-infant dyad impacted by OUD, there is a critical need to have well-defined protocols in place during antenatal, neonatal, and post discharge phases as depicted in Figure 11.5.

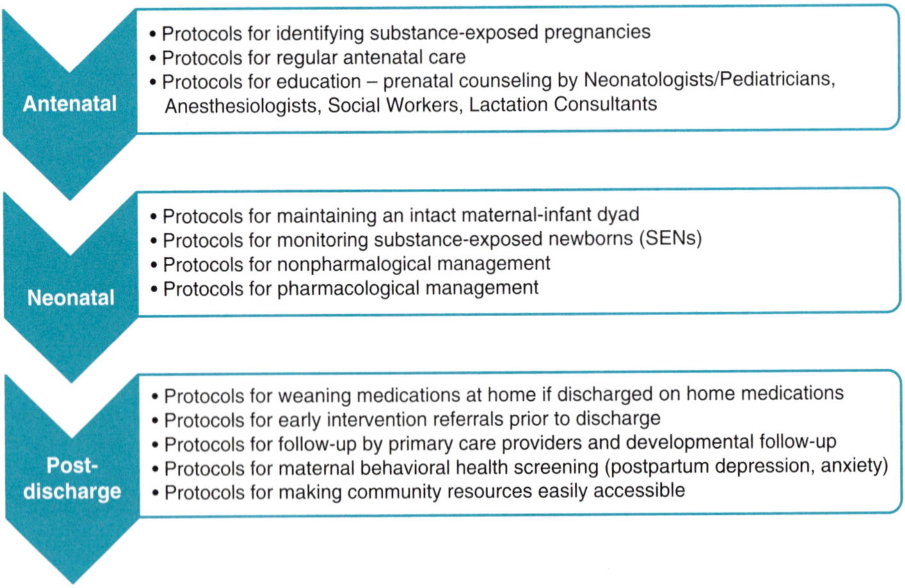

Antenatal
- Protocols for identifying substance-exposed pregnancies
- Protocols for regular antenatal care
- Protocols for education – prenatal counseling by Neonatologists/Pediatricians, Anesthesiologists, Social Workers, Lactation Consultants

Neonatal
- Protocols for maintaining an intact maternal-infant dyad
- Protocols for monitoring substance-exposed newborns (SENs)
- Protocols for nonpharmalogical management
- Protocols for pharmacological management

Post-discharge
- Protocols for weaning medications at home if discharged on home medications
- Protocols for early intervention referrals prior to discharge
- Protocols for follow-up by primary care providers and developmental follow-up
- Protocols for maternal behavioral health screening (postpartum depression, anxiety)
- Protocols for making community resources easily accessible

FIGURE 11.5 • Schematic for protocols needed to provide optimal care for pregnancies impacted by opioid use disorder.

IMPLEMENTATION OF GUIDELINE

DESCRIPTION OF IMPLEMENTATION STRATEGY

We recommend establishing written guidelines/protocols, allowing a small degree of built-in flexibility, rendering them "tailorable" to specific clinical scenarios. This process requires clinical care providers from differing disciplines (internists, OB/GYNs, pediatricians, anesthesiologists, ancillary medical staff, federal workers [Department of Child and Families, Department of Public Health, Bureau of Substance Abuse Services, Early Intervention/Head Start Programs]) to work together over an extended period of time, in order to support families affected by SUD as well as their infants affected by NAS.

QUALITY METRICS

Potential quality metrics would focus on the provision of coordinated, consistent care focusing on nonpharmacologic interventions and family support. Such metrics could include breastfeeding rates in SENs, consistency in NAS scoring, consistent use of nonpharmacologic methods prior to pharmacotherapy, time to initiation and capture of NAS symptoms, readmission rates, and engagement with early intervention after discharge. Other important measures from a community perspective that may speak to quality of care provided to this population broadly include incidence of SENs, enrollment of mothers with OUD in treatment programs that include MAT, relapse rates for mothers in MAT after delivery, and discharge disposition of SENs (home vs foster care). In general, we do not focus on hospital length of stay as a primary quality metric, although a shorter length of stay is often associated with improvements in family-centered care.

SUMMARY

In summary, we recommend that clinical care of the SENs begins with the identification of women in childbearing age who are actively abusing opioids or in stable MAT programs due to a past history of opioid abuse, and continues with close nutritional and neurodevelopmental follow-up after discharge. Best care practice–driven protocols/guidelines should be in place to provide consistent care as well as education to caregivers. This will require creating multidisciplinary teams (medical and nonmedical) to provide care for the families and infants affected by SUD over a longitudinal timeframe, and raising awareness of effective utilization of available resources.

BIBLIOGRAPHIC SOURCE(S)

Abrahams RR, Kelly SA, Payne S, Thiessen PN, Mackintosh J, Janssen PA. Rooming-in compared with standard care for newborns of mothers using methadone or heroin. *Can Fam Physician.* 2007;53(10):1722-30.

Agthe AG, Kim GR, Mathias KB, et al. Clonidine as an adjunct therapy to opioids for neonatal abstinence syndrome: a randomized, controlled trial. *Pediatrics.* 2009;123:e849-56.

American College of Obstetricians and Gynecologists. Committee Opinion No. 524. Opioid abuse, dependence, and addiction in pregnancy. *Obstet Gynecol.* 2012;119:1070-6.

Backes CH, Backes CR, Gardner D, Nankervis CA, Giannone PJ, Cordero L. Neonatal abstinence syndrome: transitioning methadone-treated infants from an inpatient to an outpatient setting. *J Perinatol.* 2012;32:425-30.

Bada HS, Sithisam T, Gibson J, et al. Morphine versus clonidine for neonatal abstinence syndrome. *Pediatrics*. 2015;135(2):e383-91.

Balain M, Johnson K. Neonatal abstinence syndrome: the role of breastfeeding. *Infant*. 2014;10(1):9-13.

Benningfield MM, Arria AM, Kaltenbach K, et al. Co-occurring psychiatric symptoms are associated with increased psychological, social and medical impairment in opioid dependent pregnant women. *Am J Addict*. 2010;19:416-21.

Bureau of Substance Abuse Services, Massachusetts Department of Public Health. Description of admissions to BSAS contracted/licensed programs FY 2014. http://www.mass.gov/eohhs/docs/dph/substance-abuse/care-principles/state-and-city-town-admissions-fy14.pdf. Accessed January 29, 2019.

Burns L, Mattick RP, Lim K, Wallace C. Methadone in pregnancy: treatment retention and neonatal outcomes. *Addiction*. 2007;102:264-70.

Cleary BJ, Donnelly J, Strawbridge J, et al. Methadone dose and neonatal abstinence syndrome-systemic review and meta-analysis. *Addiction*. 2010;105:2071-84.

Coyle MG, Ferguson A, Lagasse L, Oh W, Lester B. Diluted tincture of opium (DTO) and phenobarbital versus DTO alone for neonatal opiate withdrawal in term infants. *J Pediatr*. 2002;140:561-4.

D'Apolito KC. Assessing neonates for neonatal abstinence: are you reliable? *J Perinat Neonatal Nurs*. 2014;28:220-31.

D'Apolito K, Finnegan L. Assessing signs and symptoms of neonatal abstinence using the Finnegan scoring tool, an inter-observer reliability program. 2010. Available from http://www.neoadvances.com.

Dobkin PL, Civita MD, Paraherakis A, Gill K. The role of functional social support in treatment retention and outcomes among outpatient adult substance abusers. *Addiction*. 2002; 97:347-56.

Finnegan L, Connaughton JJ, Kron R. A scoring system for evaluation and treatment of the neonatal abstinence syndrome: a new clinical and research tool. In: Marselli P, Garanttini S, Sereni F, eds. *Basic and Therapeutic Aspects of Perinatal Pharmacology*. New York, NY: Raven. 1995:139-52.

Grim K, Harrison TE, Wilder RT. Management of neonatal abstinence syndrome from opioids. *Clin Perinatol*. 2013;40:509-24.

Grossman MR, Berkwitt AK, Osborn RR, et al. An initiative to improve the quality of care of infants with neonatal abstinence syndrome. *Pediatrics*. 2017;139:e20163360.

Grossman MR, Lipshaw MJ, Osborn RR, Berkwitt AK. A novel approach to assessing infants with neonatal abstinence syndrome. *Hosp Pediatrs*. 2018;8:1-6.

Hall ES, Wexelblatt SL, Crowly M, et al. Implementation of a neonatal abstinence syndrome weaning protocol: a multicenter cohort study. *Pediatrics*. 2015;136:e803-10.

Hall ES, Wexelblatt SL, Crowley M, et al for MOCHNAS Consortium. A multicenter cohort study of treatments and hospital outcomes in neonatal abstinence syndrome. *Pediatrics*. 2014;134:e527-34.

Heil SH, Gaalema DE, Johnston AM, Sigmon SC, Badger GJ, Higgins ST. Infant pupillary response to methadone administration during treatment for neonatal abstinence syndrome: a feasibility study. *Drug Alcohol Depend*. 2012;126:268-71.

Hudak ML, Tan RC. The American Academy of Pediatrics Committee on Drugs and the Committee on Fetus and Newborn. Neonatal drug withdrawal. *Pediatrics*. 2012;129:e540-60.

Hunt RW, Tzioumi D, Collins E, Jeffery HE. Adverse neurodevelopmental outcome of infants exposed to opiate in-utero. *Early Hum Devel*. 2008;84:29-35.

Jansson LM, DiPietro JA, Elko A, et al. Pregnancies exposed to methadone, methadone and other illicit substances, and poly-drugs without methadone: A comparison of fetal neurobehaviours and infant outcomes. *Drug Alcohol Depend*. 2012;122:213-9.

Jones HE, Fischer GH, Heil SH, et al. Maternal Opioid Treatment: Human Experimental Research (MOTHER) – approach, issues, and lessons learned. *Addiction*. 2012;107:28-35.

Jones HE, Huag N, Silverman K, Stitzer M, Svikis D. The effectiveness of incentives in enhancing treatment attendance and drug abstinence in methadone-maintained pregnant women. *Drug Alcohol Depend.* 2001;61(3):297-306.

Jones HE, Kaltenbach K, Heil SH, et al. Neonatal abstinence syndrome after methadone or buprenorphine exposure. *N Engl J Med.* 2010;363:2320-31.

Jones HE, O'Grady KE, Malfi D, Tuten M. Methadone maintenance vs. methadone taper during pregnancy: maternal and neonatal outcomes. *Am J Addict.* 2008;17:372-86.

Kaltenbach K, Holbrook AM, Coyle MG, et al. Predicting treatment for neonatal abstinence syndrome in infants born to women maintained on opioid agonist medication. *Addiction.* 2012;107:45-52.

King R, Visintainer P, Foss S, Singh R. Impact of maternal medically assisted treatment medications on neurodevelopmental outcomes of infants treated for neonatal abstinence syndrome. 2015–Abstract 314. https://www.aps-spr.org/Regions/ESPR/Meetings/Program/2015Program.pdf.

Kocherlakota P. Neonatal abstinence syndrome. *Pediatrics.* 2014,134(2):e547-61.

Kraft WK, van den Anker JN. Pharmacologic management of the opioid neonatal abstinence syndrome. *Pediatr Clin North Am.* 2012;59:1147-65.

Maguire D. Care of the infant with neonatal abstinence syndrome: strength of the evidence. *J Perinat Neonatal Nurs.* 2014;28:204-11.

Maremmani I, Pani PP, Pacini M, Parugi G. Substance use and quality of life over 12 months among buprenorphine maintenance-treated and methadone maintenance-treated heroin-addicted patients. *J Subst Abuse Treat.* 2007;33(1):91-8.

Massachusetts Department of Public Health. Data brief: opioid-related overdose deaths among Massachusetts residents. http://www.mass.gov/eohhs/docs/dph/quality/drugcontrol/county-level-pmp/overdose-deaths-by-county-including-map-may-2016.pdf. Accessed January 29, 2019.

McKnight S, Coo H, Davies G, et al. Rooming-in for infants at risk of neonatal abstinence syndrome. *Am J Perinatol.* 2016;33(5):495-501.

McQueen KA, Murphy-Oikonen J, Gerlach K, Montelpare W. The impact of infant feeding method on neonatal abstinence scores of methadone-exposed infants. *Adv Neonatal Care.* 2011;11:282-90.

Minnes S, Lang A, Singer L. Prenatal tobacco, marijuana, stimulant, and opiate exposure: outcomes and practice implications. *Addict Sci Clin Pract.* 2011;6:57-70.

Neger EN, Prinz RJ. Interventions to address parenting and parental substance abuse: conceptual and methodological considerations. *Clin Psychol Rev.* 2015;39:71-82.

Newman A, Davies GA, Dow K, et al. Rooming-in care for infants of opioid-dependent mothers: implementation and evaluation at a tertiary care hospital. *Can Fam Physician.* 2015;61:e555-61.

Paris R, Herriott A, Holt M, Gould K. Differential responsiveness to parenting intervention for mothers in substance abuse treatment. *Child Abuse Neglect.* 2015;50:206-17.

Patrick SW, Kaplan HC, Passarella M, Davis MM, Lorch SA. Variation in treatment of neonatal abstinence syndrome in US Children's Hospitals, 2004-2011. *J Perinatol.* 2011;34:867-72.

Patrick S, Schumacher R, Benneyworth B, et al. Neonatal abstinence syndrome and associated health care expenditures United States, 2000-2009. *JAMA.* 2012;307:1934-40.

Pritham UA. Breastfeeding promotion for management of neonatal abstinence syndrome. *J Obstet Gynecol Neonatal Nurs.* 2013;42:517-26.

Rudd RA, Seth P, David F, Scholl L. Increases in drug and opioid-involved overdose deaths— United States, 2010–2015. *MMWR Morb Mortal Wkly Rep.* 2016;65:1445-52. http://dx.doi.org/10.15585/mmwr.mm655051e1.

Salisbury AL, Coyle MG, O'Grady KE, et al. Fetal assessment before and after dosing with buprenorphine or methadone. *Addiction.* 2012;107:36-44.

Simpson LL. Maternal medical disease: risk of antepartum fetal death. *Semin Perinatol.* 2002;26(1):42-50.

Surran B, Visintainer PV, Chamberlain S, Kopcza K, Shah BL, Singh R. Efficacy of clonidine versus phenobarbital in reducing neonatal morphine sulfate therapy days for neonatal abstinence syndrome. A prospective randomized clinical trial. *J Perinatol.* 2012;33:954-9.

The American College of Obstetricians and Gynecologists. Committee Opinion. Smoking cessation in pregnancy. 2010. http://www.acog.org/Resources-And-Publications/Committee-Opinions/Committee-on-Health-Care-for-Underserved-Women/Smoking-Cessation-During-Pregnancy. Accessed March 21, 2018.

Tolia VN, Patrick SW, Bennett MM, et al. Increasing incidence of the neonatal abstinence syndrome in U.S. neonatal ICUs. *N Engl J Med.* 2015;372(22):2118-26.

Vela RM. The effects of severe stress on early brain development, attachment and emotions. *Psych Clin North Am* 2014;37(4):519-34.

Velez M, Jansson LM. The opioid-dependent mother and newborn dyad: nonpharmacologic care. *J Addict Med.* 2008;2(3):113-20.

Wachman EM, Hayes MJ, Brown MS, et al. Association of OPRM1 and COMT single–nucleotide polymorphisms with hospital length of stay and treatment of neonatal abstinence syndrome. *JAMA.* 2013;309:1821-7.

Wachman EM, Hayes MJ, Lester BM, et al. Epigenetic variation in the mu-opioid receptor gene in infants with neonatal abstinence syndrome. *J Pediatr.* 2014;165:472-8.

Young JL, Martin PR. Treatment of opioid dependence in the setting of pregnancy. *Psychiatr Clin N Am.* 2012;35:441-60.

Zeanah CH, Berlin LJ, Boris NW. Practitioner review: clinical applications of attachment theory and research for infants and young children. *J Child Psychol Psychiatry.* 2011;52(8):819-33.

Neonatal Transport

Caraciolo J. Fernandes, MD, MBA, FAAP • Lakshmi Katakam, MD, MPH, FAAP

SCOPE

DISEASE/CONDITION(S)

Neonatal transport.

GUIDELINE OBJECTIVE(S)

To provide an overview of important aspects of transporting neonates between healthcare facilities or to home.

BRIEF BACKGROUND

Ideally, babies should be delivered at healthcare facilities equipped with the staff and resources required for their care. Nevertheless, even in today's era of advanced antenatal fetal surveillance, neonates are occasionally born in healthcare facilities unable to care for them and require transfer to a higher-level facility. Neonatal transports may urgent or non-urgent. Urgent neonatal transport usually occurs in the first few days of life in a newborn infant with a congenital anomaly or neonatal disease resulting from failure of adaptation to extrauterine life. Occasionally, urgent transfer is needed when a hospitalized preterm neonate develops a disease state (e.g., necrotizing enterocolitis) that requires subspecialty services at a tertiary care center. In situations where the infant is clinically unstable, rapidity of transfer to a center with the appropriate resources is critical for survival. Planning for such events will increase the likelihood of a favorable patient outcome, decrease family stress, and allow for efficient transports.

Program Considerations

All hospitals that have maternity facilities, Levels I and II neonatal intensive care units (NICUs), and emergency rooms should have agreements with regional tertiary care centers about where they should transfer patients who they are unable to care for. Policies and guidelines should delineate criteria for consultation, neonatal transfer, and methods of stabilizing neonates prior to transfer. All relevant contact information and written guidelines and protocols should be easily accessible and reviewed periodically to ensure they are current. Legal counsel should be sought to ensure that the program and hospital comply with all local, state, and federal laws.

Neonatal Transport Teams

Regional neonatal transport teams should have a *medical director* who works with hospital administration to oversee and ensure efficient functioning of the transport team, develop guidelines and protocols for neonatal transfer, and monitor the quality of neonatal transport services.

Depending on the frequency of transports, transport teams may be *unit based*, where personnel (nurses, respiratory therapists, neonatal nurse practitioners, and physicians) are deployed when necessary, or *dedicated*, where selected personnel have the sole responsibility for neonatal transport. Dedicated teams often are responsible for transporting patients of a wide age range, in addition to neonates. A major advantage of dedicated teams is that they can respond rapidly when needed, as opposed to unit-based teams who are required to hand over clinical responsibilities to colleagues for the duration of the transport and for some time afterward. Regardless of the type of team, all team members should be covered by appropriate malpractice insurance for care rendered during transport.

Modes of Transport

The mode of transport chosen by the transport team will depend on the distance and terrain to be traveled and the acuity of the patient(s) to be transported. At a minimum, transport teams will have an ambulance. Some teams have rotor-wing (helicopter) and/or fixed-wing (airplane) aircraft. Ambulance and rotor-wing transport allow for rapid deployment to closer locations (up to 100–150 miles). Fixed-wing aircrafts will allow for long-range transports (greater than 150 miles) but are expensive and need an airport as well as ambulances to transport the patient to and from the airport. Regardless of the mode of transport chosen, the vehicle requires adaption to serve as a mobile medical facility and accommodate the transport incubator, tanks with medical gases, reliable electrical power supply, and storage for medical equipment and medications. Seating for personnel should allow for optimal monitoring of the patient, while preserving personnel safety. All local, state, and federal guidelines for ground and air transport should be followed in designing and equipping the transport vehicle.

Equipment

Transport teams should carry with them all necessary equipment and medications needed to stabilize and transport the neonate. Use of checklists prior to team departure ensures that essential items are not missed. Transport supply packs should be organized in a standardized manner, ideally packed by team members themselves, and restocked immediately following completion of a transport; this will help ensure required items are found promptly when needed. See Table 12.1 for representative list of equipment, supplies, and medications.

TABLE 12.1. **Equipment, Supplies, and Medications***

1. Equipment
   - Transport incubator
   - Ventilator
   - Cardiorespiratory monitor
   - Pulse oximeter
   - Suction devices
   - Tanks of oxygen, air, and nitric oxide
   - Intubation supplies (laryngoscope with 0, 00, and 1 blades; CO_2 detector)
   - Infusion pumps
   - Stethoscope
   - Gel mattress with transport restraints
2. Supplies
   - Airway and endotracheal tubes
   - Supplies for IV insertion (alcohol and betadine swabs, IV catheters, securing tape, gauze, etc.)
   - Culture tubes
   - Nasogastric and Replogle tubes
   - Umbilical catheter kits
   - Pigtail catheter kits
   - Tubes for blood specimens
   - Oxygen tubing and face mask
   - Thermometer
3. Medications
   - Antibiotics (ampicillin, gentamicin, vancomycin, etc.)
   - IV fluids (normal saline, 5% dextrose, 5% albumin, etc.)
   - Cardiac medications (atropine, dopamine, dobutamine, epinephrine, etc.)
   - Analgesics, sedatives, and neuromuscular blockade agents (morphine, fentanyl, midazolam, lorazepam, pancuronium, vecuronium, etc.)
   - Surfactant
   - Calcium
   - Sodium bicarbonate
   - Prostaglandin E_1
   - Vitamin K_1
   - Oral sucrose solution

*Representative non-exhaustive list.

RECOMMENDATIONS

MAJOR RECOMMENDATIONS

To ensure the best possible outcome, healthcare practitioners should anticipate and plan for potential scenarios that could be encountered during a transfer from a lower level of care facility to a tertiary care center. When possible, maternal transfer prior to delivery is preferable to a post-birth neonatal transport. This is particularly true for extremely premature infants or infants anticipated to be born with poor cardiorespiratory reserve (e.g., congenital diaphragmatic hernia) who might need higher-level support such as extracorporeal membrane oxygenation (ECMO). Maternity hospitals, maternal-fetal specialists, obstetricians, and pediatricians should have ready access to neonatologists at tertiary care centers for consultation prior to and after the birth of an infant who might need transfer for higher level of care. Not all congenital anomalies will need evaluation in the immediate newborn period, and this may be determined by a quick phone call to the consultant neonatologist. Efforts should be made to limit mother and infant separation when possible. Anticipatory guidance during antenatal counseling will allow prospective parents to decide whether to deliver in a tertiary care facility or opt for postnatal transfer. The transport process may broadly be divided into three phases: 1) pre-transport, 2) transport, and 3) post-transport. Safe and efficient neonatal transports occur in settings where regional or tertiary care centers work collaboratively with referring hospitals to train the front-line staff to optimize care and stabilize sick neonates for transfer. If transfer of the mother is not possible because of impending delivery, the neonatal transport team can be dispatched to the referring hospital prior to the birth of the infant and can help resuscitate and stabilize the infant there prior to transport.

PRACTICE OPTIONS

Practice Option #1: Pre-Transport/Observe and Monitor

All clinicians who care for neonates should be trained in neonatal resuscitation and have expertise necessary to stabilize newborn infants after delivery room resuscitation. The Neonatal Resuscitation Program (NRP) and sugar, temperature, airway, blood pressure, lab work, and emotional support for the family (STABLE) programs are education programs endorsed by the American Academy of Pediatrics to educate clinicians who care for neonates.

Following initial resuscitation after birth, clinicians may opt to observe and monitor a newly born infant at the local hospital while reserving the option to transfer the neonate if necessary. Discussions with consultants at the tertiary care facility can help ensure that optimal care is provided from the time of birth while allowing mother and infant to remain together. Stabilization should focus on ensuring thermoneutral environment, adequate oxygenation and ventilation, optimal cardiac function and blood pressure, and provision of fluids and nutrition (the infant should be "pink, warm, and sweet").

Pre-transport interventions may include placement of peripheral intravenous catheters or umbilical venous catheters, insertion of nasogastric tubes, obtaining appropriate laboratory samples and imaging, and administering necessary medications. If blood pressure monitoring or frequent blood sampling is needed, umbilical arterial access is preferred.

Parents should be informed about the infant's clinical condition and the possible need for transfer to a tertiary care center so that they are emotionally prepared and can provide consent when needed. The local clinician and consultant should discuss what specific triggers would mandate transfer and include parents in the decision-making process. Some parents/families might prefer earlier transfer than others. Babies who fall in this category are usually term or late preterm neonates without congenital anomalies who exhibit cardiorespiratory compromise after birth. They may have transient tachypnea of the newborn, delayed transition, transient neonatal hypoglycemia, signs of neonatal infection, jaundice, etc. Depending on the local expertise, these infants may be cared for and discharged from the local facility or transferred out.

From a program standpoint, tertiary care centers would be wise to have active outreach education programs for staff at referring hospitals. Didactic lectures on topics of interest, conferences, workshops, etc. enhance the quality of care delivered at the referring facilities and optimize care of neonates that are transferred.

Practice Option #2: Urgent Transfer of a Critically Ill Neonate

When a neonate is critically ill, timeliness and institution of appropriate therapy dictates outcome. Typical indications for urgent transfer of a newborn infant include prematurity (<32 weeks gestation), respiratory distress requiring positive pressure support, hypoxic-respiratory failure or persistent pulmonary hypertension (PPHN), congenital heart disease, severe hypoxic-ischemic encephalopathy requiring therapeutic hypothermia, seizures, and suspected inborn error of metabolism. Indications later in the neonatal period may include clinical deterioration secondary to conditions such as NEC or life-threatening infection.

Prompt consultation with tertiary care consultants will allow appropriate therapy to be instituted while the transport team is en route to pick up the neonate for transfer. Parents should be counseled about the need for transfer of their infant for higher level of care, and consent obtained for transfer. They should be allowed to spend time with their infant prior to the arrival of the transport team. Some transport teams may allow one parent to accompany the infant to the tertiary care facility. Depending on the specific circumstances, a Level I or II NICU may choose to transfer the infant to a Level III or IV NICU (see Levels of neonatal care [*Pediatrics*, 2012] in Bibliographic Sources).

Parents should be given the option to participate in the decision-making process when feasible and appropriate. While transfer to a Level III NICU may be sufficient for some infants, occasionally infants transferred to a Level III NICU may need to be transferred again. For example, neonates with hypoxic-respiratory failure at birth transferred from a Level II NICU to a Level III NICU may deteriorate clinically to the point of needing ECMO support, necessitating further transfer to a Level IV NICU.

While awaiting the team's arrival, the local facility should prepare copies of all maternal and neonatal records for the transport team. Radiographic studies are usually loaded on a compact disc with relevant software for viewing. Details of medications given, including timing of when the last dose was given, are important. For laboratory investigations that are not yet final (e.g., cultures), the phone number to the laboratory for follow-up should be provided.

In addition to the general stabilization procedures (see previous section), some infants may need specific therapy directed toward known or suspected pathophysiology. For example, a suspicion of ductal-dependent congenital heart disease could necessitate prostaglandin (PGE) infusion; pulmonary hypertension, the need for inhaled nitric oxide (iNO); and surfactant deficiency, the need for surfactant. Transport teams should carry such medications, as not all referring centers will stock them; if they do, therapy can be instituted following the initial phone call.

Telephone consultation also allows the local clinician to tailor their care of the neonate to allow for rapid and efficient transport. For example, if the team prefers that a non-intubated infant with respiratory distress be intubated and ventilated for transport, doing so would facilitate transport, whereas if the team is minutes away, delaying procedures like insertion of umbilical lines would be appropriate. In most instances, consultant neonatologists at tertiary care facilities would prefer the sick infant transported to their institution as quickly as possible, but all measures should be taken first to ensure the infant's clinical stability before transport.

When the transport team arrives at the referring facility, they should introduce themselves to the local caregivers and parents, perform a thorough assessment of the infant to determine whether the clinical status has changed, and communicate with the medical transport control at the tertiary care center to affirm plans of care during transport and/or need for modification of treatment. In some instances, therapy instituted by the transport team prior to transport will make for safer transport. For example, initiation of iNO for PPHN, evacuation of a pneumothorax, or initiation of prostaglandin E1 infusion.

Infants should not be transported if they are deemed too unstable for transport, which usually occurs in a scenario of active cardiopulmonary resuscitation. In some instances, specific therapy may be instituted or continued by the transport team during transport to ensure the transport itself does not delay required care. Examples include initiation of active cooling on transport, phototherapy for hyperbilirubinemia, and antibiotic therapy for suspected infection. A few transport teams are able to provide ECMO and high-frequency oscillation during transport. Transport by air requires consideration of the effects of barometric pressure variation on intrathoracic and/or intraabdominal gases in sick neonates. For example, as altitude increases and barometric pressure decreases, pneumothoraces will expand and abdominal gaseous distension will increase. To prevent clinical deterioration during transport, pneumothoraces should be evacuated with a chest tube connected to a Heimlich valve and the stomach vented with a nasogastric or Replogle tube. In cases of ventilated neonates, increasing abdominal distension may also make it more difficult to ventilate the neonate. Effects of barometric pressure can also be ameliorated by requesting the pilot to pressurize the cabin to sea level.

During transport, the team should have the ability to communicate with the medical control physician at the tertiary care center if the patient's clinical condition deteriorates. The use of telemedicine devices can enhance such consultation and remote monitoring. The most useful form of monitoring is direct observation of the infant. In the incubator, the infant should be secured firmly to prevent injury related to transport and to ensure tubes and lines are not dislodged. While expeditious transport is desired, use of lights and sirens are not promoted as they do not improve outcomes but add the risk of an accident for the transport team. Upon arrival at the tertiary care facility, the transport team should contact the referring facility and the infant's parents to inform them of the patient's condition on arrival, patient's location in the NICU, and the name of the physician assuming care for the infant.

Routine post-transport debriefs can help identify opportunities for improvement during future transports. Regular participation in simulation training can help transport team members maintain and enhance their skills.

There is much variation in the composition of neonatal transport teams across the country. Many neonatal transport teams in the United States are led by a specially trained nurse-respiratory therapist dyad, with the option to add a physician or nurse practitioner as team leader if the patient's illness acuity is high. In some situations, the neonate at the referring hospital is at high likelihood of dying because of critical illness unresponsive to therapy, or serious congenital anomalies. In such situations, the referring physician, the physician at the higher-level facility, the transport team, and the parents might come to a consensus that the infant should not be transported and should be provided palliative care and comfort measures only at the referring hospital. This prevents parent-infant separation and displacement of the family during the process of the infant's death.

Practice Option #3: Non-Urgent Neonatal Transports

Clinically stable neonates are sometimes transferred between hospitals or between hospital and home. Tertiary care centers may have contractual agreements to "back-transfer" preterm infants to the referring facility once the infant no longer needs the services of a tertiary care center. Reasons for non-urgent transfer to a different facility include unavailability of necessary resources at the birth hospital (such as a cardiologist or an ophthalmologist), parental request, relocation to a facility closer to family's home, or insurance company requirements.

Medical indications for non-urgent transfers between healthcare facilities are usually prompted by congenital anomalies requiring specialists' evaluation and management, such as the need for specialized imaging and/or surgery. In such instances, the infant is not critically ill, but has a condition that precludes normal care and discharge home. In these situations, it is imperative to do due diligence to ensure the infant is being transferred to the right location for the planned treatment, that the specialist is available, and approval from the insurance company is obtained prior to transfer. Families should be appropriately counseled regarding the infant's condition and what to anticipate following transfer. What medical teams may consider as non-urgent may be considered a crisis by families. Consultation with tertiary care specialists and procedures for stabilizing and preparing neonates for transfer are detailed in the section above.

Finally, transports home are usually uneventful but anxiety provoking for families as they take their technology-dependent infant home. A parent usually accompanies the team with the infant during the trip home. Families may be supported in this process by "rooming-in" a day or two prior to transport home, and by having home nursing readily available at home.

CLINICAL ALGORITHM(S)

There are no universally applicable algorithms that can be applied to neonatal transport. Institutions should create their own algorithms and guidelines based on the level of neonatal care provided at their facility and institutions within their healthcare network, as well as distances between facilities and modes of transport employed.

IMPLEMENTATION OF GUIDELINE

DESCRIPTION OF IMPLEMENTATION STRATEGY

All institutions that have maternity facilities, Level I and II neonatal intensive care units (NICUs), or emergency rooms should develop contractual agreements with regional tertiary care centers to allow for consultation as needed and transfer of patients that they are unable to care for.

QUALITY METRICS

The Ground Air Medical Quality Transport Quality Improvement Collaborative, supported in part by the American Academy of Pediatrics Section on Transport Medicine, offers the GAMUT Database as a free resource for transport teams to track, report, and analyze their performance on transport-specific quality metrics by comparing it to other programs. Some metrics that can be tracked include timeliness (dispatch time, scene time, total transport time), use of lights and sirens, the courteousness and support provided by the receiving physician and the transport team to the health professionals in the referring facility and to the parents, safety events, equipment failure, clinical adverse events during transport (including dislodgement of therapeutic devices), maintenance of physiological parameters (such as temperature) within the desirable range during transport, pain assessment and management, timeliness of clinical updates to the referring health professionals, and crew injuries.

SUMMARY

Neonatal transports, while relatively infrequent for referring facilities, require an organized and predetermined plan for transport of critically ill neonates to ensure optimal outcomes. Timely communication between clinicians at referring facilities and consultants at tertiary care centers can optimize care provided from the time of birth.

BIBLIOGRAPHIC SOURCE(S)

AAP Section of Transport Medicine; Meyer K, et al. *Field Guide for Air and Ground Transport of Neonatal and Pediatric Patients.* In: Myer KM, Fernandes CJ, Schwartz HP, eds. American Academy of Pediatrics; 2018.

Bigham MT, Schwartz HP; Ohio Neonatal/Pediatric Transport Quality Collaborative. Quality metrics in neonatal and pediatric critical care transport: a consensus statement. *Pediatr Crit Care Med.* 2013;14(5):518-24.

Campbell DM, Dadiz R. Simulation in neonatal transport medicine. *Semin Perinatol.* 2016;40(7):430-7.

Committee on Fetus and Newborn. Levels of neonatal care. *Pediatrics.* 2012;130:587-97.

Diehl BC. Neonatal transport: current trends and practices. *Crit Care Nurs Clin North Am.* 2018;30(4):597-606.

Ground Air Medical Quality Transport Quality Improvement Collaborative. GAMUT Database. http://gamutqi.org/.

Karlsen KA, Trautman M, Price-Douglas W, Smith S. National survey of neonatal transport teams in the United States. *Pediatrics.* 2011;128(4):685-91.

McNamara PJ, Mak W, Whyte HE. Dedicated neonatal retrieval teams improve delivery room resuscitation of outborn premature infants. *J Perinatol.* 2005;25(5):309-14.

Patel MM, Hebbar KB, Dugan MC, Petrillo T. A survey assessing pediatric transport team composition and training. *Pediatr Emerg Care.* 2018. doi: 10.1097/PEC.0000000000001655.

Ratnavel N. Evaluating and improving neonatal transport services. *Early Hum Dev.* 2013;89(11):851-3.

Schierholz E. Therapeutic hypothermia on transport: providing safe and effective cooling therapy as the link between birth hospital and the neonatal intensive care unit. *Adv Neonatal Care.* 2014;14 (Suppl 5):S24-31.

Stroud MH, Trautman MS, Meyer K, et al. Pediatric and neonatal interfacility transport: results from a national consensus conference. *Pediatrics.* 2013;132(2):359-66.

Nutrition, Fluids, and Electrolytes

Breastfeeding

Diane L. Spatz, PhD, RN-BC, FAAN

SCOPE

DISEASE/CONDITION(S)

Address human milk and breastfeeding for the hospitalized infant.

GUIDELINE OBJECTIVE(S)

Understand the significance of human milk and breastfeeding for vulnerable infants; identify evidence-based practice principles to ensure infants receive human milk through hospital discharge; recommendations for transition to direct breastfeeding.

BRIEF BACKGROUND

The American Academy of Pediatrics recommends human milk and breastfeeding as the preferred form of nutrition for all infants. Human milk has specific health benefits for hospitalized and vulnerable infants.

Examples of how human milk influences health and developmental outcomes:

- Decreased mortality and morbidity
- Decreased incidence and severity of infections (ear, gastrointestinal, respiratory, urinary) and sepsis
- Decreased incidence and severity of necrotizing enterocolitis
- Improved feed tolerance, advancement of feeds for vulnerable infants (decreased total parenteral nutrition days)
- Decreased retinopathy of prematurity
- Decreased bronchopulmonary disease
- Improved brain development (increase in white matter and gray matter) and improved intelligence and developmental outcomes
- Decreased risk of sudden infant death syndrome

- Improved long-term health outcomes (reduction in obesity, diabetes, heart disease)
- Enhanced long-term protection of gastrointestinal system (reduction in irritable bowel syndrome, Crohn disease, celiac disease)
- Reduced risk of childhood cancers (leukemia and lymphoma)

RECOMMENDATIONS

MAJOR RECOMMENDATIONS

Human milk is the preferred form of nutrition for all infants. All efforts should be made to help mothers make an informed decision to express milk for their infants. If mother's own milk is not available or its use is contraindicated, pasteurized donor human milk (PDHM) should be utilized during the hospital stay. PDHM should never be viewed as a replacement to mother's own milk, but rather a bridge. PDHM has a significant role in the reduction of necrotizing enterocolitis; however, does not have the same benefits as mother's own milk for other health outcomes.

PRACTICE OPTIONS

Practice Option #1

Ensure that all families make an informed decision regarding the science of human milk and how human milk is a medical intervention. All families should receive antenatal counseling regarding human milk as a medical intervention. Families should receive specific information about how human milk will protect their infant from morbidity and mortality. Consider using specific education tailored to the neonatal intensive care unit (NICU) such as the *Power of Pumping* DVD.

Practice Option #2

Initiation and maintenance of maternal milk supply throughout the hospitalization is essential. Women are prepared to make milk for their infants no matter how early they deliver, as the breasts begin to secrete milk from 16 weeks of gestation onward (Lactogenesis I). Lactogenesis I refers to the period of time in which the mother is producing colostrum. Colostrum is of vital importance to the NICU infant, and colostrum should be specially labeled and fed to the infant in the exact order that it was pumped. In order for the mother to establish a normal milk supply, early frequent pumping with a hospital-grade electric pump is essential. Mothers should be instructed to pump early and pump often (every 2–3 hours for a goal of 8 or more in 24 hours). Research demonstrates that if mothers initiate pumping with a hospital-grade electric pump within 1 hour of birth, there is a significantly earlier onset of Lactogenesis II and increased milk production at week 3. Furthermore, research demonstrates that frequency of milk expression and milk volume at day 4 are predictive of milk supply at 6 weeks and if mothers fail to achieve milk production of 500 mL by 2 weeks after delivery, they will not have good long-term breastfeeding outcomes.

Practice Option #3

Infants should receive exclusive human milk diet during hospitalization, and mothers should be provided with assistance to transition the infant to direct breastfeeding if that is the mother's goal.

Practice Option #4

Hospitals should have adequate number of refrigerators and freezers for the storage of human milk. Hospitals should have systems in place to ensure the correct infant receives the correct milk (i.e., two-healthcare provider check or barcoding systems). Hospitals should track milk and prioritize the use of a 100% fresh milk diet whenever feasible due to the bioactive components of human milk.

CLINICAL ALGORITHM(S)

The transition to breast pathway was developed to facilitate the process of a mother going from being pump dependent to be able to directly breastfeed at the breast. The positive outcomes of a Continuous Quality Improvement project utilizing this pathway have been previously published. The pathway has been refined and is included (Figure 13.1) courtesy of the Lactation Program at Children's Hospital of Philadelphia.

My mom's name is:				My name is:
				I was born on:
				I was admitted on:
				I was discharged on:
Our goal for providing human milk/breastfeeding is:				

Initiation of pumping and maintenance of milk supply	Week	Ave # of pumps per day	Average daily volume	Initiate pumping within 1 hour of birth and then pump every 2–3 hours for a goal of 8 pumps in 24 hours.
				By the end of week 1, goal = 500–1000 mL/24 hours.
				If the mother is a high producer, she may be able to decrease pumping frequency if the milk supply can be maintained.

Human milk oral care								Have the mother pump at the bedside. When fresh milk is available, use a swab to absorb some milk and then rub the swab on the infant's lips and the inside of the cheeks. **This should be done anytime fresh milk is available.**
Record every date done								
Use only freshly expressed milk and **do not** thaw frozen milk for oral care								

FIGURE 13.1 • Transition to breast pathway.

Skin-to-skin care Record every date done								As soon as the infant is stable, have the mother hold the infant skin-to-skin **as much as possible**.

Nonnutritive sucking at the breast Record every date done								Once extubated, have the mother do nonnutritive sucking at the breast with the infant **at least once daily**. **Remember to have the mother pump first to empty her breasts.**

My first feeding at the breast experience!	Date: Time: The nurse(s) who helped us: How did it go?	Initiation of oral feeds for milk transfer. Remember to do pre- and post-weights if the mother has transitioned to Lactogenesis II.

Subsequent feeds at the breast	Date	Time	Amount transferred	Pre- and post-weights for all feeds **at the breast** (once the mother has transitioned to Lactogenesis II).
				Heads-up for discharge: The mother may need a baby weigh scale for home use.

FIGURE 13.1 • (*Continued*)

SUMMARY

Human milk is an important medical intervention for hospitalized infants. All health professionals should ensure that mothers make an informed choice regarding the importance of human milk to protect their child from morbidity and mortality. Mothers need specific education to pump early and pump often in order to establish and maintain a full milk supply (ideally 700–800 mL per day). Mothers should be supported with performing human milk oral care, skin-to-skin holding of their infant, nonnutritive suckling at the breast, and support for transition to direct breastfeeding if that is the mother's goal. Provided the infant's condition is appropriate for oral feeding, the priority should be direct breastfeeding and cue-based breastfeeding prior to discharge.

BIBLIOGRAPHIC SOURCE(S)

American Academy of Pediatrics Committee on Fetus and Newborn, Section on Breastfeeding. Donor human milk for the high-risk infant: preparation, safety, and usage options in the United States. *Pediatrics.* 2017;139(1):e20163440.

American Academy of Pediatrics, Section on Breastfeeding. Policy statement on breastfeeding and the use of human milk. *Pediatrics.* 2012;129(3):e827–41.

Deoni SC, Dean DC 3rd, Piryatinsky I, et al. Breastfeeding and early white matter development: a cross sectional study. *Neuroimage.* 2013;82:77-86.

Edwards TE, Spatz DL. An innovative model for achieving breastfeeding success in infants with complex surgical anomalies. *J Perinat Neonat Nurs.* 2010;24(3):254-5.

Fugate K, Hernandez I, Ashmeade T, Miladinovic B, Spatz DL. Improving human milk and breastfeeding practices in the NICU. *J Obstet Gynecol Neonat Nurs.* 2015;44(3):426-38.

Ghandehari H, Lee ML, Rechtman DJ; H2MF Study Group. An exclusive human milk-based diet in extremely premature infants reduces the probability of remaining on total parenteral nutrition: a reanalysis of the data. *BMC Res Notes.* 2012;5:188.

Hair AB, Peluso AM, Hawthorne KM, et al. Beyond necrotizing enterocolitis prevention: improving outcomes with an exclusive human milk-based diet. *Breastfeed Med.* 2016;11(2):70-4.

Hill PD, Aldag JC. Milk volume on day 4 and income predictive of lactation adequacy at 6 weeks of mothers of non-nursing preterm infants. *J Perinat Neonatal Nurs.* 2005;19(3):273-82.

Isaacs EB, Fischl B, Quinn BT, Chong WK, Gadian DG, Lucas A. Impact of breast milk on intelligence quotient, brain size, and white matter development. *Pediatr Res.* 2010;67(4):357-62.

Parker LA, Sullivan S, Krueger C, Kelechi T, Mueller M. Effect of early breast milk expression on milk volume and timing of lactogenesis stage II among mothers of very low birth weight infants: a pilot study. *J Perinatol.* 2012;32:205-9.

Power of Pumping. DVD available from http://www.chop.edu/centers-programs/breastfeeding-and-lactation-program.

Spatz DL. Ten steps for promoting and protecting breastfeeding in vulnerable populations. *J Perinat Neonat Nurs.* 2004;18(4):412-23.

Spatz DL, Lessen R. *The Risks of Not Breastfeeding—Position Statement.* The International Lactation Consultant Association; 2011.

Victora CG, Rollins NC, Murch S, Krasevec J, Bahl R. Breastfeeding in the 21st century. *Lancet.* 2016;38:479-90.

Formula Feeding

David H. Adamkin, MD

SCOPE

Use of preterm infant formula for very low birth weight (VLBW) infants.

DISEASE/CONDITION(S)

Nutritional support for VLBW infants with preterm formula.

GUIDELINE OBJECTIVE(S)

Indications for the use of preterm formula in VLBW infants.

BRIEF BACKGROUND

The guiding principles for all nutritional strategies and products that we use in these VLBW infants is that undernutrition is by definition nonphysiologic and undesirable. Any measure that diminishes inadequate nutrition is inherently good as long as safety is not compromised. Improving nutritional status and therefore growth will optimize neurodevelopmental outcomes.

Enteral nutrition is provided to these VLBW infants with either human milk or preterm formula. The America Academy of Pediatrics (AAP) recommends human milk as the preferred feeding for all of these infants, including the use of donor milk where their own mother's milk is preferred but not available. It is also clear that human milk fortifiers are required to meet the nutritional needs of the VLBW infants receiving own mother's milk or donor milk.

Formula is an option if there is an inadequate supply of mother's milk, donor milk is unavailable, or the mother is unable for other reasons to provide milk. Premature formula meets the nutrient needs of the growing VLBW infant but is absent of many important bioactive factors in human milk.

IMPORTANCE OF NUTRITION FOR VLBW INFANTS

These VLBW infants have greater nutritional needs to achieve optimal growth during their neonatal period than any other time in their lives. The reasons for this include:

1. Birth at the beginning of the third trimester of pregnancy is often associated with growth restriction because they have not received the nutrients that are plentiful during the third trimester.
2. Critical illnesses and associated complications such as respiratory distress, acidosis, hypoxia, sepsis, and gastrointestinal complications all increase metabolic requirements.
3. Difficulty in tolerating both parenteral and enteral feedings make provision of nutrients more challenging, and drugs such as steroids may impede growth as well.

Directly linking nutrient intake and outcome was demonstrated in a study where preterm infants fed an enriched preterm formula with higher protein and energy for the first month of life had higher scores in neurodevelopmental indices at 18 months and sustained at 8 years of life than those infants receiving a standard term formula. Scores at 8 years of life are predictive of adult outcomes.

NEED FOR ADDITIONAL ENERGY AS WELL AS HIGHER PROTEIN IN HIGH-PROTEIN FORMULAS

The higher concentrations of protein in these formulas also have increased energy content. Both energy and protein are necessary for growth of body weight, length, and head circumference. Energy is required for synthesis of and depositing protein and fat. These VLBW infants probably need a minimum of 110 cal/k/day to match the adipose tissue deposition seen in the normal growing fetus. Summarizing the experience with protein energy ratios, more protein is synthesized and deposited as lean mass when protein intakes are higher versus energy, and more fat is deposited at higher energy intakes (Figure 14.1). Slightly higher amounts of energy, more than 100 cal/k/day, were needed to promote lean body mass at the in utero rate. Therefore a caloric intake of 115–120 cal/k/day will appropriately support a protein intake of 3.5–4.0 g/k/day. More energy produces a gain in fat.

There is no benefit to provide energy in excess of that necessary to assure utilization of the protein intake. Excessive energy and carbohydrate intake simply result in excessive fat deposition. There is evidence indicating changes in body composition that occur

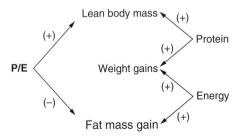

FIGURE 14.1 • Increased P/E ratio promotes lean body mass.

during the neonatal intensive care unit (NICU) stay are made of increased fat deposition versus what would have occurred in utero. The potential for such rapid gains in adiposity may lead to later-life obesity and associated complications.

PROTEIN COMPOSITION IN PRETERM FORMULA

There are two fractions of protein in human milk and preterm formula: whey and casein. They are defined by their solubility in acid. The predominance of whey in both human milk and preterm formula (70% and 60%, respectively) are beneficial for VLBW infants compared with bovine milk. Bovine milk is 82% casein. The whey is superior in promoting feeding tolerance and for human milk contains advantageous immune factors that play a role in host defense.

Most exciting is the possibility that whey predominance in preterm formula, like that in human milk, may confer benefits in brain development. Both human milk and preterm formulas contain cysteine and taurine, two amino acids that are deficient in preterm infants. Cysteine is necessary to synthesize the antioxidant glutathione, and taurine is needed for bile conjugation and brain development.

Some preterm formulas are available with 100% whey partially hydrolyzed protein and are marketed to improve enteral feeding tolerance by enhancing amino acid absorption into the circulation. However, there is some controversy, as some studies suggest that the hydrolyzed protein is not used as efficiently as intact protein. The hydrolyzed protein product formulas and fortifiers have been used primarily in gut developmental defects like gastroschisis, necrotizing enterocolitis (NEC), or inflammation of the gut associated with reactions to bovine antigen where there is limited digestive capacity. Table 14.1 contains the formulas available in North America that are marketed as either regular protein content or high protein content.

LONG-CHAIN POLYUNSATURATED FATTY ACIDS (LCPUFA) FOR VLBW INFANTS

These include arachidonic acid (AA) and docosahexaenoic acid (DHA). They are present in human milk and not in bovine milk. They are important components of phospholipids found in the brain, retina, and red cell membranes. LCPUFAs may be divided into two n-6 and w-3 fatty acids. Linoleic acid is the essential n-6 LCPUFA and linolenic acid is the essential w-3 LCPUFA. The Committee on Nutrition for the European Society for Pediatric Gastroenterology and Nutrition (ESPGHAN) suggests that the daily intake for a premature infant include linoleic acid 385–1540 mg/kg; linolenic acid 0.55 mg/kg; DHA 12–30 mg/kg; AA 18–42 mg/kg.

LCPUFAs were added to infant formulas in the early 1990s. This was done because in preterm infants, visual acuity was better in those receiving human milk. It had been hypothesized that the results may have been in part related to the differences in DHA levels in breast milk versus formula.

Results from systemic reviews evaluating the effect of LCPUFA supplementation of formulas for preterm infants have been inconsistent regarding cognitive performance, visual acuity, and growth. The results, however, are difficult to analyze because of the variations in study design, such as which products are used, dose, duration of treatment, test used for cognitive performance and visual acuity, among other issues. It does appear that supplementation may be of greatest benefit for the VLBW infant.

TABLE 14.1. Composition of Preterm Formulas

	Protein (g/100 mL)	Calcium (mg/100 mL)	Phosphorus (mg/100 mL)	Zinc (mg/100 mL)	Protein/Energy (g/100 cal)	Protein Source
Standard Preterm Formulas						
Enfamil Premature 24 with Iron (Mead Johnson Nutrition)	2.4	134	67	1.2	3	60% whey, 40% casein*
Gerber Good Start Premature 24	2.4	133	69	1.1	3	100% whey partially hydrolyzed
Similac Special Care 24 (Abbott Nutrition)	2.4	146	81	1.2	3	60% whey, 40% casein*
High-Protein Formulas						
Enfamil Premature 24 Cal High Protein	2.8	134	67	1.2	3.5	60% whey, 40% casein*
Gerber Good Start Premature 24 High Protein	2.9	133	69	1.1	3.6	100% whey partially hydrolyzed
Similac Special Care 24 High Protein	2.7	146	81	1.2	3.3	60% whey, 40% casein*
International Formulas						
Milupa Aptamil Preterm (Wiltshire, England)	2.6	94	62	1.1	3.3	60% whey, 40% casein*
Nestle Partially Hydrolyzed Premature (Nestle)	2.9	116	77	1.2	3.6	100% whey partially hydrolyzed
Cow & Gate Nutriprem 1 Low Birthweight (Cuijk, the Netherlands)	2.6	94	62	1.1	3.3	61% whey, 39% casein*

*From nonfat milk and whey protein concentrate.

There has also been recent interest in looking at the effects of w-3 because of its anti-inflammatory properties for its potential benefit with bronchopulmonary dysplasia or infections. Results are still inconclusive in the area of morbidity prevention as well.

Although most of the biochemical trials show clearly the insufficiency of DHA in the diet of these VLBW infants, the picture is not clear from the intervention studies with clinical and developmental outcomes. There is evidence that the products available for supplementation in our preterm formulas are low in toxic contaminants and are safe and with no adverse effects on growth. Supplementation in formula is based on the facts that these w-3 LCPUFAs are important components of the developing brain and retinal phospholipids during the third trimester of pregnancy and the first 6 months of life.

NUTRITIONAL GOALS FOR VLBW INFANTS AND THE NEED FOR NUTRIENT-ENRICHED FORMULAS

The generally accepted goal for nutritional management of these infants is to achieve and maintain the growth velocity and perhaps even more importantly the body composition of the normally growing, healthy human fetus of the same gestational age. Formulas have been developed to meet the additional protein, energy, and micronutrient requirements of these VLBW infants. Enteral protein feeding requirements have been reevaluated and emphasize the concept of promoting lean body mass gain. The contribution of protein to match fetal lean mass growth ex utero is even as important as protein is for growth.

DESCRIPTION OF IMPLEMENTATION STRATEGY

Figure 14.1 is a compilation of the impact of protein-to-energy ratio (protein grams per 100 kcal) on body composition. Additional protein is necessary for early catch-up growth to compensate for the cumulative protein deficit which develops in the first weeks of life. The increase in protein-energy ratio is mandatory to improve the lean body mass accretion and limit fat mass deposition. The avoidance of maldistribution of fat (visceral fat deposition) has long-term implications.

Table 14.2 shows the current recommendations for nutrient intakes for fully enteral fed VLBW infants per kilogram fed at 100 kcal energy intake. A number of reference sources are noted and rely on both the Ziegler reference fetus and the empirical approach to determine requirements.

Table 14.3 shows revised recommendations for protein intake and protein-energy ratio for preterm infants which include adjustments for postconceptional age and the need for catch-up growth. This is the best way to consider protein needs because it takes into account the dynamic requirement of protein as it changes relating to all of these variables in these VLBW infants.

Table 14.4 shows the role for higher-containing protein preterm formulas to meet the needs of these infants, as lean body mass is promoted by adhering to recommended protein-energy ratios. The higher ratios of protein to energy match up more favorably with fetal body composition. The target goal shown as 4 g/kg/day of protein can be reached with standard preterm formula but mean feeding higher volumes, excessive energy, and protein.

TABLE 14.2. Current Recommendations of Advisable Nutrient Intakes for Fully Enterally Fed Preterm VLBW Infants per Kilogram per Day and per 100 kcal Energy Intake*

Nutrient	Current Recommendation (per kg/day)	Current Recommendation (per 100 kcal)	LSRO, 2002 (formula-fed infants only, per kg/day)	Tsang et al (per kg/day)	ESPGHAN, 2010 (per kg/day)
Fluids	135–200	–	NS	150–200	135–200
Energy, kcal	110–130 (85–95 IV)	–	100–141	110–120	110–135
Protein, g	3.5–4.5	3.2–4.1	3.0–4.3	3.0–3.6	4.0–4.5 (<1 kg) 3.5–4.0 (1–1.8 kg)
Lipids, g	4.8–6.6	4.4–6	5.3–6.8		4.8–6.6 (<40% MCT)
Linoleic acid, mg	385–1540	350–1400	420–1700	(4–15 E%)	385–1540
α-Linoleic acid, mg	>55	>50	90–270	(1–4 E%)	>55
DHA, mg	(18–) 55–60	(16.4–) 50–55	NS	NS	12–30
EPA, mg	<20	<18	NS	NS	<30% of DHA
AA, mg	(18–) 35–45	(16.4–) 32–41	NS	NS	18–42
Carbohydrate, g	11.6–13.2	10.5–12	11.5–15.0 Lactose 4.8–15.0	Lactose: 3.8–11.8 Oligomers: 0–8.4	11.6–13.2
Sodium, mg	69–115	63–105	46.8–75.6	0–23	69–115
Potassium, mg	78–195	71–177	72–192	0–39	66–132
Chloride, mg	105–177	95–161	72–192	0–35	105–177
Calcium, mg	120–200	109–182	148–222	120–230	120–140
Phosphate, mg	60–140	55–127	98–131	60–140	60–90
Magnesium, mg	8–15	7.3–13.6	8.2–20.4	7.9–15	8–15
Iron, mg	2–3	1.8–2.7	2–3.6	0–2	2–3
Zinc, mg	1.4–2.5	1.3–2.3	1.32–1.8	0.5–0.8	1.1–2.0
Copper, µg	100–230	90–210	120–300	120	100–132

Selenium, µg	5–10	4.5–9	2.2–6.0	1.3	5–10
Manganese, µg	1–15	0.9–13.6	7.6–30	0.75	<22.7
Fluoride, µg	1.5–60	1.4–55	NS	NS	1.5–60
Iodine, µg	10–55	9–50	7.2–42	11–27	11–55
Chromium, µg	30–2250	27–2045	NS	50	30–1230
Molybdenum, µg	0.3–5	0.27–4.5	NS	0.3	0.3–5
Thiamin, µg	140–300	127–273	36–300	180–240	140–300
Riboflavin, µg	200–400	181–364	96–744	250–360	200–400
Niacin, mg	1–5.5	0.9–5	660–6000	3.6–4.8	0.38–5.5
Pantothenic acid, mg	0.5–2.1	0.45–1.9	360–2280	1.2–1.7	0.33–2.1
Pyridoxine, µg	50–300	45–273	36–300	150–210	45–300
Cobalamin, µg	0.1–0.8	0.09–0.73	0.096–0.84	0.3	0.1–077
Folic acid, µg	35–100	32–91	36–54	25–50	35–100
L-ascorbic acid, mg	20–55	18–50	10–45	18–24	11–46
Biotin, µg	1.7–16.5	1.5–15	1.2–44.4	3.6–6	1.7–16.5
Vitamin A, µg RE	400–1100	365–1000	245–456	700	400–1000
Vitamin D, IU	400–1000 per day, from milk + supplement	200–350 from milk only	90–324	150–400	800–1000 per day (100–350 per 100 kcal from milk only)
Vitamin E, mg α-TE	2.2–11	2–10	2.4–9.6	6–12	2.2–11
Vitamin K(1), µg	4.4–28	4–25	4.8–30	300 (bolus injection)	4.4–28
Nucleotides, mg	NS	NS	NS	NS	<5
Choline, mg	8–55	7.3–50	8.4–27.6	14.4–28	8–55
Inositol, mg	4.4–53	4–48	4.8–52.8	32–81	4.4–53

*Recommendations are compared to the previous intake recommendations of US Life Science Research Office (for formula-fed preterm infants only), Tsang et al 2005, and the European Society for Paediatric Gastroenterology, Hepatology and Nutrition, 2010.

TABLE 14.3. Revised Recommended Protein Intake and Protein-Energy Ratio for Premature Infants According to Postconceptional Age and the Need for Catch-Up

	Without Need of Catch-Up Growth	With Need of Catch-Up Growth
26–30 weeks PCA: 16–18 g/kg/day	3.8–4.2 g/kg/day	4.4 g/kg/day
LBM 14% protein retention	P/E: 3.0	P/E: 3.3
30–36 weeks pCA: 14–15 g/kg/day	3.4–3.6 g/kg/day	3.6–4.0 g/kg/day
LBM 15% protein retention	P/E: 2.8	P/E: 3.0
36–40 weeks PCA: 13 g/kg/day	2.8–3.2 g/kg/day	3.0–3.4 g/kg/day
LBM 17% protein retention	P/E: 2.4–2.6	P/E: 2.6–2.8

LBM, lean body mass; PCA, post-conceptual age; P/E, protein/energy ratio.
Based on Rigo, in Tsang. *J Pediatr.* 2006;149:s80-8.

Table 14.5 then makes the comparisons of the protein requirement for two birth-weight categories of VLBW infants versus the protein provided in human milk, fortified human milk, and preterm formulas. The standard preterm formula or standard fortifiers do not reach the requirement for the smallest babies. The numbers to the right (4.8, 4.1, and 4.3 g/kg at 120 cal/k/day, respectively) are the increased protein options that have become available more recently with the new fortified liquid concentrates and higher-protein preterm formulas.

CALORIC-DENSE FEEDINGS FOR INFANTS WITH BRONCHOPULMONARY DYSPLASIA

Caloric-dense feedings are intended for use in critically ill VLBW infants unable to tolerate sufficient feeding volumes (volume restricted) to meet their needs for growth using standard premature formulas or standardized fortified breast milk. Most of these infants requiring milk with >24 calories per ounce will be infants with bronchopulmonary dysplasia (BPD). Before ready-to-feed or concentrated liquid products became available, milks for these infants were produced as "mixtures" of powders with milk to make concentrated formulas or modified human milk. These were not sterile because of the powders and the mixing sterility issues, and they were inadequate in protein. The challenge is providing enough protein for volume-restricted infants. The recent introduction

TABLE 14.4. Preterm Formulas Reaching 4 g/kg/day Protein

	Preterm Formula 24 kcal	High Protein Preterm Formula 24 kcal
Protein/energy/g/100 kcal	3	3.3/ 3.5/ 3.6
Protein intake at 120 kcal/k/day [g/kg/day] (150 mL/k/day)	3.6	4.0/ 4.2/ 4.3
Protein intake at 144 kcal/k/day [g/kg/day] (180 mL/k/day)	4	4.7/ 4.9/ 5.2

TABLE 14.5. Comparison of Protein Requirements and Enteral Options*

Requirement	(g/kg/day)
<1000 g	3.5–4.5
1000—1500 g	3.5–4.0
Unfortified preterm breast milk	2.7
Fortified preterm breast milk	3.7–4.8
Fortified donor breast milk	3.0–4.1
Preterm formula 24	3.6
Preterm formula 24 high protein	4.0–4.5

*Includes factorial and empirical methods.

of 26–30 calorie per ounce ready-to-feed products in formula and human milk fortifier concentrates increased caloric density and protein without having to increase fluid volume. The proteins attainable at lower volumes are quite similar to those reached by VLBW infants receiving standard preterm formula or standard fortified human milk feedings. The calories from fat are increased while the carbohydrate calories are lower versus standard preterm formula. For example, the osmolarity of the 30 cal/oz formula is 325 mOsm/L versus standard preterm formula at 280 mOsm/L. There is also human milk fortification from donor milk concentrates that allows preparation of the increase protein with 26–30 calorie-per-ounce milk.

Infants with BPD demonstrate high resting energy expenditure and oxygen consumption and therefore need more energy than other preterm infants. However, without adequate protein, additional energy will not be used for lean mass. One study used a high-energy nutrient-enriched (caloric dense) formula for 3 months after discharge for patients with BPD and found that for selected infants with established BPD, energy intake may need to be increased beyond 120–130 calories per kilogram per day. We performed a study including 88 VLBW infants weighing <1000 g at birth who all had BPD and followed their growth rates in the NICU from return to birth weight through discharge. In all, 73% grew at or above the fetal growth rate of 15 g/k/day. These patients received the newly available high-protein preterm formulas, caloric-dense formulas (26–30 cal/ounce) and caloric-dense human milk fortifiers which had become available. There was less growth failure and an association with improved growth in those receiving more protein and early intravenous amino acids at higher dosage. Therefore, despite a diagnosis of BPD, nutritional strategies increasing protein and energy for these volume-restricted infants enhanced growth for patients with high risk for postnatal growth failure.

RECOMMENDATIONS

- Prevention of inadequate nutrition and therefore poor neurodevelopmental outcome is the goal of nutritional management of VLBW infants.
- Preterm formula developed specifically for these infants is provided when own mother's milk or donor human milk is not available or when a supplement is needed.
- Enriched diet, like that which is provided with a high-protein preterm formula as opposed to a standard-term formula, is associated with improved neurodevelopmental

outcomes demonstrated lasting through adolescence. Therefore, when formula is used with these infants it should be a high-protein–containing preterm formula with 24 calories per ounce. Infants receiving these high-protein preterm formulas should receive approximately 4–4.3 g/k/day of protein and require at least 100–110 calories per kilogram of energy.

- Protein-to-energy ratios of feedings for VLBW infants to promote accretion of lean body mass and limit fat deposition should be in the range of 3.3 g to 3.6 g protein to 100 calories of energy which are provided by the various preterm formulas.
- Partially hydrolyzed preterm formulas may be used in gut developmental defects like gastroschisis, NEC, or inflammatory conditions associated with bovine antigen where there is limited digestive capacity.
- The preterm high-protein formulas should be those supplemented with LCPUFAs.
- Those infants being managed with fluid restriction because of BPD should receive caloric dense feedings between 26 and 30 calories per ounce, which allows fluid restriction (120–140 mL/k/day) but still maintaining the protein and energy ratio needed to meet growth demands while promoting lean body mass accretion.

SUMMARY

A mainstay of nutrition for VLBW infants for the past 40 years has been the use of preterm formulas designed to meet the increased needs of energy, protein, and micronutrients in these infants. New generations of high-protein preterm formulas are now available that address the needs of the most immature infants. Essentially all studies have documented that inadequate protein intakes for these infants results in postnatal growth restriction and risk for long-term growth failure and neurodevelopmental impairment. Adequate protein-to-energy ratios are necessary to not only grow at similar velocities as the fetus or to catch up in growth after growth faltering, but to also have a body composition similar to the fetus.

It is possible that the addition of LCPUFAs to preterm formulas may improve neurologic and visual development during early development, and DHA and AA should be considered conditionally essential. Finally, infants requiring fluid restriction because of BPD will benefit from the use of caloric-dense feedings which permit fluid restriction while at the same time provide adequate protein and energy for lean body mass growth.

BIBLIOGRAPHIC SOURCE(S)

Agostoni C, Buonocore G, Carnielli VP, et al; ESPGHAN Committee on Nutrition. Enteral nutrient supply for preterm infants: commentary from the European Society of Paediatric Gastroenterology, Hepatology, and Nutrition Committee on Nutrition. *J Pediatr Gastroenterol.* 2010;50:85-91.

American Academy of Pediatrics Committee on Nutrition. Nutritional needs of low-birth-weight infants. *Pediatrics.* 1985;75(5):976-86.

Belfort MB, Gillman MW, Buka SL, et al. Preterm infant linear growth and adiposity gain: trade-offs for later weight status and intelligence quotient. *J Pediatr.* 2013;163(6):1564-9.

Brenna JT. Animal studies of the functional consequences of suboptimal polyunsaturated fatty acid status during pregnancy, lactation and early post-natal life. *Matern Child Nutr.* 2011;7(Suppl 2):59.

Brenna JT, Varamini B, Jensen RG, et al. Docosahexaenoic and arachidonic acid concentrations in human breast milk worldwide. *Am J Clin Nutr.* 2007;85:1457.

Brown LD, Hay WW Jr. The nutritional dilemma for preterm infants: how to promote neurocognitive development and linear growth, but reduce the risk of obesity. *J Pediatr.* 2013;163(6):1543-5.

Brunton JA, Saigal S, Atkinson SA. Growth and body composition in infants with bronchopulmonary dysplasia up to 3 month corrected age: a randomized trial of a higher-energy nutrient-enriched formula fed after hospital discharge. *J Pediatr.* 1998;133:340-5.

Carlson SE, Cooke RJ, Rhodes PG, et al. Long-term feeding of formulas high in linolenic acid and marine oil to very low birth weight infants: phospholipid fatty acids. *Pediatr Res.* 1991;30:404.

Ehrenkranz RA, Dusick AM, Vohr BR, Wright LL, Wrage LA, Poole WK. Growth in the neonatal intensive care unit influences neurodevelopmental and growth outcomes of extremely low birth weight infants. *Pediatrics.* 2006;117:1253-61.

Innis SM. Essential fatty acid transfer and fetal development. *Placenta.* 2005;26(Suppl A):S70.

Innis SM. Omega-3 Fatty acids and neural development to 2 years of age: do we know enough for dietary recommendations? *J Pediatr Gastroenterol Nutr.* 2009;48(Suppl 1):S16.

Innis SM, Foote KD, MacKinnon MJ, King DJ. Plasma and red blood cell fatty acids of low-birth-weight infants fed their mother's expressed breast milk or preterm-infant formula. *Am J Clin Nutr.* 1990;51:994.

Johnson MG, Wootton SA, Leaf AA, et al. Preterm birth and body composition at term equivalent age: a systematic review and meta-analysis. *Pediatrics.* 2012;130(3);e640-9.

Klein CJ. Nutrient requirements for preterm infant formulas. *J Nutr.* 2002;132(Suppl 1):1395S-1577S.

Lucas A, Morley R, Cole TJ. Randomised trial of early diet in preterm babies and later intelligence quotient. *BMJ.* 1998;317:1481-87.

Maggio L, Zuppa AA, Sawatzki G, et al. Higher urinary excretion of essential amino acids in preterm infants fed protein hydrolysates. *Acta Paediatr.* 2005;94(1):75-84.

Micheli JL, Schutz Y. Protein. In: Tsang RC, Lucas A, Uauy R, et al, eds. *Nutritional Needs of the Preterm Infant.* Pawling, NY: Caduceus Medical Publishers; 1993:29-46.

Rigo J, Salle BL, Picaud JC, et al. Nutritional evaluation of protein hydrolysate formulas. *Eur J Clin Nutr.* 1995;49(Suppl 1):S26-38.

Rigo J, Senterre J. Nutritional needs of premature infants: current issues. *J Pediatr.* 2006; 149:S80-8.

Schulzke SM, Patole SK, Simmer K. Long-chain polyunsaturated fatty acid supplementation in preterm infants. *Cochrane Database Syst Rev.* 2011;CD000375.

Taroni F, Liotto N, Morlacchi L, et al. Body composition in small for gestational age newborns. *Pediatri Med Chir.* 2008;30(6):296-301.

Theile AR, Radmacher PG, Anschutz TW, Davis DW, Adamkin DH. Nutritional strategies and growth in extremely low birth weight infants with bronchopulmonary dysplasia over the past 10 years. *J Perinatol.* 2012;32:117-22.

Tsang R, Uauy R, Koletzko B, Zlotkin S. *Nutrition of the Preterm Infant. Scientific Basis and Practical Application.* 2nd ed. Cincinnati: Digital Education Publishing; 2005.

Uauy R, Hoffman DR. Essential fatty acid requirements for normal eye and brain development. *Semin Perinatol.* 1991;15:449.

Uthaya S, Thomas EL, Hamilton G, Dore CJ, Bell J, Modi N. Altered adiposity after extremely preterm birth. *Pediatr Res.* 2005;57:211-5.

Valentine CJ, Morrow G, Fernandez S, et al. Docosahexaenoic acid and amino acid contents in pasteurized donor milk are low for preterm infants. *J Pediatr.* 2010;157:906.

Valentine CJ, Morrow G, Morrow AL. Promoting pasteurized donor human milk use in the neonatal intensive care unit (NICU) as an adjunct to care and to prevent necrotizing enterocolitis and shorten length of stay. In: *FDA Division of Dockets Management (HFA-305),* ed. Rockville, MD; 2010.

van Goudoever JB, Sulkers EJ, Lafeber HN, et al. Short-term growth and substrate use in very-low-birth-weight infant fed formulas with different energy contents. *Am J Clin Nutr.* 2000;71(3):816-21.

Ziegler EE, O'Donnell AM, Nelson SE, et al. Body composition of the reference fetus. *Growth.* 1976;40(4):329-41.

Parenteral Nutrition

Traci Fauerbach, MS, RD, CNSC, LDN • Michael A. Posencheg, MD
• Lori Christ, MD

SCOPE

DISEASE/CONDITION(S)

Very low birth weight (VLBW) infants are at high risk of growth failure as compared with their full-term, age-matched peers. The provision of adequate caloric intake, with proportional carbohydrates, proteins, and lipids, is crucial to optimizing growth of these fragile infants while also optimizing fluid balance. During the first days of life, these infants receive the majority of their nutrition via parenteral nutrition (PN) while enteral feedings are advanced. Careful management of the components of PN is essential to promote adequate postnatal growth and to minimize PN-related complications.

GUIDELINE OBJECTIVE(S)

To provide guidance for neonatologists and trainees rotating through the neonatal intensive care unit (NICU), advanced practitioners, neonatal dietitians, and neonatal nurses regarding management of PN for VLBW infants.

BRIEF BACKGROUND

As noted above, VLBW infants are at an increased risk for growth failure. Observational studies have noted that VLBW infants with a diagnosis of extrauterine growth failure, defined as weight less than the 10th percentile at a corrected gestational age of 36 weeks, have impaired neurodevelopmental outcomes compared with those infants without a diagnosis of growth failure. Many factors contribute to growth failure in the NICU, and these factors can be divided broadly into inadequate caloric input and excessive caloric output. Ideally, PN would mimic nutrition provided to the fetus in utero. However, during the first few days of life, the administration of optimal PN is often limited by critical illness and metabolic immaturity, combined with fluid intake restriction and limited central IV access for preterm infants, especially those <1 kg at birth. Once enteral feeding is initiated, PN is weaned as the feeding volume is advanced. This transitional period is one of the most nutritionally vulnerable time points for VLBW infants. A retrospective, observational study demonstrated that during this time, protein intake from a combination of total parenteral nutrition (TPN) and enteral feeding is often inadequate. Poor growth velocity during this transitional period is predictive of later diagnosis of growth failure. Given the constraints of administering PN to preterm infants, meticulous attention must be paid when reviewing and prescribing the content of daily PN formulations. In this chapter, we review evidence-based recommendations for early initiation of PN, provision of macronutrients and micronutrients via PN, monitoring guidelines, and considerations for weaning PN during feed advances.

RECOMMENDATIONS

EARLY PARENTERAL NUTRITION

Delay in initiation of PN contributes to the protein deficit that VLBW infants can accumulate. VLBW neonates receiving only dextrose fluids can lose 1% of body protein stores per day. The provision of calories in excess of basal metabolic rates via PN has been shown to improve weight for age to greater than the 10th percentile at 36 weeks. Providing a minimum of 50 kcal/kg, starting within 2 hours of birth, is considered safe and is equivalent to resting metabolic rates, but additional energy is needed to support growth. Neutral nitrogen balance can be achieved with an initial protein intake of 1–1.5 g/kg/day of protein, but 2.5–3 g/kg/day is recommended to promote a positive nitrogen balance and is considered safe.

MACRONUTRIENTS

Energy

The total energy requirement for a VLBW infant is determined by basal energy needs as well as the energy required for growth. VLBW infants need 90–115 kcal/kg/day from PN to support both. Provision of adequate energy intake prevents the use of protein as a fuel source and thereby increases its availability for the synthesis of lean mass.

Glucose

The fetus receives a constant transfer of glucose from the placenta, and after birth the preterm infant is at risk for hypoglycemia due to limited glycogen stores. Initial glucose infusion should begin within 30 minutes of birth at an infusion rate of 4–7 mg/kg/min to mimic basal metabolic rate and to decrease the need for endogenous glucose production.

Hyperglycemia, defined as a blood glucose >125 mg/dL, is commonly observed in VLBW infants. Immature glucose homeostasis pathways, insulin resistance, and a relative lack of insulin-dependent tissues such as fat and muscle contribute to risk for hyperglycemia in premature infants. Stress, steroid treatment, and excessive glucose infusion rates are common exogenous culprits. To optimize glycemic response, daily advancement of glucose infusion rates (GIR) should not exceed 2 mg/kg/min/day with a goal GIR of 7–10 mg/kg/min. Reducing the rate of glucose infusion to remedy hyperglycemia will also reduce caloric intake and may affect growth and development; a GIR less than 4 mg/kg/min may promote the utilization of non-carbohydrate energy to maintain euglycemia and is not recommended. The upper oxidative limit of glucose metabolism is not known and suggested upper limits vary, but excessive rate of glucose infusions (>10 mg/kg/min) should be avoided. When oxidative capacity is exceeded, excess glucose is converted to fat stores. This can play a role in the development of PN–associated cholestasis (PNAC) and contribute to excess carbon dioxide production. In a small study by Gupta, a GIR of less than 9.3 mg/kg min was shown to decrease the incidence of PNAC when caloric needs were met and euglycemia was maintained.

Protein

Protein is the primary source of energy for fetal growth and can be considered the growth-limiting factor. Provision of inadequate amounts of protein has been associated with poor growth and impaired neurodevelopment.

Fetuses receive approximately 3.5 g/kg/day of amino acid via the placenta. A fetus will accrete approximately 2.5 g/kg of protein daily with losses estimated to be 1 g/kg/day. Initial protein requirements to maintain neutral nitrogen balance have been reviewed above. Advancement to a goal protein intake of 3.5–4.0 g/kg/day should be achieved within 48 hours of life.

Blood urea nitrogen (BUN) has been used historically as a marker of amino acid tolerance. However, emerging evidence has demonstrated little to no association between BUN and protein intake and does not support limiting protein intake in response to elevated BUN, as unnecessary restriction of protein due to elevated BUN risks impeding growth velocity.

Lipids

Lipids are a required part of PN due to their provision of essential fatty acids and their calorically dense composition. Essential fatty acid deficiency (EFAD) can be prevented with as little as 0.5–1.0 g/kg/day infusion of lipids. Endogenous lipid stores of preterm infants are limited and infusions should be initiated by day of life 1. Gilberson demonstrated that initiation of 1 g/kg/day on the first day of life with a stepwise increase of 1 g/kg/day to a goal of 3 g/kg/day was well tolerated without adverse effects in VLBW infants. Ghassan suggests initiating lipids at 2–3 g/kg/day within the first 24 hours of life and notes that there is little evidence to support the often slow stepwise process of initiating and advancing lipids that is common practice in many NICUs.

Although the infusion of lipids is considered a relatively benign therapy, and the incidence of complications associated with its use in neonates is low, there is a degree of unpredictability of an infant's tolerance to fat emulsions. Complications of hyperlipidemia in the neonate include impairment of pulmonary function, hyperbilirubinemia due to displacement of albumin-bound bilirubin by plasma free fatty acids, and fat overload syndrome (fever, lethargy, liver damage, coagulopathy). Trending serum triglyceride levels is important to monitor tolerance and prevent complications from lipid infusion. Practices among units vary as to acceptable level and when to decrease or discontinue lipid infusion. A unit-wide guideline regarding how to respond to elevated triglyceride levels is necessary to avoid variation in limitation of lipid infusions and unnecessary suboptimal daily caloric intake (Table 15.1). The American Society for Parenteral and Enteral Nutrition (ASPEN) recommends that serum triglyceride concentration not exceed 200 mg/dL, while the European Society of Pediatric Gastroenterology, Hepatology, and Nutrition (ESPGHAN) and the European Society for Clinical Nutrition and Metabolism (ESPEN) recommend that serum or plasma triglyceride concentrations during infusion not exceed 250 mg/dL.

TABLE 15.1. Triglyceride Level and Suggested Interventions

Serum Triglyceride Level (mg/dL)	Intervention
<200	Continue advancement to goal or maintain goal infusion of 3 g/kg/day
201–250	Decrease lipid infusion by 0.5 g/kg/day
251–300	Decrease lipid infusion by 1 g/kg/day
>300	Discontinue lipids and resume the next day at previously tolerated rate

Limiting lipid infusions to 1 g/kg/day is a common practice for infants with direct hyperbilirubinemia. Caution is advised with this routine restriction of calories in VLBW infants who are not likely to require long-term PN, as limitation of caloric intake will contribute to growth failure.

MICRONUTRIENTS

Calcium and Phosphorus

The goal intake for calcium and phosphorus should be achieved by day of life 3–4 (Table 15.2). A calcium:phosphorus ratio of 2:1 (mEq:mMol) is optimal for bone mineralization. Regular use of calcium-wasting medications (i.e., Lasix or steroids) may increase calcium needs. Infants with a history of intrauterine growth restriction may require additional phosphorus supplementation to prevent a refeeding-like syndrome. Adequate calcium and phosphorus supplementation (to mimic in utero accretion rates) is limited by their ability to stay in solution. The risk of precipitation increases with volume restriction and lower protein provisions. The addition of cysteine will lower the pH of the PN solution and improve solubility.

Magnesium

The addition of magnesium is not necessary initially but can be added once serum levels are known to be within normal limits. Special considerations and monitoring of magnesium levels should be given to infants whose mothers received magnesium sulfate prior to delivery.

Electrolytes

Sodium intake should be carefully monitored during the postnatal diuretic phase. The sodium contribution from stock saline solutions for arterial lines will often exceed initial sodium requirements in extremely low birth weight (ELBW) infants; PN additives

TABLE 15.2. Target Mineral Dosing

Mineral	Initial Dose	Goal Dose for Preterm	Maximum Dose
Calcium (mEq/kg)	1–3	3	4–4.6
Phosphorus (mMol/kg)	0–0.5	1.5	2–2.3
Magnesium (mEq/kg)	0	0.3–0.6	1

TABLE 15.3. **Electrolyte Target Dosing**

Electrolytes	Day 1	Day 2	Day 3	Day 4	Goal (max)
Na (mEq/kg)	0–1	0–1	0–2	1–2	2–4 (7)
K (mEq/kg)	0–1	1–2	2–3	2–3	2–3
Cl (mEq/kg)	0–1	0–1	0–2	1–2	2–3 (7)
Acetate (mEq/kg)*	0–1	0–1	0–2	0–2	0–2+ (6)

*As needed to buffer.

AA solutions provide ~1 mEq acetate per gram of protein.

should factor in this additional source of sodium chloride. The addition of potassium should be minimized until urine output is established and serum potassium is within acceptable ranges. Infants with a history of growth restriction may also have increased needs for potassium in the setting of a refeeding-like response. See Table 15.3 for target electrolyte dosing.

Vitamins

Intravenous pediatric multivitamin preparations are appropriate to meet vitamin recommendations (Table 15.4) when dosed based on the weight of the infant (Table 15.5).

Trace Elements

ASPEN guidelines suggest adding individual trace elements (TE) rather than using commercial multi-trace element formulations for VLBW infants. Individual dosing of TEs will avoid the inadequate dosing of zinc, the excess provision of manganese and chromium, and provide additional selenium (Table 15.6).

TABLE 15.4. **Vitamin Dosing Recommendations**

Vitamin	Parenteral Preterm Vitamin Recommendations (All values are per kg/day)	Amount if 5 mL of Pediatric MVI Injection (Hospira) Infuvite Pediatric (Baxter)
Vitamin A	700–1500 IU	2300 IU
Vitamin D	40–160 IU	400
Vitamin E	2.8–3.5 IU	7
Vitamin K	10 µg	200
Thiamin	200–350 µg	1200
Riboflavin	150–200 µg	1400
Niacin	4–6.8 mg	17
B6	150–200 µg	1000
Folate	56 µg	140
B12	0.3 µg	1
Pantothenic acid	1–2 mg	5
Biotin	5–8 µg	20
Vitamin C	15–25 mg	80

TABLE 15.5. Suggested Parenteral Vitamin Doses by Weight

	<1 kg	1–3 kg	>3 kg
Pediatric MVI	1.5 mL	3.3 mL	5 mL

Carnitine

Carnitine is an amino acid that plays a role in long-chain fatty acid oxidation. It is not commonly added to PN, but it is a component of breast milk and preterm formulas. Infants who are exclusively parenterally fed have low levels of carnitine, but the significance of this is not known. Literature does not support regular supplementation of carnitine in parenterally fed infants; however, supplementation of 2–5 mg/kg can be considered for premature infants who do not have an enteral source.

Cysteine

The addition of cysteine to PN will decrease the overall pH of the solution and thus improve the ability of calcium and phosphorus to stay in solution. The lower pH of the PN solution may contribute to increased risk of metabolic acidosis and the infant's acid/base balance should be monitored. The recommended dose of amino acid is 40 mg/g. The addition of acetate can be considered as needed to buffer and prevent metabolic acidosis when cysteine is added to PN.

TABLE 15.6. Trace Element Recommendations

Trace Elements	Suggested TE Formulation Dosing		RDA/AI	APSEN Recommendations
	<3 kg 1 mL/kg/day	>3 kg 0.4 mL/kg/day	0–6 months	
Zinc	300 µg/kg	120 µg/kg	200 µg	450–500 µg/kg/day (preterm) 250 µg/kg/day (<3 mo) 50 µg/kg/day (>3 mo)
Copper	20 µg/kg	8 µg/kg	200 µg	20 µg/kg/day (10 µg/kg/day with cholestasis)
Manganese	5 µg/kg	2 µg/kg	3 µg	1 µg/kg/day (remove with cholestasis)
Chromium	0.17 µg/kg	0.068 µg/kg	0.2 µg	Contaminates in PN satisfy this so no additional supplementation is needed
Selenium	0	0	15 µg	2 µg/kg/day (decrease to 1 µg/kg/day or remove with renal failure)
Carnitine	0	0		2–5 mg/kg/day
Choline	0	0		125 mg/day Currently no parenteral source available

LABORATORY MONITORING

Unit-specific guidelines for lab monitoring may assist in limiting excessive blood draws. Frequent electrolyte and blood gas monitoring during the postnatal diuretic phase is often necessary. Once PN is meeting caloric goals and electrolytes and acid/base are normal, reduce monitoring of electrolytes to 1–2 times per week. Monitoring of liver function tests to assess for PN-induced cholestasis should begin when PN therapy is used for more than 2 weeks. Screening for metabolic bone disease of prematurity should begin by 6 weeks of age.

WEANING TPN DURING A FEED ADVANCE

The transitional phase of VLBW infant nutrition, which occurs as enteral feeds advance and TPN is weaned, is described by Miller and is associated with slowed growth velocity of <10 g/kg/day. This slower growth is also predictive of growth failure (weight percentile for age <10% at discharge) and is likely related to inadequate protein intake during PN weaning. NICUs should consider a feeding protocol that maintains adequate protein intake during this phase. This can be done by concentrating PN volume or customizing PN orders to maintain a targeted protein intake. Earlier fortification is also an option to improve protein intake during the transitional phase. Our unit focuses on volume-led weaning of TPN, and thus our practice is to concentrate TPN by taking into account the volume of enteral feeds until fortification of breast milk or formula occurs at 60 mL/kg/day.

IMPLEMENTATION OF GUIDELINE

QUALIFYING STATEMENTS

These recommendations are not intended to dictate an exclusive course of management or treatment. They must be evaluated with reference to individual patient needs, resources, and limitations unique to the institution and variations in local populations. It is hoped that this process of local ownership will help to incorporate these guidelines into routine practice. Attention is drawn to areas of clinical uncertainty where further research might be indicated.

DESCRIPTION OF IMPLEMENTATION STRATEGY

Our unit developed a TPN worksheet (Figure 15.1) to highlight the specific advancement of TPN components based on metabolic tolerance of GIR and lipid infusion increases. Goals for glucose infusion rate and protein/lipids were provided as well as target supplementation for electrolytes and trace elements.

QUALITY METRICS

Outcome Measures

Outcome measures should include average weight and head circumference percentile at 36 weeks corrected gestational age or discharge, whichever is first. In more recent studies, the delta Z-score (change in Z score from birth to 36 weeks corrected gestational age or hospital discharge) has been shown to be more predictive of longer-term cognitive outcomes and better accounts for growth velocity during an infant's NICU stay.

Patient name _____   Date _____   Medication weight_____kg

1. Determine TFL:_____mL/kg/day × weight kg =_____mL/day ÷ 24 = _____mL/h

2. **Calculate intravenous fat emulsion (IVFE):**
    Start dose: 1 g/kg for infants <1000 g and 2 g/kg for infants >1000 g
    Advance: 1 g/kg to goal of 3 g/kg
    Ordered dose_____g/kg × wt in kg = g/day × 5 mL/g =_____mL/d ÷ 24 = _____ **mL/h IVFE**
    2 kcal/mL/day × total mL/day =   _____ **kcal from fat**

3. **Calculate volume of TPN needed:**
    First, add up the non-TPN fluid the baby in receiving.
    _____ mL/h for IVFE
    _____ mL/h for arterial line
    _____ mL/h for UVC lumen #2 or PICC lumen #2 if applicable
    _____ mL/h for all medication infusion (e.g., dopamine, morphine, versed)
    _____ mL/h for other medications (volume for antibiotics, etc.) **See RN flow sheet at bed side**
    +_____ mL/h for feeds (may account for up to 80 mL/kg/day of feeds)
    Total_____ **mL/h non-PN fluid**
    TFL (mL/h) − non-PN fluid (mL/h)= _____ **mL/h PN rate × 24 =**_____ **mL/day PN**
    Note: Minimum total volume for compounding PN is 40 mL/kg.

4. **Determine protein intake (4 cal/g of protein)**
    Start dose: 4 g/kg for all infants <1500 g if on starter PN and 3 g/kg for infants >1500 g
    Goal: 4–4.5 g/kg for infants ≤500 g, 3–4 g/kg for infants >1500 g, and 2–3 g/kg for term infants
    Ordered dose:_____ **g/kg** × wt (kg) × 4 =   _____**kcal from protein**

5. **Determine dextrose concentration (3.4 cal/g of dextrose)**
    Access: Peripheral: max D12.5 and osmolarity ≤1000 Central: >D12.5% allowed
    Ordered concentration:_____%100 × total TPN volume × 3.4 =   _____**kcal from dextrose**

    Note: Total glucose infusion rate (GIR) should not be less than 4 mg/kg/min to prevent catabolism in ELBW infants.
    May decrease as feeds advance. Avoid GIR >14 mg/kg/min
        $\text{GIR} = \dfrac{\text{\% dextrose} \times \text{rate of PN} \times 0.167}{\text{Weight in kg}} =$ _____mg/kg/min TPN GIR

    + $\dfrac{\text{\% dextrose} \times \text{rate of carrier} \times 0.167}{\text{Weight in kg}} =$ _____mg/kg/min carrier GIR

        _____mg/kg/min Total GIR

6. **Determine total kcal/kg from TPN:**
    $\dfrac{\text{Total kcals from protein} + \text{total kcals from dextrose} + \text{total kcals from fat}}{\text{Current wt(kg)}} =$ _____**kcal/kg/day**

7. **Determine electrolyte additives:** Please refer to most recent electrolytes and discuss changes on rounds.

    Below is a guide; follow infant's labs determine specific electrolyte requirements.
    Please note that some electrolytes are ordered as mEq/kg and others mmol/kg! See conversion chart below.

	Day 1	Day 2	Day 3	Day 4	Goal
Na (mEq/kg as NaCl Na Acetate)	0–1	0–1	0–2	1–2	2–4
K (mEq/kg as KCl or KAcetate)	0–1	1–2	2–3	2–3	2–3
Acetate (as needed to buffer)	0–1	0–1	0–2	0–2	0–2+ as needed
Calcium (mEq/kg)	2	2–3	2–3	3–4	3–4
Phosphorus (mMol/kg as NaPhos)	0.5–1	1–1.5	1.5–2	1.5–2	1.5–2
Mg (mEq/kg - *unless Mg exposed*)	0–0.35	0–0.35	0.35–0.5	0.35–0.5	0.35–0.5

Note: $\frac{1}{2}$ NSS through UAC may provide significant source of NaCl; calcium may not be needed on day 1 in term infants, K and Phos should be considered in SGA infants as they are prone to hypokalemia and hypophosphatemia.

FIGURE 15.1 • Example of parenteral nutrition ordering worksheet.

Previous electrolytes: Changes:

Na: _____ mEq/kg NaCl   _____ _____ _____ _____
     _____ mEq/kg Na Acetate _____ _____ _____ _____
     _____ mMol/kg NaPhos** _____ _____ _____ _____
     **preferred Phos source
K: _____ mEq/kg KCl   _____ _____ _____ _____
     _____ mEq/kg K Acetate _____ _____ _____ _____
     _____ mMol/kg KPhos   _____ _____ _____ _____

Ca: _____ mEq/kg   _____ _____ _____ _____
Mg: _____ mEq/kg   _____ _____ _____ _____

Electrolyte conversions: 1 mmol KPhos = 1.5 mEq K   1 mmol NaPhos = 1.3 mEq Na   1 mEq Calcium = 0.5 mmol Ca

8. Determine other additives:

TPN Additives (circle)		<1 kg	1 to 3 kg	>3 kg
Heparin	(unit per mL)	0.5 unit per mL	0.5 unit per mL	0.5 unit per mL
Multivitamin	(unit per mL)	1.5 mL per day	3.3 mL per day	5 mL per day
Selenium	(all infants)	2 µg/kg		
Copper	(all infants)	20 µg/kg		
Manganese	(all infants)	1 µg/kg		
		Preterm	**Term**	**>3 months**
Zinc		400 mg/day	250 mg/day	100 mg/day

FIGURE 15.1 • (*Continued*)

Process Measures

Monitoring the average protein and caloric intake of VLBW infants in each of the nutritional stages is recommended to develop and monitor improvement in response to unit-specific interventions.

Balancing Measures

Undesired consequences of prolonged TPN administration are increased numbers of central line days and their associated complications (central line–associated bloodstream infection, catheter migration), late-onset sepsis, and TPN-related complications as noted above.

BIBLIOGRAPHIC SOURCE(S)

American Academy of Pediatrics. *Pediatric Nutrition Handbook.* Evanston, IL: American Academy of Pediatrics; 2014.

American Dietetics Association. *ADA Pocket Guide to Neonatal Nutrition.* Chicago, IL: American Dietetics Association; 2009.

Berry MA, Abrahamowicz M, Usher RH. Factors associated with growth of extremely premature infants during initial hospitalization. *Pediatrics.* 1997;100(4):640-6.

Bonsante F, Iacobelli S, Latorre G, et al. Initial amino acid intake influences phosphorus and calcium homeostasis in preterm infants—it is time to change the composition of the early parenteral nutrition. *PLoS One.* 2013;8(8):e72880.

Brans YW, Andrew DS, Carrillo DW, Dutton EP, Mechaca EM, Puelo-Scheppke BA. Tolerance of fat emulsions in very low birthweight neonates. *AJCD.* 1988;142:145-52.

Cairns PA, Stalker DJ. Carnitine supplementation of parenterally fed neonates. *Cochrane Database Syst Rev.* 2000;(4):CD000950.

Denne SC, Poindexter BB. Supporting early nutrition with parenteral amino acid infusion. *Semin Perinatol.* 2007;31(2):56-60.

Ehrenkranz RA, Dusick AM, Vohr BR, Wright LL, Wrage LA, Poole K. Growth in the neonatal intensive care unit influences neurodevelopmental and growth outcomes of extremely low birth weight infants. *Pediatrics.* 2006;117(4):1253-61.

Farrag HM, Cowett RM. Glucose homeostasis in the micropremie. *Clin Perinatol.* 2000;27(1):1-22, v.

Gilbertson N, Kovar IZ, Cox DJ, et al. Introduction of intravenous lipid administration on the first day of life in the very-low-birth-weight neonate. *J Pediatr.* 1991;119:615-23.

Gupta K, Wang H, Amin SB. Parenteral nutrition-associated cholestasis in premature infants: role of macronutrients. *JPEN J Parenter Enteral Nutr.* 2016;40(3):335-41.

Herrmann KR. Early parenteral nutrition and successful postnatal growth of premature infants. *Nutr Clin Pract.* 2010;25(1):69-75.

Innis SM. Lipids in parenteral nutrition. *NeoReviews.* 2002;3(3);e48-e55.

Miller M, Vaidya R, Rastogi D, Bhutada A, Rastogi R. From parenteral to enteral nutrition: a nutrition-based approach for evaluating postnatal growth failure in preterm infants. *JPEN J Parenter Enteral Nutr.* 2014;38(4):489-97.

Mitanchez D. Glucose regulation in preterm newborn infants. *Hormone Res.* 2007;68:265-71.

Poindexter BB, Langer JC, Dusick AM, Ehrenkranz RA. Early provision of parenteral amino acids in extremely low birth weight infants: relation to growth and neurodevelopmental outcome. *J Pediatr.* 2006;148:300-305.

Salama GS, Kaabneh MA, Almasaeed MN, Alquran MIA. Intravenous lipids for preterm infants: a review. *Clin Med Insights Pediatr.* 2015;9:25-36.

Shah PS, Wong KY, Merko S, et al. Postnatal growth failure in preterm infants: ascertainment and relation to long-term outcome. *J Perinat Med.* 2006;34(6):484-9.

Taylor SN, Kiger J, Finch C, Bizal D. Fluid, electrolytes, and nutrition: minutes matter. *Adv Neonatal Care.* 2010;10(5):248-55.

Thureen PJ, Melara D, Fennessey PV, Hay WW Jr. Effect of low versus high intravenous amino acid intake on very low birth weight infants in the early neonatal period. *Pediatr Res.* 2003;53(1):24-32.

Tsang RD. *Nutrition of the Preterm Infant Scientific Basis and Practical Guidelines.* Cincinnati, OH. Digital Educational Publishing; 2005.

Vanek VW, Borum P, Buchman A, et al; Novel Nutrient Task Force, Parenteral Multi-Vitamin and Multi–Trace Element Working Group; American Society for Parenteral and Enteral Nutrition (A.S.P.E.N.) Board of Directors. A.S.P.E.N. Position paper: recommendations for changes in commercially available parenteral multivitamin and multi-trace element products. *Nutr Clin Pract.* 2012;27(4):440-91.

Weintraub AS, Blanco V, Barnes M, Green RS. Impact of renal function and protein intake on blood urea nitrogen in preterm infants in the first 3 weeks of life. *J Perinat.* 2015;35:52-6.

Ziegler EE. Protein requirements of very low birth weight infants. *J Pediatr Gastroenterol Nutr.* 2007;45(Suppl 3):S170-4. Review. Erratum in: *J Pediatr Gastroenterol Nutr.* 2009;48(1):121-2.

Ziegler EE, O'Donnell AM, Nelson SE, Fomon SJ. Body composition of the reference fetus. *Growth.* 1976;40(4):329-41.

Hyperkalemia and Hypokalemia

Wendy A. Araya, DNP, APRN, NNP-BC • Catherine Huskins, MSN, APRN, NNP-BC • Kiersten LeBar, DNP, MMHC, CPNP-AC • Colleen Moss, MSN, APRN, NNP-BC • Helen L. Nation, MSN, APRN, NNP-BC, C-NPT • Charlotte Ramieh, DNP, APRN, NNP-BC

SCOPE

DISEASE/CONDITION(S)

Treatment and evaluation of hypokalemia and hyperkalemia in the neonate.

GUIDELINE OBJECTIVE(S)

Review causes of hypokalemia and hyperkalemia; identify ways to evaluate for hypokalemia and hyperkalemia; recommendations for evaluation and treatment of hypokalemia and hyperkalemia.

BRIEF BACKGROUND

Electrolyte abnormalities are a recognized problem in the neonatal population that health care providers face on a daily basis; specifically, hypokalemia and hyperkalemia. Knowing how to assess and verify for potassium abnormalities prior to initiating treatment is invaluable. Prior to treating electrolyte abnormalities, it is important to evaluate the causes, which can range from a sampling error to effects of medications to a syndrome. The following is a guideline with recommendations on treatment of hypokalemia and hyperkalemia based on the severity and condition of the neonate.

RECOMMENDATIONS

HYPERKALEMIA RECOMMENDATIONS

Hyperkalemia is defined as a serum potassium value >6 mmol/L. Immediate intervention is necessary if cardiac changes are present.

PRACTICE OPTIONS

Practice Option #1

If sample was obtained from heel stick the specimen should be analyzed for hemolysis. If no hemolysis is present and the value is >6.5 mmol/L, a repeat venous or arterial specimen should be sent to the laboratory for analysis. Falsely elevated capillary specimens are commonly due to hemolysis.

Practice Option #2

In the first 48 hours of life, potassium should be withheld from intravenous fluids until urine output is well established and potassium level is decreasing; this is especially important for extremely low birth weight (ELBW) infants. Check all intravenous fluids to ensure that potassium has not been added to the solution. When potassium is added to fluids, maintenance requirements are 1–2 mEq/kg/day.

Practice Option #3

If hyperkalemia is present in the very low birth weight (VLBW) or ELBW infant in conjunction with low urine output, this is nonoliguric hyperkalemia. Goal is to promote the movement of potassium from the extracellular fluid into the cells by *one* of three ways:

1. Administering IV glucose (2 mL/kg of D10) with insulin (0.05 units/kg), followed by a continuous infusion of insulin (0.1 units/kg/h with 2–4 mL/kg/h of D10).
    a. Recheck K 30–60 minutes after starting infusion. Wean insulin drip as the K drops to <6 mmol/L, since there will be a drift downward after stopping.
2. Administering IV sodium bicarbonate (1–2 mEq/kg/dose) over 30–60 minutes.
3. Administering albuterol via nebulization (2.5 mg) or IV (4–5 µg/kg/dose over 20 minutes).

Practice Option #4

If hyperkalemia is severe and/or life threatening, administer 10% calcium gluconate (0.5–1 mL/kg IV) over 5 minutes.

Practice Option #5

The above interventions do not eliminate potassium from the body. Additional therapy is needed to excrete potassium; in infants with adequate urine output, administer furosemide 1 mL/kg/dose IV.

Practice Option #6

In infants with severe oliguria or anuria, administer cation exchange resin (Kayexalate) in one of two ways: 1 g/kg dissolved in saline (rectal solution), or 1 g/kg/dose in D10% (enteral solution). Resins are not recommended in the preterm population, as obstruction and intestinal necrosis have been reported. Monitor sodium closely, as this intervention may result in hypernatremia.

Practice Option #7

Infants receiving oral supplementation of potassium chloride due to chronic diuretic therapy, with potassium value >6 mmol/L should have oral supplementation stopped and value repeated in 48 hours.

HYPOKALEMIA RECOMMENDATIONS

Hypokalemia can result from potassium loss due to renal dysfunction, diuretic therapy (specifically with furosemide or hydrochlorothiazide), diarrhea, nasogastric secretions, and ostomy output. The underlying etiology of hypokalemia can be compounded by inadequate potassium intake through enteral or parental nutrition. Additionally, altered acid-base status resulting in the presence of alkalosis causes intracellular shifting of potassium ions leading to hypokalemia. The treatment of hypokalemia should address the underlying etiology while preventing and treating cardiac and muscular complications.

Practice Option #1: Potassium Supplementation

Treatment for hypokalemia should be considered for serum potassium <3.0 mEq/L or if patient is symptomatic. If additional potassium supplementation is required, administration can be through intravenous or oral/enteral routes. Titration should be based on serum, non-hemolyzed potassium samples. The normal daily requirement of K+ is 1–2 mEq/kg/day in three to four divided doses, preferably with feeds. The safest method is oral/enteral route. Replacement therapy through intravenous administration should be given slowly, usually by replacement of potassium through adjustment of daily fluid concentrations given over 24 hours. The potassium concentration in intravenous fluids should not exceed 40 mEq/L. If potassium infusion is required, dosing needs to be limited to 0.3 to a maximum rate of 1 mEq/kg/h for life-threatening hypokalemia. Intravenous potassium ideally is administered via a central line under continuous cardiac monitoring. Potassium chloride infusion needs to be given over 30–60 minutes.

Choosing the type of replacement K salt depends on the underlying situation. During episodes of hypovolemia, K chloride is usually preferred versus during times of metabolic acidosis, when K bicarbonate, K citrate, and K acetate may be utilized. While K phosphate is not readily utilized in the neonatal population during times of phosphate depletion, K phosphate may be a better supplement of choice. Some cases of hypokalemia may be resistant to treatment, therefore requiring additional treatment of magnesium levels as well.

Practice Option #2: Utilize Potassium-Sparing Diuretics

In neonates at risk or who have already developed chronic lung disease requiring continued diuretic therapy, hypokalemia can be a direct result of prolonged use. Certain diuretics such as furosemide have a high potential for renal excretion of potassium. In these cases, potassium-sparing diuretics such as spironolactone, potentially in addition to oral supplementation–based serum values, should be considered to improve diuretic-induced alkalosis.

Practice Option #3: Monitor Glucose Infusion Rates

Intravenous fluids with dextrose may result in increased insulin secretion resulting in a further decrease in serum potassium levels.

Practice Option #4: Monitor Gastrointestinal Losses

1) Replace nasogastric drainage each 12-hour shift with milliliter for milliliter with ½ normal saline with 20 mEq of potassium chloride and 2) utilize oral supplementation of 2–3 mEq/kg/day for patients with Bartter syndrome.

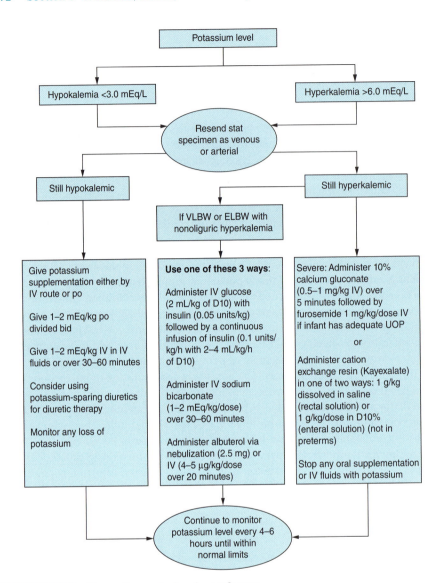

FIGURE 16.1 • Hypo-/hyperkalemia pathway.

IMPLEMENTATION OF GUIDELINE

DESCRIPTION OF IMPLEMENTATION STRATEGY

Recommend written guidelines/protocols for monitoring potassium levels in neonates. Provide written recommendations for when the potassium level is not within normal limits of 3.5 and 5.5 mEq/L. The recommendation for the ELBW infant is to leave the potassium out of the IV fluids until 48 hours after birth, until renal function is established. Develop written protocols for treatment plans and monitoring potassium levels for both hypokalemia and hyperkalemia. Provide the recommended amount of potassium for the daily requirements of 1–2 mEq/kg per day. Send stat repeat specimen to lab either as a venous or arterial sample; if hyperkalemia, stop IV fluids with potassium and hang clear fluids without potassium. See Figure 16.1 for detailed treatment options.

QUALITY METRICS

Monitor rates of treatment plans used; monitor length of time to bring the potassium level back to within the normal limits, severity of the out-of-range value (i.e., abnormal cardiac rhythms), and monitor cause of the hypokalemia or hyperkalemia.

SUMMARY

Once an abnormal potassium level is observed it is important to verify the value prior to initiating treatment. Once the value is verified there are several recommended treatment options based on the severity of abnormality and the patient's condition. Reviewing the neonate's gestational age, day of life, current potassium supplementation, urinary output, and medications the neonate is receiving are important factors to be evaluated prior to starting treatment for hypokalemia or hyperkalemia.

BIBLIOGRAPHIC SOURCE(S)

Bockenjauer D, Zieg J. Electrolyte disorders. *Clin Perinatol.* 2014;41(3):575-90.

Daly K, Farrington E. Hypokalemia and hyperkalemia in infants and children: pathophysiology and treatment. *J Pediatr Health Care.* 2013;27(6):486-96.

Gomella T, Cunningham M. *Neonatology: Management, Procedures, On-Call Problems, Diseases, and Drugs.* 7th ed. New York, NY: McGraw Hill; 2013.

Kerr B, Starbuck A, Block, S. Fluid and electrolyte management. In: Merenstein G, Gardner S, eds. *Handbook of Neonatal Intensive Care.* 6th ed. St. Louis, MO: Elsevier; 2006:351-67.

Nash P. Potassium and sodium homeostasis in the neonate. *Neonatal Network.* 2007;26(2):125-8.

Oh W. Fluid and electrolyte management of very low birth weight infants. *Pediatr Neonatol.* 2012;53:329-33.

Posencheg MA, Evans JR. *Avery's Diseases of the Newborn.* 9th ed. 2016. Retrieved from https://www.clinicalkey.com/#!/content/book/3-s2.0-B9781437701340100319.

Profit J. Fluid and electrolyte therapy in newborns. UpToDate. 2016. Accessed June 6, 2016.

Sarici D, Sarici SU. Neonatal hypokalemia. *Res Reports Neonatol.* 2012;(2):15-19.

Shah S, Catallozzi M, Zaoutis L, Frank G. *The Philadelphia Guide: Inpatient Pediatrics.* 2nd ed. New York, NY: McGraw-Hill Education; 2016.

Skorecki K, Chertow GM, Marsden PA, Taal MW, Yu ASL, eds. *Brenner & Rector's The Kidney.* 10th ed. Philadelphia, PA: Elsevier; 2016:2365-401.

Zenk KE, Sills JH, Koeppel RM. *Neonatal Medications & Nutrition: A Comprehensive Guide.* 2nd ed. Santa Rosa, CA: NICU Ink Book Publishers; 2000.

Hypernatremia and Hyponatremia

Andrew C. Bowe, DO, MS, FAAP

SCOPE

DISEASE/CONDITION(S)

Both hyponatremia and hypernatremia are common problems within the newborn intensive care unit. Hyponatremia, defined by a serum sodium less than 130 mEq/L, frequently occurs as a result of an inability to secrete a water load, increasing sodium losses, or poor sodium intake. Hypernatremia, defined as serum sodium greater than 150 mEq/L, frequently occurs as a result of increased losses of free body water, insufficient water intake, or inadvertent excess sodium administration.

GUIDELINE OBJECTIVE(S)

To provide guidance for neonatologists, pediatricians, advanced practitioners, and nurses on management of disorders of sodium equilibrium in the neonatal period.

BRIEF BACKGROUND

Treatment of hyponatremia (serum sodium <130 mEq/L) and hypernatremia (serum sodium >150 mEq/L) in newborn infants continues to be problematic. There is a significant lack of evidence to support specific management guidelines, and physiologic changes of the developing premature infant further confound treatment. These guidelines were developed with the intention to assemble and distribute more specific treatment methodologies to guide the clinician.

RECOMMENDATIONS

MAJOR RECOMMENDATIONS

Hyponatremia (Serum Sodium <130 mEq/L)

Hypovolemia. Defined by decreased total body sodium and total body water.

- If the **urine sodium <20 mEq/L**, one should consider *extra-renal losses* (i.e., vomiting, diarrhea, drainage tubes or fistulas, pleural effusions, ascites, ileus, and necrotizing enterocolitis).
  - Sodium content (mmol/L) of various body fluids:
    - Stomach: 20–80
    - Small intestine: 100–140
    - Bile: 120–140
    - Ileostomy: 45–135
    - Diarrheal stool: 10–90
- If the **urine sodium >20 mEq/L**, one should consider *renal losses* (i.e., diuretics, osmotic diuresis, contraction alkalosis, mineralocorticoid deficiency, mineralocorticoid resistance, Fanconi syndrome, Bartter syndrome, or obstructive uropathy).

Treatment. Volume expansion.

Recommendations:

1. Treat underlying cause.
2. In cases of symptomatic hyponatremia or Na <120 mEq/L, correction to a serum sodium above 120 mEq/L with 3% saline solution (0.513 mEq of sodium per milliliter) is recommended over 4–6 hours in addition to ongoing maintenance fluids at the appropriate rates suggested below. Calculation of the sodium deficit (mEq) and the use of fluids with the applicable sodium concentration may aid the clinician in more appropriate replacement of sodium deficits (Table 17.1).

$$\text{Total sodium deficit (mEq)} = (\text{ideal Na} - \text{actual Na}) \times 0.6 \times \text{weight in kg}$$

   a. Term infants: 60–80 mL/kg/day.
   b. Preterm infants 1250 g to 2000 g: 80–100 mL/kg/day, advancing by 20 mL/kg/day up to 140 mL/kg/day.
   c. Preterm infants <1250 g: 120 mL/kg/day, advancing by 20 mL/kg/day up to 140 mL/kg/day or higher depending on persistent insensible losses.

TABLE 17.1. **Free Water Content as a Volume of Common Intravenous Fluids**

Intravenous Fluid	Serum Sodium Concentration			
	145 mEq/L		195 mEq/L	
	Isotonic (%)	Water (%)	Isotonic (%)	Water (%)
Water	0	100	0	100
¼ saline	22	78	17	83
½ saline	50	50	39	61
Normal saline	100	0	79	21
Lactated Ringer's	86	14	68	32

3. Asymptomatic hyponatremia above 120 mEq/L can be corrected more slowly over 24–48 hours with 0.45% (0.077 mEq of sodium per milliliter) and 0.9% (0.154 mEq of sodium per milliliter) saline solutions.
4. Follow serum sodium concentrations closely at a minimum of every 6–12 hours until normal levels are achieved.

Euvolemia. Defined by variable body sodium concentrations and increased total body water.
- In this case, the **urine sodium is usually >20 mEq/L** and related to thyroid or glucocorticoid deficiencies or antidiuretic hormone (ADH) excess.

Treatment. Water restriction.

Recommendations:
1. Treat underlying cause.
2. Restriction of free water intake by decreasing total daily fluids by 15–20 mL/kg/day.
3. Repeat serum sodium in 12–24 hours until normalized.

Hypervolemia. Defined by increased total body sodium and increased total body water.
- If the **urine sodium <20 mEq/L**, one should consider *systemic etiologies of edema*, such as congestive heart failure, liver failure or cirrhosis, nephrotic syndrome, or indomethacin therapy.
- If the **urine sodium >20 mEq/L**, the likely cause is *renal failure* (either, acute or chronic).

Treatment. Sodium and water restriction.

Recommendations:
1. Treat underlying cause.
2. Restriction of free water intake by decreasing total daily fluids by 15–20 mL/kg/day.
3. Repeat serum sodium in 12–24 hours until normalized.
4. In instances of poor renal perfusion as determined by decreased urine output and/or elevated creatinine in the setting of hypervolemic hyponatremia (i.e., congestive heart failure or a hemodynamically significant patient ductus arteriosus), the use of low-dose dopamine to promote adequate renal function or medications furosemide and hydrocortisone can promote excretion of water. However, there is limited data to support these medications in infants and their use is highly situation-specific.

Hypernatremia (Serum Sodium >150 mEq/L)

Hypovolemia. Defined by decreased total body water.
- Hypernatremia in the very low birth weight infant during the first 24 hours is almost always due to water deficits. Also consider increased renal and insensible water losses or antidiuretic hormone (ADH) deficiency secondary to intraventricular hemorrhage (IVH).

Treatment. Replace free water deficit.

Recommendations:

1. If infant is a VLBW infant (<1500 g BW), correct insensible losses to the environment with polyethylene wrap, double-walled incubator, or the use of humidity.
2. Calculate free water deficit using the following equation:

$$\text{Free water deficit (L)} = 0.75 \times \text{weight in kg} \times \frac{(1 - \text{current Na concentration})}{145}$$

3. Replace free water deficits, in addition to maintenance fluids, at such a rate to decrease the serum sodium concentration by no more than 12 mEq/kg/day (see Table 17.1 for free water content estimates).
4. For term infants who are clinically stable with serum sodium values >120 mEq/L, oral fluid replacement with breast milk or formula may be safe and effective.
5. There are no data to support the use of enteral feeds using sterile water, especially for extremely low birth weight infants.

Euvolemia. Defined as increased total body sodium concentration, often related to the iatrogenic supplementation of high sodium–containing fluids.
- Sodium concentration of commonly used fluids (adapted from Molteni)
  - Sodium bicarbonate: mEq of sodium equals dose per kilogram.
  - Normal saline: 1.5 mEq of sodium for every 10 mL/kg administered.
  - Arterial line fluids using sodium chloride or acetate: 1 mEq/kg/d of sodium if using ½ normal saline (77 mEq/L) at 0.5 mL/kg/h.

Treatment. Decrease supplemental sodium.

Recommendations:

1. Review all fluids for excessive sodium and remove, particularly fluids through arterial lines and secondary ports of peripherally inserted central catheters (PICCs) or umbilical lines.
2. Consider increasing free water volume by 10–15 mL/kg/day to facilitate urinary excretion sodium.

Hypervolemia. Related to excessive administration of isotonic or hypertonic fluids.

Treatment. Restrict sodium administration and/or fluid administration.

Recommendations:

1. Review all fluids for excessive sodium and remove, particularly fluids through arterial lines and secondary ports of PICCs or umbilical lines.
2. Decrease total fluid volume by 10–15 mL/kg/day.
3. There is no evidence to support the use or disuse of furosemide for the reduction of hypervolemic hypernatremia. However, a short course over 2–3 days with serial measurements of electrolytes may be considered.

CLINICAL ALGORITHM(S)

As above.

IMPLEMENTATION OF GUIDELINE

QUALIFYING STATEMENTS

These recommendations are not intended to dictate an exclusive course of management or treatment. They must be evaluated with reference to individual patient needs, resources, and limitations unique to the institution and variations in local populations. It is hoped that this process of local ownership will help to incorporate these guidelines into routine practice. Attention is drawn to areas of clinical uncertainty where further research might be indicated.

SUMMARY

While the treatment of hyponatremia and hypernatremia in newborn infants can be problematic due to lack of evidence, the guidelines above are meant to provide a simple approach to this dilemma. In most cases, adjustment of total daily fluids and knowledge of basic daily sodium requirements and sodium concentrations of fluids can help maintain normal serum sodium concentrations. Further research is needed to provide more concise treatment strategies.

BIBLIOGRAPHIC SOURCE(S)

Avner ED. Clinical disorders of water metabolism: hyponatremia and hypernatremia. *Pediatr Ann.* 1995;24:23-30.

Erdemir A, Kahramaner Z, Cosar H, et al. Comparison of oral and intravenous fluid therapy in newborns with hypernatremic dehydration. *J Matern Fetal Neonatal Med.* 2014;27(5):491-4.

Fanaroff AA, Martin RJ, Walsh MC. *Fanaroff and Martin's Neonatal-Perinatal Medicine: Diseases of the Fetus and Infant.* 9th ed. Philadelphia, PA: Mosby Elsevier; 2011.

Gleason CA, Juul SE. *Avery's Diseases of the Newborn.* Elsevier Health Sciences; 2011.

Huston RK, Dietz AM, Campbell BB, Dolphin NG, Sklar RS, Wu YX. Enteral water for hypernatremia and intestinal morbidity in infants less than or equal to 1000 g birth weight. *J Perinatol.* 2007;27(1):32-8.

Molteni KH. Initial management of hypernatremic dehydration in the breastfed infant. *Clin Pediatr.* 1994;33:731-40.

Olney CJ, Huseby V, Kennedy KA, Morris BH. Sterile water gastric drip in extremely low birthweight infants: a randomized trial. *Am J Perinatol.* 2005;22(5):253-8.

Parish A, Bhatia J. Nutritional considerations in the intensive care unit: neonatal issues. In: Shikora SA, Martindale RG, Schwaitzberg SD, eds. *Nutritional Considerations in the Intensive Care Unit: Science, Rationale and Practice.* Dubuque, IA: Kendall/Hunt; 2002:297-309.

Acidosis and Alkalosis

Alejandro Frade Garcia, MD • Saima Aftab, MD

SCOPE

DISEASE/CONDITION(S)

Neonatal acidosis and alkalosis.

GUIDELINE OBJECTIVE(S)

Physiology, pathology, diagnosis, and management of acid-base pathology.

BRIEF BACKGROUND

Acid-base homeostasis is the regulation of the pH in the extracellular space of the body and is crucial for physiologic cellular function. The pH at which proteins optimally function is very narrow (7.35–7.45); therefore, very complex mechanisms are in place to control it. In the immediate postnatal period as the baby is transitioning to extrauterine life, the body is susceptible to numerous conditions that may disturb the balance in the pH. In addition, in the newborn period, the adaptive responses to reach equilibrium of acid base balance are still maturing, making the newborn more susceptible to these changes in the pH homeostasis. At the time of delivery, the baby experiences an abrupt increase in the sensitivity of the central respiratory control to changes in pH compared to that of fetal life. There is also a steady but gradual increase in the intracellular compartment after birth which enhances the body's buffering system. In general, the body's pH is tightly regulated by three basic systems: the respiratory system, the renal system, and the chemical buffers. Imbalance in this balance or homeostasis is known as acidosis when the acidity is high (low pH), or alkalosis when the acidity is low (high pH). Soon after delivery, there are a series of changes in the cardiac and respiratory systems that allow the lungs to serve for gas exchange, establishing their role as the end organ of respiratory compensation for acid-base homeostasis. The respiratory cycle controls the carbonic acid concentration in the extracellular fluid by blowing off or retaining carbon dioxide (CO_2) and ultimately, carbonic acid from the plasma. Respiratory acidosis implies an elevated CO_2 level in the plasma. This may be due to respiratory distress, as seen in pneumonia, or surfactant deficiency or poor respiratory drive due to medications or perinatal depression. The respiratory acidosis triggers an immediate increase in ventilation, as CO_2 will diffuse freely across the blood-brain barrier and stimulates the respiratory drive center in the central nervous system. Metabolic acidosis implies a net low level of base in the plasma. This can be due to loss of bicarbonate in the kidneys or gastrointestinal tract, or increased levels of fixed acids such as lactate, etc. in the plasma, as seen in states of shock. When acidosis is metabolic in origin, the compensation is delayed for hours due to the time needed to equilibrate plasma and cerebrospinal fluid bicarbonate. Neonates with an immature pulmonary system, especially premature infants, have a decreased capacity for respiratory compensation of the acid-base balance. The renal system's role in maintaining the acid-base balance is through adding or removing bicarbonate ions from the extracellular fluid. The renal tubular cells enzymatically convert CO_2 into carbonic acid, which dissociates into bicarbonate (HCO_3) and hydrogen ions. With acidosis, the kidney excretes hydrogen ions into the urine and secretes the bicarbonate ions into the blood plasma in an effort to raise the pH. The opposite happens with alkalosis. The renal compensatory mechanism is immature in the neonatal period, decreasing the ability to maintain homeostasis. Glomerular filtration rate is low in the immediate postnatal period and increases exponentially with time, which again predisposes the newborn period to acid-base imbalance. Of note, preterm neonates are prone to bicarbonate losses in the urine due to immaturity of the renal tubular system. That is why they are prone to metabolic acidosis in the first few days of life. Lastly, the chemical buffers that minimize abrupt changes in pH are the bicarbonate buffer system, the phosphate buffer system, and the protein buffer system. These chemical buffers do not correct pH deviations but stabilize the pH, making imbalance less likely.

Metabolic Acidosis

Metabolic acidosis is defined as acidosis with a base deficit greater than 5 mEq/L. In metabolic acidosis it is useful to calculate the anion gap, which is the result of the difference between sodium and the sum of chloride and bicarbonate. The normal value is 8–16 mEq/L. The most common causes of increased anion-gap metabolic acidosis in this patient population are hypoxemia or ischemia secondary to perinatal asphyxia, hypovolemia, vasoregulatory disturbances, myocardial dysfunction from immaturity, metabolic disorders, and sepsis. All these conditions may result in an elevated lactate level and hence a wide anion gap acidosis. Premature neonates tend to develop mild to moderate non-anion-gap acidosis due to the premature kidneys' low threshold for bicarbonate. Metabolic acidosis has several major consequences, including pulmonary vasoconstriction with risk of persistent pulmonary hypertension, decreased myocardial contractility, shift of oxygen hemoglobin dissociation to the right, neurological damage, and respiratory compensation which can cause respiratory distress.

Respiratory Acidosis

Respiratory acidosis is defined as acidosis associated with an elevated plasma CO_2 level, or partial pressure of carbon dioxide ($PaCO_2$). The normal range for $PaCO_2$ is 35 to 45. In this age group, the most common cause of respiratory acidosis is respiratory distress syndrome, as any pulmonary pathology that may compromise ventilation will subsequently lead to a buildup of CO_2 leading to respiratory acidosis.

Metabolic Alkalosis

Metabolic alkalosis is a disturbance in acid base balance caused by a primary increase in serum bicarbonate (HCO_3^-) concentration. The most common cause of metabolic alkalosis in the neonatal period is iatrogenic, as a result of diuretic treatment that may be used in treatment of bronchopulmonary dysplasia in premature newborns.

Respiratory Alkalosis

Respiratory alkalosis is a disturbance in acid-base balance caused by a decreased plasma CO_2 level or $PaCO_2$, due to alveolar hyperventilation. This may be seen in neonates with fever, pain, or inborn errors of metabolism such as urea cycle disorders and so forth.

The utilization of a venous, capillary, or arterial blood gas is an important laboratory test in the evaluation of a newborn's acid-base status. The gasometry has four basic components: the pH, $PaCO_2$, partial pressure of oxygen (PaO_2), and the HCO_3. The pH is a numeric scale used to determine if an aqueous solution is acidic or basic; it is a logarithmic expression of hydrogen ion concentration. Normal pH in arterial samples is 7.4 ± 0.05, where a pH less than 7.35 indicates acidosis and one more than 7.45 indicates alkalosis. Both conditions can be caused by respiratory or metabolic processes. $PaCO_2$ in the blood measures adequate minute ventilation; the normal value in an arterial sample ranges from 35 to 45 mmHg. For every 10 mmHg change from baseline, the pH changes by 0.08. PaO_2 in the blood measures oxygenation; the normal value ranges from 80 to 100 mmHg in a patient breathing room air. HCO_3 is an ion which helps measure the metabolic component of the acid-base status ventilation; the normal value in an arterial sample ranges from 22 to 28 mEq/L. Base excess is defined as the amount of acid required to normalize the pH on a liter of blood at a baseline $PaCO_2$ of 40 mmHg. The base excess increases in metabolic alkalosis and decreases in metabolic acidosis. In the 1950s, it was recognized that sampling the umbilical cord for evaluation of gas analysis could be an indication of preceding fetal hypoxia. It has since been common practice to evaluate cord gases if there is suspected neonatal distress or for high-risk deliveries. Analyzing the pH, base excess, and $PaCO_2$ from arterial blood in the umbilical cord can help evaluate the metabolic condition of a neonate at the moment of birth.

Pathway for work-up is summarized in Figure 18.1.

RECOMMENDATIONS

MAJOR RECOMMENDATIONS

Acid-base imbalance has to be suspected in critically ill newborns despite no clear signs and symptoms to suggest acidosis or alkalosis. The diagnosis is made with a blood gas, preferably arterial. When analyzing an arterial blood gas, a systematic approach while reading the results will help understand the etiology of the imbalance and therefore where to target treatment. First, determine if the pH is normal or abnormal (7.35–7.45).

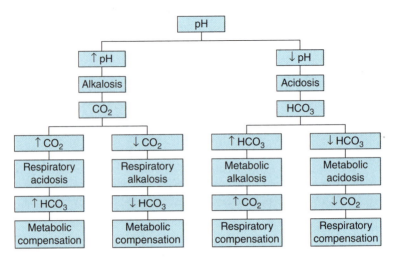

FIGURE 18.1 • Blood gas analysis algorithm.

Remember, a low pH indicates acidosis and a high pH alkalosis. However, values may normalize once compensatory mechanisms from the respiratory or renal systems have taken place. Second, determine if the $PaCO_2$ is high (>45 mmHg) or low (<35 mmHg). A gas with a high $PaCO_2$ and low pH suggests respiratory acidosis. Third, evaluate the HCO_3. If it is low with a low pH, this indicates metabolic acidosis, and conversely if the HCO_3 is high and the pH is high, this indicates metabolic alkalosis. If these conditions have been present for several hours or days, the compensatory mechanisms have already initiated. Often the abnormalities are mixed, having components of both respiratory and metabolic origin. Management of acid-based disorders should be aimed toward treating the underlying cause when possible. For treatment of severe metabolic acidosis, volume resuscitation may be the first-line treatment when elevated lactate levels are due to shock, perinatal depression, or poor perfusion. Use of an alkali such as sodium bicarbonate ($NaHCO_3$) is highly controversial. This is generally discouraged for use in the neonate, as sick neonates often have inadequate ventilation, which supplementation of $NaHCO_3$ will worsen due to liberation of CO_2. It is only used in severe cases due to risks of hyperosmolality, intracranial hemorrhage, hypocalcemia, paradoxical central nervous system acidosis, among other side effects. Hyperventilation should be avoided, as it can cause deleterious effects on cardiac output and pulmonary blood flow. In critically ill neonates on parenteral nutrition, maximization of acetate and minimizing chloride will help correct the acidosis. Alkalosis due to hyperventilation is corrected by appropriate adjustments to ventilation. If alkalosis is secondary to diuretic use, adequate chloride repletion or addition of a potassium-sparing agent to the regimen to replace potassium and chloride deficits may be helpful. If the loss is via vomiting or diarrhea, rehydration is key in order to keep up with loses. Bartter syndrome, an inherited defect in electrolyte regulation in the thick ascending tubule, is corrected by replacing electrolytes. Respiratory etiologies of acid-base imbalances are usually treated with managing the baseline condition and improving ventilation.

PRACTICE OPTIONS

Practice Option #1: Respiratory Acidosis Gasometry: pH 7.29, CO$_2$ 57, HCO$_3$ 24, PaO$_2$ 70

The first step is to analyze the pH, which in this case is low, meaning acidosis (less than 7.35); also note that CO$_2$ is elevated (more than 45). The combination of a low pH with a high CO$_2$ corresponds to respiratory acidosis; the normal HCO$_3$ with abnormal pH indicates that the abnormality is acute, hence the renal compensatory mechanisms have not started. PaO$_2$ is low, meaning not only is ventilation compromised, but also oxygenation has been affected.

When evaluating the patient in this case it is important to have a complete assessment, starting with evaluation of the airway and breathing as well as the circulation. Once those are established, individual case assessment will be based on the concomitant symptoms. A complete physical examination will point toward the etiology of the abnormal gas, which in this case points to the respiratory system. Based on acuity, associated pathology, and clinical context, a decision will be made on how to correct the respiratory problem. This may begin with adequate positioning of the head or possibly escalate to providing respiratory support through CPAP, noninvasive ventilation, or advanced airway placement with mechanical ventilation.

Practice Option # 2: Metabolic Acidosis Gasometry: pH 7.22, CO$_2$ 32, HCO$_3$ 12, PaO$_2$ 90

The first step is to analyze the pH, which in this case is low, meaning acidosis (less than 7.35); CO$_2$ is low normal (35–45), HCO$_3$ is low (less than 22). The combination of low pH with low HCO$_3$ indicates a metabolic acidosis. Treatment of neonatal metabolic acidosis consists of supportive care and specific measures dependent upon the cause. Treatment of hypothermia, dehydration, hypoxia, and electrolyte disturbances will usually be needed in the NICU setting.

Practice Option #3: Metabolic Alkalosis Gasometry: pH 7.49, CO$_2$ 42, HCO$_3$ 38, PaO$_2$ 89

The first step is to analyze the pH, which in this case is high, meaning alkalosis (more than 7.45), CO$_2$ is within normal limits (35–45), HCO$_3$ is high (more than 28). The combination of high pH with high HCO$_3$ gives a diagnosis of metabolic alkalosis. Evaluation of the possible etiology and correcting the cause is the ideal management in cases of metabolic alkalosis.

BIBLIOGRAPHIC SOURCE(S)

Benaron DA, Yorgin PD, Lapuk S, Gibson R, Dennery PA. Alkalemia in a newborn infant. *J Pediatr.* 1992;120:489-94.

Brouillette RT, Waxman DH. Evaluation of the newborn's blood gas status. *Clin Chem.* 1997;43:1.

Delivoria-Papadopoulos M, McGowan JE. Oxygen transport and delivery. In: Polin RA, Fox WW, Abman SH, eds. *Fetal and Neonatal Physiology*. Philadelphia, PA: Saunders; 2004:880-9.

Farmand M. Blood gas analysis and the fundamentals of acid-base balance. *Neonatal Netw.* 2009;28(2):125-8.

Fencl V, Jabor A, Kazda A, Figge J. Diagnosis of metabolic acid base disturbances in critically ill patients. *Am J Respir Crit Care Med.* 2000;162:2246-51.

Gomella TL, Cunningham MD. *Neonatology*. 7th ed. McGraw-Hill; 2013.

Henderson LJ. The theory of neutrality regulation in the animal organism. *Am J Physiol*. 1908;21:427-48.

Kellum JA. Clinical review: reunification of acid-base physiology. *Crit Care*. 2005;9:500-7.

Lekhwani S, Shanker V, Gathwala G, Vaswani ND. Acid-base disorders in critically ill neonates. *Indian J Crit Care Med*. 2010;14(2):65-9.

Malley WJ. *Clinical Blood Gases: Assessment and Intervention*. 2nd ed. Philadelphia, PA: Saunders; 2005.

Morrison RS. Metabolic acidosis and alkalosis. *N Engl J Med*. 1966;274:1195-7.

Yeomans ER, Hauth JC, Gilstrap LC III, Strickland DM. Umbilical cord pH, PCO_2, and bicarbonate following uncomplicated term vaginal deliveries (146 infants). *Am J Obstet Gynecol*. 1985;151:798-800.

Young DG. Neonatal acid-base disturbances. *Arch Dis Child*. 1966;41:201.

Respiratory Distress

Surfactant Therapy

Megan Lagoski, MD • Aaron Hamvas, MD

SCOPE

DISEASE/CONDITION(S)

Neonatal respiratory distress syndrome (RDS).

GUIDELINE OBJECTIVE(S)

Surfactant administration: indications, types of surfactant, timing, and route of administration.

BRIEF BACKGROUND

Pulmonary surfactant is a phospholipid-protein complex that decreases surface tension at the air-liquid interface of the alveolus, thus maintaining alveolar expansion at end expiration. This complex is comprised of phospholipid, primarily phosphatidylcholine, and surfactant-associated proteins that facilitate the surface tension lowering properties (surfactant proteins B and C [SP-B, SP-C]) and provide immunologic functions (surfactant proteins A and D).

Clinical use of exogenous surfactant products began with the FDA approval in 1990 in the United States after many international trials. Since that earliest approval for Exosurf, a synthetic phospholipid preparation, several additional preparations have been approved for clinical use worldwide. All trials have shown consistent results: decrease in the risk of death from RDS and a decrease in the incidence of pneumothorax. These trials have investigated the early and later use of surfactant, the type of surfactant, and the dosing regimen. However, as neonatal and obstetrical practice has changed, with up to 90% of women with threatened preterm labor receiving antenatal corticosteroids and the increasingly prevalent use of noninvasive ventilation, new questions are arising that have not been answered by large multicenter, randomized clinical trials. In this guideline we attempt to answer some of these questions based on available literature and clinical experience.

RECOMMENDATIONS

MAJOR RECOMMENDATIONS

To formulate recommendations for the various aspects of surfactant administration, one must consider the conditions under which the evidence was gathered and the constant advances made in medicine. Over the past 25 years since surfactant first received FDA approval and became more widely available, perinatal practices have evolved significantly. The most significant change in antenatal management was the accepted use of antenatal steroids for fetuses 24–34 weeks: any woman qualifying for tocolytics is also a candidate for corticosteroids. As corticosteroids have been shown to decrease the risk of RDS by accelerating fetal lung maturation, short-term respiratory outcomes have improved. Many of the initial randomized controlled trials (RCTs) involving surfactant administration (prophylactic vs late selective/rescue treatment) were performed prior to this widespread use of corticosteroids.

Resuscitation guidelines have also changed within this time period with emphasis in establishing functional residual capacity (FRC), the use of noninvasive ventilation, and gentler ventilation strategies. In combination with the use of antenatal steroids, these approaches have led to more success in avoiding intubation.

One must also consider the environment where the resuscitation is taking place and the availability of resources. Most studies are conducted at Level III(+) NICUs where other modes of noninvasive ventilation are readily available, as are support staff who are comfortable with these techniques. In non-tertiary or quaternary facilities, these resources are often not available. Also, the patient population is often very different from that studied—maternal or fetal conditions often preclude the ability to transfer, and deliveries are often precipitous; thus steroid treatment is either not able to be given or is provided shortly before delivery.

TIMING OF SURFACTANT ADMINISTRATION

Before deciding when to give surfactant, one must determine who should get surfactant. Those with the most immature lungs are also surfactant deficient and are at highest risk for lung injury from the force required to maintain adequate oxygenation and ventilation. As exogenous surfactant increases compliance and permits easier establishment of FRC, this group would be the most likely to respond. However, not all neonates at risk for RDS need to be intubated. With careful, gentle resuscitation, many of the neonates may be supported with less invasive modes of respiratory support. Those that go on to require intubation, with or without mechanical ventilation, appear to be at the highest risk for further lung injury, so should receive surfactant. Below, we examine the independent yet intrinsically linked decision-making for when to intubate and when to administer surfactant. An algorithm for the approach to decision-making for administration is shown in Figure 19.1.

Decision to Intubate

The decision to intubate in the delivery room is not a simple one and depends on the stability of the baby, the equipment available, and the comfort level of all team members

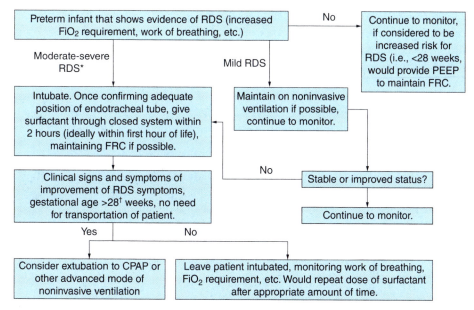

FIGURE 19.1 • Algorithm for decision-making for intubation and surfactant administration. *Moderate RDS in the lower gestational ages or worsening RDS despite adequate resuscitation efforts and noninvasive respiratory support would be signs that intubation should be performed. †Some centers may feel more comfortable extubating patients at earlier gestational ages shortly after giving surfactant if they have reliable methods of providing noninvasive ventilation.

involved in the care. The patients at highest risk for severe RDS are those that are extremely premature (<28 weeks), were not exposed to antenatal steroids, were exposed to maternal chorioamnionitis, and those with maternal/placental/fetal conditions causing fetal distress. In these cases, it is likely that these patients will require a higher level of respiratory support, so early surfactant administration should be considered. We recommend that any neonate exhibiting any signs of respiratory failure as listed in Table 19.1 should be intubated shortly after delivery and treated with surfactant.

TABLE 19.1. Clinical Signs of Respiratory Failure that Warrant Intubation and Surfactant Administration

Ongoing bradycardia

Apnea or poor respiratory drive

Ongoing requirement for positive pressure ventilation to maintain heart rate and SpO_2

Increased work of breathing despite adequate level PEEP

Elevated or rising FiO_2 requirement

Lack of reliable equipment to maintain stable respiratory status on noninvasive ventilation

Concern for airway stability on noninvasive ventilation if requiring transport

Conversely, if a neonate shows clinical improvement with noninvasive ventilation, the evidence supports the continuation of this mode and closely monitoring for signs of worsening respiratory distress. The risk of air leak and BPD is decreased when using a lower threshold to intubate and give surfactant (FiO_2 <0.45). In addition to FiO_2, increased work of breathing and hemodynamic instability (apnea, bradycardia, and/or ongoing desaturations) should also be indicators of need for intubation and surfactant administration. Those at the highest risk for lung damage from volu-/atelecto-trauma should be resuscitated carefully with a low threshold for intubation and surfactant administration.

Once the decision to intubate has been made, especially in the delivery room, many providers feel comfortable giving surfactant with confidence that the endotracheal tube is in appropriate position, as indicated by symmetric breath sounds and an estimate of the depth of the tube relative to the gums (alveolar ridge): approximately 6 cm plus the estimated weight of the infant in kilogram. For example, a 1-kg infant should have the tube placed at 7 cm at the gum line. Other providers only feel comfortable administering surfactant after verifying adequate endotracheal tube positioning with a chest radiograph.

Early versus Late Administration

To define timing of surfactant administration, studies have examined two major strategies: 1) prophylaxis in which surfactant is administered as close to the first breath as possible in an effort to improve compliance rapidly and minimize alveolar injury, and 2) rescue treatment, in which surfactant is administered once an infant demonstrates development of RDS and the need for intubation. Early studies demonstrated that surfactant administration immediately or shortly after birth (20 minutes) improved short-term respiratory outcomes, decreased complications (i.e., pneumothorax, pulmonary interstitial emphysema, etc.), and resulted in shorter duration of mechanical ventilation when compared to waiting until development of clinical/radiologic signs of worsening RDS. However, these studies also estimated that up to 50% of infants who were treated at delivery might not have required intubation. These trials failed to consistently demonstrate any decrease in the risk for bronchopulmonary dysplasia (BPD) or chronic lung disease (CLD). In more recent trials where neonates were randomized to receive either prophylactic intubation and surfactant administration or noninvasive ventilation via continuous positive airway pressure (CPAP) (SUPPORT, COIN, VON DRM, Curpap, Neocosur, and Columbian network trials), the superiority of giving prophylactic surfactant was no longer demonstrated, with evidence that avoiding intubation, surfactant, and mechanical ventilation when possible may be preferable. In the SUPPORT trial, including neonates at 24 weeks, outcomes were significantly improved in those 24–25 weeks that were able to remain on CPAP.

Thus evidence does not support the prophylaxis approach, but data suggest that consideration of intubation and early surfactant administration within the first 2 hours in a neonate with developing RDS provides an advantage over later administration. A Cochrane review examining the outcomes of early versus late surfactant administration demonstrated clear benefits of giving surfactant earlier. Both short- and long-term outcomes (decreased risk of mortality and trend toward decreased risk for BPD) were improved when giving surfactant earlier for patients requiring mechanical ventilation. In the newer studies, the early INSURE (INtubate, SUrfactant, Rapid Extubation) method decreased need for reintubation, subsequent surfactant doses, and reduced time of mechanical ventilation. Of note, the time period for "rapid" extubation varies from immediately to 6 hours after surfactant administration.

After surfactant administration, management should be based on the degree of respiratory distress prior to and after the surfactant is administered in addition to the availability of reliable noninvasive ventilation. In studies of the INSURE method, predictors of failure included low gestational age, birth weight <750 g, hemoglobin <8.5 g/dL, high FiO_2/low paO_2, and a/ApO_2 <0.44 on first blood gas. Thus it may be beneficial to maintain mechanical ventilation for a longer period of time (>2 hours). In contrast, the INSURE method is more effective in higher gestational ages and would be an ideal method to use if practicing in a hospital without a tertiary NICU to attempt to avoid transfer of neonates >32 weeks, 1500 g, etc. if a skilled practitioner is readily available. In these cases, the standard of care is to extubate to nasal CPAP. If a patient requires transport to a tertiary facility, the most reasonable option is to maintain a secure airway and mechanical ventilation for stability on transport.

The Golden Hour Initiative, in which a bundle of care focused on thermoregulation, cardiovascular stability, respiratory support, and fluid management in the initial phases of care, is increasing in popularity and has, in small retrospective studies, shown some improvement in short- and long-term outcomes. A goal of giving surfactant within this time frame allows adequate time to stabilize in the delivery room, transport to NICU, and confirm correct placement of the endotracheal tube.

In summary, if a patient with increased risk for or signs of RDS needs to be intubated, it follows that surfactant should be given. For patients under 26 weeks, minimal data exist about whether to intubate and give surfactant prophylactically or attempt to maintain noninvasive ventilation (excluding the SUPPORT trial). In these cases, and especially if combined with risk factors increasing the likelihood of more severe or complex RDS, prophylactic intubation and surfactant administration can still be performed and may decrease the risk of short-term complications such as air leak or pneumothorax and may decrease the duration of mechanical ventilation.

ROUTE OF SURFACTANT ADMINISTRATION

Four formulations of surfactant are commercially available in the United States (Table 19.2). Natural surfactants, that is, those derived from porcine or bovine lungs, contain small amounts of surfactant proteins B and C in addition to the phospholipid, and thus tend to work more quickly and are the most widely used preparations. The recent approval of lucinactant, a synthetic phospholipid with a synthetic hydrophobic peptide that mimics the biophysical effects of SP-B, provides an alternative to the animal-derived products. Although some studies have demonstrated small differences in mortality, each preparation has relatively similar short- and long-term outcomes.

Currently, the only widely approved method of giving surfactant is through an endotracheal tube. Ideally, this should be a closed sterile system via a 5 or 8 French feeding tube or suction catheter or a side port in the circuit where a constant level of positive pressure is flowing to maintain FRC. In animal models, distribution of surfactant is more uniform with quick administration. The most common/easiest method of administering is in two separate aliquots, turning the neonate from midline to one side, administering the surfactant, returning to midline for a short (1–2 minutes) recovery period, and then turning to the other side and administering the second aliquot. The problem with administering in less than two aliquots is a transient blockage of the endotracheal tube or reflux of surfactant into the tubing.

Other, less invasive methods of surfactant have been studied with attempts to avoid intubation. A technique whereby a thin catheter is visually inserted into the trachea

TABLE 19.2. Surfactant Preparations Available in the United States

Name of Surfactant	Derivation	Components and Concentration per mL	Dosage	Maximum Number of Doses	Frequency
Beractant (Survanta)	Bovine minced lung extract	25 mg phospholipids (11–15.5 mg DPPC) <1 mg SP-B + SP-C	4 mL/kg	4	Every 6 hours
Calfactant (Infasurf)	Bovine lavage extract	35 mg phospholipids (16 mg DPPC) 0.7 mg SP-B + SP-C	3 mL/kg	4	Every 6–12 hours
Poractant Alfa (Curosurf)	Porcine minced lung extract	76 mg/mL phospholipids (30 mg DPPC) 1 mg SP-B + SP-C	2.5 mL/ kg (1st dose) 1.25 mL/kg (2nd/3rd doses)	3	Every 12 hours
Lucinactant (Surfaxin)	Synthetic	30 mg/mL phospholipids (22.5 mg DPPC) 0.862 mg SP-B analog	5.8 mL/kg	4	Every 6 hours

All information obtained from package inserts of products.

and surfactant is administered while the patient remains on CPAP has been gaining favor. Studies using this technique for infants with worsening RDS demonstrate a decreased need for subsequent intubation and mechanical ventilation. Of note, aerosolized surfactant administration is currently being studied in a phase II trial. Table 19.3 describes other modes of noninvasive surfactant instillation that have been studied in small pilot trials.

REPEATED DOSES

Early trials of single versus multiple doses of surfactant demonstrated a reduced risk of morbidity and mortality of premature neonates where multiple doses of surfactant were given. In a Cochrane review performed in 2009, the results of three studies from the 1990s were analyzed. In each of the studies (two using animal-derived surfactant and one using synthetic protein-free surfactant), infants were randomized to receive either a single dose of surfactant or multiple doses of surfactant at set intervals. When combining the results, a trend toward reduction of pneumothorax and decreased risk of mortality was demonstrated. Also, a more sustained response was obtained, a lower FiO_2 was required, and decreased need for mechanical ventilation was shown. In addition, the risk of pulmonary hemorrhage was not increased in multiple versus single doses of surfactant.

TABLE 19.3. Approved and Experimental Modes of Surfactant Administration

Mode of Surfactant Administration	FDA Approved/Level of Studies Completed	Brief Description	Advantages	Disadvantages
Intratracheal via endotracheal tube	Approved Multiple phase 3 RCTs	Surfactant is given most commonly through 5/8F catheter threaded through ETT in bolus dosing with or without administration of positive pressure.	Most evidence Easiest way to insure dose is administered Uniform distribution	Airway trauma Needing adequate ETT placement to ensure uniform distribution Difficult to maintain FRC depending on method of instillation Hemodynamic instability
Thin catheter/less invasive surfactant administration (LISA)	Experimental Multiple RCTs, observational studies	5F catheter is threaded into trachea via forceps under direct laryngoscopy; surfactant administered through catheter.	Less risk of airway trauma May avoid mechanical ventilation and volu-/barotrauma	Slower instillation of surfactant Increased incidence of reflux of surfactant Dependent on adequately spontaneous breathing
Aerosolized	Experimental 2 RCTs One pilot study, one active phase II study	Aerosolized surfactant is given while patient is on CPAP. Dose and frequency varies.	Theoretical avoidance of intubation and ventilation	Small number of patients enrolled No significant difference in amount progressing to intubation No decrease in RDS
Laryngeal mask airway (LMA) instillation	Experimental Several RCTs in past 3 years with ~200 total patients	Patients on CPAP had LMA placed. Surfactant administered via 5f tube through LMA and then given 2 minutes PPV.	Avoidance of intubation Does not require spontaneous breathing May decrease need for mechanical ventilation	Size limitation for LMAs Risk of baro-/volutrauma from manual PPV still present
Nasopharyngeal instillation	Experimental Small observational studies	After delivery of the head, surfactant administered into nasopharynx. Patients placed on CPAP afterward.	Avoids intubation/risk of airway trauma May avoid unnecessary PPV	Difficult to perform if breech delivery, precipitous delivery Dose administered is unknown

Drawing conclusions and basing practices off of these results is difficult, as further studies to address this question have not been performed since clinical practices have evolved. Retrospective studies demonstrate that more premature patients with risk factors or signs of worse RDS require multiple doses of surfactant but do not clearly or consistently identify what parameters are used to make these decisions.

When considering the known causes of lung injury, largely based on animal data, we can extrapolate the factors that can potentially induce that injury in neonates with RDS: oxygen toxicity, atelecto-trauma, volutrauma, stretch, etc. As surfactant administration may be able to decrease the chance of lung injury in those most susceptible, it would be beneficial to base guidelines for repeat dosing on surfactant on multiple criteria. Many use the cutoff of FiO_2 of 0.4 for repeating surfactant administration. However, regardless of the mode of ventilation (i.e., noninvasive or invasive), we recommend using multiple parameters for making this decision, including increasing FiO_2 requirement, increasing ventilator support, and increasing work of breathing as indications for additional doses of surfactant.

The benefits of exogenous surfactant administration tend to decline after 48–72 hours when endogenous production of surfactant increases. Thus, additional doses beyond this time period are unlikely to provide significant benefits.

OFF-LABEL USES OF SURFACTANT

Since the benefits of exogenous surfactant replacement in neonates with RDS have been identified and repeatedly validated through multiple RCTs and meta-analyses, other uses of surfactant have been investigated. Multiple medical conditions specific to neonates have been shown to displace and/or deactivate surfactant (i.e., meconium aspiration syndrome, pulmonary hemorrhage, neonatal pneumonia) or create deficiency of and impair the function of surfactant (i.e., SP-B deficiency). As these ideas are relatively newer, fewer studies have been performed.

Meconium Aspiration Syndrome

Multiple pilot studies have demonstrated the relative safety of surfactant use. Four RCTs used bolus dosing of surfactant and four RCTs used a surfactant lavage. Two Cochrane reviews analyze these studies and, although no difference in mortality was reported, both demonstrated a statistically significant decrease in the risk for extracorporeal membrane oxygenation (ECMO). Although no other statistically significant outcomes were affected, this reduction in need for ECMO supports the use of surfactant. Currently, bolus dosing of surfactant is the most widely accepted method of administration for this disease condition. Specific parameters for use in meconium aspiration are not given. However, in absence of air leak and evidence of decreased or worsening compliance, a dose of surfactant seems to be a reasonable therapy for these infants with respiratory distress.

Pulmonary Hemorrhage

No RCTs have been performed to date, but retrospective analysis demonstrates that clinical course is improved by giving surfactant. In one study including 15 infants (diagnoses split between underlying RDS with pulmonary hemorrhage, meconium aspiration with pulmonary hemorrhage, and isolated pulmonary hemorrhage), an improvement in the oxygenation index was noted as well as no deterioration after surfactant administration. Another retrospective analysis of 27 neonates noted that outcomes also improved after surfactant therapy, particularly if given early after pulmonary hemorrhage had been diagnosed. More recently, a trial comparing effects of two different surfactants (beractant and poractant) in the treatment of pulmonary hemorrhage was conducted. The use of both surfactants noted an improvement in oxygenation but no significant differences were noted between the two groups. Although no parameters have been defined for when or how to treat neonates, it can be extrapolated that surfactant therapy can acutely improve the course of pulmonary hemorrhage.

Bacterial Pneumonia/Neonatal Sepsis

As neonates with bacterial pneumonia have reduced surfactant production, surfactant dysfunction, inactivation, or peroxidation, it is postulated that providing exogenous surfactant would be beneficial to these neonates. In addition, in animal studies, the administration of exogenous surfactant may enhance bacterial clearance. However, implementation of a study in neonates has not been performed to date due to the difficulty in definitive diagnosis of pneumonia versus respiratory distress secondary to sepsis. A study by Herting evaluated the effects of surfactant therapy on 28 patients that had been diagnosed with group B strep infection via culture (blood, urine, cerebrospinal fluid, tracheal aspirate, gastric aspirate, and/or skin swab) and respiratory failure. The results demonstrated reduced FiO_2 requirement but approximately 25% of patients did not respond to surfactant therapy. With this limited evidence, strong recommendations cannot be made, but it appears that benefits outweigh risks in treating with surfactant if intubating due to worsening respiratory distress.

Congenital Diaphragmatic Hernia

Studies suggesting a diminished surfactant pool in the presence of a diaphragmatic hernia led to small trials of surfactant replacement but without clear success. Thus there is no evidence to recommend surfactant replacement in this setting.

Inherited Disorders of Surfactant Metabolism

Mutations in the genes encoding SP-B and SP-C and the ATP-binding cassette member A3 (ABCA3) result in severe neonatal surfactant deficiency, primarily in late preterm or term newborns. The surfactant synthesized in these disorders has diminished function, due to either abnormal phospholipid composition or inhibition by incompletely processed prosurfactant peptides. Theoretically surfactant replacement should help; however, since surfactant metabolism is a dynamic process, with a turnover of the surfactant pool in a period of 8–24 hours, the exogenously administered surfactant is rapidly replaced by the native dysfunctional surfactant. One published experience of using surfactant replacement for SP-B deficiency demonstrated this phenomenon in that over 80 doses were administered over 3 weeks and resulted in only transient and increasingly shorter responses to treatment. Other case reports have also mentioned these transient responses. Thus data do not suggest that routine surfactant replacement be used in these situations, although if an infant's clinical condition deteriorates and a temporizing measure is needed, especially if the infant is awaiting lung transplantation, an occasional dose might provide that bridge to respiratory stability.

Late Surfactant for the Prevention of BPD

Clinical trials are underway to determine if surfactant administration to premature infants who still require mechanical ventilation after 7 days will prevent or decrease the severity

TABLE 19.4. Equipment Required for Surfactant Administration

Endotracheal tubes (and stylet)
Tape or other securing device
End tidal CO_2 detector (Pediacap)
Means to provide positive pressure ventilation
• Anesthesia bag
• Self-inflating bag
• NeoPuff
Suction
Closed ventilation/suction system, if available
If a closed system is not available:
• Sterile gloves
• Sterile suction catheters or feeding tubes cut to the length of the endotracheal tube
• Sterile scissors to cut feeding tube
Syringe and needle to draw up surfactant

of BPD (Trial Of Late SURFactant [TOLSURF]; ClinicalTrials.gov NCT00569530). The trial has completed enrollment, and data analysis and follow-up are underway.

IMPLEMENTATION OF GUIDELINE AND QUALITY METRICS

For a hospital that does not regularly care for premature babies, the decision to have surfactant available depends on several factors, including the number of premature births, the expertise and comfort level of the newborn care team, the expense and limited shelf life of the surfactant preparations, and the proximity to a tertiary center. For example, if it will be more than 6 hours until a baby has access to tertiary care, either through a transport team or admission to the NICU, then developing the skills and having surfactant available would be a reasonable effort to develop. The necessary equipment is listed in Table 19.4.

These discussions require multidisciplinary involvement of nursing, pharmacy, and respiratory care for development of indications, protocols, and regular training experiences for the team to maintain familiarity with the equipment and procedures. Also important to this process is developing evaluation tools to measure outcomes such as the number of training sessions, number of attempts at intubation, number of doses administered, timeliness of surfactant administration, and untoward events (bradycardia, endotracheal tube obstruction, pneumothorax).

SUMMARY

Once making the decision to intubate a patient based on risk factors or signs and symptoms of RDS, we recommend that surfactant should be given shortly after intubation is complete as long as the endotracheal tube is in proper position. Ideally, administration should be within the first 2 hours, if not earlier, of life. Although the evidence no longer supports routine use of prophylactic intubation and surfactant administration, the data are limited regarding gestational ages below 26 weeks; thus the decision may be made at the discretion of the provider. The decision on whether to extubate or remain on the ventilator should be based on history, risk factors, and gestational age of the patient, as well as the equipment available to the provider. If the patient develops signs and symptoms of worsening RDS, repeat dosing of surfactant should be given. A lower threshold for repeat administration, not necessarily focused only on FiO_2 requirement but increased work of breathing or escalation of ventilatory support may be used, especially if the patient remains intubated. Trials have been performed regarding alternate less invasive methods of administering surfactant but strong evidence to support these methods is currently lacking, thus the recommended way to give surfactant is via the endotracheal tube.

Currently, RDS is the only FDA-approved indication for giving surfactant. Surfactant has been studied in other conditions (i.e., meconium aspiration, pulmonary hemorrhage, sepsis/pneumonia, congenital diaphragmatic hernia, inherited disorders involving surfactant dysfunction/deficiency, and lastly, late administration for BPD prevention). However, the lack of strong evidence precludes the ability to give specific recommendations, although a trial of surfactant administration appears to be beneficial in most of these conditions.

BIBLIOGRAPHIC SOURCE(S)

Ashmeade TL, Haubner L, Collins S, Miladinovic B, Fugate K. Outcomes of a Neonatal Golden Hour Implementation Project. *Am J Med Qual.* 2016;31(1):73-80.

Bahadue FL, Soll R. Early versus delayed selective surfactant treatment for neonatal respiratory distress syndrome. *Cochrane Database Syst Rev.* 2012;11:CD001456.

Ballard PL, Ballard RA. Scientific basis and therapeutic regimens for use of antenatal glucocorticoids. *Am J Obstet Gynecol.* 1995;173(1):254-62.

Barbosa RF, Simões E Silva AC, Silva YP. A randomized controlled trial of the laryngeal mask airway for surfactant administration in neonates. *J Pediatr (Rio J).* 2017;93:343-50.

Batenburg JJ. Surfactant phospholipids: synthesis and storage. *Am J Physiol.* 1992;262(4 Pt 1): L367-85.

Bohlin K, Merchak A, Spence K, Patterson BW, Hamvas A. Endogenous surfactant metabolism in newborn infants with and without respiratory failure. *Pediatr Res.* 2003;54:185-91.

Bousleiman S, Rice MM, Moss J, et al. Use and attitudes of obstetricians toward 3 high-risk interventions in MFMU Network hospitals. *Am J Obstet Gynecol.* 2015;213(3):398.e1-11.

Brix N, Sellmer A, Jensen MS, Pedersen LV, Henriksen TB. Predictors for an unsuccessful INtubation-SURfactant-Extubation procedure: a cohort study. *BMC Pediatr.* 2014;14:155.

Carlo WA. Gentle ventilation: the new evidence from the SUPPORT, COIN, VON, CURPAP, Colombian Network, and Neocosur Network trials. *Early Hum Dev.* 2012;88 (Suppl 2):S81-3.

Castrodale V, Rinehart S. The golden hour: improving the stabilization of the very low birth-weight infant. *Adv Neonatal Care.* 2014;14(1):9-14; quiz 15-6.

Cogo PE, Zimmermann LJ, Meneghini L, et al. Pulmonary surfactant disaturated-phosphatidylcholine (DSPC) turnover and pool size in newborn infants with congenital diaphragmatic hernia (CDH). *Pediatr Res.* 2003;54:653-8.

Dani C, Corsini I, Poggi C. Risk factors for intubation-surfactant-extubation (INSURE) failure and multiple INSURE strategy in preterm infants. *Early Hum Dev.* 2012;88(Suppl 1):S3-4.

Dunn MS, Shennan AT, Zayack D, Possmayer F. Bovine surfactant replacement therapy in neonates of less than 30 weeks' gestation: a randomized controlled trial of prophylaxis versus treatment. *Pediatrics.* 1991;87(3):377-86.

Effect of corticosteroids for fetal maturation on perinatal outcomes. *NIH Consens Statement.* 1994;12(2):1-24.

El Shahed AI, Dargaville PA, Ohlsson A, Soll R. Surfactant for meconium aspiration syndrome in term and late preterm infants. *Cochrane Database Syst Rev.* 2014;12:CD002054.

Fernandez-Ruanova MB, Alvarez FJ, Gastiasoro E, et al. Comparison of rapid bolus instillation with simplified slow administration of surfactant in lung lavaged rats. *Pediatr Pulmonol.* 1998;26(2):129-34.

Finer NN, Merritt TA, Bernstein G, Job L, Mazela J, Segal R. An open label, pilot study of Aerosurf(R) combined with nCPAP to prevent RDS in preterm neonates. *J Aerosol Med Pulm Drug Deliv.* 2010;23(5):303-9.

Garmany TH, Moxley MA, White FV, et al. Surfactant composition and function in patients with ABCA3 mutations. *Pediatr Res.* 2006;59(6):801-5.

Gower WA, Nogee LM. Surfactant dysfunction. *Paediatr Respir Rev.* 2011;12(4):223-9.

Hahn S, Choi HJ, Soll R, Dargaville PA. Lung lavage for meconium aspiration syndrome in newborn infants. *Cochrane Database Syst Rev.* 2013;4:CD003486.

Hamvas A, Cole FS, deMello DE, et al. Surfactant protein B deficiency: antenatal diagnosis and prospective treatment with surfactant replacement. *J Pediatr.* 1994;125(3):356-61.

Hayes D Jr, Feola DJ, Murphy BS, Shook LA, Ballard HO. Pathogenesis of bronchopulmonary dysplasia. *Respiration.* 2010;79(5):425-36.

Herting E, Gefeller O, Land M, van Sonderen L, Harms K, Robertson B. Surfactant treatment of neonates with respiratory failure and group B streptococcal infection. Members of the Collaborative European Multicenter Study Group. *Pediatrics.* 2000;106(5):957-64; discussion 1135.

Jobe AH. Pulmonary surfactant therapy. *N Engl J Med.* 1993. 328(12):861-8.

Jobe AH, Ikegami M. Surfactant metabolism. *Clin Perinatol.* 1993;20:683-96.

Kattwinkel J, Robinson M, Bloom BT, Delmore P, Ferguson JE. Technique for intrapartum administration of surfactant without requirement for an endotracheal tube. *J Perinatol.* 2004;24(6):360-5.

Keller RL, Merrill JD, Black DM, et al. Late administration of surfactant replacement therapy increases surfactant protein-B content: a randomized pilot study. *Pediatr Res.* 2012;72(6):613-9.

Langhammer K, Roth B, Kribs A, Göpel W, Kuntz L, Miedaner F. Treatment and outcome data of very low birth weight infants treated with less invasive surfactant administration in comparison to intubation and mechanical ventilation in the clinical setting of a cross-sectional observational multicenter study. *Eur J Pediatr.* 2018;177:1207-17.

Li J, Ikegami M, Na CL, et al. N-terminally extended surfactant protein (SP) C isolated from SP-B-deficient children has reduced surface activity and inhibited lipopolysaccharide binding. *Biochemistry.* 2004;43(13):3891-8.

Micaglio M, Zanardo V, Ori C, Parotto M, Doglioni N, Trevisanuto D. ProSeal LMA for surfactant administration. *Paediatr Anaesth.* 2008;18(1):91-2.

More K, Sakhuja P, Shah PS. Minimally invasive surfactant administration in preterm infants: a meta-narrative review. *JAMA Pediatr.* 2014;168(10):901-8.

Pinheiro JM, Santana-Rivas Q, Pezzano C. Randomized trial of laryngeal mask airway versus endotracheal intubation for surfactant delivery. *J Perinatol.* 2016;36:196-201.

Polin RA, Carlo WA, Committee on Fetus and Newborn, American Academy of Pediatrics. Surfactant replacement therapy for preterm and term neonates with respiratory distress. *Pediatrics.* 2014;133(1):156-63.

Ramanathan R. Choosing a right surfactant for respiratory distress syndrome treatment. *Neonatology.* 2009;95(1):1-5.

Ramanthan R, Kamholz K, Fujii AM. Is there a difference in surfactant treatment of respiratory distress syndrome in premature neonates? A review. *J Pulmon Resp Med.* 2013;S13:004.

Ramos-Navarro C, Sánchez-Luna M, Zeballos-Sarrato S, González-Pacheco N. Three-year perinatal outcomes of less invasive beractant administration in preterm infants with respiratory distress syndrome. *J Matern Fetal Neonatal Med.* 2018;9:1-171.

Roberts KD, Brown R, Lampland AL, et al. Laryngeal mask airway for surfactant administration in neonates: a randomized, controlled trial. *J Pediatr.* 2018;193:40-46.e1.

Rojas-Reyes MX, Morley CJ, Soll R. Prophylactic versus selective use of surfactant in preventing morbidity and mortality in preterm infants. *Cochrane Database Syst Rev.* 2012;3:CD000510.

Segerer H, van Gelder W, Angenent FW, et al. Pulmonary distribution and efficacy of exogenous surfactant in lung-lavaged rabbits are influenced by the instillation technique. *Pediatr Res.* 1993;34(4):490-4.

Singh N, Hawley KL, Viswanathan K. Efficacy of porcine versus bovine surfactants for preterm newborns with respiratory distress syndrome: systematic review and meta-analysis. *Pediatrics.* 2011;128(6):e1588-95.

Stevens TP, Harrington EW, Blennow M, Soll RF. Early surfactant administration with brief ventilation vs. selective surfactant and continued mechanical ventilation for preterm infants with or at risk for respiratory distress syndrome. *Cochrane Database Syst Rev.* 2007;(4):CD003063.

SUPPORT Study Group of the Eunice Kennedy Shriver NICHD Neonatal Research Network, Early CPAP versus surfactant in extremely preterm infants. *N Engl J Med.* 2010;362(21):1970-9.

Tan K, Lai NM, Sharma A. Surfactant for bacterial pneumonia in late preterm and term infants. *Cochrane Database Syst Rev.* 2012;2:CD008155.

Trevisanuto D, Grazzina N, Ferrarese P, Micaglio M, Verghese C, Zanardo V. Laryngeal mask airway used as a delivery conduit for the administration of surfactant to preterm infants with respiratory distress syndrome. *Biol Neonate.* 2005;87(4):217-20.

Vannozzi I, Ciantelli M, Moscuzza F, et al. Laryngeal mask endotracheal surfactant therapy: the CALMEST approach as a novel MIST technique. *J Matern Fetal Neonatal Med.* 2017;30:2375-7.

Zhang JP, Wang YL, Wang YH, Zhang R, Chen H, Su HB. Prophylaxis of neonatal respiratory distress syndrome by intra-amniotic administration of pulmonary surfactant. *Chin Med J (Engl).* 2004;117(1):120-4.

Conventional Ventilation

Eduardo Bancalari, MD • Nelson Claure, MSc, PhD

SCOPE

DISEASE/CONDITION(S)

Mechanical ventilatory support for neonates in respiratory failure.

GUIDELINE OBJECTIVE(S)

The objectives of this chapter are to review the concepts of mechanical ventilatory support in the neonate according to the various indications, describe the most common modalities of mechanical ventilation, and discuss their advantages and limitations.

BRIEF BACKGROUND

Mechanical ventilation remains the main supportive therapy for neonates in severe respiratory failure. This is more common in premature infants because of the structural and functional immaturity of their respiratory system.

Although mechanical ventilation is necessary to maintain adequate gas exchange, serious complications associated with this therapy make the decision to initiate mechanical ventilation very important and should be done considering all available alternatives. The severity of respiratory failure is usually assessed by the clinical presentation of the infant plus evaluation of respiratory function and arterial blood gases.

Mechanical ventilation is indicated based on the severity of respiratory failure and the underlying lung disease. In the extreme premature infant, mechanical ventilation is often initiated shortly after birth due to poor respiratory effort leading to hypoxemia and bradycardia. In the preterm infant, mechanical ventilation is frequently started because of recurrent episodes of apnea and hypoxemia. Alveolar hypoventilation with hypercapnia and respiratory acidosis is another common indication for mechanical ventilation to support the infant's failing respiratory pump. In preterm infants with respiratory distress syndrome (RDS), mechanical ventilation contributes to the recruitment of distal air spaces with improvement in ventilation perfusion matching and gas exchange.

In full-term infants, the indication for mechanical ventilation is usually more conservative since these infants are better able to cope with the increased work of breathing. In term infants with lung hypoplasia, mechanical ventilation is usually initiated early after birth, whereas in infants with congenital pneumonia or meconium aspiration a more conservative approach can be adopted. These decisions are driven by the degree of hypoxia and hypercapnia.

Mechanical ventilation consists of the alternation of two levels of positive pressure at the infant's airway. The positive end-expiratory pressure (PEEP) provides a continuous distending pressure that maintains lung volume. The pressure is increased intermittently to a set peak inspiratory pressure (PIP) during a predetermined inspiratory time (Ti). This produces a gradient with respect to the alveolar pressure that generates gas flow into the lung. The flow and the tidal volume (V_T) during each cycle for a given pressure gradient is determined by the compliance of the respiratory system, the resistance of the airways, and the infant's inspiratory effort when the positive pressure is provided in synchrony with the effort.

The neonate's respiratory system mechanical properties, that is, compliance and airway resistance, determine its time constant. The respiratory time constant, which is a measure of the time to achieve equilibrium between the applied pressure and the alveolar pressure, varies with different types of lung diseases and their severity.

In restrictive lung diseases such as RDS, lung compliance is decreased, and the infant's respiratory pump is often not strong enough to produce the pressure required to achieve an adequate V_T. Hence the need for higher PIP levels is common. In obstructive diseases characterized by increased airway resistance, there is tendency to gas trapping because of reduced expiratory flow rates; therefore the timing of the respiratory cycles must be managed to allow a full expiration and avoid gas trapping.

Modalities of Mechanical Ventilation

Intermittent mandatory ventilation (IMV) is a modality where the PIP and Ti is set by the clinician, and ventilator cycles are delivered at constant intervals determined by the ventilator rate. In IMV, total minute ventilation is produced by the ventilator breaths plus the infant's spontaneous breathing. The PIP is adjusted to maintain an adequate V_T and the ventilator rate is reduced when the infant's ability to contribute to the total ventilation increases as the lung condition improves.

During IMV, cycles may be delivered toward the end of the infant's spontaneous inspiration or during exhalation. These asynchronous ventilator cycles can disrupt the infant's breathing pattern and lead to agitation and reduced ventilatory efficacy, especially at higher ventilator rates.

Synchronized intermittent mandatory ventilation (SIMV) is similar to IMV except that ventilator cycles are synchronous to the beginning of the spontaneous inspiration. The interval between cycles is continuously adjusted by the ventilator to achieve synchrony but the total number of ventilator cycles is set by the clinician. The ventilator management in SIMV is similar to that during IMV. However, SIMV can produce a greater and more consistent V_T than IMV because of the synchrony between the positive pressure and the infant's inspiratory effort. As the lung disease improves and the infant's spontaneous breathing effort becomes more consistent, PIP is decreased gradually to maintain V_T. During the initial phase of severe respiratory failure, SIMV rates above 40 per minute are likely to assist almost every spontaneous breath. Later, the SIMV rate is reduced as spontaneous breathing contributes more to the maintenance of ventilation.

Assist-control AC ventilation is a modality where each spontaneous inspiration is assisted by the ventilator. The ventilator only initiates a backup ventilator rate during apnea. During AC, PIP is set to maintain V_T within an adequate target range and is gradually decreased as lung mechanics improve and the infant's respiratory effort increases. In AC, PIP should be adjusted to avoid a large V_T that can produce hyperventilation while the backup rate should be just sufficient to prevent hypoventilation during periods of apnea. Auto-cycling must be monitored to avoid hyperventilation or gas trapping because neonatal ventilators may not have an upper limit on cycling rate.

Pressure support ventilation (PSV) is a modality similar to AC where the ventilator provides a cycle with each spontaneous inspiration. The start and end of the ventilator cycle are in synchrony with the infant's breath. PSV can be used as a stand-alone mode with a backup ventilator rate for apnea or as an adjunct to SIMV to assist spontaneous breaths between SIMV cycles. During PSV, auto-cycling should also be monitored to avoid hyperventilation.

SCOPE

DISEASE/CONDITION(S)

Respiratory depression/apnea.

GUIDELINE OBJECTIVE(S)

To identify and review approaches to initiate and manage conventional mechanical ventilation in infants with respiratory depression or apnea.

BRIEF BACKGROUND

Infants with respiratory depression or apnea frequently require mechanical ventilatory support to maintain stable ventilation and blood gases. Many of these infants have normal lung function and therefore do not need high ventilator settings to maintain normal gas exchange.

RECOMMENDATIONS

MAJOR RECOMMENDATIONS

Management of Conventional Ventilation

When the infant's respiratory effort is insufficient or inconsistent, the settings in the ventilator should be adjusted to supplement the spontaneous breathing effort but avoiding hyperventilation and hypocapnia that can further inhibit spontaneous respiration. The use of SIMV at a relatively low rate, alone or combined with pressure support, can meet these objectives. Modalities such as AC or PSV can also be used to assist the spontaneous breathing effort, but these require setting a backup mechanical rate to maintain ventilation during periods of apnea.

In infants with poor respiratory effort, the ventilator settings must be adjusted at ventilator rates sufficient to provide normal alveolar ventilation and keep $PaCO_2$ within adequate ranges. In doing this, ventilator rate and V_T should not be excessive to avoid hyperventilation that leads to more inhibition of respiratory drive.

The infant's spontaneous respiratory drive must be continuously monitored, and ventilator settings must be decreased as the infant's breathing effort becomes more consistent and effective.

Respiratory stimulants should be started before extubation and maintained thereafter to increase extubation success.

In infants with good respiratory effort and normal lung function but frequent episodes of apnea, gas exchange may be adequately maintained without intubation by using nasal intermittent positive-pressure ventilation (NIPPV) or nasal continuous positive airway pressure (NCPAP) alone. The use of respiratory stimulants, for example, caffeine, in these infants, at adequate dosing is effective in improving respiratory drive and decreasing apnea.

IMPLEMENTATION OF GUIDELINE

QUALIFYING STATEMENTS

- Maintenance of lung volume by continuous positive airway pressure (CPAP) to achieve adequate oxygenation and respiratory stimulants to prevent apnea are often effective in reducing the need for mechanical ventilation. This is more likely at more advanced gestational ages.
- No advantage has been demonstrated with any specific modality of mechanical ventilation in preterm infants with apnea or respiratory depression.
- Administration of respiratory stimulants to mechanically ventilated preterm infants without immediate plans for extubation has not been examined in clinical trials.

DESCRIPTION OF IMPLEMENTATION STRATEGY

- The use of center consensus guidelines on the initiation, management, and weaning from mechanical ventilation in preterm infants with respiratory depression is recommended.
- Close observation and monitoring of the spontaneous respiratory drive is recommended.
- Respiratory depression can be induced by factors other than prematurity (e.g., infection, drugs, alkalosis). Identification of the root problem is important to select the best treatment strategy.

QUALITY METRICS

- Monitoring and benchmarking for the rates of intubation for respiratory depression; monitoring for the actual indications for intubation and for factors other than prematurity that could lead to respiratory depression
- Documenting short- and long-term respiratory and neurologic outcomes of infants with respiratory depression

SCOPE

DISEASE/CONDITION(S)

Respiratory distress syndrome.

GUIDELINE OBJECTIVE(S)

To describe the basis for respiratory support in infants with RDS and review the most common strategies to manage these infants.

BRIEF BACKGROUND

A large proportion of preterm infants born before 32 weeks of gestation have RDS. The underlying pathophysiology of this condition is surfactant insufficiency that leads to low functional residual capacity (FRC) and lung compliance, airspace collapse, low ventilation-to-perfusion ratio with pulmonary shunting. These factors combined with an unstable chest wall and poor respiratory drive frequently result in respiratory failure with hypoxemia and hypercapnia.

The severity of the respiratory failure can vary from mild, requiring only supplemental oxygen, to severe, requiring mechanical ventilation.

RECOMMENDATIONS

PRACTICE OPTIONS

Practice Option #1

Infants with mild RDS and good respiratory drive can be supported with NCPAP or NIPPV and supplemental oxygen without invasive mechanical ventilation.

Continuous maintenance of the distending pressure is necessary to avoid lung volume loss.

Close vigilance of their respiratory course is important to determine if a higher level of support is needed.

Practice Option #2

Infants with more severe RDS and poor respiratory effort, who fail NCPAP or NIPPV, may need to be intubated, given surfactant, and supported with intermittent positive-pressure ventilation (IPPV).

The level of PEEP is usually set between 4 cm H_2O and 6 cm H_2O depending on the severity of the lung disease. Continued provision of PEEP is key in maintaining FRC and assuring adequate oxygenation.

The modality of ventilation can be AC, SIMV, or SIMV plus pressure support. There is no clear evidence that any one mode is superior to the others but in one study SIMV plus pressure support was associated with shorter duration of ventilation in infants 750–1000 g compared to SIMV.

In any of these modalities, PIP is adjusted to maintain V_T between 4 mL/kg and 6 mL/kg. In SIMV, the ventilator rate is adjusted to keep $PaCO_2$ between 40 mmHg and 50 mmHg. In AC, or PSV, the rate is determined by the infant except for a backup rate that must be set in case the infant becomes apneic.

In infants with RDS, the time constant of the respiratory system is usually short due to the low lung compliance and resistance and therefore it is recommended to use short Ti, ranging 0.25–0.35 seconds.

The ventilator rate and PIP are reduced as the infant's condition improves and spontaneous breathing effort is sufficient to maintain acceptable levels of ventilation and gas exchange.

Extubation is usually considered as soon as the infant is able to maintain a $PaCO_2$ <50 mmHg and PaO_2 >50 mmHg or SpO_2 >90% with a mechanical rate <15 per minute, PIP <16 cm H_2O and FiO_2 <0.40.

IMPLEMENTATION OF GUIDELINE

QUALIFYING STATEMENTS

- Although avoidance of mechanical ventilation by providing noninvasive support is recommended, unnecessary delays in administration of surfactant in infants with severe RDS may be counterproductive.
- Clinical trials in infants with RDS have not demonstrated advantages of one modality of mechanical ventilation compared to others.
- In the acute phase of respiratory failure, assistance of every spontaneous inspiration with modalities such as AC or PSV or providing higher mandatory rates with SIMV provide similar levels of support.
- Maintenance of synchrony between the infant and the ventilator has been shown to facilitate reducing the level of support and in accelerating weaning from mechanical ventilation.
- Extubation after a period of endotracheal CPAP is not recommended because it decreases success rate.

DESCRIPTION OF IMPLEMENTATION STRATEGY

- The use of center consensus guidelines on the initiation, management, and weaning from mechanical ventilation in preterm infants with RDS is recommended.
- Close monitoring is important to avoid excessive or insufficient V_T.
- Monitoring the contribution of the infant to minute ventilation is recommended to reduce the ventilatory support as soon as possible.

QUALITY METRICS

- Benchmarking by monitoring the rates of intubation for RDS, monitoring for the actual indication for intubation, and monitoring for factors other than RDS that could lead to respiratory failure
- Benchmarking by monitoring the duration of mechanical ventilation and for any period of time that the infant remains on the ventilator at minimal settings that may be considered unnecessary
- Monitoring of extubation failure rates
- Benchmarking for mortality and respiratory outcomes of infants with RDS

SCOPE

DISEASE/CONDITION(S)

Respiratory distress syndrome + pulmonary hemorrhage.

GUIDELINE OBJECTIVE(S)

To identify and review the strategies to manage the mechanical ventilatory support in infants with RDS complicated by pulmonary hemorrhage.

BRIEF BACKGROUND

In infants with RDS increased pulmonary blood flow (PBF) due to a patent ductus arteriosus can lead to pulmonary edema and hemorrhage.

RECOMMENDATIONS

MAJOR RECOMMENDATIONS

When pulmonary hemorrhage complicates RDS, a higher mean airway pressure can be used to reduce PBF and attenuate the pulmonary hemorrhage. This can be achieved by increasing PEEP, PIP, and the ventilator rate. Airway patency should be monitored and maintained by careful suctioning.

IMPLEMENTATION OF GUIDELINE

See RDS section earlier.

SCOPE

DISEASE/CONDITION(S)

Respiratory distress syndrome + pulmonary interstitial emphysema.

GUIDELINE OBJECTIVE(S)

To describe the ventilatory strategies in cases of RDS complicated by pulmonary interstitial emphysema (PIE).

BRIEF BACKGROUND

Infants with RDS, especially when treated with positive pressure ventilation, can develop PIE. This is a severe complication that is correlated with higher risk of pneumothorax and also bronchopulmonary dysplasia (BPD).

RECOMMENDATIONS

PRACTICE OPTIONS

Practice Option #1

When PIE is detected, ventilator settings of PIP and Ti should be reduced to avoid lung overexpansion and limit the progression of PIE. In infants with RDS, a Ti of 0.20–0.25 seconds is sufficient and may help reducing PIE.

Practice Option #2

In severe cases of PIE, infants can be switched to high frequency ventilation.

IMPLEMENTATION OF GUIDELINE

See RDS section earlier.

SCOPE

DISEASE/CONDITION(S)

Neonatal pneumonia.

GUIDELINE OBJECTIVE(S)

To describe the ventilatory strategies in infants with respiratory failure associated with neonatal pneumonia.

BRIEF BACKGROUND

Neonatal pneumonia can occur in term or preterm infants and may be associated with respiratory failure of variable severity. In the more severe cases it may be necessary to use mechanical ventilation to maintain gas exchange. These infants are also at increased risk of gas leak and pulmonary interstitial emphysema and pneumothorax, and also pulmonary hypertension with right-to-left shunting.

RECOMMENDATIONS

PRACTICE OPTION

Practice Option #1

Because the underlying mechanism of respiratory failure is the inflammatory process with edema and exudate, the response to IPPV is less predictable than in infants with RDS due to surfactant deficiency. For this reason, the indication of mechanical ventilation is more questionable and more conservative in infants with suspected pneumonia than in infants with RDS, especially in the more mature infants.

In these infants a higher threshold for FiO_2 (e.g., >0.50 or 0.60) may be used before intubation and initiating mechanical ventilation. Otherwise, the basic principles for mechanical ventilation are similar to those for infants with RDS—that is, trying to maintain relatively normal arterial blood gases with the lowest possible settings and trying to preserve spontaneous respiratory activity by using patient triggered ventilation.

IMPLEMENTATION OF GUIDELINE

See RDS section earlier.

SCOPE

DISEASE/CONDITION(S)

Chronic lung disease.

GUIDELINE OBJECTIVE(S)

To describe the mechanical ventilatory strategies for infants with chronic respiratory failure.

BRIEF BACKGROUND

Many preterm infants who receive mechanical ventilation develop chronic lung disease that requires the use of prolonged respiratory support. Under this condition, the aim is to maintain adequate gas exchange while minimizing the progression of the lung damage and limit as much as possible the duration of invasive support.

RECOMMENDATIONS

MAJOR RECOMMENDATIONS

Use SIMV combined with PS to maintain the infant's respiratory drive and provide sufficient support to keep gas exchange and arterial blood gases within acceptable range.

The ventilator settings are adjusted to keep $PaCO_2$ 40–70 mmHg and pH >7.25.

The PIP and rate of SIMV breaths are adjusted to maintain blood gas as above. These larger mandatory breaths can help maintaining unstable areas of the lung open. The PS is titrated to maintain V_T between 5 mL/kg and 8 mL/kg.

Because infants with chronic lung disease have increased airway resistance and heterogeneous distribution of ventilation, high inspiratory flow rates and short inspiratory time should be avoided. Ventilator cycles of Ti ranging 0.4–0.5 seconds are generally adequate. Caution should be used if Ti is increased while the ventilator rate is high due to the risk of gas trapping.

Weaning is accomplished by gradually reducing SIMV rate to 10–15/min and reducing PS to 6–8 cm H_2O while monitoring $PaCO_2$ and oxygenation.

PRACTICE OPTION

Practice Option #1

In cases of chronic hypercapnia and metabolic compensation, it may be acceptable to allow higher $PaCO_2$ as long as the pH remains >7.25.

IMPLEMENTATION OF GUIDELINE

QUALIFYING STATEMENTS

- The ventilatory support and supplemental oxygen should be minimized to the least required to avoid perpetuating the cycle of lung injury and increased need for support.
- In infants with severe chronic lung disease and prolonged mechanical ventilator support, normal blood gases are difficult to achieve and higher $PaCO_2$ levels must be tolerated.
- The use of patient-triggered ventilation is aimed at assisting the infant's spontaneous breathing to maintain an acceptable total minute ventilation and gas exchange.

DESCRIPTION OF IMPLEMENTATION STRATEGY

- The use of center consensus guidelines on the management and weaning from mechanical ventilation in preterm infants with chronic ventilator dependency is advisable.
- Monitoring patient-ventilatory synchrony and avoidance of excessive or insufficient V_T or ventilator rates are recommended.
- Extubation to slightly higher CPAP levels or NIPPV can reduce the risk of post extubation failure.

QUALITY METRICS

- Benchmarking by monitoring the duration of mechanical ventilation and supplemental oxygen
- Monitoring for the factors and indications that determine long-term ventilator dependency in these infants
- Monitoring of extubation failure rates and the use of strategies to prevent failure
- Benchmarking for long-term respiratory and neurologic outcomes of infants with BPD

SCOPE

DISEASE/CONDITION(S)

Meconium aspiration.

GUIDELINE OBJECTIVE(S)

To describe the ventilatory approach to be used in infant with different severities of respiratory failure due to meconium aspiration.

BRIEF BACKGROUND

Meconium aspiration syndrome (MAS) is seen less commonly today because of improvements in obstetrical care and a higher rate of births by cesarean section. When it occurs, the presentation can range from mild respiratory distress to severe respiratory failure with serious complications such as pneumothorax and pulmonary hypertension. The type of respiratory support must be adapted to the mechanism and severity of the respiratory failure and associated complications.

RECOMMENDATIONS

PRACTICE OPTIONS

Practice Option #1

In mild cases of MAS, supplemental oxygen and maintenance of nutrition, hydration, and acid-base balance are sufficient to support these infants.

Practice Option #2

In cases with more severe respiratory failure, mechanical respiratory support with IPPV may be necessary to maintain normal gas exchange.

Both AC and SIMV + PS may be used adjusting PIP to generate adequate tidal volumes and keep $PaCO_2$ levels between 35 mmHg and 45 mmHg. The level of PEEP and FiO_2 are adjusted to achieve SpO_2 between 95% and 99%.

Maintenance of oxygenation, $PaCO_2$, and pH within normal range are important to minimize the risk of pulmonary hypertension in these infants.

These infants are at increased risk for pneumothorax. Excessive V_T must be avoided. Infants with MAS often have increased airway resistance. Long Ti or high ventilator rates should be avoided to reduce the risk of inverse I:E ratio and gas trapping.

Use of synchronized ventilation is important in infants with MAS because they are frequently agitated and may be maladapted to the ventilator. In some cases, the use of mild sedation is helpful to achieve better adaptation to the ventilator.

Practice Option #3

High frequency ventilation (HFV) is indicated in cases with severe respiratory failure where conventional mechanical respiratory support cannot achieve adequate ventilation despite the provision of V_T in the recommended range.

HFV should also be considered when there is evidence of pulmonary hypertension with right-to-left shunting. In this situation, maintenance of normal $PaCO_2$ and pH levels becomes critical to reduce pulmonary vascular resistance.

IMPLEMENTATION OF GUIDELINE

QUALIFYING STATEMENTS

- Infants with MAS often have vigorous spontaneous breathing effort and seem to be "air hungry." Use of patient-triggered ventilation that assists every spontaneous effort is often more effective than lower ventilator rates.
- Infants with MAS can improve rapidly. Monitoring the adequacy of the ventilatory support is important for timely weaning from the ventilator.
- Long inspiratory times and high ventilator rates should be avoided due to the high risk for gas trapping if there is not sufficient time for exhalation.

DESCRIPTION OF IMPLEMENTATION STRATEGY

- The use of center consensus guidelines on the initiation and management and weaning from the ventilator in infants with MAS is recommended.
- Monitoring for conditions that lead to gas trapping or lead to agitation of these infants is recommended.

QUALITY METRICS

- Benchmarking by monitoring the rates of intubation and duration of mechanical ventilation in infants with MAS
- Monitoring the incidence of pneumothorax and pulmonary hypertension in infants with MAS
- Benchmarking for survival and respiratory outcomes of infants with MAS

SCOPE

DISEASE CONDITION(S)

Persistent pulmonary hypertension of the neonate.

GUIDELINE OBJECTIVE(S)

To describe the approach to provide ventilatory support to preterm infants presenting with persistent pulmonary hypertension of the neonate (PPHN).

BRIEF BACKGROUND

Infants with perinatal asphyxia, MAS, pneumonia, or lung hypoplasia are susceptible to develop severe pulmonary hypertension. When the pulmonary artery pressure becomes suprasystemic, it leads to right-to-left shunting through the foramen ovale or a patent ductus arteriosus, aggravating the arterial hypoxemia.

The management of these infants is complex and requires a clear understanding of the interactions between the respiratory and cardiovascular systems.

RECOMMENDATIONS

PRACTICE OPTION

Practice Option #1

The mechanical ventilatory support in these infants must be guided by the same general principles that apply to infants with MAS or neonatal pneumonia. The goal is to achieve relatively normal gas exchange but minimize the potential detrimental effects of high mean airway pressures on venous return and pulmonary vascular resistance.

PIP must be adjusted to achieve adequate V_T in the range of 4 mL/kg to 7 mL/kg. Preferably, mechanical ventilation should be provided using modes such as AC or SIMV+PS that preserve spontaneous respiratory activity and provide sufficient assistance to neonates making vigorous inspiratory effort.

Maintenance of an optimal lung volume is critical in these infants because over- or underinflation of the lungs can be associated with further increase in pulmonary vascular resistance (PVR) and pulmonary artery pressure aggravating the right-to-left shunting. For this, the PEEP level is adjusted to maintain normal end-expiratory lung volume reflected by optimal arterial oxygen levels and normal lung expansion on chest radiographs.

IMPLEMENTATION OF GUIDELINE

See MAS section earlier.

SCOPE

DISEASE/CONDITION(S)

Pulmonary hypoplasia.

GUIDELINE OBJECTIVE(S)

To describe the ventilatory approach in neonates born with pulmonary hypoplasia.

BRIEF BACKGROUND

A number of conditions can interfere with normal lung development and result in variable degrees of lung hypoplasia. Mass occupying lesions such as congenital diaphragmatic hernia, large pleural effusions, and tumors represent some of these conditions. Premature prolonged rupture of membranes can lead to oligohydramnios that is also associated with impaired lung development.

Infants with severe lung hypoplasia have poor adaptation after birth and severe respiratory failure with CO_2 retention and severe hypoxemia that is frequently aggravated by cardiac right-to-left shunting due to pulmonary hypertension.

RECOMMENDATIONS

PRACTICE OPTIONS

Practice Option #1

Infants with severe lung hypoplasia are some of the most difficult to support with mechanical ventilation, particularly if they are also born preterm. It is very difficult to achieve adequate ventilation and keep $PaCO_2$ within acceptable ranges with conventional ventilation without producing additional lung damage. Because of this, these infants are frequently managed with HFV, which is more effective in removing CO_2.

Practice Option #2

When HFV is not available, ventilator settings should be adjusted to achieve small V_T, for example, in the range of 2 mL/kg to 4 mL/kg, to avoid alveolar overdistention and further lung damage.

Use the lowest mean airway pressure necessary to achieve adequate oxygenation while minimizing the negative effects on the cardiovascular systems. This is aimed at assuring adequate venous return and avoiding a further increase in PVR that can occur with pulmonary overdistention.

High pressures and volumes in these infants also increase the risk of airspace rupture, PIE, and pneumothorax, all frequent complications in infants with pulmonary hypoplasia.

IMPLEMENTATION OF GUIDELINE

QUALIFYING STATEMENTS

- In infants with pulmonary hypoplasia, achievement of normal blood gases by use of high ventilator settings should be avoided. Less aggressive levels of support have been shown to result in better outcomes.

DESCRIPTION OF IMPLEMENTATION STRATEGY

- The use of consensus guidelines on the initiation and management of the ventilatory support in infants with pulmonary hypoplasia is recommended. These should include the indications to initiate HFV.
- Monitoring for excessive expansion of the hypoplastic lung.
- Close monitoring of cardiovascular function is important to avoid side effects.

QUALITY METRICS

- Benchmarking by monitoring the rates of intubation, level of support, and duration of ventilatory support in infants with lung hypoplasia
- Benchmarking for hospital and long-term respiratory outcome

SCOPE

DISEASE/CONDITION(S)

Infants with congenital cardiac malformations.

GUIDELINE OBJECTIVE(S)

To describe the ventilatory support strategy in neonates with congenital cardiac anomalies.

BRIEF BACKGROUND

Infants with congenital heart disease and single ventricle physiology can develop severe pulmonary over circulation and low systemic perfusion. In these cases, mechanical respiratory support can be used to induce a higher PVR and reduce pulmonary blood flow while increasing systemic flow.

RECOMMENDATIONS

PRACTICE OPTION

Practice Option #1

The ventilator settings must be adjusted to avoid hyperventilation and maintain normal or high $PaCO_2$ levels to increase PVR. This can be accomplished by using relatively high MAP with PEEP levels of 6–10 cm H_2O and low PIP to induce hypoventilation.

It is also critical to avoid hyperoxemia that can reduce PVR increasing PBF and reducing systemic flow. This is done by maintaining low normal values of PaO_2 by closely titrating FiO_2. In general, if ABP and systemic flow are adequate one should try to keep PaO_2 between 50 mmHg and 60 mmHg or SpO_2 between 75% and 85%.

IMPLEMENTATION OF GUIDELINE

QUALIFYING STATEMENTS

- In infants with cardiac malformations the level of ventilatory support must be carefully managed to optimize PVR.

DESCRIPTION OF IMPLEMENTATION STRATEGY

- The development and use of center consensus guidelines on the initiation and management of the ventilatory support in infants with cardiac anomalies is recommended.

QUALITY METRICS

- Benchmarking by monitoring the rates of intubation, level of support and duration of ventilatory support in this population of infants
- Benchmarking survival, and respiratory, neurologic, and other neonatal outcomes

SUMMARY

Mechanical ventilation is used to maintain adequate gas exchange in neonates with severe respiratory failure and is more frequently needed in premature infants. Because of the multiple indications for mechanical ventilation, the ventilatory support must be adjusted to match the pathophysiologic conditions that lead to respiratory failure. Ventilator settings must be carefully managed and ventilation continuously monitored to assure efficacy and avoid complications. For this, the goals of mechanical ventilatory support should be to assist the infant's spontaneous effort and minimize the support as much as possible. A conservative approach is recommended to reduce the risk of lung injury.

BIBLIOGRAPHIC SOURCE(S)

Bancalari E, Claure N. The evidence for non-invasive ventilation in the preterm infant. *Arch Dis Child Fetal Neonatal Ed.* 2013;98:F98-102.

Bancalari E, Wilson-Costello D, Iben SC. Management of infants with bronchopulmonary dysplasia in North America. *Early Hum Dev.* 2005;81:171-9.

Buzzella B, Claure N, D'Ugard C, Bancalari E. A randomized controlled trial of two nasal CPAP levels after extubation in preterm infants. *J Pediatr.* 2014;164:46-51.

Chan V, Greenough A. Comparison of weaning by patient triggered ventilation or synchronous mandatory intermittent ventilation. *Acta Paediatr.* 1994;83:335-7.

Claure N, Bancalari E. New modalities of mechanical ventilation in the preterm newborn: evidence of benefit. *Arch Dis Child Fetal Neonatal Ed.* 2007;92:F508-12.

Davis PG, Henderson-Smart DJ. Extubation from low-rate intermittent positive airways pressure versus extubation after a trial of endotracheal continuous positive airways pressure in intubated preterm infants. *Cochrane Database Syst Rev.* 2000;CD001078.

Davis PG, Lemyre B, de Paoli AG. Nasal intermittent positive pressure ventilation (NIPPV) versus nasal continuous positive airway pressure (NCPAP) for preterm neonates after extubation. *Cochrane Database Syst Rev.* 2001;(3):CD003212.

Di Fiore JM, Martin RJ, Gauda EB. Apnea of prematurity--perfect storm. *Respir Physiol Neurobiol.* 2013;189:213-22.

Dimitriou G, Greenough A, Giffin FJ, et al. Synchronous intermittent mandatory ventilation modes versus patient triggered ventilation during weaning. *Arch Dis Child.* 1995; 72:F188-90.

Gittermann MK, Fusch C, Gittermann AR, Regazzoni BM, Moessinger AC. Early nasal continuous positive airway pressure treatment reduces the need for intubation in very low birth weight infants. *Eur J Pediatr.* 1997;156:384-8.

Goldsmith JP. Continuous positive airway pressure and conventional mechanical ventilation in the treatment of meconium aspiration syndrome. *J Perinatol.* 2008;28:S49-55.

Greenough A, Dimitriou G, Prendergast M, Milner AD. Synchronized mechanical ventilation for respiratory support in newborn infants. *Cochrane Database Syst Rev.* 2008;(1):CD000456.

Greenough A, Morley C, Davis J. Interaction of spontaneous respiration with artificial ventilation in preterm babies. *J Pediatr.* 1983;103:769-73.

Gregory GA, Kitterman JA, Phibbs RH, Tooley WH, Hamilton WK. Treatment of the idiopathic respiratory-distress syndrome with continuous positive airway pressure. *N Engl J Med.* 1971;284:1333-40.

Ho JJ, Subramaniam P, Henderson-Smart DJ, Davis PG. Continuous distending pressure for respiratory distress syndrome in preterm infants. *Cochrane Database Syst Rev.* 2002;CD002271.

Jonsson B, Katz-Salamon M, Faxelius G, Broberger U, Lagercrantz H. Neonatal care of very-low-birthweight infants in special-care units and neonatal intensive-care units in Stockholm. Early nasal continuous positive airway pressure versus mechanical ventilation: gains and losses. *Acta Paediatr Suppl.* 1997;419:4-10.

Kim EH. Successful extubation of newborn infants without preextubation trial of continuous positive airway pressure. *J Perinatol.* 1989;9:72-6.

Locke R, Greenspan JS, Shaffer TH, Rubenstein SD, Wolfson MR. Effect of nasal CPAP on thoracoabdominal motion in neonates with respiratory insufficiency. *Pediatr Pulmonol.* 1991;11:259-64.

Logan JW, Cotten CM, Goldberg RN, Clark RH. Mechanical ventilation strategies in the management of congenital diaphragmatic hernia. *Semin Pediatr Surg.* 2007;16:115-25.

Martin RJ, Nearman HS, Katona PG, Klaus MH. The effect of a low continuous positive airway pressure on the reflex control of respiration in the preterm infant. *J Pediatr.* 1977;90:976-81.

Miller MJ, Carlo WA, Martin RJ. Continuous positive airway pressure selectively reduces obstructive apnea in preterm infants. *J Pediatr.* 1985;106:91-4.

Reyes ZC, Claure N, Tauscher MK, D'Ugard C, Vanbuskirk S, Bancalari E. Randomized, controlled trial comparing synchronized intermittent mandatory ventilation and synchronized intermittent mandatory ventilation plus pressure support in preterm infants. *Pediatrics.* 2006;118:1409-17.

Sweet DG, Carnielli V, Greisen G, et al; European Association of Perinatal Medicine. European consensus guidelines on the management of neonatal respiratory distress syndrome in preterm infants–2013 update. *Neonatology.* 2013;103:353-68.

Verder H, Albertsen P, Ebbesen F, et al. Nasal continuous positive airway pressure and early surfactant therapy for respiratory distress syndrome in newborns of less than 30 weeks' gestation. *Pediatrics.* 1999;103:E24.

High-Frequency Ventilation

Martin Keszler, MD

SCOPE

DISEASE/CONDITION(S)

Newborn infants with a variety of underlying causes of respiratory failure who require invasive respiratory support.

GUIDELINE OBJECTIVE(S)

Outline the best clinical practice of high-frequency ventilation (HFV) based on an understanding of the indications, benefits, risks, and optimal implementation strategies for different modalities of HFV.

BRIEF BACKGROUND

High-frequency ventilation (HFV) is a group of ventilation techniques that share in common the basic characteristics of rapid ventilator rate and very small tidal volume (V_T). These techniques were developed several decades ago in an effort to minimize lung injury and to treat existing lung damage, in particular airleak. There are three types of HFV available for clinical use. Although similar in the basic principles of ventilation, each HFV modality has its own unique features. With high-frequency oscillatory ventilation (HFOV), gas within the large airways is moved in and out by pressure oscillations generated by a piston, diaphragm, or an intermittent expiratory venturi. Irrespective of how the oscillations are generated, the key feature of a true oscillator is that at 1:1 inspiratory: expiratory ratio, the negative pressure deflection is equal to the positive deflection, and therefore both the inspiration and expiration phases are active. The only HFOV currently approved for use in newborn infants in the United States is the Sensormedics 3100A (Vyaire Medical, Chicago, IL). Several more modern oscillators are available throughout the rest of the world and include the Humming V, the Flowline Dragonfly, the Stephan SHF 3000, the SLE 5000, the Leoni Plus, and the Babylog VN500. The latter is currently being evaluated in a clinical trial and may become available in the United States (the VN500 and the Leoni HFOV are already available in Canada). Unlike the Sensormedics, modern oscillators have the ability to measure, and in some cases automatically regulate, delivered V_{T}, which should substantially reduce the risk of inadvertent hypocapnia.

High-frequency jet ventilation (HFJV) delivers short pulses of pressurized gas directly into the upper airway via a special endotracheal tube adaptor containing an HFJV injector port and a pressure monitoring port. In contrast to HFOV, exhalation is passive, resulting in somewhat lower optimal operating frequencies. The mean airway pressure is primarily generated by applying positive end-expiratory pressure via a conventional ventilator used in tandem, sometimes combined with very low rate conventional mechanical ventilation to provide periodic sigh as a means of lung volume recruitment. The inspiratory time is very short, and this characteristic appears to make HFJV uniquely suitable for treatment of airleak. The only jet ventilator available in the United States is the Bunnell LifePulse (Bunnell Inc. Salt Lake City, UT).

High-frequency flow interruption (HFFI) also known as high-frequency percussive ventilation (HFPV) generates short bursts of gas delivered directly into the ventilator circuit without the narrow injector cannula used in HFJV. For many years, the Infant Star 950 ventilator was widely used in the United States, Europe, and elsewhere. It is no longer manufactured but remains in use in some parts of the world. In this device, a venturi system on the exhalation valve was applied to assist expiration. However, the negative deflection was much smaller than the positive deflection, leading to air-trapping and increased risk of airleak. The Bronchotron (Bird Corporation, Sand Point, ID), a portable pneumatically powered high-frequency flow interrupter developed in the 1980s, has gained acceptance as a neonatal transport ventilator because of its light weight, low gas consumption, and ability to function as both a conventional and high-frequency ventilator. The Volumetric Diffusive Respirator (VDR 4) is a time-cycled, pressure-limited, pneumatically driven high-frequency flow interrupter device similar to the Bronchotron, but more complex and designed for hospital use. The Bronchotron and VDR 4 have been "grandfathered" by the US Food and Drug Administration and thus have not undergone rigorous clinical evaluation.

Preclinical studies comparing HFV to conventional mechanical ventilation in surfactant-depleted or premature animal models have shown that HFV attenuates acute lung injury, but only when combined with an optimal lung volume or open lung ventilation strategy. Elegant studies in preterm baboons demonstrated better preservation of lung architecture and better gas exchange after prolonged exposure to HFOV compared to conventional ventilation. Other animal studies showed effectiveness of HFJV in models of respiratory distress syndrome (RDS) and meconium aspiration syndrome (MAS).

Rescue use of various forms of HFV in infants failing conventional ventilation became widely accepted in the 1990s, based on mostly anecdotal evidence and early randomized trials of HFOV and HFJV that used relatively crude conventional ventilation strategies as controls. Results of studies to evaluate benefits of HFV as first-line treatment in infants with uncomplicated RDS have been more equivocal, and the evidence in support of HFV as a first-line treatment remains weak.

SCOPE

DISEASE/CONDITION(S)

Respiratory distress syndrome (RDS).

GUIDELINE OBJECTIVE(S)

To outline indications and approaches to initiation and management of high-frequency ventilation in infants with respiratory distress syndrome.

BRIEF BACKGROUND

RDS is characterized by surfactant deficiency and a tendency of the lung to undergo microatelectasis, leading to loss of aeration of substantial portions of the terminal saccules. Positive pressure ventilation of infants with RDS may result in atelectrauma if care is not taken to achieve adequate lung volume recruitment and thus uniform distribution of tidal volume into a well-expanded lung. Atelectrauma includes overexpansion of the more compliant non-dependent portion of the lung resulting in volutrauma, sheer stress, and repeated collapse and re-expansion of terminal air sacs. HFV may be uniquely suited to facilitate lung volume recruitment, and the open lung strategy of HFOV has been widely accepted. All forms of HFV are suitable for the treatment of infants with atelectasis-prone lung conditions such as RDS as long as the open lung strategy is employed. Whether all extremely low birth weight infants with uncomplicated RDS should be treated with HFV as a *first-line treatment* remains an open question.

RECOMMENDATIONS

PRACTICE OPTIONS

Practice Option #1

Infants with RDS should initially be managed with noninvasive support and only be intubated and mechanically ventilated when adequate respiratory effort is lacking or when noninvasive support is insufficient to maintain adequate gas exchange without excessively high FiO_2. Following surfactant administration, most such infants can be successfully managed with relatively low level of conventional positive pressure ventilation and extubated as expeditiously as possible. If peak inflation pressure (PIP) or mean airway pressure (MAP) reach levels above the practitioner's comfort level (typically PIP >25 cm H_2O, MAP >10–12 cm H_2O), or if a high oxygen requirement persists despite adequate positive end-expiratory pressure (PEEP), changing to HFV should be considered. There is no clear advantage of one form of HFOV over another in the treatment of uncomplicated RDS, as long as an open lung strategy is followed. However, if airleak is present, HFJV is preferred (see below).

Practice Option #2

A relatively small minority of neonatologists utilize HFV as first-line therapy in extremely preterm infants with RDS who require invasive respiratory support. This approach is based largely on the lung-protective characteristics of HFV documented in preclinical studies. All modalities of HFV are being used in this fashion in NICUs in North America and elsewhere. It should be pointed out that this practice is not strongly evidence-based;

convincing evidence of the superiority of HFV over state-of-the-art conventional ventilation is lacking and thus we cannot recommend this practice as a first option.

IMPLEMENTATION OF GUIDELINE

QUALIFYING STATEMENTS

- Like all modes of ventilation, HFV is a powerful and potentially life-saving tool that can be used safely and effectively, or not. Significant adverse effects on the hemodynamics, lungs, and brain can occur if HFV is not used with care and a clear understanding of the safe and effective strategy to be used in a given patient.
- The key to obtaining the best results is to carefully consider the underlying pathophysiology and chose an appropriate strategy that addresses the underlying disease process.
- RDS evolves over time from a disease with short time constants and a relatively homogeneous lung (when adequately recruited) to chronic lung disease with longer time constants, which makes the lungs more prone to air-trapping with high frequencies, especially when using modes that rely on passive exhalation (i.e., HFJV and HFFI).
- No advantage has been demonstrated for any specific modality of HFV in preterm infants with RDS. The choice of the mode of HFV is thus largely based on personal preference and training.
- An essential element of optimal use of any HFV device in infants with RDS is lung volume recruitment, using oxygen requirement as a proxy for adequacy of lung inflation. When adequate recruitment has been achieved, FiO_2 should be <0.30. Recruitment with HFOV is achieved by stepwise increments in MAP. With HFJV, this is achieved by increasing the PEEP. Because the inspiratory time is very short with HFJV, the MAP is only a few cm H_2O above the PEEP level; thus PEEP settings that are substantially higher than those used with conventional ventilation are needed to achieve adequate MAP and optimal lung volume. At equal MAP, HFJV, HFOV, and HFFI result in comparable improvement in oxygenation. Once the lung is open, it becomes more compliant and MAP needs to be decreased until just above where oxygenation begins to deteriorate.
- Failure to wean MAP once lung compliance improves may result in impaired venous return and cardiac output, impaired ventilation, and lung injury. Thus, frequent reassessment of the appropriateness of MAP (clinical and, if needed, radiographic) is recommended.
- Because of the nature of gas flow with HFJV, endotracheal tube position is critical to effective use. The tube should not be too close to the carina to avoid inadvertently directing the gas flow down one or the other mainstem bronchus. Equally important is to maintain midline head position to direct the gas flow down the center of the airway, rather than hitting the tracheal wall.
- HFJV is quite sensitive to endotracheal tube malposition or accumulation of secretions. Thus if an acute increase in PCO_2 is noted, tube position should be verified. Secretions are not normally a problem in the first few days in infants with RDS but begin to increase as chronic lung disease develops.

DESCRIPTION OF IMPLEMENTATION STRATEGY

- HFV should only be used after all relevant NICU staff have received adequate training in its use.
- The medical providers and respiratory therapists should become familiar with the capabilities and limitations of the HFV device to be used.
- Ideally, each center should develop consensus guidelines for the criteria for the use of HFV, its initiation, management, and weaning from HFV.
- Close observation of chest wall movement and transcutaneous CO_2 monitoring is recommended when HFV is initiated. Because with HFV, CO_2 elimination is proportional to frequency $\times V_T^2$, even modest increase in V_T can lead to marked hypocapnia.
- Nursing and respiratory therapy staff must be taught to maintain midline head position when using HFJV.

QUALITY METRICS

- Surveillance for the occurrence of hypocapnia is recommended.
- Benchmarking of survival rates, incidence of severe intraventricular hemorrhage, periventricular leukomalacia, and chronic lung disease against NICUs with similar patient populations is highly desirable.

SCOPE

DISEASE/CONDITION(S)

Airleak syndromes (pulmonary interstitial emphysema [PIE], pneumothorax, bronchopleural fistula).

GUIDELINE OBJECTIVE(S)

To describe the basis for the use of HFV in infants with airleak syndromes and review the most effective strategies to manage these difficult infants.

BRIEF BACKGROUND

Both invasive and noninvasive respiratory support may be complicated by airleak. Tidal breathing in the presence of extensive atelectasis predisposes infants to airleak complications as described in the section on RDS. Airleak syndrome includes PIE, pneumothorax, and pneumomediastinum. All forms of HFV may offer advantages over conventional ventilation because of the small V_T used, but HFJV is uniquely suited for this task, presumably because of its extremely short inspiratory time and the nature of the gas flow in the large airways: the gas emerging from the jet cannula streams down the center of the airway with essentially no pressure on the lateral wall. HFOV has been shown to decrease the risk of new airleak, but not specifically to promote resolution of existing airleak. HFJV has been shown to lead to faster resolution of PIE, lower flow of gas through bronchopleural and trachea-esophageal fistulas, and improved gas exchange in all these conditions and thus is the treatment of choice in NICUs that have access to the Bunnell Jet ventilator.

RECOMMENDATIONS

PRACTICE OPTIONS

Practice Option #1

Infants with significant airleak should be treated with HFJV using a strategy of mild permissive hypercapnia and moderate MAP with the goal of minimizing further lung injury and allowing the tissue disruption to heal. Previously, a low-pressure strategy using PEEP ≤5 cm H_2O was used, but in infants with coexisting RDS, this led to worsening atelectasis, deteriorating oxygenation, and ultimately higher ventilator settings. Because leakage of gas through airway disruption occurs predominantly at peak pressure, it is safe and preferable to employ an end-expiratory pressure that is sufficient to maintain alveolar recruitment. Because of the extremely short inspiratory time, there is minimal, if any, leakage, allowing faster resolution of airleak. Infants should remain on HFJV until at least 24 hours after complete resolution of airleak, or until extubation.

Practice Option #2

When HFJV is not available, other forms of HFV may offer some similar benefits, but the evidence for their efficacy in airleak is largely anecdotal. A strategy of just adequate but not excessive MAP should be used with the lowest amplitude consistent with acceptable $PaCO_2$ level.

IMPLEMENTATION OF GUIDELINE

QUALIFYING STATEMENTS

- Ventilation of infants with coexisting RDS and airleak requires the clinician to carefully balance the competing imperatives of the two conditions. When RDS predominates with only localized or mild PIE, the ventilation strategy should focus on maintaining optimal lung volume while avoiding progression of airleak by targeting less ambitious gas exchange targets and avoiding lung overexpansion.
- When airleak is the predominant pathophysiology, the strategy needs to change to one that prioritizes resolution of airleak, even if that compromises gas exchange to some extent.
- Frequent reassessment is needed to detect evolution of the lung pathology over time.
- When using HFJV for treating unilateral airleak, such as severe PIE involving one lung, it is possible to direct the flow of gas preferentially to the contralateral lung by placing the endotracheal tube close to the carina and turning the head in the opposite direction (i.e., toward the involved lung). This is usually tolerated better than the alternative, which is selective mainstem bronchus intubation.

DESCRIPTION OF IMPLEMENTATION STRATEGY

- Development of center consensus guidelines for the initiation, management, and discontinuation of HFV in infants with airleak syndromes is recommended.
- Close monitoring of chest wall vibration and transcutaneous CO_2 monitoring is desirable to avoid hypo- or hypercapnia.
- Monitoring lung expansion and progression/resolution of airleak by periodic chest radiographs is important.

QUALITY METRICS

- Benchmarking of important neonatal outcomes in infants requiring rescue HFV because of airleak is recommended.

SCOPE

DISEASE/CONDITION(S)

Respiratory distress syndrome complicated by pulmonary hemorrhage.

GUIDELINE OBJECTIVE(S)

To identify and review HFV strategies to manage respiratory support in infants with RDS complicated by pulmonary hemorrhage.

BRIEF BACKGROUND

True parenchymal pulmonary hemorrhage is quite uncommon. What is commonly termed "pulmonary hemorrhage" is hemorrhagic pulmonary edema due to acute increase in pulmonary blood flow (PBF) secondary to a patent ductus arteriosus (PDA). The typical presentation is an acute respiratory deterioration in an extremely low birth weight infant with copious bloody fluid welling up from the airway and a whiteout chest radiograph. Hemorrhagic pulmonary edema must be distinguished from tracheal mucosal bleeding, which is characterized by a small amount of blood-streaked endotracheal secretions without severe respiratory deterioration or corresponding radiographic change. When hemorrhagic pulmonary edema is diagnosed, the most effective intervention is a large increase in MAP designed to increase pulmonary vascular resistance and promote edema fluid movement into the pulmonary interstitium. This goal is often best achieved with HFOV or HFJV. In addition, blood and protein in the alveolar spaces rapidly inactivate both endogenous and exogenous surfactant; thus a substantial increase in MAP is needed to restore lung volume. Suctioning should be avoided because it leads to loss of distending pressure and recurrence of hemorrhage. Iced saline and topical epinephrine may be useful for mucosal hemorrhage but *have no place in the treatment of hemorrhagic pulmonary edema.*

RECOMMENDATIONS

PRACTICE OPTION

Practice Option #1

When hemorrhagic pulmonary edema complicates RDS, rapid initiation of HFV with a high MAP is often life saving. The MAP needs to be titrated up to arrest the welling up of edema fluid and improve gas exchange. Both HFOV and HFJV have been used effectively in this condition.

IMPLEMENTATION OF GUIDELINE

QUALIFYING STATEMENTS

- See RDS section earlier.
- With hemorrhagic pulmonary edema, it is critical that ventilation is not interrupted for suctioning. The edema fluid is thin and will not clot the endotracheal tube.

The edema fluid will disappear from the endotracheal tube and upper airways once sufficient distending pressure is applied, to literally push the fluid back into the pulmonary interstitium.

- Transiently, it may be necessary to use very high MAP/PEEP to achieve these goals (MAP 15–20, PEEP with HFJV 12–15). These should then be gradually reduced once lung compliance begins to improve.
- Hemorrhagic edema is often a manifestation of a large PDA, which should be addressed once the infant's condition has stabilized.

DESCRIPTION OF IMPLEMENTATION STRATEGY

- See RDS section earlier.
- Clinicians should be comfortable with the use of HFV in less critical situations prior to applying the technique in these challenging circumstances.

QUALITY METRICS

- This condition is rare; thus metrics, other than adherence to protocol are difficult to perform.

SCOPE

DISEASE/CONDITION(S)

Meconium aspiration syndrome (MAS).

GUIDELINE OBJECTIVE(S)

To describe the rationale for the use of HFV and the appropriate ventilatory strategies in infants with MAS.

BRIEF BACKGROUND

Most infants born through meconium stained amniotic fluid are well or turn out only to have transient tachypnea, but infants with true MAS often require invasive respiratory support. The pathophysiology of MAS is complex and includes surfactant inactivation, inflammation, and a variable obstructive component. In many infants, the problem is compounded by their altered pulmonary vascular reactivity related to both inflammation and prenatal/postnatal hypoxia-ischemia. The phenotype of MAS is highly variable; in some infants the clinical features of MAS may be predominantly that of surfactant inactivation and inflammation, giving rise to a relatively homogeneous lung pathophysiology well suited for treatment with HFV. Other infants have heterogeneous lung aeration with prominent air-trapping due to aspiration of particulate meconium. This combination of airway obstruction and surfactant dysfunction results in a non-homogeneous lung disease that makes managing severe MAS quite difficult. Persistent pulmonary hypertension (PPHN) is a frequent complication in infants with severe MAS and may be effectively addressed by optimizing lung inflation and normalizing PCO_2/pH with HFV in infants who are difficult to ventilate conventionally.

The goal of respiratory support is to optimize lung inflation by recruitment and maintenance of underinflated airspaces while attempting to minimize overinflation of the more compliant regions of the lung and air-trapping. Acquired surfactant dysfunction may be treated with exogenous surfactant, and lung volume is optimized through judicious application of distending airway pressure. Appreciation of the prolonged time constants present in MAS is critical to choosing appropriate ventilation strategies. Coexisting conditions, such as infection, hypovolemia, and multiple organ dysfunction, must be addressed as necessary.

Both HFOV and HFJV may offer benefit in infants with MAS. The key to safe and effective use of HFOV in this condition characterized by long time constants is the use of lower ventilation rate, typically 6–8 Hz with HFOV and 240–300 cycles/min with HFJV. The MAP should be set based on the overall pattern of lung inflation. For infants with significant air-trapping, the low end of the frequency range (6 Hz) is recommended with a MAP similar to that on conventional ventilation. Amplitude (ΔP) is adjusted to generate adequate chest vibration. If using a modern HFOV device with V_T measurement or targeting, expect to use a relatively large V_T of 2.5–3.5 mL/kg because of increased alveolar dead space. For those infants with MAS who have relatively poor lung inflation, the MAP is typically started at 2–4 cm H_2O above that on conventional ventilation. Subsequent adjustments are made based on the FiO_2 response and radiographic assessment of lung inflation. Lower rate (240–300 cycles/min, 4–5 Hz) is even more critical with HFJV, which depends on passive exhalation. Air-trapping could be aggravated if adequacy of expiratory time is not ensured.

RECOMMENDATIONS

PRACTICE OPTIONS

Practice Option #1

When severe MAS is present, especially when complicated by PPHN and/or airleak, HFV should be considered as an early rescue modality to optimize lung volume and ventilation. There is good evidence for the use of HFV when PPHN is present and treatment with inhaled nitric oxide is considered. Both HFJV and HFOV are used extensively in infants with severe MAS with apparently similar success.

Practice Option #2

Although not strongly evidence-based, the use of HFJV or HFOV as a first-line strategy in infants with MAS who require mechanical ventilation is practiced in many institutions in an effort to minimize complications of MAS.

IMPLEMENTATION OF GUIDELINE

QUALIFYING STATEMENTS

- Frequent clinical and radiographic assessment is needed because the predominant pathophysiology often changes rapidly. Attention to cardio-respiratory interactions is an important component of management of these infants.
- Transcutaneous CO_2 monitoring is advisable when initiating HFV, because of the rapidity with which PCO_2 may drop.
- It may be necessary to increase the I-time from 0.02 sec to 0.03 sec to generate a larger V_T with these lower rates when approaching the upper limits of PIP setting. A sigh rate of 2–5/min may be helpful in improving gas exchange with HFJV.

- When initiating HFJV early on, it is common to see an increased amount of meconium-stained secretions coming up the endotracheal tube, being swept out by the expiratory flow. Be prepared to suction.
- When particulate meconium and/or copious secretions are present, clinicians must be alert to the possibility of interference of the secretions with the jet stream. This is usually manifested by decreased chest wall movement, and rising $TCCO_2$ and must be quickly corrected by suctioning.

DESCRIPTION OF IMPLEMENTATION STRATEGY

- Development of center consensus guidelines for the use of HFV in infants with MAS is recommended.
- Close monitoring of chest wall vibration and transcutaneous CO_2 monitoring is desirable when V_T measurement is not available.
- Monitoring of lung expansion periodic chest radiographs is important to recognize air-trapping or loss of inflation as the disease evolves.

QUALITY METRICS

- Monitoring the incidence of pneumothorax and pulmonary hypertension in infants with MAS.
- Monitoring for occurrence of inadvertent overventilation.
- Benchmarking for survival and respiratory outcomes of infants with MAS.

SCOPE

DISEASE/CONDITION(S)

Neonatal pneumonia.

GUIDELINE OBJECTIVE(S)

To describe the high-frequency ventilatory strategies in infants with respiratory failure associated with neonatal pneumonia.

BRIEF BACKGROUND

Neonatal pneumonia may be seen in both term and preterm infants. In preterm infants, it may coexist with and be radiographically indistinguishable from RDS. Pneumonia may lead to respiratory failure of variable severity and is often associated with a poor response to exogenous surfactant. Infants with neonatal pneumonia are at increased risk of PPHN as well as hemodynamic instability. Treatment should be directed at the underlying infection, addressing circulatory derangements, normalizing gas exchange, and treating PPHN, if present. Because these infants may be difficult to ventilate, HFV may be of benefit if relatively high ventilator settings are required.

RECOMMENDATIONS

PRACTICE OPTION

Practice Option #1

All forms of HFV may be indicated when high conventional ventilator settings are needed or refractory PPHN is present.

IMPLEMENTATION OF GUIDELINE

QUALIFYING STATEMENTS

- The ventilation strategy should be tailored to address the predominant pathophysiology and the size of the patient.
- Larger term infants have longer time constants and thus may benefit from slower ventilator frequency.
- If severe pneumonia is present, lung volume may not be easily recruitable. Thus caution should be exercised in escalating MAP, due to potential adverse hemodynamic effects.
- Also see RDS section earlier.

DESCRIPTION OF IMPLEMENTATION STRATEGY

See RDS section earlier.

QUALITY METRICS

See RDS section earlier.

SCOPE

DISEASE/CONDITION(S)

Chronic lung disease.

GUIDELINE OBJECTIVE(S)

To describe high-frequency ventilatory strategies for infants with chronic ventilator dependency.

BRIEF BACKGROUND

Some extremely preterm infants develop chronic lung disease that requires prolonged mechanical ventilation. Often these are the sickest extremely preterm infants who were treated with HFV during their acute illness and remain on HFV as the disease evolves to a more chronic form. There is paucity of data on the use of HFV of any sort in this population of infants. Because increased airway resistance is an inherent part of chronic lung disease of prematurity, HFV is not necessarily appropriate in these infants, but clinicians often find it hard to know if and when to transition these infants to conventional ventilation modes. Because infants with the simplified lung of new bronchopulmonary dysplasia have poorly supported small airways, they are more prone to air-trapping with the active exhalation of HFOV. There is limited evidence from small crossover studies suggesting that HFJV may be more effective in these infants, provided adequate expiratory time is provided with slower rates.

RECOMMENDATIONS

PRACTICE OPTIONS

Practice Option #1

Transition infants to conventional mechanical ventilation when they are unable to be extubated from HFV and remain ventilator-dependent past 3–4 weeks of age.

Practice Option #2

If continuing HFV is desired, consider transitioning to HFJV with slower rate (~360 cycles/min–6 Hz) to allow adequate time for passive exhalation.

IMPLEMENTATION OF GUIDELINE

QUALIFYING STATEMENTS

- If continuing HFOV, recognize that overexpansion of the lungs is likely due to air-trapping and resist the knee-jerk response of lowering MAP. In fact, the overexpansion is likely the result of small airway collapse with active exhalation and will be relieved by increasing, not decreasing the MAP.
- Permissive hypercapnia is commonly used and is an appropriate strategy.
- Thick secretions become a common problem as chronic lung disease develops and can acutely affect ventilation.
- In chronically ventilated infants, the reason for continuation of HFV should be periodically reassessed. A trial of conventional ventilation often shows that adequate gas exchange can be achieved with lower settings than with HFV.

DESCRIPTION OF IMPLEMENTATION STRATEGY

- Development of consensus guidelines for the management of infants requiring prolonged mechanical ventilation, including criteria for changing to conventional ventilation, is recommended.
- Monitoring periodically for evidence of air-trapping is advisable.
- Increased awareness of airway obstruction with secretions is important.

QUALITY METRICS

- Benchmarking by monitoring the duration of mechanical ventilation and supplemental oxygen.
- Monitoring the use/misuse of HFV in infants with chronic ventilator dependence is advised.
- Benchmarking for long-term respiratory and neurologic outcomes of infants with BPD.

SCOPE

DISEASE/CONDITION(S)

Pulmonary hypoplasia.

GUIDELINE OBJECTIVE(S)

To describe the ventilatory approach in neonates with pulmonary hypoplasia, including congenital diaphragmatic hernia (CDH).

BRIEF BACKGROUND

Both term and preterm infants may develop pulmonary hypoplasia as a result of low amniotic fluid volume, space-occupying intrathoracic lesions, lack of spontaneous respiration, or asphyxiating thoracic dystrophy. Oligohydramnios from prolonged premature rupture of the membranes or lack of urine production from a variety of renal lesions and CDH are the most common conditions associated with pulmonary hypoplasia. The degree of hypoplasia is variable, but in extreme cases may be so severe as to preclude adequate gas exchange despite all efforts. Persistent pulmonary hypertension often complicates the picture. Infants with CDH additionally have varying degrees of ventricular dysfunction and respond poorly to inhaled nitric oxide.

Infants with severe lung hypoplasia may present with severe respiratory failure, with CO_2 retention and hypoxemia soon after birth. Aggressive efforts to correct respiratory acidosis may result in early development of airleak. Excessive application of distending airway pressure may aggravate pulmonary hypertension and should be avoided.

HFV has long been used to attempt to improve ventilation with a gentle approach designed to avoid overexpansion and minimize lung injury. There is limited evidence from a series of small, mostly anecdotal observations of a beneficial effect of HFV combined with inhaled nitric oxide in preterm infants with pulmonary hypoplasia related to oligohydramnios. While a number of observational studies strongly suggested benefits of gentle HFOV in infants with CDH, a recent randomized controlled trial conducted in Europe (the VICI trial) failed to document any advantage of HFOV and indeed found better outcomes in the conventional arm. However, the trial has been criticized for the use of excessively high MAP in the HFOV arm and other aspects of design and execution. Thus the study conclusions should be specific to HFOV used with the particular strategy used. Other strategies of HFOV may be more beneficial, but likely will never be formally studied. Although it is used frequently to treat infants with CDH, there are limited published data on the benefits of HFJV in this population.

RECOMMENDATIONS

PRACTICE OPTIONS

Practice Option #1

Infants with CDH or other forms of pulmonary hypoplasia should be initially stabilized with gentle conventional ventilation, accepting some degree of permissive hypercapnia. If low ventilator settings are unable to provide adequate gas exchange, early change to HFJV or HFOV should be considered. If airleak develops, a change to HFJV (preferable), or HFOV is indicated (see Airleak section earlier).

Practice Option # 2

HFJV or HFOV may be used as a first-line therapy for CDH in centers that are experienced and comfortable with HFV. Preterm infants with pulmonary hypoplasia probably benefit from first-line treatment with HFV. The lowest mean airway pressure necessary to achieve adequate but not excessive lung expansion and oxygenation should be used.

IMPLEMENTATION OF GUIDELINE

QUALIFYING STATEMENTS

- As with most complex interventions, it is not just *what* we do but *how well* we do it that determines the outcome. Thus the specific strategy and focus on gentle support with avoidance of excessive lung inflation is probably more critical than whether conventional or high-frequency ventilation is used.

- Attention to cardio-respiratory interactions are especially important in these infants. Decreased venous return and systemic hypotension resulting from high distending airway pressure are particularly dangerous in these infants prone to pulmonary hypertension.
- High MAP should be avoided, because overexpansion of hypoplastic lungs worsens PPHN.
- Inhaled nitric oxide and other approaches to managing pulmonary hypertension are often required in combination with gentle ventilation.

DESCRIPTION OF IMPLEMENTATION STRATEGY

- The development of consensus guidelines for management of the ventilatory support in infants with pulmonary hypoplasia is essential. These should include the indications to initiate HFV and the specific strategies to be used, including target blood gas values.
- Monitoring lung expansion and hemodynamic status is critical.
- Close monitoring of signs of pulmonary hypertension and prompt intervention to correct circulating blood volume, lung expansion, and sedation is recommended.

QUALITY METRICS

- Benchmarking by monitoring survival in infants with lung hypoplasia.
- Benchmarking for long-term respiratory outcome.

SUMMARY

High-frequency ventilation includes several related modalities that provide the clinician with powerful but potentially dangerous tools for the management of the sickest newborns who require invasive respiratory support. Safe and effective use of HFV requires adequate training and experience with meticulous attention to avoidance of complications. Achievement of optimal lung volume recruitment with improved oxygenation and prevention/treatment of airleak are the most common indications for its use. Inadvertent hyperventilation remains a common and serious adverse effect, which can be minimized by the use of transcutaneous CO_2 monitoring. When available, modern HFV devices that can measure and regulate directly the tidal volume should substantially reduce this risk.

BIBLIOGRAPHIC SOURCE(S)

AlKharfy TM. High-frequency ventilation in the management of very-low-birth-weight infants with pulmonary hemorrhage. *Am J Perinatol*. 2004;21:19-26.

Chock VY, Van Meurs KP, Hintz SR, et al. Inhaled nitric oxide for preterm premature rupture of membranes, oligohydramnios, and pulmonary hypoplasia. *Am J Perinatol*. 2009;26:317-22.

Clark RH, Yoder BA, Sell MS. Prospective, randomized comparison of high-frequency oscillation and conventional ventilation in candidates for extracorporeal membrane oxygenation. *J Pediatr*. 1994;124(3):447-54.

Cools F, Askie LM, Offringa M, et al. Elective high-frequency oscillatory versus conventional ventilation in preterm infants: a systematic review and meta-analysis of individual patients' data. *Lancet* 2010;375:2082-91.

Cools F, Henderson-Smart DJ, Offringa M, Askie LM. Elective high frequency oscillatory ventilation versus conventional ventilation for acute pulmonary dysfunction in preterm infants. *Cochrane Database Syst Rev (Online)*. 2009;CD000104.

Engle WA, Yoder MC, Andreoli SP, Darragh RK, Langefeld CD, Hui SL. Controlled prospective randomized comparison of high-frequency jet ventilation and conventional ventilation in neonates with respiratory failure and persistent pulmonary hypertension. *J Perinatol*. 1997;17(1):3-9.

Friedlich P, Subramanian N, Sebald M, Noori S, Seri I. Use of high-frequency jet ventilation in neonates with hypoxemia refractory to high-frequency oscillatory ventilation. *J Matern Fetal Neonatal Med*. 2003;13:398-402.

Froese AB. Role of lung volume in lung injury: HFO in the atelectasis-prone lung. *Acta Anaesthesiol Scand*. 1989;90:126.

Keszler M. High-frequency jet ventilation. In: Donn S, Sinha S, eds. *Manual of Neonatal Respiratory Care*. 4th ed. Switzerland: Springer International; 2017:329-35.

Keszler M, Donn S, Buciarelli R, et al. Multi-center controlled trial comparing high-frequency jet ventilation and conventional ventilation in newborn infants with pulmonary interstitial emphysema. *J Pediatr*. 1991;119:85-93.

Keszler M, Pillow JJ, Courtney S. High-frequency ventilators. In: Rimensberger P, ed. *Pediatric and Neonatal Mechanical Ventilation: From Basics to Clinical Practice*. Springer; 2015:221-39.

Kuluz MA, Smith PB, Mears SP, et al. Preliminary observations of the use of high-frequency jet ventilation as rescue therapy in infants with congenital diaphragmatic hernia. *J Pediatr Surg*. 2010;45:698-702.

Lakshminrusimha S, Keszler M. Persistent pulmonary hypertension of the newborn. *NeoReviews*. 2015;16:e680-92.

Migliazza L, Bellan C, Alberti D, et al. Retrospective study of 111 cases of congenital diaphragmatic hernia treated with early high-frequency oscillatory ventilation and presurgical stabilization. *J Pediatr Surg*. 2007;42:1526-32.

Peliowski A, Finer NN, Etches PC, Tierney AJ, Ryan CA. Inhaled nitric oxide for premature infants after prolonged rupture of the membranes. *J Pediatr*. 1995;126:450-3.

Snoek KG, Capolupo I, van Rosmalen J, et al; CDH EURO Consortium. Conventional mechanical ventilation versus high-frequency oscillatory ventilation for congenital diaphragmatic hernia: a randomized clinical trial (the VICI-trial). *Ann Surg*. 2016;263(5):867-74.

Vain NE, Batton DG. Meconium "aspiration" (or respiratory distress associated with meconium-stained amniotic fluid?). *Semin Fetal Neonatal Med*. 2017;22:214-9.

Yoder BA, Siler-Khodr T, Winter VT, Coalson JJ. High-frequency oscillatory ventilation: effects on lung function, mechanics, and airway cytokines in the immature baboon model for neonatal chronic lung disease. *Am J Respir Crit Care Med*. 2000;162:1867-76.

Noninvasive Ventilation and High-Flow Nasal Cannula Therapy

Bradley A. Yoder, MD • Kevin Crezee, BS, RRT-NPS

SCOPE

DISEASE/CONDITION(S)

Post extubation support of neonatal respiratory insufficiency.

GUIDELINE OBJECTIVE(S)

Review important mechanisms of action; identify detrimental approaches to high-flow nasal cannula (HFNC) therapy; recommendations for initiation, adjusting, and weaning HFNC.

BRIEF BACKGROUND

High-flow nasal cannula (HFNC) support, more properly termed heated humidified high-flow nasal cannula (HHHFNC), has also been described as nasal high-flow therapy (nHFT). The shorter term, HFNC, will be used throughout this chapter, but the importance of proper heating and humidification must not be forgotten when using HFNC. First used in NICUs in the early 2000s, HFNC is now almost universally available in NICUs around the world, despite the fact the first randomized trial was not published until December 2012. In many clinical units, HFNC has nearly completely superseded the application of nasal CPAP. Important mechanisms of action for HFNC support of respiratory function include: 1) optimal heating and humidification of inspired gas to reduce metabolic work, improve airway mechanics, and maintain epithelial cell integrity; 2) increased gas flow rates equal to or greater than normal peak inspiratory flow to augment inspired tidal volume, offload diaphragmatic muscle activity, and enhance gas washout of respiratory dead space; 3) provision of minimal to moderate level of positive airway pressure that contributes to increased end expiratory lung volume.

RECOMMENDATIONS

MAJOR RECOMMENDATIONS

1. When properly applied, randomized trials demonstrate that HFNC has similar efficacy to nasal CPAP in post-extubation support of preterm infants (Figure 22.1). To date there are limited data from randomized controlled trials defining safety and efficacy for preterm infants below 28 weeks' gestation. Nonetheless, large retrospective and prospective observational studies have not found evidence for increased adverse events associated with HFNC in this population, while reporting effective noninvasive respiratory support.
2. Randomized controlled trials demonstrate that HFNC, as compared to nasal CPAP, is inferior as the initial respiratory support mode for the primary treatment of neonatal respiratory distress syndrome (RDS) (Figure 22.2).
3. Use only HFNC systems that allow proper heating (35–37°C) and humidification (100%) of gas; ensure that adequate gas egress is maintained from the nares by limiting nasal cannula (NC) diameter to approximately 50% and no more than 80% of the

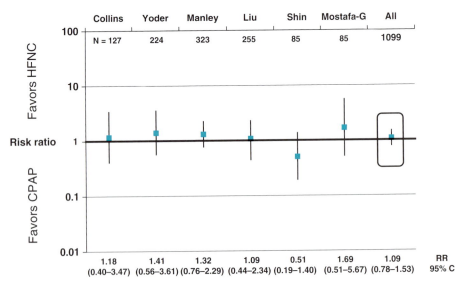

FIGURE 22.1 • Simplified meta-analysis comparing the use of high-flow nasal cannula (HFNC) to nasal CPAP for post-extubation respiratory support in neonates. (Yoder B, University of Utah, January 2019.)

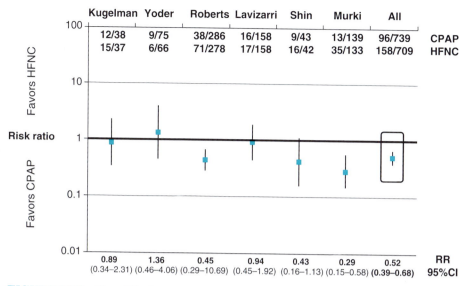

FIGURE 22.2 • Simplified meta-analysis comparing the use of high-flow nasal cannula (HFNC) to nasal CPAP as initial respiratory support mode for neonates with RDS. (Yoder B, University of Utah, January 2019.)

diameter of the nares; recognize that at flow rates equal to or greater than weight in kilogram, the blended FiO_2 is equal to the FiO_2 delivered to the infant.

4. Manage HFNC with an approach similar to other advanced modes for noninvasive respiratory support; specifically, wean FiO_2 initially until <30%, then wean flow as tolerated to a level acceptable for transition to room air or standard NC support; escalation in flow rates should be considered for increasing FiO_2 needs and for signs of increasing work of breathing or respiratory distress.

Initiation of HFNC (Table 22.1)

1. Regardless of weight, initiate at flow rates = 4–8 L/min.
2. There is no evidence to suggest higher flow rates are accompanied by increased adverse event rates, nor is there evidence to support improved efficacy at higher starting flow rates.
3. Consider higher flows (6–8 L/min) for infants extubated from ventilator support with mean airway pressure >6 cm H_2O and/or FiO_2 >30%.

Escalation of HFNC (Table 22.1)

1. Do not exceed 8 L/min in neonates.
2. Increase flow rates by 1–2 L/min based on increasing FiO_2 (>30–35%), increasing respiratory rate (>60 bpm), and/or signs of increasing work of breathing.
3. Flow rates may be increased every 15–30 minutes as needed to achieve effect or to maximum flow rate of 8 L/min.

Weaning of HFNC (Table 22.1)

1. Similar to mechanical ventilation (MV)/nasal intermittent mandatory ventilation/ CPAP, wean FiO_2 to <30% before weaning flow rate.
2. For stable infants, review on a regular basis to determine if flow rates can be reduced.

TABLE 22.1. Heated Humidified High-Flow Nasal Cannula: Basic Considerations for Initiation and Management in Neonates with Respiratory Dysfunction

Weight	Initiation of Flow	Escalation of Flow	Weaning Flow	Discontinuing HHFNC
<1500 g	4–5 L/min	FiO$_2$ >35% and/or ↑ RR, WOB	↓ by 0.5 L/min q12–24h	Typically at flow = weight (kg)
1500–3000 g	5–6 L/min	FiO$_2$ >35% and/or ↑RR, WOB	↓ by 0.5–1 L/min q6–12h	Typically at 2 L/min
> 3000 g	6–7 L/min	FiO$_2$ >35% and/or ↑RR, WOB	↓ by 0.5–1 L/min as indicated	Typically at 2 L/min
Comments	Maximum flow 8 L/min	↑by 1–2 L/min q15–20min PRN	Typically slower; wean with BPD	

3. Use FiO$_2$ needs, respiratory rates, and work of breathing to determine if flow can be reduced.
4. For infants weighing <1000 g, consider weaning by flow rates of 0.5–1.0 L/min no more frequently than every 24 hours.

Discontinuation of HFNC (Table 22.1)

1. Randomized trials have discontinued HFNC at flow rates of 2–4 L/min.
2. Currently we typically wean off HFNC to standard NC therapy at 2 L/min; however, in infants weighing <1000 g we may continue HFNC to as low as 1 L/min in order to minimize the effects of cool, dry gas flow on airway of such small infants.
3. In general, there is no consensus on when to stop HFNC.

CLINICAL ALGORITHM(S)

The algorithm developed for initiation, escalation and weaning of HFNC at the University of Utah NICU is shown in Figure 22.3. Other algorithms may exist and or be developed per local practice guidelines.

IMPLEMENTATION OF GUIDELINE

QUALIFYING STATEMENTS

1. No studies have compared optimal flow rate for initiation of HFNC.
2. There are limited data from randomized controlled trials (RCTs) regarding use of HFNC at <28 weeks.

DESCRIPTION OF IMPLEMENTATION STRATEGY

1. Recommend written guidelines for extubation from MV.
2. Provide written guidelines for initiation, escalation, weaning, and discontinuing HFNC. Include details related to high-flow delivery system, heating/humidification, NC-to-nares ratio, clinical parameters for change, timing of change, and flow rate change.

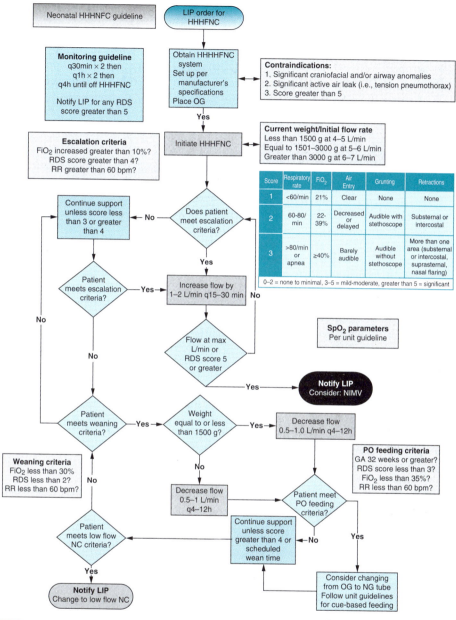

FIGURE 22.3 • Algorithm for management of heated humidified high-flow nasal cannula (HHHFNC). (Yoder B, Crezee K, University of Utah, June 2015.)

QUALITY METRICS

Monitor rates for intubation/re-intubation, delivery system failure, nasal trauma, feeding tolerance, length of stay, BPD rates, duration of MV/noninvasive support/supplemental oxygen therapy.

SUMMARY

When used with systems specifically designed for the application of heated humidified high-flow nasal cannula therapy, HHHFNC is a safe, effective therapy for the post-extubation support of premature infants using flow rates up to 8 L/min. Wide-scale use of HHHFNC suggests it may also be safe and effective for noninvasive support of neonates with other respiratory problems. Additional studies are needed to optimize the application of this therapy in neonates.

BIBLIOGRAPHIC SOURCE(S)

Al-Alaiyan S, Dawoud M, Al-Hazzani F. Positive distending pressure produced by heated, humidified high flow nasal cannula as compared to nasal continuous positive airway pressure in premature infants. *J Neonatal Perinatal Med*. 2014;7:119.

Benaron DA, Benitz WE. Maximizing the stability of oxygen delivered via nasal cannula. *Arch Pediatr Adolesc Med*. 1994;148:294.

Chidekel A, Zhu Y, Wang J, et al. The effects of gas humidification with high-flow nasal cannula on cultured human airway epithelial cells. *Pulm Med*. 2012;2012:380686.

Collaborative Group for the Multicenter Study on Heated Humidified High-flow Nasal Cannula Ventilation. Efficacy and safety of heated humidified high-flow nasal cannula for prevention of extubation failure in neonates. *Zhonghua Er Ke Za Zhi*. 2014;52:271-6. [Chinese]

Collins CL, Barfield C, Horne RS, et al. A comparison of nasal trauma in preterm infants extubated to either heated humidified high-flow nasal cannulae or nasal continuous positive airway pressure. *Eur J Pediatr*. 2014;173:181.

Collins CL, Holberton JR, Barfield C, et al. A randomized controlled trial to compare heated humidified high-flow nasal cannulae with nasal continuous positive airway pressure postextubation in premature infants. *J Pediatr*. 2013;162:949.

Collins CL, Holberton JR, König K. Comparison of the pharyngeal pressure provided by two heated, humidified high-flow nasal cannulae devices in premature infants. *J Paediatr Child Health*. 2013;49:554.

de Jongh BE, Locke R, Mackley A, et al. Work of breathing indices in infants with respiratory insufficiency receiving high-flow nasal cannula and nasal continuous positive airway pressure. *J Perinatol*. 2014;34:27.

Dysart K, Miller TL, Wolfson MR, et al. Research in high flow therapy: mechanisms of action. *Respir Med*. 2009;103:1400.

Frizzola M, Miller TL, Rodriguez ME, et al. High-flow nasal cannula: impact on oxygenation and ventilation in an acute lung injury model. *Pediatr Pulmonol*. 2011;46:67.

Greenspan JS, Wolfson MR, Shaffer TH. Airway responsiveness to low inspired gas temperature in preterm infants. *J Pediatr*. 1991;118:443.

Hasani A, Chapman TH, McCool D, et al. Domiciliary humidification improves lung mucociliary clearance in patients with bronchiectasis. *Chron Respir Dis*. 2008;5:81.

Hochwald O, Osiovich H. The use of high flow nasal cannulae in neonatal intensive care units: Is clinical practice consistent with the evidence? *J Neo Perinatal Med*. 2010;3:187.

Holleman-Duray D, Kaupie D, Weiss MG. Heated humidified high-flow nasal cannula: use and a neonatal early extubation protocol. *J Perinatol*. 2007;27:776.

Hough JL, Pham TM, Schibler A. Physiologic effect of high-flow nasal cannula in infants with bronchiolitis. *Pediatr Crit Care Med*. 2014;15:e214.

Kopelman AE, Holbert D. Use of oxygen cannulas in extremely low birthweight infants is associated with mucosal trauma and bleeding, and possibly with coagulase-negative staphylococcal sepsis. *J Perinatol*. 2003;23:94.

Kubicka ZJ, Limauro J, Darnall RA. Heated, humidified high-flow nasal cannula therapy: yet another way to deliver continuous positive airway pressure? *Pediatrics*. 2008;121:82.

Kugelman A, Riskin A, Said W, et al. A randomized pilot study comparing heated humidified high-flow nasal cannulae with NIPPV for RDS. *Pediatr Pulmonol.* 2015;50:576.

Lavizzari A, Ciuffini F, Colnaghi M, Veneroni C, Matassa P, Mosca F. Heated, humidified high flow nasal cannula versus nasal CPAP for respiratory distress syndrome in preterm infants: a randomized clinical trial. Pediatric Academic Society; 2015, Abstract #1675.1.

Manley BJ, Owen L, Doyle LW, et al. High-flow nasal cannulae and nasal continuous positive airway pressure use in non-tertiary special care nurseries in Australia and New Zealand. *J Paediatr Child Health.* 2011;48:16.

Manley BJ, Owen LS, Doyle LW, et al. High-flow nasal cannulae in very preterm infants after extubation. *N Engl J Med.* 2013;369:1425.

McQueen M, Rojas J, Sun SC, et al. Safety and long term outcomes with high flow nasal cannula therapy in neonatology: A large retrospective cohort study. *J Pulm Respir Med.* 2014;4:216.

Mostafa-Gharehbaghi M, Mojabi H. Comparing the effectiveness of nasal continuous positive airway pressure (NCPAP) and high flow nasal cannula (HFNC) in prevention of post extubation assisted ventilation. *Zahedan J Res Med Sci.* 2015;17(6):e984.

Murki S, Singh J, Khant C, et al. High-flow nasal cannula versus nasal continuous positive airway pressure for primary respiratory support in preterm infants with respiratory distress: a randomized controlled trial. *Neonatology.* 2018;113(3):235-41.

Ojha S, Gridley E, Dorling J. Use of heated humidified high-flow nasal cannula oxygen in neonates: a UK wide survey. *Acta Paediatr.* 2013;102:249.

Pham TM, O'Malley L, Mayfield S, et al. The effect of high flow nasal cannula therapy on the work of breathing in infants with bronchiolitis. *Pediatr Pulmonol.* 2015;50(7):713-20.

Roberts CT, Owen LS, Manley BJ, Frøisland DH, Donath SM, Dalziel KM for the HIPSTER Trial Investigators. Nasal high-flow therapy for primary respiratory support in preterm infants. *N Engl J Med.* 2016;375(12):1142-51.

Saslow JG, Aghai ZH, Nakhla TA, et al. Work of breathing using high-flow nasal cannula in preterm infants. *J Perinatol.* 2006;26:476.

Schmalisch G, Wilitzki S, Wauer RR. Differences in tidal breathing between infants with chronic lung diseases and healthy controls. *BMC Pediatr.* 2005;5:36.

Shin J, Park K, Lee EH, Choi BM. Humidified high flow nasal cannula versus nasal continuous positive airway pressure as an initial respiratory support in preterm infants with respiratory distress: a randomized, controlled non-inferiority trial. *J Korean Med Sci.* 2017;32(4):650-5.

Shoemaker MT, Pierce MR, Yoder BA, et al. High flow nasal cannula versus nasal CPAP for neonatal respiratory disease: a retrospective study. *J Perinatol.* 2007;27:85.

Sivieri EM, Gerdes JS, Abbasi S. Effect of HFNC flow rate, cannula size, and nares diameter on generated airway pressures: an in vitro study. *Pediatr Pulmonol.* 2013;48:506.

Spence KL, Murphy D, Kilian C, et al. High-flow nasal cannula as a device to provide continuous positive airway pressure in infants. *J Perinatol.* 2007;27:772.

Waugh JB, Granger WM. An evaluation of 2 new devices for high-flow gas therapy. *Respir Care.* 2004;49:902.

Woodhead DD, Lambert DK, Clark JM, et al. Comparing two methods of delivering high-flow gas therapy by nasal cannula following endotracheal extubation: a prospective, randomized, masked, crossover trial. *J Perinatol.* 2006;26:481.

Yoder BA, Stoddard RA, Li M, et al. Heated, humidified high-flow nasal cannula versus nasal CPAP for respiratory support in neonates. *Pediatrics.* 2013;131:e1482.

Nasal CPAP

Kathleen Brennan, MD • Richard A. Polin, MD, FAAP

SCOPE

DISEASE/CONDITION(S)

Prevention/reduction of bronchopulmonary dysplasia.

GUIDELINE OBJECTIVE(S)

Recommendations for initiation of continuous positive airway pressure (CPAP); define CPAP failure and identify strategies to prevent failure; recommendations for weaning of CPAP.

BRIEF BACKGROUND

In the past decade, the incidence of bronchopulmonary dysplasia (BPD) has remained relatively unchanged despite improvements in neonatal intensive care, which have enhanced survival. Since the earliest identification of BPD by Northway et al. in 1967, development of BPD has been associated with exposure to mechanical ventilation. A seminal paper by Avery et al. in 1987 reported a decreased incidence of BPD at Babies Hospital in New York compared with seven similar centers; they hypothesized that this decreased incidence resulted in part from avoidance of mechanical ventilation through the use of CPAP. Consequently, several randomized controlled trials and meta-analyses have sought to answer the question of whether CPAP use compared to standard intubation and surfactant administration can prevent BPD.

RECOMMENDATIONS

MAJOR RECOMMENDATIONS

Randomized trials and meta-analyses demonstrate that early, routine CPAP use significantly reduces the combined outcome of BPD or death in preterm infants. However, the treatment effect remains disappointingly small with an incidence of BPD in survivors still at ~40%. This lack of treatment effect may result from a high proportion of CPAP failures, which result in need for mechanical ventilation. Thus work is ongoing to investigate how to improve implementation of CPAP and prevent CPAP failure.

INITIATION OF CPAP

1) Provided that the neonate demonstrates spontaneous respiratory effort, CPAP can be initiated in the delivery room via nasal prongs or mask in any weight infant. 2) Distending pressures of 5–8 mmHg and flow rates of 5–10 L/min of warmed, humidified gasses are sufficient.

IDENTIFYING CPAP FAILURE

CPAP failure may be defined as FiO_2 requirement >60% (controversial) to maintain SpO_2 >89%, pCO_2 >65 mmHg, pH <7.2, or apneic episodes requiring positive pressure ventilation or frequent stimulation. Strategies to avoid CPAP failure are targeted at delivering effective distending pressure and include appropriate size nasal prongs, proper positioning of nasal device to infant's nose and face, use of chin straps and pacifiers to minimize air leak, placement of feeding tube to permit gastric decompression, and frequent monitoring of device, device positioning, and infant's respiratory status by neonatal nurses and physicians.

WEANING CPAP

Three weaning methods are commonly used in clinical practice—sudden removal of CPAP, gradual reduction of pressure, and gradual reduction in time off CPAP (aka "sprinting"). No significant benefits of any one strategy have been demonstrated. Infants >30 weeks post menstrual age with stable respiration on CPAP (4–6 mmHg vs <9 mmHg) with 21% FiO_2 should be considered for CPAP wean.

IMPLEMENTATION OF GUIDELINE

DESCRIPTION OF IMPLEMENTATION STRATEGY

Institutions should provide written guidelines for the use of nasal CPAP. These guidelines should include: 1) Early application of CPAP in the delivery room; 2) ongoing monitoring of CPAP safety and effectiveness; 3) criteria for defining CPAP failure; 4) criteria for identifying infants ready for CPAP wean; and 5) methods to wean CPAP.

QUALITY METRICS

CPAP failure rates, nasal trauma, BPD rates, duration of CPAP, duration of mechanical ventilation.

SUMMARY

Noninvasive continuous positive airway pressure is a safe and effective therapy for respiratory distress syndrome in preterm infants. When used early and effectively, CPAP can decrease rates of BPD or death. The treatment effect of CPAP remains small in current randomized, controlled trials but this appears to be in part due to a high incidence of CPAP failures. Attempts to limit CPAP failure through increased experience with CPAP and more successful delivery of continuous pressure should enhance the effectiveness of this therapy.

BIBLIOGRAPHIC SOURCE(S)

Amatya S, Rastogi D, Bhutada A, Rastogi S. Weaning of nasal CPAP in preterm infants: who, when and how? a systematic review of the literature. *World J Pediatr*. 2014;1(11):7-13.

Avery ME, Tooley WH, Keller JB, et al. Is chronic lung disease in low birth weight infants preventable? A survey of eight centers. *Pediatrics*. 1987;79:26-30.

Dunn MS, Kaempf J, de Klerk A, et al. Randomized trial comparing 3 approaches to the initial respiratory management of preterm neonates. *Pediatrics*. 2011;128:e1069-76.

Finer NN, Carlo WA, Walsh MC, et al. Early CPAP versus surfactant in extremely preterm infants. *N Engl J Med*. 2010;362:1970-9.

Jenson CF, Sellmer A, Ebbesen F, et al. Sudden vs pressure wean from nasal continuous positive airway pressure in infants born before 32 weeks of gestation: a randomized clinical trial. *JAMA Pediatr*. 2018;9(172):824-31.

McMorrow A, Millar D. Methods of weaning preterm babies <30 weeks off CPAP: a multicenter randomized controlled trial. *J Clin Neonatol*. 2012;1(4):176-8.

Morley CJ, Davis PG, Doyle LW, Brion LP, Hascoet JM, Carlin JB; COIN Trial Investigators. Nasal CPAP or intubation at birth for very preterm infants. *N Engl J Med*. 2008;358:700-8.

Northway WH, Rosan RC, Porter DY. Pulmonary disease following respiratory therapy of hyaline membrane disease: bronchopulmonary dysplasia. *N Engl J Med*.1967;276-357.

Rojas-Reyes MX, Morley CJ, Soll R. Prophylactic versus selective use of surfactant in preventing morbidity and mortality in preterm infants. *Cochrane Database Syst Rev* 2012;3:CD000510.

Sahni R, Schiaratura M, Polin RA. Strategies for the prevention of continuous positive airway pressure failure. *Semin Fetal Neonatal Med*. 2016;21(3):196-203.

Schmolzer GM, Kumar MK, Pichler G, et al. Non-invasive versus invasive respiratory support in preterm infants at birth: systematic review and meta-analysis. *BMJ*. 2013;347:f5980.

Stoll BJ, Hansen NI, Bell EF, et al. Trends in care practices, morbidity, and mortality of extremely preterm neonates, 1993-2012. *JAMA*. 2015;314:1039-51.

Todd DA, Wright A, Broom M, et al. Methods of weaning preterm babies <30 weeks gestation off CPAP: a multicenter randomized controlled trial. *Arch Dis Child Fetal Neonatal Ed*. 2012;97(4):F236-40.

Pneumothorax

Sarah D. Keene, MD, FAAP

SCOPE

DISEASE/CONDITION(S)

Pneumothorax in neonates.

GUIDELINE OBJECTIVE(S)

Review risk factors and at-risk populations; symptoms and diagnosis; clinical management options and outcomes.

BRIEF BACKGROUND

A pneumothorax occurs when air enters the pleural space, typically becoming trapped there. In neonates it is most often secondary to a pulmonary process such as respiratory distress syndrome (RDS) or transient tachypnea of the newborn (TTN) and typically occurs after the application of positive airway pressure. Pneumothorax can also occur spontaneously in newborn infants; this is thought to be related to unequal distribution of air in the partially liquid-filled lungs as they are expanding and the infant is crying and generating its own positive expiratory pressure.

The clinical spectrum of neonatal pneumothorax includes the term infant exhibiting only mild tachypnea who has a pneumothorax seen on chest x-ray (CXR), to the critically ill infant with a tension pneumothorax resulting in cardiac arrest, and a broad spectrum of illness in between. Pneumomediastinum may also occur, and in rare cases is large enough to result in cardiac compression.

Incidence

Existing population data are quite old, but the incidence of pneumothorax may be as high as 1–2% in newborn infants, though the vast majority are asymptomatic. Symptomatic

TABLE 24.1. Risk Factors for Pneumothorax

Prematurity
Lung disease (RDS, TTN, MAS)
Congenital lung malformation (CDH, CPAM)
Pulmonary interstitial emphysema
Male gender
Cesarean delivery
Positive pressure ventilation
Mechanical ventilation
High oxygen requirement

CDH, congenital diaphragmatic hernia; CPAM, congenital pulmonary airway malformation; MAS, meconium aspiration syndrome; RDS, respiratory distress syndrome; TTN, transient tachypnea of the newborn.

pneumothorax is much more rare on a population basis, estimated at 0.1% though much more common in patients requiring treatment in the neonatal intensive care unit (NICU) (1.6–4.4%), especially in the most premature infants (<28 wk, 4–14%). Pneumothorax most typically occurs in the first 72 hours after birth, though later ones occur, especially in infants with severe lung disease. Once a common NICU event, pneumothoraces are much less frequent with current neonatal respiratory care including prenatal steroids, volume-targeted ventilation, and surfactant administration.

Risk Factors

As with the majority of neonatal conditions, prematurity is the most important risk factor for pneumothorax (see Table 24.1). Smaller, sicker infants, particularly those requiring significant mechanical ventilation and high fraction of inspired oxygen, are at the greatest risk. Randomized trial data have shown this risk is lower when volume-targeted ventilation and early surfactant administration are used. However, early use of continuous positive airway pressure (CPAP) may obviate the need for surfactant in patients that can be appropriately supported without intubation.

Late preterm and term infants are also at risk, especially those receiving positive pressure ventilation or CPAP either during delivery resuscitation or NICU care. Pneumothorax has become more common in this population as use of CPAP has risen.

Outcomes

Small pneumothoraces, especially in larger, fairly well infants, have an excellent prognosis and minimal if any mortality risk. However, in premature infants, pneumothorax caries a several-fold increase in the risk of death, likely related to both the severity of lung disease and the pneumothorax itself. Mortality can be as high as 30–45% in these patients, and is highest in those with a large pneumothorax and limited response to treatment. Likewise, in less preterm but more ill infants (such as those with severe pneumonia or meconium aspiration syndrome [MAS]) or with congenital anomalies of the pulmonary system (as in congenital diaphragmatic hernia [CDH]), pneumothorax is associated with prolonged intubation, need for extracorporeal membrane oxygenation (ECMO), and mortality.

Diagnosis

Unlike in adults or older patients, symptoms in neonates are often fairly nonspecific. There may be a slow progressive increase in work of breathing, respiratory rate, and oxygen requirement or increase in ventilator pressures if the patient is mechanically ventilated. The rapid development of desaturation unresponsive to increases in oxygen or ventilation, with development of hypotension and ultimately bradycardia, can be indicative of a tension pneumothorax, but also many other processes. In babies, the small chest and bronchotubular type of breath sounds mean air flow can often be heard throughout the chest, even in the case of a large pneumothorax. A deviated trachea or point of maximal impulse are infrequently seen so the diagnosis must be considered based on nonspecific signs, but additional diagnostic tools (such as transillumination and CXR) are necessary for confirmation.

Transillumination with a fiberoptic light is a rapid bedside test that can allow prompt diagnosis and treatment, especially of a tension pneumothorax causing cardiac destabilization or arrest. When the room is darkened and a light is placed either in the axilla or on the anterior chest, the affected side will glow more than the unaffected side—the "Chinese lantern sign" (Figure 24.1). This works best for small infants with large pneumothoraces, though false negatives and more rarely false positives occur, and sensitivity and specificity data are not established. In emergency this can allow rapid lateralization and treatment for a neonate that is arresting or in near-arrest.

CXR is the primary method by which pneumothoraces are diagnosed, though because neonatal CXR are taken supinely, smaller air collections may be subtle and difficult to see, as they are spread across the anterior chest. A large pneumothorax causing collapse of the affected side and mediastinal shift is easy to detect (Figure 24.2). However, subtle radiographic indications such as hyperlucency of the abdomen, the deep sulcus sign (a deep and lucent costophrenic angle, as in Figure 24.3), double diaphragm

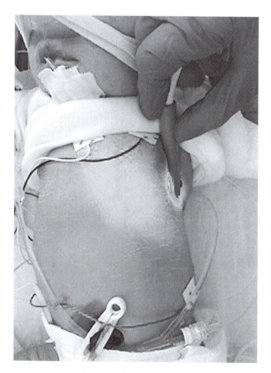

FIGURE 24.1 • Transillumination with a fiberoptic light demonstrates extensive light transmission causing a glowing chest indicative of a left pneumothorax in this patient on CPAP.

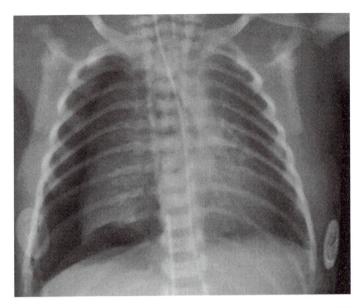

FIGURE 24.2 • CXR demonstrates a large right pneumothorax in this mechanically ventilated patient. Note also tracheal and mediastinal deviation resulting from the enlarging right hemithorax. This patient required thoracostomy tube placement.

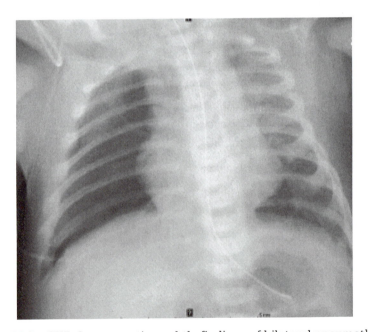

FIGURE 24.3 • CXR demonstrating subtle findings of bilateral pneumothoraces in a term infant on CPAP. Note right sulcus sign (right lateral sulcus is deep and hyperlucent) and over-distinct cardiac border on the left. This infant had relatively mild lung disease, was taken off CPAP, and did not require treatment.

sign, and increased sharpness of the cardiomediastinal border (see also Figure 24.3) may be present in smaller pneumothoraces but can also be missed without close attention. In patients requiring mechanical ventilation, these may present subtly initially but will often expand over time and require treatment (Figure 24.4). It can be difficult to distinguish between a hyperlucent or hyperinflated hemithorax and contralateral atelectasis or opacification, making the chest appear relatively hyperlucent. In these cases, a cross-table lateral CXR or lateral decubitus film may help in differentiating the two conditions.

Computed tomography (CT) scan can pick up small pneumothoraces not seen on CXR, but is infrequently used in the neonate for initial evaluation. It may be useful in infants with cystic lung disease or recurrent pneumothoraces as part of a more detailed evaluation. Lung ultrasound (US) has also been used to make a bedside diagnosis, but this practice is currently uncommon.

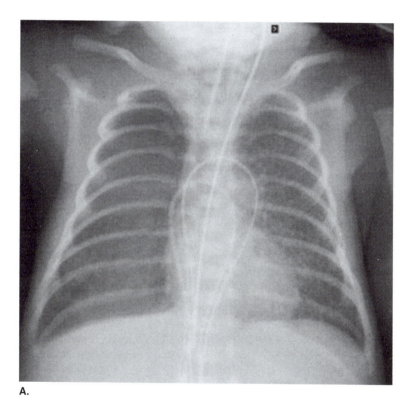

A.

FIGURE 24.4 • Progressively more apparent right pneumothorax in a ventilated infant. Note subtle hyperinflation and a nearly imperceptible double diaphragm sign in (A), with progression to increasing inflation, hyperlucency, and a deep sulcus (B) and then a very large pneumothorax causing compression of the right lung and mediastinum (C). Because of the supine positioning, lung markings are seen out to the periphery until the pneumothorax is quite advanced. Figure (D) demonstrates evacuation of the pneumothorax and reinflation of the lung after pigtail catheter placement. Note lower than normal entry site (7th intercostal space) because this patient also had a basilar empyema.

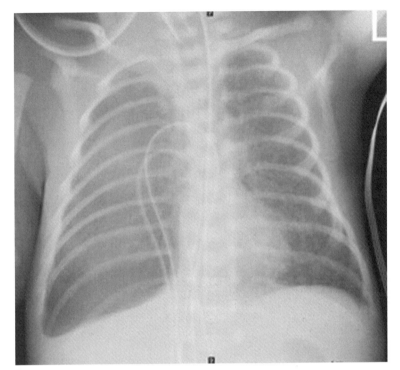

B.

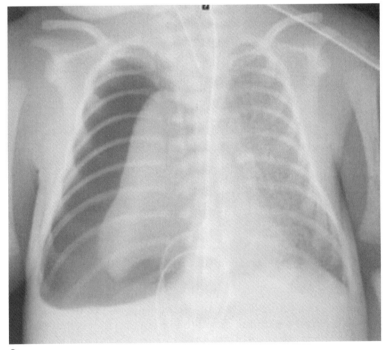

C.

FIGURE 24.4 • (Continued)

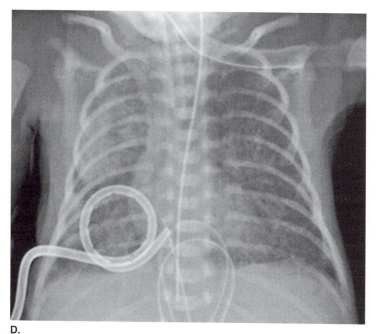

D.

FIGURE 24.4 • (*Continued*)

RECOMMENDATIONS

MAJOR RECOMMENDATIONS

Treatment should be individualized based on the degree of respiratory distress, extent of lung disease, and clinical course. Current data suggest that the so-called "nitrogen wash-out method," which necessitates placing the infant in an oxyhood with 100% oxygen to aid the resorption of the pneumothorax, is ineffectual and exposes the infant to hyperoxia unnecessarily. This technique is based on fairly small adult and animal studies and has very little neonatal data. Recent knowledge about the dangers of hyperoxia and this lack of evidence has led to questions about this practice regarding both safety and efficacy. Indeed, two recent studies, though nonrandomized and retrospective, showed that time to resolution of clinical symptoms of pneumothorax was no shorter when patients were treated with 100% oxygen than when oxygen was titrated based on saturations or patients were followed in room air. Those in the 100% oxygen group, unsurprisingly, had a longer time on oxygen treatment and intravenous fluids.

Special consideration should also be given to neonates with a smaller pneumothorax who need to be transported by air. The lower oxygen content can have an effect, resulting in the expansion of the pneumothorax. Thus the threshold for treatment should be lowered in these infants.

PRACTICE OPTIONS

Practice Option #1: Observation/Increased Monitoring

Infants who evidence only tachypnea or slightly increased work of breathing and are able to maintain ventilation and oxygenation with only modest support (such as nasal cannula oxygen titrated as needed) will often have spontaneous resolution of the pneumothorax over time. These infants are more likely to be term, have mild lung disease, and have small and/or moderate-sized pneumothoraces rather than large. These patients should be closely observed in regard to respiratory rate, work of breathing, and pulse oximetry, and blood gases should be done as needed. If the infant initially required positive pressure ventilation (e.g., CPAP) but has improved and no longer requires this support, it should be removed to decreased the likelihood of the pneumothorax enlarging.

Supportive care, including intravenous fluids or orogastric feeds, should also be supplied as appropriate. Symptom resolution usually occurs in 12–24 hours. This is much less likely to be successful for infants who continue to need positive pressure ventilation (CPAP or mechanical ventilation) or with large pneumothoraces. Infants with congenital anomalies or pulmonary hypoplasia will also usually fail conservative management.

Practice Option #2: Needle Thoracentesis

Needle aspiration of the pneumothoraces is undertaken in two specific settings. For infants with a tension pneumothorax causing compression of the mediastinum and cardiac arrest, this emergency treatment is an absolute necessity. Symptomatic infants with a moderate to large pneumothorax who are cardiovascularly stable may also be treated with thoracentesis initially, with close follow-up by CXR to see if the pneumothorax recurs.

The procedure can be performed with either a large-bore angiocatheter (16- to 20-gauge) or a butterfly needle. In the supine infant, thoracentesis should be undertaken in the midclavicular line in the second, third, or fourth intercostal space, just above the rib. This is the most anterior portion of the chest and should be the site of collection of air. Sterile technique should be used to whatever degree is possible given the emergent nature of the procedure. A "whoosh" of air may be heard, and neonates with a tension pneumothorax should show rapid improvement. Extension tubing and a syringe should be connected to measure the amount of air evacuated and assess for continuous air leak.

The main advantages of this procedure are that it is quick and is less invasive than thoracostomy tube placement. Most infants requiring mechanical ventilation, particularly those with a continuous air leak, will require subsequent placement of a thoracostomy tube.

Practice Option #3: Thoracostomy/Chest Tube Placement

Thoracostomy tubes are used to allow continuous evacuation of a pneumothorax, and as stated, are needed for continuous air leak, and for the majority of patients requiring mechanical ventilation with a pneumothorax. Patients with loculated pneumothorax or bilateral air leak may require several chest tubes. Placement should be undertaken by an experienced clinician following sterile procedure and with appropriate analgesia, sedation, and immobilization of the patient. Both traditional PVC chest tubes (with or without trocar) and pigtail catheters have been used extensively, and either is appropriate. Choice is often made on clinician experience; there is no trial data comparing the two, though those preferring a pigtail drain have described faster insertion time and a smaller incision. However, they may be more prone to kinking and obstructing, given their smaller size.

The usual recommended insertion site is in the lateral chest (mid axillary line) in the fourth, fifth, or sixth intercostal space just above the rib, and directed anteriorly to allow optimal evacuation of air. The patient should be positioned so the site of insertion is the most anterior, and air collects there. Chest tubes may also be placed anteriorly, or higher or lower if conditions necessitate this (e.g., additional fluid collection, anatomic abnormalities); ultrasound guidance may be useful in such cases. Position should be confirmed on CXR; a lateral CXR may also be useful to determine if the tube has been placed anteriorly as desired. It is important that all evacuation holes are inside the chest for the tube to work effectively. Even with excellent technique, perforation of the lung can occur with all types of chest tubes.

Once in place, the chest tube should be secured and connected to an evacuation chamber, usually under slight negative pressure—a recommended starting point is 10 cm H_2O. If possible, pressures should be lowered on the ventilator, which can decrease the amount of air leak. Subsequently, the output and patient should be monitored continuously. Usually there is a substantial release of air followed by intermittent air evacuation, which may be minimal, although continuous air leaks also occur. Patients with a continuous air leak are very tenuous, and any change in status (e.g., increased work of breathing, desaturation) should prompt evaluation of the chest tube, especially for patency and position.

In rare cases of persistent and continuous air leak—often lasting several weeks— measures such as unilateral ventilation or surgical treatment (either pleurodesis or removal of the affected part of the lung) have been attempted with varying degrees of success. There are case reports only of such therapies, which should be attempted at specialty centers.

CLINICAL ALGORITHM(S)

Although there is general agreement on the management of pneumothorax, a society-supported algorithm is not available and full consensus does not exist. Many clinical practice guidelines exist that have been developed by various institutions and are published online (http://www.adhb.govt.nz/newborn/Guidelines/Respiratory/Pneumothorax/PneumothoraxOverview.htm; http://www.asph.mobi/Guidelines_Neonatal/Pneumothorax.pdf). These can be used as guides when institutions are developing their own algorithms, but are based on expert opinion alone and none have been validated.

IMPLEMENTATION OF GUIDELINE

DESCRIPTION OF IMPLEMENTATION STRATEGY

It is recommended that institutions develop and agree on clinical guidelines for both initial and continuing management of pneumothorax in neonates. These are rarer in the modern era of neonatology, and staff caring for infants with a pneumothorax or thoracostomy tube may do so infrequently, so guidelines and frequent training are essential.

QUALITY METRICS

There are no published quality metrics regarding pneumothorax, either prevention or treatment. However, NICUs should monitor their incidence of pneumothorax and evaluate each occurrence. For very low birth weight (VLBW) infants, best practices such as volume-driven ventilation and appropriate use of surfactant have been shown to decrease the incidence significantly. Close attention should be paid to use of positive pressure applied during resuscitation and judicious use of CPAP, especially for term infants.

Treatment should be individualized based on the degree of respiratory distress, extent of lung disease, and clinical course. Use of 100% oxygen should be avoided unless necessary for maintaining saturations.

SUMMARY

Though much less common with modern neonatal care, pneumothorax remains a significant concern and is associated with high mortality in VLBW infants. Preventive measures are key, but pneumothoraces still occur and prompt diagnosis and thoughtful management are essential. Prognosis varies widely depending on etiology.

BIBLIOGRAPHIC SOURCE(S)

Aly H, Massaro A, Acun C, Ozen M. Pneumothorax in the newborn: clinical presentation, risk factors and outcomes. *J Matern Fetal Neonatal Med.* 2014;27(4):402-6.

Bahadue FL, Soll R. Early versus delayed selective surfactant treatment for neonatal respiratory distress syndrome. *Cochrane Database Syst Rev.* 2012;14;11:CD001456.

Benterud T, Sandvik L, Lindemann R. Cesarean section is associated with more frequent pneumothorax and respiratory problems in the neonate. *Acta Obstet Gynecol Scand.* 2009;88(3):359-61.

Bhat YR, Ramdas V. Predisposing factors, incidence and mortality of pneumothorax in neonates. *Minerva Pediatr.* 2013;65(4):383-8.

Bhatia R, Davis PG, Doyle LW, Wong C, Morley CJ. Identification of pneumothorax in very preterm infants. *J Pediatr.* 2011;159(1):115-20.

Clark SD, Saker F, Schneeberger MT, Park E, Sutton DW, Littner Y. Administration of 100% oxygen does not hasten resolution of symptomatic spontaneous pneumothorax in neonates. *J Perinatol.* 2014;34(7):528-31.

Cizmeci MN, Akin K, Kanburoglu MK, et al. The utility of special radiological signs on routinely obtained supine anteroposterior chest radiographs for the early recognition of neonatal pneumothorax. *Neonatology.* 2013;104(4):305-11.

Cizmeci MN, Kanburoglu MK, Akelma AZ, Andan H, Akin K, Tatli MM. An abrupt increment in the respiratory rate is a sign of neonatal pneumothorax. *J Matern Fetal Neonatal Med.* 2015;28(5):583-7.

Duong HH, Mirea L, Shah PS, Yang J, Lee SK, Sankaran K. Pneumothorax in neonates: trends, predictors and outcomes. *J Neonatal Perinatal Med.* 2014;7(1):29-38.

Hishikawa K, Goishi K, Fujiwara T, Kaneshige M, Ito Y, Sago H. Pulmonary air leak associated with CPAP at term birth resuscitation. *Arch Dis Child Fetal Neonatal Ed.* 2015;100(5):F382-7.

Joseph LJ, Bromiker R, Toker O, Schimmel MS, Goldberg S, Picard E. Unilateral lung intubation for pulmonary air leak syndrome in neonates: a case series and a review of the literature. *Am J Perinatol.* 2011;28(2):151-6.

Ozer EA, Ergin AY, Sutcuoglu S, Ozturk C, Yurtseven A. Is pneumothorax size on chest x-ray a predictor of neonatal mortality? *Iran J Pediatr.* 2013;23(5):541-5.

Peng W, Zhu H, Shi H, Liu E. Volume-targeted ventilation is more suitable than pressure-limited ventilation for preterm infants: a systematic review and meta-analysis. *Arch Dis Child Fetal Neonatal Ed.* 2014;99(2):F158-65.

Shaireen H, Rabi Y, Metcalfe A, et al. Impact of oxygen concentration on time to resolution of spontaneous pneumothorax in term infants: a population based cohort study. *BMC Pediatr.* 2014;14:208.

Smith J, Schumacher RE, Donn SM, Sarkar S. Clinical course of symptomatic spontaneous pneu-mothorax in term and late preterm newborns: report from a large cohort. *Am J Perinatol.* 2011;28(2):163-8.

Wei YH, Lee CH, Cheng HN, Tsao LT, Hsiao CC. Pigtail catheters versus traditional chest tubes for pneumothoraces in premature infants treated in a neonatal intensive care unit. *Pediatr Neo-natol.* 2014;55(5):376-80.

Wheeler KI, Klingenberg C, Morley CJ, Davis PG. Volume-targeted versus pressure-limited ventilation for preterm infants: a systematic review and meta-analysis. *Neonatology.* 2011;100(3):219-27.

Apnea

Mitali Pakvasa, MD • Ravi M. Patel, MD, MSc

SCOPE

DISEASE/CONDITION(S)

Apnea of prematurity, bronchopulmonary dysplasia.

GUIDELINE OBJECTIVE(S)

The objective of this care path is to summarize current evidence and provide guidance on the use of caffeine in preterm infants as it relates to the management of apnea of prematurity.

BRIEF BACKGROUND

Apnea of prematurity, defined as a cessation of breathing for 20 seconds or longer, or a shorter pause accompanied by bradycardia, cyanosis, or pallor, is one of the most common diagnoses in the neonatal intensive care unit. Apnea is traditionally classified into three categories: central, obstructive, and mixed, with the majority of apneic episodes in preterm infants being mixed events. The incidence of apnea increases with decreasing gestational age, occurring in nearly all infants born at or before 28 weeks' gestation and 85% of infants who are born at 30 weeks' gestation. The frequency of hypoxemic episodes, which can be related to apnea, are associated with a higher risk of death or disability at 18 months corrected age. Methylxanthines, including aminophylline, theophylline, or caffeine, have been the mainstay of pharmacologic therapy to treat and prevent apnea of prematurity for more than 30 years. Caffeine is currently the preferred and most commonly used methylxanthine because of its wide therapeutic index, longer half-life, and lack of need for drug-level monitoring.

RECOMMENDATIONS

MAJOR RECOMMENDATIONS

Treatment with caffeine in the first 10 days after birth in a large, multicenter, multinational, placebo-controlled, and blinded randomized trial was demonstrated to reduce the risk of bronchopulmonary dysplasia (BPD) (adjusted odds ratio 0.63; 95% CI 0.52–0.76) and decrease the risk of death or disability at 18–21 months (adjusted odds ratio 0.77; 95% CI 0.64–0.93) without any significant short- or long-term safety concerns. Further, a systematic review and meta-analysis of five studies enrolling 192 preterm infants demonstrated methylxanthine treatment effectively reduces apnea 2 to 7 days after treatment (pooled relative risk 0.44; 95% CI 0.32–0.60; I^2 10%).

- *Recommendation:* In patients weighing 500 to 1250 g at birth, caffeine citrate should be initiated at a loading dose of 20 mg/kg followed by 5 mg/kg daily to either treat apnea, prevent apnea, or to facilitate extubation. *Strong recommendation, high quality evidence.*
- *GRADE assessment:* No significant downgrades to the quality of evidence were identified, based on the cumulative evidence from a systematic review and meta-analysis of five trials evaluating the effect of methylxanthines on apnea as well as a single, large, multicenter randomized trial evaluating the effect of caffeine on short- and long-term outcomes. In addition, future randomized, placebo-controlled trials of caffeine are unlikely to be conducted given the efficacy and safety of caffeine demonstrated in studies to date.

Practice Option #1: Should Caffeine be Used to Increase the Success of Extubation?

Several randomized trials have evaluated the use of caffeine in mechanically ventilated neonates. The Caffeine for Apnea of Prematurity trial demonstrated that caffeine-treated infants had a shorter duration of mechanical ventilation by approximately 1 week with this group having a younger postmenstrual age at extubation (median [interquartile range] 29.1 weeks [28.0–31.0] among caffeine treated infants compared to 30.0 weeks [28.7–31.9] among placebo-treated infants; P <0.001). A Cochrane review of six trials evaluating the use of methylxanthines (caffeine or theophylline) in 197 patients on the outcome of failed extubation concluded that treatment with methylxanthines significantly reduced failure of extubation within 1 week of treatment (pooled relative risk 0.48; 95% CI 0.32–0.71; I^2 0%).

- *Recommendation:* In mechanically ventilated very low birth weight infants (<1500 g), caffeine use should be considered to increase the success of extubation. *Weak recommendation, moderate quality evidence.*
- *GRADE assessment:* Quality of evidence was downgraded from high to moderate for imprecision (small studies with wide confidence intervals) and indirectness (generalizability to the population of ventilated preterm infants in current neonatal care).

Practice Option #2: Use of Early Caffeine in Infants on Positive Airway Pressure Respiratory Support

Four observational studies have evaluated the association between early initiation of caffeine in the first 2 days after birth, compared to later initiation, and neonatal outcomes. Pooled estimates obtained from confounder-adjusted associations including 37,262 infants from these four studies indicate that early initiation of caffeine is associated with a decreased risk of BPD when compared to later initiation (pooled adjusted odds ratio 0.74; 95% CI 0.69–0.78 fixed-effects; I^2 12%). Additional potential benefits of early initiation of caffeine include a reduction in the duration of ventilation, decreased treatment of retinopathy of prematurity, and a decreased treatment of a patent ductus arteriosus. However, results from adequately powered randomized trials are lacking to confirm the benefit of early caffeine treatment on important neonatal outcomes, including BPD. In addition, one study reported a small but statistically significant increased risk of mortality associated with early caffeine, which was not reported in any of the other observational studies. This association was thought to be biased from survival bias related to late caffeine treatment.

- *Recommendation:* In very low birth weight infants who are receiving positive airway pressure respiratory support (e.g., invasive or noninvasive ventilation, continuous positive airway pressure therapy), consider early initiation of caffeine in the first 2 days after birth as part of a strategy to decrease the duration of ventilation and risk of BPD. *Weak recommendation, low quality evidence.*
- *GRADE assessment:* Quality of evidence was based on observational studies and therefore was low. The risk of bias was high due to potential for confounding by indication for early caffeine, although studies used various approaches to adjust for confounding, including covariate adjustment and propensity matching. In addition, the findings of the association between early caffeine and decreased BPD were consistent across studies and the estimates were precise owing to the large sample sizes of studies. It is possible that ongoing clinical trials (clinicaltrials.gov identifiers NCT02524249 and NCT01751724) may change the recommendation, and therefore this possibility along with the low quality of evidence led to a weak recommendation.

Practice Option #3: Should High Dose Maintenance Therapy with Caffeine Citrate (20 mg/kg/day) Be Used in Patients with Persistent Apnea?

Caffeine citrate is labeled in the United States for maintenance dosing of 5–10 mg/kg/day. Studies suggest higher maintenance doses of caffeine citrate (20 mg/kg/day) are more effective in reducing apneic episodes and decreasing extubation failure compared to standard doses of caffeine citrate (5 mg/kg/day). In a multicenter randomized, blinded trial, high-dose caffeine decreased the risk of extubation failure (relative risk 0.51; 95% CI 0.31–0.85) and the median number (IQR) of apnea episodes per day (four episodes [1–12] among high-dose infants compared to seven episodes [2–22] among standard-dose infants; P <0.01). However, there are safety concerns with the use of high-dose caffeine owing to an increased frequency of cerebellar hemorrhage reported in a single-center randomized trial of high-dose caffeine citrate (80 mg/kg loading dose followed by 20 mg/kg/day) compared with standard-dose caffeine citrate (20 mg/kg loading dose followed by 5–10 mg/kg/day) (36% vs 10%, P = 0.03). Of note, as preterm infants get older, they may require increases in caffeine dose to maintain therapeutic effects.

- *Recommendation:* In patients with persistent apnea on maintenance caffeine citrate of 5 mg/kg/day, the dose can be safely increased to a maximum daily dose of 10 mg/kg/day. *Strong recommendation, moderate quality evidence.*
- *GRADE assessment:* Quality of evidence was based on randomized trials and therefore started as high. However, the indirectness of the evidence with regard to the lack of assessment of the effect of increases in the dose of caffeine on apnea in a large,

multicenter clinical trial led evidence to be downgraded to moderate. Given the extensive long-term follow-up and safety assessment of caffeine citrate with doses up to 10 mg/kg/day, this was given a strong recommendation.

- *Recommendation:* In patients with persistent apnea, high-dose caffeine (20 mg/kg/day of maintenance caffeine citrate) should *not* be routinely used because of a potential for increased risk of cerebellar hemorrhage. *Weak recommendation, low quality evidence.*
- *GRADE assessment:* Quality of evidence was based on randomized trials and therefore started as high. However, the inconsistency across studies and imprecision with regard to the risk of intracranial hemorrhage with high-dose caffeine and the bias from multiple hypothesis testing of a secondary outcome led to the evidence being downgraded to low quality. Because some studies suggest potential benefit from high-dose caffeine, which must be weighed against the potential for an increased risk of intracranial hemorrhage, a weak recommendation against high-dose caffeine was provided.

CLINICAL ALGORITHM(S)

Figure 25.1 is a suggested algorithm that was developed as a quick reference summation of the previously mentioned practice options and recommendations.

IMPLEMENTATION OF GUIDELINE

DESCRIPTION OF IMPLEMENTATION STRATEGY

Strategies for implementation include incorporation of caffeine in admission order sets. Clinical decision support could be utilized to ensure infants with documented apnea are receiving caffeine. Development of local guidelines for use, with allowance for variation utilizing practice options in this care path, could be employed.

QUALITY METRICS

No current quality metrics for caffeine are available. Given the effect of caffeine on BPD, the local incidence of BPD among very low birth weight infants during relevant time periods (e.g., quarterly, yearly) could be considered as an outcome metric.

SUMMARY

Apnea of prematurity remains a common problem in preterm infants. Caffeine citrate is a safe and effective treatment for apnea of prematurity when using routine dosing of a loading dose of 20 mg/kg followed by daily maintenance dose of 5 mg/kg. Caffeine should be considered in mechanically ventilated preterm infants as caffeine treatment within the first 10 days after birth has been shown to decrease the duration of invasive ventilation. In addition, caffeine increases the success of extubation. Early initiation of caffeine therapy in the first 2 days after birth may be considered in those infants who are likely to require caffeine, as observational studies suggest that caffeine may reduce the duration of mechanical ventilation or decrease the risk of BPD. If the patient continues to experience symptoms despite pharmacologic therapy, increasing the maintenance dose to 10 mg/kg/day may be considered. However, there are currently safety concerns for the use of caffeine citrate doses that exceed 10 mg/kg/day.

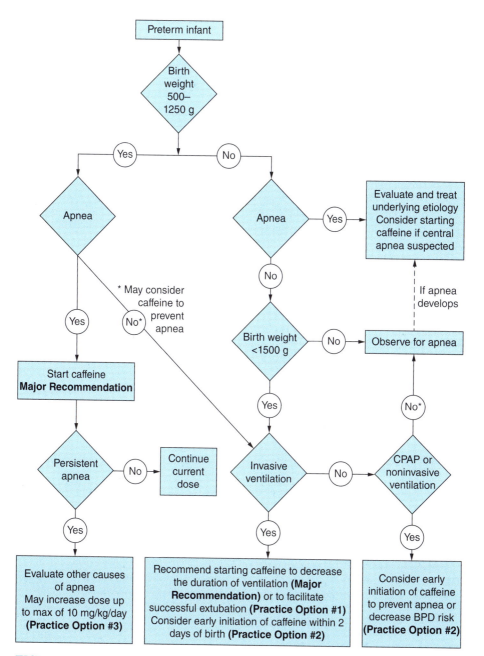

FIGURE 25.1 • Clinical algorithm for use of caffeine. *Disclaimer*: Additional factors beyond this algorithm should be taken into account in deciding on caffeine treatment. These include individual patient circumstances, the quality of evidence and strength of recommendation, and the balance of potential risks and benefits.

BIBLIOGRAPHIC SOURCE(S)

Charles BG, Townsend FR, Steer PA, Flenady VJ, Grady PH, Sherman A. Caffeine citrate treatment for extremely premature infants with apnea: population pharmacokinetics, absolute bioavailability, and implications for therapeutic drug monitoring. *Ther Drug Monit.* 2008;30(6):709-16.

Dobson NR, Hunt CE. Pharmacology review: caffeine use in neonates: indications, pharmacokinetics, clinical outcomes. *NeoReviews.* 2003;14:e54-550.

Dobson NR, Patel RM, Smith PB, et al. Trends in caffeine use and association between clinical outcomes and timing of therapy in very low birth weight infants. *J Pediatr.* 2014;164(5):992-8.e3.

Eichenwald EC, Committee on Fetus and Newborn. Apnea of prematurity. *Pediatrics.* 2016;137(1):e1-6.

Henderson-Smart DJ, Davis PG. Prophylactic methylxanthines for endotracheal extubation in preterm infants. *Cochrane Database Syst Rev.* 2010;(12):CD000139.

Henderson-Smart DJ, De Paoli AG. Methylxanthine treatment for apnoea in preterm infants. *Cochrane Database Syst Rev.* 2010;(12):CD000140.

Lodha A, Seshia M, McMillan DD, et al. Association of early caffeine administration and neonatal outcomes in very preterm neonates. *JAMA Pediatr.* 2015;169(1):33-8.

Martin JR, Abu-Shaweesh JM, Baird TM. Pathophysiologic mechanisms underlying apnea of prematurity. *NeoReviews.* 2002;3:e59-64.

McPherson C, Neil JJ, Tjoeng, Pineda R, Inder TE. A pilot randomized trial of high-dose caffeine therapy in preterm infants. *Pediatr Res.* 2015;78(2):198-204.

Park HW, Lim G, Chung SH, Chung S, Kim KS, Kim SN. Early Caffeine use in very low birth weight infants and neonatal outcomes: a systematic review and meta-analysis. *J Korean Med Sci.* 2015;30(12):1828-35.

Patel RM, Leong T, Carlton DP, Vyas-Read S. Early caffeine therapy and clinical outcomes in extremely preterm infants. *J Perinatol.* 2013;33(2):134-40.

Poets CF, Roberts RS, Schmidt B, et al. Association between intermittent hypoxemia or bradycardia and late death or disability in extremely preterm infants. *JAMA.* 2015;314(6):595-603.

Schmidt B, Anderson PJ, Doyle LW, et al. Caffeine for apnea of prematurity (CAP) trial investigators. Survival without disability to age 5 years after neonatal caffeine therapy for apnea of prematurity. *JAMA.* 2012;307(3):275-82.

Schmidt B, Roberts RS, Davis P, et al. Caffeine therapy for apnea of prematurity. *N Engl J Med.* 2006;354(20):2112-21.

Schmidt B, Roberts RS, Davis P, et al. Long-term effects of caffeine therapy for apnea of prematurity. *N Engl J Med.* 2007;357(19):1893-1902.

Steer P, Flenady VJ, Shearman A, et al. High dose caffeine citrate for extubation of preterm infants: a randomized control trial. *Arch Dis Child Fetal Neonatal Ed.* 2004;89(6):F499-503.

Taha D, Kirkby S, Nawab U, et al. Early caffeine therapy for prevention of bronchopulmonary dysplasia in preterm infants. *J Matern Fetal Neonatal Med.* 2014;27(16):1698-702.

Subglottic Stenosis

Roy Rajan, MD • Paula Harmon, MD

SCOPE

DISEASE/CONDITION(S)

Narrowing of the subglottic airway leading to respiratory distress in the neonate.

GUIDELINE OBJECTIVE(S)

Identify the condition and describe the nature and severity of the problem; identify means to avoid subglottic stenosis; review medical and surgical treatment options for subglottic stenosis.

BRIEF BACKGROUND

The subglottic airway is the narrowest portion of the childhood airway due to the complete ring of the cricoid cartilage at that site. Subglottic stenosis is defined as narrowing of the normal diameter of this area just below the vocal cords. In a full-term newborn, this is considered an airway that measures less than 4 mm in diameter. Preterm infants have normal airway diameters of 3 or 3.5 mm or larger. Stenoses can be either congenital or acquired, though at times it can be difficult to differentiate, as the airway may have been instrumented prior to discovery. Subglottic stenosis is usually suggested with either insertion of a smaller than expected endotracheal tube or failure to maintain stable respiratory status after extubation.

RECOMMENDATIONS

MAJOR RECOMMENDATIONS

When the neonate presents with respiratory distress and stridor, an otolaryngology consultation is warranted to evaluate the airway for potential causes. Should intubation be needed more urgently, insert the smallest endotracheal tube to allow adequate ventilation. One should see an air leak at 20 cm H_2O, and if this is not found, a smaller tube should be placed. The etiology of most acquired stenosis is from injury related to either infection or trauma. Size of the tube, duration of intubation, movement of the tube, and the need for repeated intubations are all contributing factors for stenosis. Gastroesophageal reflux disease (GERD) may play an adjuvant role in development in subglottic stenosis, as acid reflux may irritate an inflamed area further.

PRACTICE OPTIONS

Practice Option #1

Full-term newborns that require intubation should be intubated with a 3.5 endotracheal tube as the first attempt. Smaller-sized tubes should be available in case there is narrowing below the vocal cords. Premature newborns should have an attempt with a 3.0 or smaller endotracheal tube as deemed appropriate.

Practice Option #2

Stridor in the neonate should warrant an otolaryngology consultation. Subglottic stenosis should be suspected with biphasic stridor that may worsen with exertion. Direct laryngoscopy and bronchoscopy under anesthesia is the gold standard for diagnosis and staging. PA and lateral neck x-rays can identify subglottic stenosis. Airway fluoroscopy can be used to identify this and other abnormalities, such as tracheal stenosis or tracheomalacia. The best test for identifying and quantifying the severity of reflux is a dual-channel pH-impedance probe.

Practice Option #3

Medical management of subglottic stenosis includes use of systemic steroids and racemic epinephrine. Animal studies have shown steroids and antibiotics have improved granular or immature subglottic stenosis, but duration of treatment is unknown and must be considered on a case-by-case basis. Use of heliox may allow better delivery of oxygen. GERD control will prevent worsening of existing irritation and stenoses and may improve the success of reconstruction. Mild or immature stenosis may be observed or dilated serially with or without local steroid injection. Dilation may be done with incisions made in the airway, dilatation, or a combination of the two. Mitomycin-C is an adjunctive topical medication that may be of benefit after dilation of an immature stenosis. Management of early or mild subglottic stenosis with balloon dilation, laser, steroids, and reflux therapy has been found to be effective in 92% of Grade I stenosis patients, 46% in Grade II stenosis, and 13% in Grade III stenosis. Severe stenoses will benefit from either a tracheostomy to bypass the obstruction or an open reconstruction procedure.

CLINICAL ALGORITHM(S)

Table 26.1 contains the Cotton-Myer grading scale of subglottic stenosis. Figure 26.1 shows representative subglottic pictures of the stenoses.

TABLE 26.1. Cotton-Myer Grading Scale of Subglottic Stenosis

Grade I: <50% obstruction	Grade II: 51–70% obstruction
Grade III: 71–99% obstruction	Grade IV: 100% obstruction

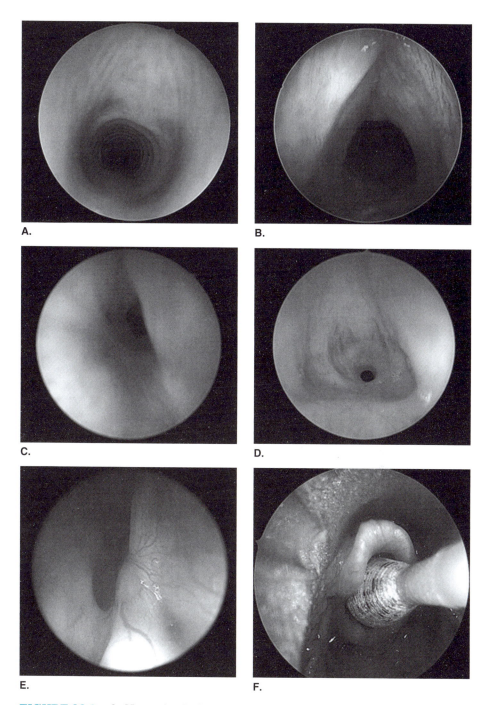

FIGURE 26.1 • A. Normal subglottis; **B.** Grade I stenosis; **C.** Grade II stenosis; **D.** Grade III stenosis; **E.** Grade IV stenosis; **F.** Balloon dilation.

IMPLEMENTATION OF GUIDELINE

QUALIFYING STATEMENTS

Most studies on management of subglottic stenosis in children are based on retrospective data.

DESCRIPTION OF IMPLEMENTATION STRATEGY

Initial management depends on initial patient presentation and findings. Mild to moderate subglottic stenosis (Grade I or II) can undergo medical and endoscopic management with serial clinic visits and interval direct laryngoscopy and bronchoscopy to assess patency. Severe subglottic stenosis patients often require open surgical management, which can include anterior and posterior cricoid split, laryngotracheal reconstruction, combined endoscopic and open surgical management, and/or tracheostomy.

QUALITY METRICS

Monitor rates of identification of subglottic stenosis, number of procedures necessary, failure to extubate, length of hospital stay, and complications.

SUMMARY

Subglottic stenosis can be either congenital or acquired. Diagnosis of subglottic stenosis should be performed in a timely fashion via airway evaluation with an otolaryngologist. This challenging condition is usually managed surgically with endoscopic or open surgical approaches and medical adjunctive treatments.

BIBLIOGRAPHIC SOURCE(S)

Blumin JH, Johnson N. Evidence of extraesophageal reflux in idiopathic subglottic stenosis. *Laryngoscope.* 2011;121:1266-73.

Lindholm CE. Prolonged endotracheal intubation. *Acta Anaesthesiol Scand Suppl.* 1970;33:1.

Maresh A, Preciado DA, O'Connell AP, Zalzal GH. A comparative analysis of open surgery vs endoscopic balloon dilation for pediatric subglottic stenosis. *JAMA Otolaryngol Head Neck Surg.* 2014;140(10):901-5.

Monnier P, George M, Monod ML, Lang F. The role of the CO_2 laser in the management of laryngotracheal stenosis: a survey of 100 cases. *Eur Arch Otorhinolaryngol.* 2005;262(8):602-8.

Myer CM, O'Connor DM, Cotton RT. Proposed grading system for subglottic stenosis based on endotracheal tube sizes. *Ann Otol Rhinol Laryngol.* 1994;103(4 Pt 1):319-23.

Yellon RF, Goyal A. What is the best test for pediatric gastroesophageal reflux disease? *Laryngoscope.* 2013;123:2925-7.

Inhaled Nitric Oxide

Bobby Mathew, MBBS • Satyan Lakshminrusimha, MD

SCOPE

Use of inhaled nitric oxide in persistent pulmonary hypertension and hypoxemic respiratory failure in newborn infants.

DISEASE/CONDITION(S)

Persistent pulmonary hypertension of the newborn (PPHN) and hypoxemic respiratory failure (HRF) are common conditions in the neonatal intensive care unit (NICU) and affect both term and preterm infants. In term infants, pulmonary hypertension can be idiopathic, but is more commonly secondary to lung pathologies such as meconium aspiration syndrome (MAS), pneumonia, respiratory distress syndrome (RDS), perinatal asphyxia, congenital diaphragmatic hernia (CDH), and as a complication of congenital heart disease (CHD), usually in the postoperative period. Pulmonary hypertension is also observed in preterm infants either as a complication of RDS or bronchopulmonary dysplasia (BPD). The severity of HRF is commonly assessed by oxygenation index (OI). Oxygenation index (OI = mean airway pressure [MAP] in cm $H_2O \times FIO_2/PaO_2$ in mmHg) is commonly used to assess severity and response to therapy in HRF. HRF is classified as mild (OI $\leq$15), moderate (OI >15 to $\leq$25), severe (OI >25 to $\leq$40), and very severe (OI >40).

BRIEF BACKGROUND

Infants with PPHN and HRF are commonly managed with mechanical ventilation, surfactant (in the presence of parenchymal lung disease), and supplemental oxygen to correct hypoxemia. If this conventional therapy is not effective, patients are treated with inhaled nitric oxide (iNO). Patients who fail to demonstrate sustained improvement in oxygenation with iNO and/or have persistent hypoxemia or evidence of cardiorespiratory compromise may need extracorporeal membrane oxygenation (ECMO). This chapter provides a framework for the indications, dosing, monitoring, contraindications, and side effects of iNO, the only FDA-approved pulmonary vasodilator in the newborn period.

RECOMMENDATIONS

The goal of therapy in HRF and PPHN is to improve oxygenation and reduce the stress on the right ventricle by reducing pulmonary vascular resistance. Specific pulmonary vasodilators such as iNO and oxygen reduce pulmonary vascular resistance and reduce right ventricular afterload.

INDICATIONS FOR iNO

Severe HRF with PPHN

Inhaled nitric oxide is a pulmonary vasodilator approved for use in post-term, term, and late preterm infants (>34 weeks' gestation at birth) for management of severe HRF (OI >25) associated with clinical or echocardiographic evidence of pulmonary hypertension in conjunction with ventilator support and other appropriate agents and reduces the need for ECMO (Class I; level of evidence A).

Moderate HRF with PPHN

Inhaled NO is indicated in term and late preterm infants with moderate HRF (OI >15 to ≤25) associated with evidence of PPHN to prevent further progression of disease (OI >30) (Class I; level of evidence B).

Non-Approved Uses of iNO

Preterm Infants. Rare instances of HRF associated with PPHN pathophysiology and suspected pulmonary hypoplasia secondary to prolonged rupture of membranes (PROM) (Class IIa; level of evidence B).

Bronchopulmonary Dysplasia. Treatment of established BPD associated symptomatic pulmonary hypertension (Class IIA; level of evidence C). The use of iNO as prophylaxis for prevention of BPD is not recommended.

Congenital Diaphragmatic Hernia. Inhaled NO is commonly used to improve oxygenation in infants with CDH and severe PPHN but was not shown to reduce the need for ECMO in a randomized trial. It should be used cautiously in subjects with suspected left ventricular dysfunction (Class IIb; level of evidence B).

Congenital Heart Disease. Inhaled NO can be used as the initial therapy for pulmonary hypertensive crisis and right-sided heart failure during the postoperative period (Class I; level of evidence B).

MECHANISM OF ACTION AND METABOLISM

The vasodilatory effect of iNO is mediated through the second messenger cyclic GMP that reduces cytosolic ionic calcium leading to vascular smooth muscle relaxation. Once NO enters the vascular system it is scavenged by hemoglobin and rapidly inactivated, thereby limiting the vasodilatory effect to the pulmonary vasculature. Cyclic GMP is degraded by phosphodiesterase 5 (PDE 5) enzyme, terminating the vasodilatory effect (Figure 27.1). iNO is a selective pulmonary vasodilator, as it does not reach the systemic circulation. It is also "microselective" as it only dilates blood vessels coupled to alveoli that are well ventilated. Hence iNO improves ventilation-perfusion matching by selectively increasing blood flow to the well-ventilated portions of the lungs.

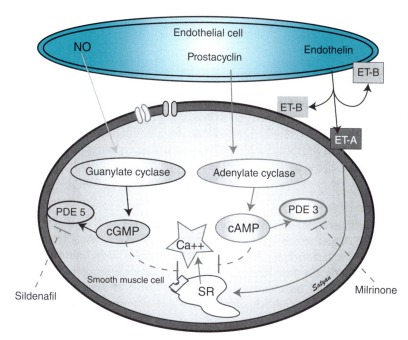

FIGURE 27.1 • Regulation of pulmonary vascular tone. Nitric oxide (NO), prostacyclin (PGI$_2$), and vasoconstrictor endothelin (ET) are the three main pathways regulating pulmonary vasculature. Endothelial nitric oxide synthase (eNOS) produces NO, which diffuses from the endothelium to the smooth muscle cell and stimulates soluble guanylate cyclase (sGC) enzyme to produce cyclic guanosine monophosphate (cGMP). Cyclic GMP is broken down by PDE 5 enzyme in the smooth muscle cell. Sildenafil inhibits PDE5 and increases cGMP levels in pulmonary arterial smooth muscle cells. Prostacyclin acts on its receptor in the smooth muscle cell and stimulates adenylate cyclase (AC) to produce cyclic adenosine monophosphate (cAMP). Cyclic AMP is broken down by phosphodiesterase 3 (PDE 3) in the smooth muscle cell. Milrinone inhibits PDE 3 and increases cAMP levels in pulmonary arterial smooth muscle cells. Cyclic AMP and cGMP reduce cytosolic ionic calcium concentrations and induce smooth muscle cell relaxation and pulmonary vasodilation. Endothelin is a powerful vasoconstrictor and acts on ET-A receptors in the smooth muscle cell and increases ionic calcium concentration and promotes pulmonary vasoconstriction. (Modified from Nair J, Lakshminrusimha S. Update on PPHN: mechanisms and treatment. *Semin Perinatol.* 2014;38(2):78-91. Copyright Satyan Lakshminrusimha.)

CLINICAL AND ECHOCARDIOGRAPHIC EVIDENCE OF PULMONARY HYPERTENSION

The hallmark of PPHN is labile oxygen saturations due to shunting of deoxygenated blood from the pulmonary artery into the systemic circulation through the patent ductus arteriosus (PDA) or across the patent foramen ovale (PFO). The lability is due to the varying amount of the shunt because of changing blood pressure differential between the pulmonary and systemic circulations. Pre- and postductal saturation gradient of

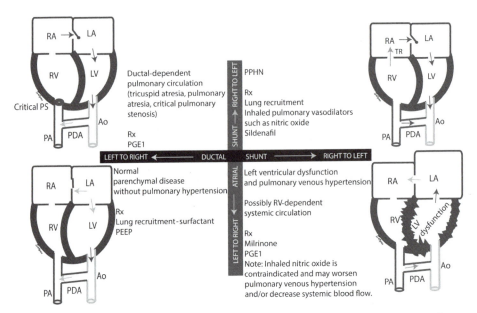

FIGURE 27.2 • Echocardiographic evaluation of neonatal hypoxemic respiratory failure. Left-to-right shunt at the ductal and atrial level is normal but can also be seen in the presence of parenchymal lung disease resulting in hypoxemia in the absence of PPHN (lower left quadrant). The presence of right-to-left shunt at the atrial and ductal level is associated with PPHN (upper right quadrant). Right-to-left shunt at the ductal level with left-to-right shunting at the atrial level is associated with left ventricular dysfunction, pulmonary venous hypertension, and ductal-dependent systemic circulation (lower right quadrant) and is a contraindication for the use of iNO. In patients with right-sided obstruction (such as critical pulmonary stenosis [PS]), right atrial blood flows to the left atrium through the PFO. Pulmonary circulation is dependent on a left-to-right shunt at the PDA (upper left quadrant). Ao, aorta; LA, left atrium; LV, left ventricle; PA, pulmonary artery; PDA, patent ductus arteriosus; PGE1, prostaglandin E1. RA, right atrium; RV, right ventricle; TR, tricuspid regurgitation. (Modified from Nair J, Lakshminrusimha S. Update on PPHN: mechanisms and treatment. *Semin Perinatol.* 2014;38(2):78-91. Copyright Satyan Lakshminrusimha.)

greater than 5% is also a feature of PPHN with shunting at the PDA level (Figure 27.2). Echocardiographic findings include elevated pulmonary arterial pressure (as assessed from tricuspid regurgitant jet velocity) in the systemic or suprasystemic range, bowing or flattening of the interventricular septum into the left ventricle, and the pattern of flow across the fetal channels PFO and PDA. The direction of shunt flow, and ventricular function dictate the choice of therapy in HRF (Figure 27.2).

ADJUVANT THERAPY

Oxygen

Oxygen is a specific and potent pulmonary vasodilator. Hypoxia causes pulmonary vasoconstriction and normoxia produces vasodilation; however, hyperoxia does not cause further vasodilation but can cause oxidative stress and impair response to iNO. A practical approach would be to maintain preductal SpO_2 between 90% and 97% or PaO_2 between 60 mmHg and 80 mmHg.

Ventilation

Respiratory acidosis exacerbates hypoxic vasoconstriction. If the pH is maintained >7.25, pulmonary vasoconstrictor response to hypoxia was attenuated in newborn calves. We recommend maintaining pH in the 7.25–7.40 range with $PaCO_2$ between 40 mmHg and 55 mmHg. Respiratory alkalosis leads to cerebral vasoconstriction and is associated with sensorineural deafness and is not recommended.

Metabolic Acidosis

Maintaining adequate perfusion and systemic blood pressure is an important factor in the management of PPHN. Correction of severe metabolic acidosis with small doses of sodium bicarbonate (1–2 mEq/kg in a diluted solution by slow infusion) may be required to maintain pH >7.25. Metabolic alkalosis with continuous infusions of sodium bicarbonate should be avoided.

Volume and Inotropic Support

Systemic hypotension is common in PPHN and can worsen right-to-left shunt. Judicious use of volume boluses (usually one or two 10 mL/kg of normal saline or lactated Ringers solution) followed by vasopressor therapy (dopamine, norepinephrine, and/or vasopressin) to keep systemic blood pressure in the physiological range is important.

Nutrition

The goal is to provide adequate parenteral calories and maintain adequate serum glucose and calcium levels for optimal cardiac function. This can be achieved by providing a parenteral nutrition solution with calcium gluconate and initiating enteral feeds when stable.

Lung Recruitment

The lung recruitment with the use of positive end-expiratory pressure (PEEP), MAP to achieve lung expansion to functional residual capacity (functional residual capacity [FRC]—usually 8–9 rib expansion on an anteroposterior chest x-ray) should be achieved prior to iNO therapy. iNO reaches only the well-ventilated alveoli; hence, it is very important to have optimal lung recruitment for iNO to reach its site of action. Surfactant administration in the presence of parenchymal lung disease (RDS, MAS, pneumonia) prior to initiation of iNO improves outcome and reduces the need for ECMO.

DOSE

Starting Dose

The starting dose of iNO is typically 20 ppm. Infants with HRF who do not respond to this dose are unlikely to benefit from higher dosing. Also, at this dose the risk of methemoglobinemia is low and increases with higher doses. The use of lower doses (2–5 ppm) of iNO can improve oxygenation but may not lead to sustained decrease in pulmonary arterial pressure. Once an oxygenation response is achieved, iNO dose can be rapidly weaned (see weaning protocol in Figure 27.3).

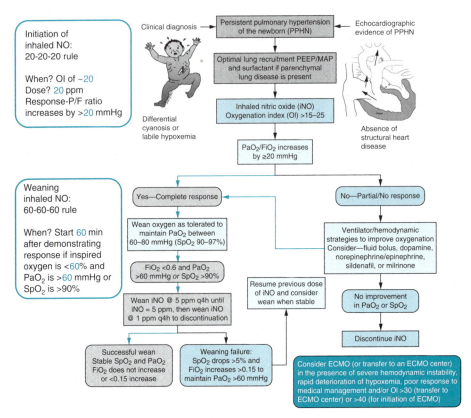

FIGURE 27.3 • Suggested guidelines for initiation and weaning iNO in PPHN/ HRF in NICU. (Adapted from Women & Children's Hospital of Buffalo.) The recommended starting dose of iNO is 20 parts per million (ppm). Improvement in $PaO_2 \geq 20$ mmHg or $SpO_2 \geq 5\%$ is considered complete response. In patients who fail to respond iNO, measures to optimize lung recruitment and hemodynamics need to be undertaken, failing which iNO should be promptly discontinued. In responders, wean FiO_2 initially while maintaining PaO_2 between 60 mmHg and 80 mmHg. Once PaO_2 is stable and FiO_2 is below 0.6, start weaning iNO by 5 ppm every 4 hours until 5 ppm. Below 5 ppm, wean iNO by 1 ppm every 4 hours. During weaning, >5% drop in SpO_2 or sustained increase in FiO_2 >0.15 to maintain $PaO_2 \geq 60$ mmHg is considered weaning failure, and previous dose of iNO should be resumed. Weaning should be restarted when oxygenation is stable. (Modified from Sharma V, Berkelhamer SK, Lakshminrusimha S. Persistent pulmonary hypertension of the newborn. *Matern Health Neonatol Perinatol BMC*. 2015;1(14):1-18. Copyright Satyan Lakshminrusimha.)

The 20-20-20 Rule for Initiation of iNO

- The typical starting dose of iNO is 20 ppm.
- The OI at which iNO is indicated in HRF with PPHN is 20 ± 5.
- Response is often defined as an increase in PaO_2 of 20 mmHg.

MONITORING
Oxygenation
Clinical response to iNO is defined in randomized trials as an improvement in PaO_2 by 20 mmHg at the same FiO_2 within 30–60 min following initiation of therapy. A significant improvement in SpO_2 enabling weaning of inspired oxygen is also considered an adequate response if there is no arterial line access. If there is no oxygenation response or a partial or ill-sustained response, ventilation, lung recruitment, and hemodynamic and inotropic support should be optimized. In spite of these efforts, if there is no oxygenation response it is important to discontinue iNO promptly to prevent downregulation of endogenous nitric oxide production and prevent further injury by formation of free radicals. In patients without arterial access, oxygen saturation index (OSI) can be measured.

$$OSI = \text{mean airway pressure} \times FiO_2 \times 100/SpO_2$$

The approximate relationship of OI and OSI is OI = 2 × OSI.

Hemodynamics
Systemic blood pressure, heart rate, and urine output are closely monitored during iNO therapy. If there is a concern about systemic compromise, base deficit and lactate levels should be monitored.

Methemoglobin and Nitrogen Dioxide
Monitoring of methemoglobin and nitrogen dioxide levels is required during treatment with iNO. High levels of methemoglobin impair the ability of hemoglobin to transport oxygen. Nitrogen dioxide hydrolyses to nitrous and nitric acid in the lung and can cause chemical pneumonitis and pulmonary edema. Nitrogen dioxide level is continuously presented as a readout on the iNO delivery device. Methemoglobin levels should be measured prior to initiation of therapy at 2 hours, 8 hours, and then every 24 hours while on iNO.

Echocardiogram
Periodic echocardiographic evaluation of pulmonary artery pressure and ventricular function is needed to evaluate the response to therapy, and this is especially important in infants with partial response to iNO. Right or left ventricular dysfunction is a very common reason for failure to respond to therapy and subsequent need for ECMO.

WEANING iNO
Abrupt withdrawal of iNO can lead to rebound pulmonary hypertension. However, there is no evidence or consensus-based approach to weaning iNO.

The 60-60-60 Rule for Weaning iNO
The approach practiced in our center is shown in Figure 27.3.
- When to wean? Following a positive oxygenation response, we recommend weaning inspired oxygen first (until it is <60%), and then initiate weaning iNO. If there is no response to iNO and ventilation and hemodynamics are optimized, consider discontinuing iNO by 60 min.

- Indication for weaning: If the patient is on <60% of inspired oxygen with a PaO_2 >60 mmHg (or preductal SpO_2 >90%), we recommend weaning iNO by 5 ppm every 4 hours. Once the patient is on 5 ppm, wean at 1 ppm every 2–4 hours until discontinuation.
- If oxygenation worsens with weaning iNO as evidenced by an increase in FiO_2 or decrease in SpO_2 or PaO_2 (Figure 27.3), resume the previous dose of iNO.

PRECAUTIONS AND CONTRAINDICATIONS

Left Ventricular Dysfunction

Patients with left ventricular dysfunction may have pulmonary venous hypertension. When treated with iNO these patients may experience pulmonary edema and worsening of oxygenation. The increased pulmonary arterial blood flow due to decreased pulmonary vascular resistance with iNO cannot be drained effectively by pulmonary veins due to high left atrial pressure. Interestingly, these patients present with a left-to-right shunt at the PFO level and a right-to-left shunt at the PDA level on echocardiography (Figure 27.2). In these patients, an inodilator such as milrinone might be a preferred pulmonary vasodilator.

Methemoglobinemia

Patients with congenital or acquired methemoglobin reductase deficiency and high levels of methemoglobin are at risk of hypoxemia secondary to methemoglobinemia following therapy with iNO. For this reason, some centers obtain a methemoglobin level prior to initiating iNO.

Congenital Heart Disease Dependent on Right-to-Left Shunting of Blood

In patients with congenital heart disease such as hypoplastic left heart syndrome, critical aortic stenosis, systemic blood supply is dependent on a right-to-left shunt across the PDA. If pulmonary vascular resistance decreases due to iNO, there will be decreased shunting across the ductus leading to systemic hypoperfusion.

SUMMARY

The approval of iNO has led to a significant reduction in need for ECMO for neonatal respiratory indications. However, only two-thirds of patients have a sustained improvement in oxygenation with iNO. Lung recruitment, surfactant use, early initiation of iNO before hemodynamic and respiratory decompensation, high-frequency ventilation, and optimal hemodynamic management can potentially enhance the efficacy of nitric oxide. Pulmonary vasodilator therapy for conditions such as HRF in preterm infants, CDH, and BPD complicated by pulmonary hypertension requires further study. Combination therapy with other vasodilators such as prostacyclins, PDE 5 and PDE 3 inhibitors, and endothelin receptor antagonists (Figure 27.1) may be required to manage intractable pulmonary hypertension associated with these conditions.

BIBLIOGRAPHIC SOURCE(S)

Abman SH, Hansmann G, Archer SL, et al. Pediatric pulmonary hypertension: guidelines from the American Heart Association and American Thoracic Society. *Circulation.* 2015; 132(21):2037-99.

Aschner JL, Gien J, Ambalavanan N, et al. Challenges, priorities and novel therapies for hypoxemic respiratory failure and pulmonary hypertension in the neonate. *J Perinatol.* 2016;36(Suppl 2): S32-6.

Atz AM, Wessel DL. Inhaled nitric oxide in the neonate with cardiac disease. *Semin Perinatol.* 1997;21(5):441-55.

Campbell BT, Herbst KW, Briden KE, Neff S, Ruscher KA, Hagadorn JI. Inhaled nitric oxide use in neonates with congenital diaphragmatic hernia. *Pediatrics.* 2014;134(2):e420-6.

Davidson D, Barefield ES, Kattwinkel J, et al. Inhaled nitric oxide for the early treatment of persistent pulmonary hypertension of the term newborn: a randomized, double-masked, placebo-controlled, dose-response, multicenter study. The I-NO/PPHN Study Group. *Pediatrics.* 1998;101(3 Pt 1):325-34.

Davidson D, Barefield ES, Kattwinkel J, et al. Safety of withdrawing inhaled nitric oxide therapy in persistent pulmonary hypertension of the newborn. *Pediatrics.* 1999;104(2 Pt 1):231-6.

Golombek SG, Young JN. Efficacy of inhaled nitric oxide for hypoxic respiratory failure in term and late preterm infants by baseline severity of illness: a pooled analysis of three clinical trials. *Clin Ther.* 2010;32(5):939-48.

Kinsella JP, Steinhorn RH, Krishnan US, et al. Recommendations for the use of inhaled nitric oxide therapy in premature newborns with severe pulmonary hypertension. *J Pediatr.* 2016;170:312-4.

Konduri GG, Sokol GM, Van Meurs KP, et al. Impact of early surfactant and inhaled nitric oxide therapies on outcomes in term/late preterm neonates with moderate hypoxic respiratory failure. *J Perinatol.* 2013;33(12):944-9.

Lakshminrusimha S, Keszler M. Persistent pulmonary hypertension of the newborn. *Neoreviews.* 2015;16(12):e680-92.

Lakshminrusimha S, Swartz DD, Gugino SF, et al. Oxygen concentration and pulmonary hemodynamics in newborn lambs with pulmonary hypertension. *Pediatr Res.* 2009;66(5):539-44.

Nair J, Lakshminrusimha S. Update on PPHN: mechanisms and treatment. *Semin Perinatol.* 2014;38(2):78-91.

NINOS. Inhaled nitric oxide in full-term and nearly full-term infants with hypoxic respiratory failure. The Neonatal Inhaled Nitric Oxide Study Group. *N Engl J Med.* 1997;336(9):597-604.

NINOS. Inhaled nitric oxide and hypoxic respiratory failure in infants with congenital diaphragmatic hernia. The Neonatal Inhaled Nitric Oxide Study Group (NINOS). *Pediatrics.* 1997;99(6):838-45.

Rawat M, Chandrasekharan PK, Williams A, et al. Oxygen saturation index and severity of hypoxic respiratory failure. *Neonatology.* 2015;107(3):161-6.

Roberts JD Jr, Fineman JR, Morin FC 3rd, et al. Inhaled nitric oxide and persistent pulmonary hypertension of the newborn. The Inhaled Nitric Oxide Study Group. *N Engl J Med.* 1997;336(9):605-610.

Sharma V, Berkelhamer SK, Lakshminrusimha S. Persistent pulmonary hypertension of the newborn. *Matern Health Neonatol Perinatol BMC.* 2015;1(14):1-18.

Steinhorn RH. Advances in neonatal pulmonary hypertension. *Neonatology.* 2016;109(4):334-44.

Pulmonary Hypertension Associated with BPD

Usama Kanaan, MD • Dawn Simon, MD

SCOPE

DISEASE/CONDITION(S)

Pulmonary hypertension, pulmonary artery hypertension, bronchopulmonary dysplasia, chronic lung disease, prematurity.

GUIDELINE OBJECTIVE(S)

Provide screening recommendations including population, mode of screening, timing, and frequency of screening. Provide recommendations for evaluation of infant with concern for bronchopulmonary dysplasia (BPD)-associated pulmonary hypertension (PH) based on screening test. Provide recommendations for treatment (general and PH-specific) of the infant with BPD-associated PH.

BRIEF BACKGROUND

Pulmonary hypertension is an increasingly recognized complication of BPD and chronic lung disease (CLD) of prematurity. Prevalence in retrospective studies of infants with moderate to severe BPD is reported as high as 37%; however, a prospective study reported a lower rate of 17.9%. Pulmonary hypertension in this population has been shown to be an independent risk factor for increased morbidity and mortality and mortality rates are impacted by PH severity. Two-year survival in those with systemic to suprasystemic pulmonary artery pressures was only 25% in one series.

There is significant variability in screening practices, evaluation of affected patients, and treatment of BPD-associated PH. Level of evidence is low for most recommendations, which are largely based on expert opinion.

RECOMMENDATIONS

Infants with moderate to severe BPD are at increased risk for PH. Intrauterine growth restriction is an important risk factor over and above prematurity and BPD. Other factors such as maternal pre-eclampsia, infection, and duration of ventilation may also play disease-modifying roles. These risk factors should be considered when deciding on frequency of screening assessment. The suggested guidelines below are based on a standard-risk infant with moderate to severe BPD. Signs that suggest that PH may be present include labile oxygen saturations, failure to thrive, and need for respiratory support out of proportion to the perceived degree of lung disease. Presence of any of these signs should prompt consideration of assessment for PH outside of a screening paradigm, as there is clinical suspicion for that disease based on more than risk factors.

Screening for BPD-associated PH is largely done by echocardiogram given its widespread availability and ability to noninvasively assess heart function and estimate pulmonary artery pressure as well as evaluate for patent ductus arteriosus (PDA), atrial septal defect (ASD), and other common congenital heart diseases that can mimic or contribute to PH and lung disease. Due to the complexity in interpreting infant echocardiograms in the setting of shunt lesions and other confounders, testing should be performed by sonographers experienced in pediatric cardiac ultrasound and interpreted by pediatric cardiologists.

There is a wide degree of variability in screening, diagnosis, and treatment of this condition across centers. Below are some options obtained from several centers and from published protocols. We have added an asterisk after the guidelines we recommend at our institution.

SCREENING

Whom to Screen

- Based on BPD severity
  - Moderate (O_2 for >28 days plus O_2 <30% at 36 weeks post-menstrual age) or greater BPD
  - All premature infants with BPD requiring any degree of respiratory support beyond 32 weeks post-menstrual age until they come off of respiratory support*
- Based on gestational age
  - Extremely low birth weight infants (<1000 g)
  - Very low birth weight (<1500 g) or smaller
  - Very preterm or less (less than 32 weeks gestational age at birth)
- Based on risk factors or clinical features
  - Only those with identifiable risk factors such as prolonged ventilation, intrauterine growth restriction, exposure to maternal substance abuse, etc.
  - Only those with concerning signs such as growth failure, cyanotic spells, hepatomegaly, increased right ventricular (RV) impulse, hypotension, "black lungs" on chest x-ray (CXR) (this overlaps with the section Evaluation of Patient with Known or Suspected PH later)
  - Any infant with unexplained progressive worsening of respiratory status despite conventional support*

Timing

- When to start
  - At any time that a patient has clinical features suggestive of possible PH[*]
  - 32 weeks corrected gestational age (CGA) or 6 weeks postnatal age, whichever comes second[*]
  - 32 weeks CGA
  - At 36 weeks CGA
  - At term
- When to stop
  - Off of oxygen, with most recent screen having been normal[*]
  - At 2 years of life if still requiring O_2 but preceding screens all normal[*]
  - For centers using one or two set screening times (see below); if screen is normal, no additional testing may be pursued
- Inpatient screening frequency
  - Monthly while in the NICU on respiratory support[*]
  - Twice at 32 weeks CGA and at term or discharge
  - Once at 36 weeks or at term
- Outpatient screening frequency
  - None if inpatient screen is negative
  - Every 6 months until off O_2 or age 2 years[*]

Modality

Echocardiogram. As noted above, interpretation of echocardiogram involves synthesis of information from multiple parts of the study, so giving strict cutoffs for diagnosing PH is not possible (e.g., a tricuspid regurgitant [TR] gradient of 50 mmHg may not suggest elevated pulmonary vascular resistance in the setting of an unrestrictive ductal shunt, whereas a TR gradient of 40 mmHg in the absence of a shunt can be concerning for PH). Consultation with a pediatric cardiologist is recommended to aid in the interpretation of these data. Though frequently cited throughout the literature, we recommend *against* using pulmonary-to-systemic ratio in defining PH (e.g., PH is greater than 50% systemic pressure) as this can lead to both underdiagnosing and overdiagnosing PH. Below are some general guidelines, though many exceptions exist.

- Evidence of right ventricular strain
  - RV hypertrophy
  - RV dilation (in the absence of an atrial shunt)
  - RV dysfunction
    - Depressed tricuspid annular plane systolic excursion (TAPSE) or qualitatively depressed function
  - Right-to-left atrial level shunt
- Evidence of elevated RV and PA pressure in the absence of a significant shunt or RV outflow obstruction
  - Elevated TR gradient
    - TR gradient >32 mmHg—possible elevation in RV/PA systolic pressure
    - TR gradient >40 mmHg—likely RV hypertension
  - Elevated pulmonary regurgitant end-diastolic gradient
    - > 6 mmHg—possible elevation in PA diastolic pressure
    - > 9 mmHg—likely elevation in PA diastolic pressure

- Septal flattening—subjective and poorly repeatable, depends on systemic pressure
  - Low sensitivity in setting of systemic hypertension
  - Low specificity in setting of low systemic pressure
- Evidence of elevated pulmonary vascular resistance
  - PA Doppler notching
  - Shortened pulmonary outflow acceleration time
  - Right-to-left ductal or ventricular shunt

B-Type Natriuretic Peptide. Increasingly, B-type natriuretic peptide (BNP) is used as a screening tool, a marker of PH severity and prognosis, and an indicator of response to therapy. Note that normal range may vary depending on institution and which test (NT-proBNP vs BNP) is performed.

- At our institution, we use BNP mainly if PH is suspected by echocardiogram to gauge severity and assess for response to treatment.
- At some institutions, BNP plays a more central role in the screening process; for example, BNP >35 prompts ongoing monitoring every 2–4 weeks and BNP >50 prompts change in management.
- BNP >220 is predictive of mortality in this population.

Physical Examination. While daily physical examination remains an important part of NICU care, the findings of PH may be subtle and confounded by monitoring equipment, oscillatory ventilation, and other impediments and is therefore a relatively insensitive marker in practice. Clinicians should, however, be familiar with typical signs that should prompt further investigation.

- Hepatomegaly
- Increased RV (parasternal) impulse
- High-pitched TR murmur
- Right-sided S3 gallop

Electrocardiogram. Inadequately sensitive for a screening test in this population. Abnormalities in this population include:

- Right atrial enlargement
- Right ventricular hypertrophy, right axis deviation
- QTc prolongation (in setting of RV strain, a poor prognostic finding)

EVALUATION OF PATIENT WITH KNOWN OR SUSPECTED PH

The first step in treating BPD-associated PH is to optimize chronic lung disease management through a multidisciplinary approach involving evaluations by neonatology, pulmonology, cardiology, gastroenterology, otolaryngology, and speech language pathology.

Pulmonary Evaluation
Blood Gases

- Chronic respiratory failure and acidosis increases pulmonary vascular resistance. Measurement of pH and PCO_2 via blood gas is important to minimize these effects.
- Central venous or "arterialized" capillary blood gas sample should be sufficient to reliably assess these. Pulse oximetry is generally adequate and accepted as a means to measure oxygen saturation. Arterial blood gases are generally not necessary in stable infants.

CXR

- CXR may be useful to assess overall degree of lung disease and assess for cyst formation, degree of pulmonary edema if present as well as presence of atelectasis, which may worsen ventilation-perfusion mismatch.

Computed Tomography

- High resolution computed tomography (CT) with computer-assisted reconstruction can be helpful to investigate airway abnormalities as well as identify more confidently areas of heterogeneous disease. The application of angiography allows visualization of vascular structures in relation to the airway, such as in a child with suspected airway compression due to innominate artery, vascular ring, or hypertensive pulmonary artery. CT angiography also allows for imaging of the pulmonary veins and may help identify pulmonary vein stenosis, an increasingly recognized cause of PH and respiratory worsening in this patient population.

Laryngoscopy/Bronchoscopy

- Should be considered in any infant who develops stridor after intubation to assess for vocal cord paresis or injury, glottic webs or cysts, subglottic or tracheal stenosis, and/or granulation tissue. The risk of laryngeal or subglottic complications is associated with longer duration, multiple episodes of intubation, or use of inappropriately large endotracheal tubes. This examination may be done with rigid or flexible bronchoscopy. Rigid bronchoscopy allows for intervention, however requires a deeper level of anesthesia, making dynamic evaluation for vocal cord mobility and airway collapsibility impossible.
- Tracheobronchomalacia is common in preterm infants and may present as wheezing, respiratory distress, and/or cyanotic spells. Airway evaluation with flexible bronchoscopy should be considered in these infants to identify the presence, extent, and severity of malacia as well as rule out alternative etiologies such as vascular compression.
- Airway causes of recurrent atelectasis, lobar emphysema, and failure to wean from mechanical ventilation are similarly important to evaluate via flexible bronchoscopy.

Cardiac Evaluation

Cardiac evaluation should be part of the care of infants with PH whether as the PH expert or as a consultant to neonatology and pulmonology.

- Evaluation for any shunts including those that can easily be missed (partial anomalous pulmonary venous return, systemic arteriovenous malformation such as vein of Galen malformation, etc.)
- Evaluation for pulmonary venous hypertension, especially pulmonary vein stenosis and LV diastolic dysfunction related to systemic hypertension
- Consider cardiac catheterization
  - Confirm PH, distinguish causes of PH (elevated PVR vs pulmonary venous hypertension), shunt evaluation, angiography for AP collaterals and pulmonary vein stenosis, assessment of cardiac output, assessment of vasoreactivity
  - Whom to catheterize
    - All infants with evidence of PH by noninvasive testing
    - All infants in whom pulmonary vasodilators may be used
    - Infants not showing improvement with supportive measures and PDE5 inhibitor*
    - Infants where diagnosis of PH is in question due to imaging limitations, shunts, or other confounders*

Gastroesophageal Reflux Evaluation

Gastroesophageal reflux (GER) is a normal phenomenon in both preterm and term infants, and while its role in the pathogenesis of BPD is controversial, it is agreed that it may complicate the management of existing BPD.

Therapeutic Trial of Transpyloric Feeds

- Transpyloric feeds reduce apnea/bradycardia events and frequency of GER events and reduce symptoms. It is a reasonable, noninvasive, and nonpharmacologic means to reduce GER in a patient with significant lung disease.

Therapeutic Trial of GER Therapy, Acid Blockade, Motility Agents

- While the addition of a proton pump inhibitor (PPI) does not necessarily reduce the total number of GER events, it is effective at reducing the number of acidic GER events.
- There is emerging evidence that PPI or H_2 blocker use in children may increase the risk of respiratory infections, including pneumonia, and gastrointestinal infections such as *Clostridium difficile* infections and possibly necrotizing enterocolitis. Therefore, it is important to use these medications selectively in preterm infants.
- The use of motility agents is generally not indicated.
  - It is against recommendation to use metoclopramide as monotherapy or adjunctive therapy with evidence that it is ineffective, and the harms outweigh the benefits.
  - Erythromycin may improve enteral feeding tolerance.

Impedance/pH Probe

- Impedance probe assessment of GER is preferable in infants as it measures non-acid GER, which is prevalent in this population due to frequent small feedings.
- Impedance probe monitoring can also measure height of refluxate, which has a high correlation with symptoms.

Nuclear Scan (Milk Scan)

- Some institutions offer a nuclear medicine study involving ingestion of milk containing a radioactive tracer and then assessing for the presence of radioactivity in the lungs.

Aspiration Evaluation

Chronic pulmonary soiling can contribute to persistence and severity of lung disease. Sufficient suck-and-swallow coordination does not develop until at least 34 weeks corrected gestation and therefore preterm infants are at risk for dysphagia and aspiration. Even in mechanically ventilated preterm infants, aspiration can be detected.

Therapeutic Trial of NPO with Tube Feeds

- In infants with significant lung disease that is more severe, is not improving as expected, or has developed significant PH, it is a reasonable first step to trial enteral tube feeds and eliminate or limit oral feedings.

Bedside Swallow Evaluation/Speech and Language Pathology Consultation

- Relying on signs/symptoms of aspiration may be misleading in preterm infants who may quickly develop silent aspiration. Therefore, it is important to consult experienced feeding specialists to assess the preterm infant's readiness and ability to safely feed orally.

Oropharyngeal Motility Swallowing Studies

- Oropharyngeal motility swallowing (OPMS) studies (also known as video fluoroscopic swallowing studies) allow experienced speech language pathologists and radiologists to identify the presence of dysphagia and aspiration. It is important to determine the liquid consistency with which infants with dysphagia can safely feed orally.

Direct Laryngoscopy

- Direct laryngoscopy can be used to assess for vocal cord paresis/paralysis in a preterm infant with a history of intubation or PDA ligation where the recurrent laryngeal nerve may be injured.

Quantification of Lipid-Laden Macrophages (LLM)

- Alveolar macrophages may be recovered from bronchoalveolar lavage sampling which, when stained by oil red O, allows for quantification of lipid ingestion by the macrophages. This has been reported to have high sensitivity and moderate specificity for aspiration; however, the practice remains controversial, as subsequent studies have been inconclusive or contradictory.
- Elevated indices of LLM may be seen in patients receiving intralipids and those with bronchial obstruction, chemotherapy, and endogenous lipoid pneumonias.
- The results must be considered within the context of the remainder of the evaluation.

Airway Evaluation

- Sleep study.
- Assess for obstructive sleep apnea, sleep disordered breathing which may contribute to hypoxemia and/or hypercarbia.

Laryngoscopy. See above.

TREATMENTS: GENERAL

Pulmonary Management

Steroids

- Antenatal steroids do not consistently decrease the development of BPD in survivors; however, they do improve survival.
- Postnatal steroid use is controversial, however is generally not recommended as standard treatment of BPD.
  - Systemic corticosteroids may facilitate extubation and decrease mortality in evolving BPD.
  - Inhaled corticosteroids are generally not effective, however may allow for less systemic corticosteroid use.
  - There are significant short- and long-term risks to use of corticosteroids in preterm infants:
    - Impaired alveolar septation
    - Gastrointestinal bleeding
    - Gastric or intestinal perforation
    - Hyperglycemia
    - Systemic hypertension
    - Hypertrophic cardiomyopathy
    - Growth failure
    - Impaired neurodevelopmental outcome

Ventilator Strategies

- Ventilator strategies to reduce work of breathing, reduce energy requirements, and minimize/avoid hypercarbia and acidosis are optimal, however may require excessive airway pressures that have been shown to result in pressure-induced deformation of the airway and resultant tracheobronchomalacia and tracheomegaly.

O_2 Recommendations

- Supplemental O_2 therapy in infants with BPD has been shown to reduce central apnea, promote growth, improve exercise tolerance, reduce pulmonary artery pressure, and reverse hypoxic vasoconstriction.
- The optimal O_2 saturation is controversial given the risks of both hypoxia and oxygen free radical-mediated damage to the lung, both of which can worsen PH. When PH is established, we recommend maintaining physiologic levels of 95–100%; however, lower ranges of 90–95% may be sufficient to achieve the goals above.
- Historically there have been concerns that excessive supplemental oxygen use and oxygen saturations contributed to the development of retinopathy of prematurity (ROP). The STOP-ROP trial found no difference in progression of ROP in at-risk infants when higher (96–99%) compared to lower (89–94%) O_2 saturations were targeted.
- In our institution, when there are signs of significant PH, we recommend maintaining O_2 saturations above 94% to protect against transient desaturations that may occur in the lower saturation range. The exception is in BPD-PH patients known to have significant CO_2 retention where we titrate the supplemental O_2 to maintain O_2 saturation 93–97% to avoid blunting of the hypoxic respiratory drive.
- We advise caregivers to monitor the infant's oxygen saturation via pulse oximetry during wakefulness, with feeding, and with sleep.
- Weaning of supplemental O_2 begins after a period of stability, improvement in their PH, and demonstration of adequate O_2 saturation in the acceptable range with decreasing O_2 flow rates. At our institution, we wean to room air (RA) during wakefulness first and then obtain either a downloadable oximeter or polysomnogram during sleep on RA to ensure adequate O_2 saturation during prolonged periods of sleep before discontinuing supplemental O_2.

CO_2 Recommendations

- While a cutoff has not been determined, it is recognized that elevated capillary PCO_2 is associated with subsequent adverse events including death, reintubation, and pulmonary hypertension.
- At our institution we strive to maintain capillary PCO_2 <60 when possible.

Cardiac Management

Diuretics. Diuretics are helpful in a number of situations, including the following:

- Improve pulmonary performance in setting of significant left to right shunts
- Improve ventricular performance in setting of dilated RV
- Improve pulmonary edema related to BPD, elevated pulmonary venous pressure, or shunt

Eliminating Shunts. Consider eliminating shunts if it is felt to be significant contributor to PH or pulmonary status and it is considered safe from procedural and PH perspective (i.e., "pop-off" not needed for pulmonary hypertensive crises).

- PDA medical, surgical, or device closure
- ASD device or surgical closure
- Other shunts

Treat Systemic Hypertension in Attempt to Normalize Left Ventricular End-Diastolic Pressure

- Goal of normal to mildly elevated SBP in setting of significant RV hypertension
- Overtreatment of systemic hypertension in the setting of severe PH can have an adverse effect on septal mechanics (and therefore cardiac output)

Support Struggling RV. Also see the section Hemodynamic Compromise later.

- Milrinone is effective in supporting failing RV—inotrope, pulmonary and systemic vasodilator, aids cardiac relaxation.
- Digoxin used in some centers.

GERD Management

Medications. While there is a role for reflux medications listed below, it is important to consider the risks and benefits as described above.

- H_2 blockers
- Proton pump inhibitors
- Motility agents

Gastrojejunostomy or Nissen Fundoplication with Gastrostomy Tube

- Antireflux surgery via fundoplication can improve symptoms in patients with symptomatic GER and those with presence of full column GER as demonstrated by impedance probe.
- GJ tube placement appears to have similar effectiveness in reducing symptoms and maintaining time free of pneumonia.

Aspiration Management

Avoiding soiling of the lung is important in the growth and repair of preterm lungs. While it is important to introduce oral feedings as early and safely as possible in preterm infants, one must remain cautious if the child is not doing well or has an intercurrent illness.

Thickened Feeds

- Many patients with oral and/or pharyngeal dysphagia may have improvement in the safety of their swallow with various degrees of thickening agent applied. An OPMS allows the speech language pathologist to assess the swallow with different consistencies and make recommendations based on those findings.
- It is not advised to empirically thicken milk unless that consistency is known to be safe by OPMS, as the risk of aspiration of thickening agents is unknown.
- It is also important to consider that it is more laborious for an infant to extract thickened formula from a bottle so they may experience more rapid fatigue with bottling, which may place them at risk for aspiration.

Slow Flow Nipple

- Use of a slow flow nipple in infants with oral and/or pharyngeal dysphagia may slow the rapidity with which the milk is extracted and therefore improve coordination to reduce dysphagia and aspiration.

NPO with Tube Feeds

- Full NPO status with reliance on tube feedings may be required in those with severe dysphagia and severe lung disease and PH. Maintenance of oral skills through small amounts (e.g., 5–10 mL) of water or puree food trials should be attempted when deemed safe.

Airway Management

Flow/O_2

- A low flow nasal cannula system providing 100% oxygen is the preferred method for delivering oxygen supplementation in the outpatient setting.
- The flow rate is determined by the minimal amount needed to achieve goal O_2 saturation.

Noninvasive Positive Pressure Ventilation

- High flow nasal cannula systems are generally not used in the outpatient setting, as the equipment is not widely available and children who require such high flow rates likely have more severe airway or lung disease where noninvasive positive pressure ventilation (NIPPV) or tracheostomy and chronic mechanical ventilation should be considered.
- Similarly, the use of continuous positive airway pressure or bilevel positive airway pressure (i.e., NIPPV) in the outpatient setting in small infants is difficult. This is often due to limited appropriate interface availability and the relative instability of the respiratory modality in a child with presumably severe airway or lung disease.

Tracheostomy +/− Ventilator

- Tracheostomy may be required when significant airway problems exist, such as sub-glottic stenosis or severe tracheomalacia, where other interventions, such as surgical correction or NIPPV have failed to achieve adequate resolution.
- Tracheostomy may also be required to apply prolonged positive airway pressure for treatment of tracheomalacia or chronic respiratory failure due to severe lung disease. The goal is to minimize work of breathing and achieve normal/near-normal O_2 saturation and PCO_2 levels as described above.

TREATMENTS: PH-SPECIFIC MEDICATIONS

The decision of whether or not to treat BPD-associated PH with PH-specific medications should be made on an individual basis. No drugs are currently approved by the FDA for treatment in this context. General considerations are the severity of the PH, whether contributing causes have already been optimized, and the overall trajectory of the patient. In cases where treatment is thought to be beneficial, below are some options.

Hemodynamic Compromise

In the setting of hemodynamic compromise due to severe PH, it is recommended to use pulmonary vasodilators acutely to lower PA pressure and cardiac performance.

Pulmonary Vasodilators

- iNO can be used in the ICU setting via endotracheal tube, CPAP/BiPAP, or nasal cannula
  - Typically started at 20 ppm.
  - If no therapeutic benefit, discontinue.
  - If a benefit is realized, periodic attempts to wean are important to lowest dose with benefit.
  - Rebound PH can be noted with abrupt withdrawal after prolonged use. Wean with prolonged tail is generally advisable. Phosphodiesterase inhibitors have been shown to blunt rebound pulmonary hypertension.
  - Routine iNO monitoring including methemoglobin levels.
  - May help oxygenation by improving ventilation-perfusion matching in addition to its effect on PVR.

- Epoprostenol is a systemically administered, potent, continuously infused intravenous pulmonary vasodilator with very short half-life which can rapidly be up- and down-titrated.
  - Adverse effect of systemic hypotension; may need concurrent pressor
- Intravenous sildenafil is also an option for the critically ill patient with hemodynamically unstable PH.

Inodilators

- Milrinone is a phosphodiesterase type 3 inhibitor which has multiple positive effects including improved cardiac contractility, reduction in pulmonary vascular resistance, and systemic afterload reduction.
  - Adverse effect of hypotension; may need concurrent pressor
- Dobutamine has a similar hemodynamic profile though through a catecholaminergic mechanism—β_1 and to a lesser extent, β_2 stimulation. Similar to milrinone, it causes increase in contractility, pulmonary and systemic vasodilation, and can cause hypotension.

Pressors/Inotropes

- Vasopressin is a systemic vasoconstrictor which causes little if any pulmonary vasoconstriction and is therefore a promising agent for combatting systemic hypotension in the setting of PH.
- Norepinephrine is a vasoconstrictor acting on α_1 and α_2 receptors to increase systemic vascular resistance. There is associated increase in pulmonary vascular resistance and pressure.
- Epinephrine is a nonselective adrenergic agonist resulting in increased cardiac contractility and heart rate as well as increased systemic vascular resistance. There is a modest associated increase in pulmonary vascular resistance.
- Dopamine is widely used in treating hypotension in infants but should be used with caution in the setting of PH as it can cause a significant increase in pulmonary resistance and increases systemic oxygen consumption, perhaps more than the associated increase in cardiac output.

Diuretics. Judicious use of diuretics can be very important in stabilizing an unstable infant with PH. RV function can improve (and commensurately cardiac output and systemic blood pressure) if a dilated RV is unloaded via diuretics. Intravenous furosemide via infusion or periodic injection is typically the first line. Caution must be taken to avoid intravascular volume depletion.

Hemodynamically Stable

Use of PH-specific medications to treat chronic, stable BPD-associated PH continues to be controversial. At our institution, we typically consider treating it if the PH is moderate or greater, if it is affecting RV function, if it is felt to be inhibiting the progress of the patient, or if it is failing to improve with time and lung growth. With all systemically administered pulmonary vasodilators, there is the risk of worsening oxygenation in the setting of parenchymal lung disease due to loss of the physiologic vasoconstriction in poorly aerated lung regions.

Phosphodiesterase Inhibitors. Phosphodiesterase inhibitors are the first-line enteral therapy at most centers.

- Sildenafil is dosed 3–4 times per day at doses not to exceed 3 mg/kg/day. Therapy-limiting side effects are rare, but include priapism, hypoxemia, and hypotension.
  - Data from a hyperoxia-induced lung injury BPD animal model suggest that sildenafil may have an anti-inflammatory effect in the lung as well as promote alveolar and vessel growth.
- Tadalafil is similar to sildenafil, though dosed once daily. There is less experience with this drug in small infants but use is increasing.
  - At our center, we often start patients on sildenafil while in the hospital, but in outpatient follow-up consider a switch to tadalafil for ease of administration and to improve compliance if it is anticipated that the patient will require prolonged treatment (e.g., greater than 6 months).
- Phosphodiesterase inhibitors may worsen GERD, complicating management.

Endothelin Receptor Antagonists. Endothelin receptor antagonists have been available longer than phosphodiesterase inhibitors (PDEIs) but are often used as second-line agents due to the need for monthly liver monitoring (bosentan), absence of a liquid formulation (ambrisentan), or lack of published pediatric experience (macitentan). We add bosentan if there is inadequate response to supportive measures and sildenafil.

- Bosentan
  - Dosed twice daily. Liver testing required prior to initiation and monthly while on the medication. Due to teratogenicity, precautions must be taken in handling medication for mothers, female nurses, and other female care providers. Adverse reactions other than reversible liver toxicity are rare.
- Ambrisentan
- Macitentan

Prostanoids. Prostanoids are the oldest and most potent pulmonary vasodilators but also have the most adverse reactions and most complex delivery systems. Adverse reactions for this class include hypotension, bone pain, vomiting, and diarrhea.

- Epoprostenol—short acting, titratable, needs dedicated central venous line.
- Treprostinil—longer acting, available intravenously via dedicated central venous line as well as subcutaneously. Oral and inhaled forms not used to date in this population.
  - Several series suggest lower incidence subcutaneous therapy-limiting site pain in infants compared older children and adults.
  - Subcutaneous route obviates problems with vascular access and associated risk of bloodstream infection.
- Iloprost—available for inhalation and has been used in this population with positive effect. Need for frequent dosing 6–9 times per day or more can be a limiting factor. There is some concern for significant swings in pulmonary artery pressures with peaks and troughs of this medication.

Soluble Guanylate Cyclase Stimulators. Soluble guanylate cyclase stimulators have not been used to treat this condition to date and are contraindicated if a PDEI is in use.

- Riociguat

CLINICAL ALGORITHM(S)

Figure 28.1 is a sample algorithm similar to what is done at our institution. Variations are possible as outlined in the text.

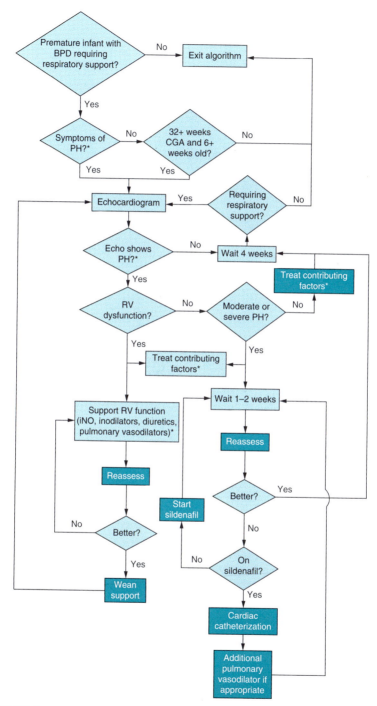

FIGURE 28.1 • BPD-PH screening and management algorithm for infants <32 weeks GA at birth. *See text for details. BPD, bronchopulmonary dysplasia; CGA, corrected gestational age; Echo, echocardiogram; PH, pulmonary hypertension; RV, right ventricular.

IMPLEMENTATION OF GUIDELINE

QUALIFYING STATEMENTS

Prospective data are largely lacking to inform decision-making in regard to BPD-associated PH management. The observations and recommendations above are largely based on experience at our center and expert opinion combined with small series, some animal data, and data extrapolated from other conditions.

DESCRIPTION OF IMPLEMENTATION STRATEGY

Institutions are encouraged to standardize screening, evaluation, and treatment of PH in this population.

QUALITY METRICS

Adherence to screening protocol, appropriate additional testing performed in those who screen positive, appropriate us of PH-specific medication, mortality rate for BPD-associated PH.

SUMMARY

BPD-associated PH is a severe condition with high associated morbidity and mortality. Evidence-based guidelines are lacking. Treatment is largely geared toward identifying and optimizing contributing causes such as airway, gastrointestinal, cardiac, and pulmonary comorbidities. Many centers use PH-specific medications in selected patients.

BIBLIOGRAPHIC SOURCE(S)

ATS Documents. Statement on the care of the child with chronic lung disease of infancy and childhood. *Am J Respir Crit Care Med*. 2003;168:356-96.

Baker CD, Abman SH, Mourani PM. Pulmonary hypertension in preterm infants with BPD. *Pediatr Allergy Immunol Pulmonol*. 2014;27(1):8-16.

Bhat R, Salas AA, Foster C, et al. Prospective analysis of pulmonary hypertension in extremely low birth weight infants. *Pediatrics*. 2012;129(3):e682-9.

Cohen S, Bueno de Mesquita M, Mimouni FB. Adverse effects reported in the use of gastroesophageal reflux disease treatments in children: a 10 years literature review. *Br J Clin Pharmacol*. 2015;80(2):200-8.

Cuna A, Kandasamy J, Sims B. B-type natriuretic peptide and mortality in extremely low birth weight infants with pulmonary hypertension: a retrospective cohort analysis. *BMC Pediatrics*. 2014;14:68.

deVisser Y, Walther FJ, Laghmani el H, et al. Sildenafil attenuates pulmonary inflammation and fibrin deposition, mortality and right ventricular hypertrophy in neonatal hyperoxic lung injury. *Respir Res*. 2009;10:30.

Farhath S, He Z, Nakhla T, et al. Pepsin, a marker of gastric contents, is increased in tracheal aspirates from preterm infants who develop bronchopulmonary dysplasia. *Pediatrics*. 2008;121;e253.

Giuffre RM, Rubin S, Mitchell I. Antireflux surgery in infants with bronchopulmonary dysplasia. *Am J Dis Child*. 1987;141(6):648-51.

Jadcherla SR, Gupta A, Fernandez S, et al. Spatiotemporal characteristics of acid refluxate and relationship to symptoms in premature and term infants with chronic lung disease. *Am J Gastroenterol.* 2008;103(3):720-8.

Khemani E, McElhinney DB, Rhein L, et al. Pulmonary artery hypertension in formerly premature infants with bronchopulmonary dysplasia: clinical features and outcomes in the surfactant era. *Pediatrics.* 2007;120:1260-9.

Kim DH, Kim HS, Choi CW, et al. Risk factors for pulmonary artery hypertension in preterm infants with moderate or severe bronchopulmonary dysplasia. *Neonatology.* 2012;101:40-6.

Kovesi T, Abdurahman A, Blayney M. Elevated carbon dioxide tension as a predictor of subsequent adverse events in infants with bronchopulmonary dyplasia. *Lung.* 2006; 184:7-13.

Ladha F, Bonnet S, Eaton F, et al. Sildenafil improves alveolar growth and pulmonary hypertension in hyperoxia-induced lung injury. *Am J Respir Crit Care Med.* 2005;172:750-6.

Mourani PM, Sontag MK, Younoszai A, et al. Early pulmonary vascular disease in preterm infants at risk for bronchopulmonary dysplasia. *Am J Respir Crit Care Med.* 2015;191(1):87-95.

Ng PC, So KW, Fung KS, et al. Randomised controlled study of oral erythromycin for treatment of gastrointestinal dysmotility in preterm infants. *Arch Dis Child Fetal Neonatal Ed.* 2001;84(3):F177-82.

Rosen R, Levine P, Lewis J, Mitchell P, Nurko S. Reflux events detected by pH-MII do not determine fundoplication outcome. *J Pediatr Gastroenterol Nutr.* 2010;50(3):251-5.

Slaughter JL, Pakrashi T, Jobes DE, et al. Echocardiographic detection of pulmonary hypertension in extremely low birth weight infants with bronchopulmonary dysplasia requiring prolonged positive pressure ventilation. *J Perinatol.* 2011;31(10):635-40.

St Cyr JA, Ferrara TB, Thompson T, Johnson D, Foker JE. Treatment of pulmonary manifestations of gastroesophageal reflux in children two years of age or less. *Am J Surg.* 1989;157(4):400-3.

Valat C, Demont F, Pegat MA, et al. Radionuclide study of bronchial aspiration in intensive care newborn children. *Nucl Med Commun.* 1986;7(8):593-8.

Vela MF, Camacha-Lobato L, Srinivasan R, Tutuian R, Katz PO, Castell DO. Intraesophageal impedance and pH measurement of acid and nonacid reflux: effect of omeprazole. *Gastroenterology.* 2001;120:1599-1606.

Extracorporeal Membrane Oxygenation

Robert J. DiGeronimo, MD

SCOPE

DISEASE/CONDITION(S)

Rescue therapy following failed conventional support of severe neonatal respiratory failure.

GUIDELINE OBJECTIVE(S)

Review criteria for patient selection; timing of referral and type of extracorporeal membrane oxygenation (ECMO) support; routine ECMO procedures and management; weaning and discontinuation of ECMO; complications and outcomes.

BRIEF BACKGROUND

ECMO is a modified form of cardiopulmonary bypass used to provide prolonged extracorporeal support to critically ill-term or near-term neonates with severe but potentially reversible respiratory and/or cardiac failure. Despite the complexity and risks associated with this modality, ECMO is an accepted and proven rescue therapy that has been routinely used for over two-and-a-half decades in neonates failing standard conventional treatments, including high-frequency ventilation (HFV) and inhaled nitric oxide (iNO). In the setting of life-threatening respiratory disease and persistent pulmonary hypertension (PPHN), ECMO allows for temporary lung rest by augmenting oxygenation and ventilation. If veno-arterial (VA) ECMO is selected, cardiovascular support is additionally provided, while veno-venous (VV) ECMO provides only respiratory support.

The Extracorporeal Life Support Organization (ELSO) provides an international registry that tracks neonatal ECMO cases. To date, over 27,000 neonates with respiratory failure have been treated with ECMO in the ELSO registry with an overall survival to discharge or transfer of 74%. Survival varies based on the severity of the underlying disease process range from 94% for neonates with a primary diagnosis of meconium aspiration syndrome to 51% with congenital diaphragmatic hernia (CDH). While VV ECMO is preferred and its use has increased in many centers over the past decade with improvements in circuit and cannula technology, VA ECMO continues to represent approximately two-thirds of cases historically.

RECOMMENDATIONS

MAJOR RECOMMENDATIONS

In appropriately selected patients, the use of ECMO provides life-saving support, resulting in one additional survivor for every three to four neonates treated, without increasing morbidity. ECMO is most effective in mature neonates with severe reversible lung disease secondary to meconium aspiration, respiratory distress syndrome, PPHN, and/or pneumonia/sepsis. Although commonly used in newborns with CDH, the benefit of ECMO in this population remains less certain. For hemodynamically stable neonates with adequate cardiac function, VV ECMO is the modality of choice for neonatal respiratory failure.

PRACTICE OPTION

Practice Option #1

ECMO Patient Selection

1. Basic patient selection criteria for neonatal ECMO are well established, as outlined in Table 29.1. Low birth weight is considered a relative contraindication based on the technical limitations of cannulation. Corrected chronologic age should be taken into account, as this more accurately reflects bleeding risks in premature infants as compared to gestational age alone.
2. Surgical cannulation for VV ECMO typically requires a minimum weight of 2 kg given that the smallest dual-lumen VV cannula is 12 French, while VA single-lumen catheters are available in sizes as small as 6 French.

TABLE 29.1. Neonatal Selection Criteria for ECMO

1. Birth or current weight ≥2.0 kg
2. Corrected gestational age ≥34 weeks
3. Absence of lethal malformations or anomalies
4. Absence of severe irreversible brain injury
5. Cranial ultrasound showing no evidence of significant intracranial hemorrhage (Grade II or higher)
6. No evidence of uncontrolled bleeding or known major bleeding diathesis
7. Reversible lung disease and/or PPHN
8. Meet respiratory failure criteria (Table 29.2)

TABLE 29.2. Respiratory Failure Criteria

1. **Oxygenation index (OI)**
   a. OI = Ventilator MAP × FiO_2 × 100/post ductal PaO_2
   b. > 35 to 60 for 0.5 to 6 hours[†]
2. **Alveolar-arterial oxygen difference ($AaDO_2$)**
   a. $AaDO_2 = (P_{atm} - 47) \times FiO_2 - PaO_2 - PaCO_2/R$
   b. > 605 to 620 torr for 4 – 12 hours[*]
3. **Severe, refractory hypoxic respiratory failure** with persistent PaO_2 <50 mmHg unresponsive to optimal medical and ventilator management
4. **Hemodynamic failure** despite optimal vasopressor support and intravascular fluid replacement resulting in inability to maintain arterial pH >7.25 with worsening metabolic and/or lactic acidosis

[*]Predicts 80% mortality with historical conventional management (i.e., predates routine use of HFV, iNOm and surfactant).

MAP, mean airway pressure, P_{atm}, atmospheric pressure (760 mmHg at sea level); $PaCO_2$, partial pressure of arterial carbon dioxide; PaO_2, partial pressure of arterial oxygen; R, respiratory quotient (0.8).

3. Absolute contraindications to ECMO include: 1) lethal congenital anomalies and malformations, 2) irreversible severe brain injury or hemorrhage, and 3) irreversible cardiopulmonary failure.

4. Table 29.2 outlines standard respiratory failure criteria to initiate ECMO. Traditional measures used to predict mortality in neonates have included both oxygenation index (OI) and alveolar-arterial oxygenation difference ($AaDO_2$). However, the availability of adjunct therapies such as iNO and HFV optimizing medical management have made it more difficult to use single measures of disease severity to predict outcome. Many centers now use more simplified but less precise criteria when considering ECMO, including severe hypoxic respiratory failure or hemodynamic failure refractory to medical management. Currently, only limited data from uncontrolled trials and retrospective reviews support recommendations regarding optimal timing for ECMO cannulation.

5. Congenital diaphragmatic hernia: ECMO continues to be routinely offered as a rescue therapy in approximately one-third of CDH cases in the United States. In non-randomized trials, ECMO has been shown to improve survival in CDH patients. While uniform protocols for management do not exist and vary by center, a strategy of delayed surgery, gentle ventilation, and permissive hypercapnia is typically employed to limit ventilator-induced lung injury and allow for improvement in PPHN. In general, ECMO is reserved for CDH patients who fail maximum medical management as evidenced by: 1) poor systemic perfusion, 2) non-reassuring blood gases, or 3) intolerable ventilator settings. Given the potential irreversible nature of lung hypoplasia, a number of centers additionally require minimum criteria to demonstrate survivable lung function. At our institution, patients need to have a best pre-ductal oxygen saturation of >85% or $PaCO_2$ <75 to qualify for ECMO.

Timing of ECMO Referral. Given the potential benefit of prenatal diagnosis and improved survival associated with delivery at an experienced tertiary center, families with a known fetus with CDH or other condition with a high likelihood of requiring ECMO should be offered the choice of where to deliver, with the risks and benefits clearly outlined. Early (<24 hours) versus delayed transport of outborn CDH patients

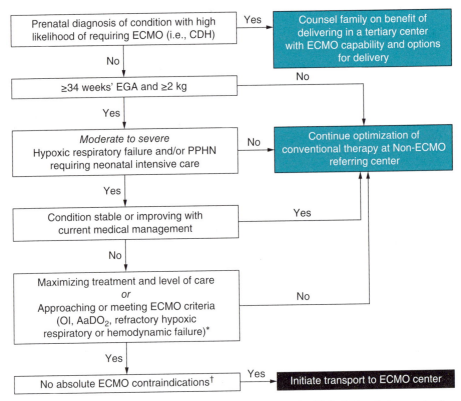

FIGURE 29.1 • Timing of ECMO referral. *See Table 29.2. †Absolute contraindications: lethal malformations/congenital anomalies, severe irreversible brain injury, Grade II intracranial hemorrhage or greater.

to ECMO referral centers has additionally been shown to be associated with improved survival. Early and continued communication with an ECMO referral center regarding appropriate timing of transfer is critical, especially in those patients requiring escalating support. It has been estimated that up to 25% of potential neonatal ECMO candidates may die prior to or during transport. Therefore, referring providers need to carefully consider continued treatment of potential ECMO patients in non-ECMO centers with specific regard to their center's capabilities and distances needed to transport (see Figure 29.1).

Mode of ECMO Support. VV ECMO is the preferred modality in hemodynamically stable neonates with respiratory failure. Access requires a single cannulation with a double-lumen catheter surgically placed into the right internal jugular vein with the tip positioned in the mid to lower right atrium. Potential benefits of VV ECMO include less risk of ischemic-reperfusion brain injury and adverse effects on cerebral oxygenation and blood flow. Additional physiologic benefits include: 1) return of pump-arterial blood to the right side of the heart, 2) improved coronary oxygenation, 3) no effect on cardiac afterload, and 4) maintenance of normal pulsatile flow.

There is not a predefined amount of pre-ECMO vasopressor support that precludes the use of VV ECMO. Many patients have improved cardiac function and significantly wean vasopressors following initiation of VV ECMO. Disadvantages of VV ECMO include: 1) no cardiac support, 2) more challenging cannula placement, 3) potential for recirculation, 4) lower oxygen delivery capacity, and 5) possibility of need to convert to VA.

VV to VA ECMO conversion rates are relatively low in our experience, ranging from 10% to 20%, which is consistent with other reports in the literature. Compared to VV, VA ECMO requires cannulation and ligation of the right carotid artery in addition to the jugular vein. Advantages include improved oxygenation and hemodynamic support. To date, there are no published follow-up data from randomized controlled trials in neonates that demonstrate superior survival or neurologic outcomes with VV compared to VA ECMO.

ECMO Procedures and Management. Evidence supporting routine ECMO care in neonates is based primarily on published guidelines from ELSO as well as recommendations from various literature reviews of best practices and expert panel consensus statements.

Initiation and Circuit Considerations. Pre-ECMO evaluation of all neonates should include a thorough medical history and physical examination, head ultrasound, echocardiogram, measurement of coagulation parameters, and renal ultrasound if indicated. Recent advances in technology have made ECMO safer, focusing on 1) improved cannula design providing better flow and less recirculation, 2) simpler, more concise circuits, 3) noninvasive monitoring, and 4) more efficient and reliable oxygenators and circuit pumps. Standard venous ECMO cannulas for neonates range from 12 to 15 French (both single and double lumen) and arterial from 8 to 12 French in size. Circuits for neonates up to 10 kg use ¼-inch tubing, have a volume of 200–300 mL, and are routinely primed with saline, albumin, and type-specific blood, respectively. If cannulation is emergent, O-negative emergency release blood can be used. For VV ECMO, blood should be fresh (less than 5 days old) or washed to reduce potassium concentration prior to priming. Hollow-fiber lungs coated with polymethylpentene have replaced membrane style silicon oxygenators. They have the advantage of a much smaller priming volume, lower risk of leakage, and a much lower pre- versus post-membrane pressure gradient. ECMO centers continue to use both roller and centrifugal pumps for neonates, even though the latter have become increasingly popular due to their simpler operation, minimized blood surface contact, and potential for less hemolysis. However, no definitive published literature currently exists demonstrating the superiority of either technology.

Oxygen Sufficiency and Monitoring. Adequate oxygenation and blood pressure support (if on VA ECMO) typically is provided with pump flows of 100–120 mL/kg/min. Higher pump flows may be needed in neonates with sepsis or significant intravascular leak up to 150 or even 200 mL/kg/min. Target oxygen saturation goals for VV typically are >85% and between 92% and 99% for VA ECMO. Oxygen sufficiency, or the balance between systemic oxygen delivery versus consumption, can be assessed by monitoring mixed venous oxygen saturations (SVO_2, goal 65% or greater) as well as other measures of perfusion including lactate levels and near-infrared spectroscopy. For centers that use cephalad drains, cerebral venous oxygen saturations can additionally be monitored. With VV ECMO, recirculation can occur but is a less common problem with recent improvements in cannula design. Recirculation should be suspected in the face of rising venous circuit oxygen saturations coupled with decreasing patient oxygenation, and is routinely managed by adjusting cannula position, maintaining adequate pre-load, and limiting circuit pump flow as necessary.

Anticoagulation. Bleeding is the most frequent complication associated with ECMO. Systemic anticoagulation with unfractionated heparin is used to prevent the extracorporeal circuit from clotting but presents significant bleeding risks to patients. While bleeding at the cannulation or other surgical sites is common, intracranial hemorrhage is the major cause of morbidity associated with ECMO. Serious intracranial bleeding is seen more frequently in neonates compared to older children, with an incidence of 7–10% reported in the ELSO registry. Known risk factors include prematurity, carotid artery ligation, sepsis, moderate to severe coagulopathy and pre-ECMO hypoxia, acidosis, and hemodynamic instability. Current consensus guidelines regarding how best to monitor anticoagulation therapy during ECMO vary by center and have minimal evidence-based support. Most centers use a combination of activated clotting time (ACT), activated partial thromboplastin time (APTT), antithrombin activity, and antifactor Xa to titrate anticoagulation. Of interest, a number of centers are now using thromboelastography (TEG) as an additional measure of anticoagulation to help guide management. At cannulation, a heparin bolus of 50–100 units/kg is given followed by the initiation of a continuous heparin infusion at 15–20 units/kg/h once the ACT drops below 300 seconds. Usual maintenance heparin range falls between 20 and 50 units/kg/h in patients with standard bleeding risks. For those patients at high risk or with active bleeding, lower anticoagulation levels are targeted in an effort to limit bleeding. For planned surgeries while on ECMO (e.g., CDH repair), pretreatment with antifibrinolytic agents such as aminocaproic acid may help reduce surgical site bleeding. Adequate platelet levels are known to reduce bleeding on ECMO and therefore are routinely maintained in the range of 80,000 to 100,000 cells/mm³. In addition, ECMO circuits are now available with heparin bonding (or other similarly active biologic surface treatment) to prevent platelet activation, inflammation, and/or fibrinolysis. While most centers now routinely use coated circuits, their utility in prolonging circuit life and function is unproven.

Lung Rest and Ventilator Management. Ventilator support is typically weaned following ECMO initiation to "rest settings" to allow lung recovery and avoid ventilator-induced lung injury and oxygen toxicity. For VV ECMO, patients typically require a greater degree of lung inflation given the more limited oxygenation support provided as compared to VA ECMO. Lung rest can be accomplished with either conventional or HFV ventilation, using primarily positive end-expiratory pressure (6–12 cm H_2O) or mean airway pressure (8–12 cm H_2O) to provide inflation, coupled with minimal tidal volume or amplitude. Neonates with respiratory failure complicated by air leak may require minimal to no pressure support until the air leak resolves with gradual reinflation of the lung over 48–72 hours to prevent recurrence. Severe air leak preferably should be managed with HFV and may necessitate the use of VA ECMO to provide adequate support during lung rest.

Fluid Balance and Nutrition. The degree of fluid overload in ECMO patients, including neonates, is associated with higher morbidity and mortality, leading to more complicated and prolonged ECMO runs. Every effort should therefore be made to avoid significant volume overload prior to ECMO. Given that neonates are often exposed to prolonged periods of poor perfusion and hypoxia during failing conventional therapy, it is not uncommon to have acute renal injury and/or failure by the time ECMO is initiated. Following intravascular stabilization on ECMO (typically 24–48 hours post cannulation), inadequate urine output may necessitate diuretic use and/or hemofiltration to remove excessive volume. Furosemide and bumetanide are loop diuretics commonly used either intermittently or as a continuous infusion. Convective hemofiltration (or ultrafiltration) uses a semipermeable membrane filter connected within the ECMO circuit to remove fluid, and can be coupled with dialysate to additionally balance solutes if necessary. Careful monitoring of fluid balance is critical with adjunct renal therapies to avoid intravascular volume depletion and potential worsening of renal function.

Total Parenteral Nutrition. Total parenteral nutrition is typically provided per unit protocol and can be given directly to the ECMO circuit or patient at a volume of 120–150 mL/kg/day depending on overall fluid balance goals. Enteral feeds have historically not been given to neonates on ECMO due to concerns for intestinal hypoperfusion. Some centers, however, will consider enteral feeds in hemodynamically stable non-CDH neonates with careful monitoring for intolerance; however, supporting literature to guide this practice is lacking.

Weaning and Discontinuation of ECMO Support. Most neonatal respiratory failure ECMO runs last 3–7 days for non-CDH etiologies, while CDH cases often are more prolonged, requiring 10–14 days or longer. As respiratory function improves over time, weaning of ECMO support is gradually initiated. Lung reinflation can be achieved as needed with escalation of conventional or HFV settings in preparation for coming off bypass. Since VV ECMO does not provide cardiac support, trialing off is simpler and only requires disconnecting sweep gas flow to the circuit oxygenator to allow assessment of native pulmonary function. Circuit pump flow typically does not need to be decreased. Patients can be challenged with increasing ventilator FiO_2 while trialing off to assess oxygenation as a marker of lung recovery. Generally, if adequate oxygenation and ventilation can be maintained on minimal to moderate ventilator settings and FiO_2 <0.60, this is considered a successful trial to discontinue ECMO. For VA ECMO, determining exact timing for coming off is more difficult. Unlike VV, since VA ECMO provides cardiac support, it is necessary to wean circuit pump flow in 10–20 mL/kg/min increments until a minimum flow of 40–50 mL/kg/min is tolerated. Most patients can then idle at this minimum flow and if they remain stable for 1–2 hours on acceptable ventilator and vasopressor support, ECMO can be discontinued. Historically, before coming off VA ECMO, both the venous and arterial cannulas are additionally clamped to completely eliminate ECMO flow to the patient (a circuit "bridge" is necessary for this technique to provide continued flow to the circuit). The disadvantage of this approach is that it requires intermittent unclamping of the cannulas every 10–15 minutes to prevent clotting, which alters cerebral blood flow and theoretically increases risk for cerebral emboli. For this reason, many centers have abandoned this step, considering it unnecessary.

Additional Considerations. Additional considerations to help facilitate the transition from ECMO back to conventional support include: 1) serial echocardiograms to assess cardiac function and degree of residual PPHN; 2) initiation or escalation of pulmonary vasodilator therapies including iNO, sildenafil, milrinone, and/or prostacyclin (epoprostenol) as necessary to improve pulmonary blood flow; and 3) flexible bronchoscopy with or without surfactant replacement therapy to assist lung recruitment. For CDH neonates placed on ECMO, the question of when to surgically repair the diaphragmatic defect, that is, either during or after ECMO, remains unanswered. Many centers still elect to repair on ECMO following physiologic stabilization given improved anticoagulation protocols that have demonstrated fewer bleeding complications. More recent evidence, however, suggests that surgical repair after ECMO may increase survival.

Complications and Outcome. Due to the high-risk nature of ECMO support and degree of critical illness necessary to meet ECMO criteria, all surviving neonates treated with ECMO require appropriate long-term follow-up through early childhood. Neurodevelopment outcomes in survivors treated with neonatal ECMO have shown equivalent or less morbidity compared to conventionally supported patients with similar disease severity. Central nervous system complications represent the major morbidities seen with ECMO and include cerebral bleeding, infarction, and seizures. Significant neurodevelopmental impairment has been reported to occur in 15–25% of ECMO-treated neonates; however, severe or profound impairment is uncommon, and is seen in <5% of survivors. Many centers routinely perform post-ECMO imaging, as 10–15% will have moderate to severe injury noted on head CT or MRI.

CLINICAL ALGORITHM(S)

See Figure 29.1.

IMPLEMENTATION OF GUIDELINE

QUALIFYING STATEMENTS

1. Small numbers of patients with CDH have been included in randomized controlled trials comparing ECMO to conventional therapy.
2. Limited follow-up data are available concerning outcomes with VV versus VA-ECMO.
3. The majority of existing evidence supporting routine ECMO management is based primarily on clinical experience and expert consensus opinion.

DESCRIPTION OF IMPLEMENTATION STRATEGY

1. Create institutional ECMO guidelines based on consensus standards and existing reliable published literature.
2. Establish multidisciplinary ECMO teams of experienced clinical providers to deliver highly specialized ECMO care to critically ill newborns.
3. Create a quality improvement infrastructure to continually identify best practices and track outcomes.
4. Provide ongoing education and promote future research.

QUALITY METRICS

1. Define optimal timing for initiating ECMO.
2. Identify risk factors for CDH survival and improved criteria for ECMO.
3. Describe best candidates for VV versus VA support.
4. Compare ECMO versus conventional therapy with regard to cost-benefit analysis.
5. Validate anticoagulation treatment algorithms.
6. Track long-term outcomes to determine risk factors for neurodevelopmental impairment in survivors.

SUMMARY

For neonatal patients with severe respiratory failure facing a high risk of mortality, ECMO can be a life-saving treatment despite its invasive nature, risk, and expense. Decades of experience with ECMO have demonstrated its utility, and improvements in technology have made it safer and more efficacious over time. ECMO survival is highest in neonates with reversible lung disease and PPHN but also may improve outcomes in selected patients with CDH. Early referral of ECMO candidates to centers with ECMO capability improves survival. Despite advances in care, however, neonates with severe respiratory failure treated with ECMO or conventional therapy remain at significant risk for death or neurodevelopmental impairment. Future studies therefore need to focus on advancements that continue to decrease mortality as well as lessen disability in survivors.

BIBLIOGRAPHIC SOURCE(S)

Bulas D, Glass P. Neonatal ECMO: neuroimaging and neurodevelopmental outcome. *Semin Perinatol.* 2005;29(1):58-65.

Extracorporeal Life Support Organization. ECLS Registry Report. Ann Arbor, MI. 2015.

Guner YS, Khemani RG, Qureshi FG, et al. Outcome analysis of neonates with congenital diaphragmatic hernia treated with venovenous versus venoarterial extracorporeal membrane oxygenation. *J Pediatr Surg.* 2009;44(9):1691.

Hoffman SB, Massaro AN, Gingalewski C, Short BL. Predictors of survival in congenital diaphragmatic hernia patients requiring extracorporeal membrane oxygenation: CNMC 15-year experience. *J Perinatol.* 2010;30(8):546.

Letourneau PA, Lally KP. Congenital diaphragmatic hernia and ECMO. In: Annich GM, Lynch WR, MacLaren G, Wilson JM, Bartlett RH, eds. *ECMO: Extracorporeal Cardiopulmonary Support in Critical Care.* 4th ed. Ann Arbor, MI: Extracorporeal Life Support Organization; 2012:251-9.

Logan JW, Rice Goldberg HE, Goldberg RN, Cotten CM. Congenital diaphragmatic hernia: a systemic review and summary of best-evidence practice strategies. *J Perinatol.* 2007;27(9):535.

Mugford M, Elbourne D, Field D. Extracorporeal membrane oxygenation for severe respiratory failure in newborn infants. *Cochrane Database Syst Rev.* 2008;16(3).

Radhakrishnan RS, Lally PA, Lally KP, Cox CS. ECMO for meconium aspiration syndrome: support for relaxed entry criteria. *ASAIO J.* 2007;53(4):489.

Reiss I, Schaibel T, van den Hout L, et al. Standardized protocol management of infants with congenital diaphragmatic hernia in Europe: The CDH EURO Consortium Consensus. *Neonatology.* 2010;98(4):354.

Saini A, Spinella PC. Management of anticoagulation and hemostasis for pediatric extracorporeal membrane oxygenation. *Clin Lab Med.* 2014;34(3):655.

Schaible T, Hermle D, Loersch F, Demirakca S, Reinshagen K, Varnholt V. A 20-year experience on neonatal extracorporeal membrane oxygenation in a referral center. *Intensive Care Med.* 2010;36(7):1229.

Selewski DT, Cornell TT, Blatt NB, et al. Fluid overload and fluid removal in pediatric patients on extracorporeal membrane oxygenation requiring continuous renal replacement therapy. *Crit Care Med.* 2012;40(9):2694.

Suttner DM, Short BL. Neonatal respiratory ECLS. In: Annich GM, Lynch WR, MacLaren G, Wilson JM, Bartlett RH, eds. *ECMO: Extracorporeal Cardiopulmonary Support in Critical Care.* 4th ed. Ann Arbor, MI: Extracorporeal Life Support Organization; 2012:225-44.

Cardiovascular Disorders

Approach to the Cyanotic Infant

David W. Bearl, MD, MA • Kevin Hill, MD, MS

SCOPE

DISEASE/CONDITION(S)

Cyanosis can be classified as central and peripheral, or acrocyanosis. Acrocyanosis is bluish discoloration of the distal extremities and is often benign and normal in the newborn period. Central cyanosis reflects deoxygenated hemoglobin in the blood and is generally detectable when there is >3 g/dL of deoxygenated hemoglobin in arterial blood or >5 g/dL in capillary blood. Frequently the "cyanotic neonate" is diagnosed upon detection of desaturation by pulse oximetry. This chapter focuses on the evaluation and treatment of cardiac causes of cyanosis or desaturation in the newborn. Approximately one out of every five heart defects are "cyanotic" lesions with an estimated prevalence of 16 out of every 10,000 live births.

GUIDELINE OBJECTIVE(S)

To provide guidance for neonatologists, pediatricians, advanced practitioners, and nurses on evaluation and treatment of the infant with known or suspected cyanotic congenital heart disease.

BRIEF BACKGROUND

The first step in assessing an infant with cyanosis is to determine the mechanism of desaturation. Cyanosis or desaturation associated with heart disease is due to a right-to-left shunt leading to mixing of deoxygenated blood from the venous circulation with the oxygenated blood of the arterial circulation. There are other potential causes of desaturation that may also require evaluation including: 1) respiratory desaturation due to lung disease with ventilation-perfusion mismatch; 2) pulmonary hypertension which causes desaturation when there is a coexisting source of intracardiac shunting (e.g., atrial septal defect, patent ductus arteriosus, or even a patent foramen ovale); 3) central desaturation due to hypoventilation usually secondary to central nervous system depression or injury; and 4) methemoglobinemia, a very rare cause of neonatal cyanosis, due to decreased affinity of hemoglobin for oxygen.

RECOMMENDATIONS

DIAGNOSTIC EVALUATION

Fetal Diagnosis

- Published guidelines outline indications for fetal echocardiography including:
  - High-risk maternal factors (e.g., maternal diabetes mellitus, teratogen exposure)
  - An immediate family history of structural heart defects
  - Concerns identified on an obstetrics screening ultrasound
- Almost half of all cardiac defects requiring surgery within the first 6 months of life (excluding patent ductus arteriosus [PDA]) in the United States are diagnosed prenatally.
  - There is variability depending on defect type with low rates of prenatal detection for defects such as:
    a. Total anomalous pulmonary venous return (~9% prenatal diagnosis rate)
    b. Ventricular septal defects (~12% prenatal diagnosis rate)
    c. Isolated coarctation of the aorta (~22% prenatal diagnosis rate).

Postnatal Diagnosis

- Physical examination remains critical to accurately diagnose life-threatening heart disease including identification of central cyanosis and features associated with specific lesions (see below).
- Pulse oximetry screening is recommended in the United States and in other nations in term neonates.
  - Healthy newborns are screened at 24 hours of life or prior to discharge with pulse oximetry readings obtained from the right hand and one foot.
  - An infant with a reading of ≥95% in either extremity and ≤3% absolute difference between the upper and lower extremity readings is unlikely to have cyanotic heart disease.
  - Confirmed desaturation should prompt further evaluation with an echocardiogram.
- The hyperoxia test can be used to differentiate respiratory from cardiac cyanosis.
  - The test is performed by comparing a baseline arterial blood gas with an arterial blood gas performed after the infant has been exposed to 100% oxygen for 10 minutes.
  - If the partial pressure of oxygen is <50 mmHg at baseline and does not increase by more than 100 mmHg with oxygen, then cyanosis is more likely to be cardiac in origin and an echocardiogram is warranted.
- Chest x-ray (CXR) can be helpful to delineate between respiratory and cardiac etiologies for desaturation. CXR features that might suggest congenital heart disease include:

- Increased or decreased pulmonary vascularity
- Cardiomegaly
- Cardiac malposition
- Electrocardiogram (ECG) may demonstrate characteristic electrical patterns depending on the cardiac lesion (see below).
- Transthoracic echocardiogram is the gold standard for noninvasive detection of most cyanotic congenital heart diseases.
  - Routine echocardiography is not cost-effective in all neonates and echocardiography is only indicated in those neonates where there is clinical suspicion.

INITIAL MANAGEMENT

- To stabilize the severely cyanotic neonate with known or suspected congenital heart disease one should:
  - Ensure stable airway management
  - Establish vascular access
  - Initiate prostaglandin therapy to maintain a patent ductus arteriosus
    a. Initial prostaglandin dosing is typically 0.05 µg/kg/min.
      i. Doses up to 0.1 µg/kg/min can be used when saturations fail to improve and there is reason to believe the ductus is not responding.
      ii. Lower doses (0.01–0.02 µg/kg/min) can be considered for initial dosing when the ductus is large by echocardiography and the objective is simply to maintain patency.
      iii. Once effective ductal patency has been established, prostaglandins can be titrated down to 0.01–0.02 µg/kg/min.
    b. Prostaglandin side effects are dose dependent and include:
      i. Apnea
        ◦ May necessitate intubation with mechanical ventilation.
        ◦ Due to apnea risk, most infants on prostaglandins are intubated prior to transfer.
          - Exceptions may be considered in patients on low-dose prostaglandins who have been clinically stable on this dose for a prolonged period of time (i.e., days).
      ii. Fever
      iii. Hypotension
        ◦ May require volume expansion
      iv. Hypoglycemia
    c. Very rarely, patients can acutely decompensate with initiation of prostaglandin therapy.
      i. This is usually due to the presence of rare congenital heart defects associated with obstruction to pulmonary venous return or left atrial drainage.
      ii. All of these lesions represent surgical or interventional emergencies, and immediate echocardiography should be obtained.
- Oxygen can improve desaturation but should be used cautiously in lesions where there is a need to balance pulmonary and systemic blood flow (e.g., single ventricle lesions).
  - A saturation target of 75–85% is typically appropriate to ensure adequate systemic oxygen delivery with a balanced pulmonary-to-systemic flow ratios.

- Echocardiography should be performed as soon as possible to establish a definitive diagnosis so that management can be tailored to the specifics of the underlying anatomy and physiology.

SURGICAL EMERGENCIES

- A subset of defects may present with severe cyanosis and/or systemic hypoperfusion with no alternative other than surgical or sometimes transcatheter intervention. Specific examples include:
  - Obstructed total anomalous pulmonary venous return (TAPVR)
  - Severe Ebstein's anomaly
  - Any congenital heart defect that requires mixing where the atrial septum is intact or restrictive (e.g., transposition of the great arteries and hypoplastic left heart syndrome)
- These lesions can all be lethal within hours of birth if not intervened upon invasively.
  - Early diagnosis is critical.
  - Prenatal diagnosis by fetal echocardiogram allows for planned delivery at a tertiary care center to facilitate rapid intervention if necessary.

LESION-SPECIFIC EVALUATION AND MANAGEMENT

Numerous cardiac diagnoses cause cyanosis, and management must be tailored to the unique anatomic and physiologic features. Some of the more common cardiac defects are summarized below, including unique diagnostic findings and management considerations.

Truncus Arteriosus

In this lesion, a single great vessel arises from the base of the heart and gives rise to the aorta, pulmonary arteries, and coronary arteries. There is an obligatory, often large ventricular septal defect (Figure 30.1). Truncus is associated with an interrupted aortic arch in approximately 10–20% of cases. Truncus is also associated with 22q-deletion syndromes (e.g., DiGeorge syndrome) in approximately 40% of cases. Severity of cyanosis in truncus is directly related to the amount of blood flow to the lungs. If there is branch pulmonary artery stenosis or persistently high pulmonary vascular resistance, then cyanosis will be more pronounced. On cardiovascular examination, there is a normal S1 often followed by an ejection click (opening of the truncal valve) and a single S2. If there is significant truncal valve insufficiency, then a high-pitched diastolic murmur can be heard on the left sternal border. ECG is usually normal, with possible biventricular hypertrophy. CXR often shows cardiomegaly and increased pulmonary vascular markings, except in the case of pulmonary stenosis, and severe cyanosis, where there might be decreased markings. Also, one-third of patients with truncus arteriosus have a right-sided aortic arch, which can be seen by CXR. The natural history of truncus without surgery is very poor, and thus the preferred management is complete surgical correction in the first weeks of life.

Transposition of the Great Arteries

Transposition of the great arteries (TGA) is characterized by ventriculoarterial discordance. In a general sense, this means that the aorta arises from the right ventricle and the pulmonary artery arises from the left ventricle. This creates a physiologic state of parallel circulation, with all of the oxygenated blood recirculating back to the lungs and all

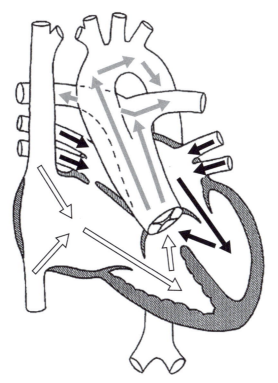

FIGURE 30.1 • Truncus arteriosus features a single great vessel that gives rise to the aorta, pulmonary arteries, and coronary arteries. The white arrow with black border represent the course of desaturated blood, black arrows represent the course of completely saturated blood, and grey arrows represent the course of mixed saturated and desaturated blood.

of the deoxygenated blood recirculating back to the systemic circulation. TGA accounts for 5–7% of congenital heart defects and is accompanied by a ventricular septal defect in slightly less than half of cases and systemic outflow obstruction (subvalvar, valvar, supravalvar aortic stenosis or coarctation of the aorta) in about one-quarter. The typical physical examination is notable for progressive and severe cyanosis. Other examination findings will reflect associated lesions (e.g., a murmur associated with outflow tract obstruction). ECG and CXR may be normal during the neonatal period, although the classic CXR description of the heart gives the appearance of an "egg on a string." Severity of cyanosis in TGA is determined by the amount of mixing of saturated and desaturated blood that is permitted by associated defects (e.g., atrial septal defect [ASD], PDA, or intact ventricular septum [VSD]). The atrial septum is typically the most stable source of mixing; if there is a restrictive or small atrial septal defect, a balloon atrial septostomy is indicated to increase mixing. Increased pulmonary vascular resistance can also exacerbate cyanosis and pulmonary vasodilator therapy (e.g., oxygen and/or inhaled nitric oxide) is often indicated in the deeply cyanotic neonate with TGA. Surgical correction is performed during the neonatal period and typically involves an arterial switch operation with correction of other associated cardiac anomalies.

Tetralogy of Fallot

Tetralogy of Fallot (TOF) lesion consists of an overriding aorta, ventricular septal defect, pulmonary stenosis (subvalvar, valvar, and/or supravalvar), and right ventricular hypertrophy. TOF is the most common form of cyanotic heart disease, with an estimated incidence of 577 per 1,000,000 live births. Approximately 20% of infants with TOF have an associated syndrome such as 22q-deletion or trisomy 21. Physical examination typically includes a normal S1, single S2 with a loud systolic ejection murmur at the left lower sternal border that radiates to the back. The severity of right ventricular outflow obstruction dictates the degree of cyanosis. An infant with minimal obstruction may be acyanotic (i.e., the "pink Tet"), while an infant with severe obstruction will be markedly cyanotic. The ECG shows right axis deviation with right ventricular hypertrophy. The CXR shows the classic "boot-shaped heart." A major and potentially life-threatening concern in unrepaired TOF is the possibility of a hypercyanotic spell ("Tet spell") marked by profoundly worsened cyanosis that is precipitated by suddenly increased subpulmonic muscular obstruction to pulmonary blood flow. Surgical management of TOF usually involves complete repair, with the typical age between 2 and 6 months. In some cases, there is profound baseline cyanosis and neonatal intervention is needed either with complete neonatal repair or a systemic-to-pulmonary artery shunt.

Total Anomalous Pulmonary Venous Return

This lesion involves anomalous drainage of all four pulmonary veins to the systemic venous side of the heart (Figure 30.2). The incidence is 1–3% of all congenital heart disease. TAPVR can be categorized as supracardiac (via the superior vena cava), cardiac (to the right atrium), infracardiac (via the inferior vena cava), or mixed. Desaturation in TAPVR occurs because systemic blood flow requires a right-to-left shunt typically across an ASD or patent foramen ovale. Some children are only mildly desaturated; however, more severe desaturation and a more critical presentation often occur in children with obstruction to pulmonary venous return. Obstruction is most common in the infradiaphragmatic type but can be seen in any form of TAPVR. Cardiovascular examination in TAPVR is typically normal except for cyanosis. ECG is also normal for age. CXR can be normal or can show signs of pulmonary edema, sometimes mimicking respiratory distress syndrome if there is significant obstruction. In one type of TAPVR, with anomalous drainage via a vertical vein to the left innominate vein, the CXR can show a classic "snowman" or "figure-8" appearance. *When TAPVR is diagnosed, consultation with a pediatric cardiologist prior to starting prostaglandin (PGE) therapy is advised, as it is possible for PGE to improve or worsen the infant's clinical condition.* Mortality without surgery is high, and obstructed TAPVR represents a true surgical emergency; relief of obstruction is the only means to restore hemodynamic stability. Even without obstruction, surgical correction is typically performed in the neonatal period, with reimplantation of the pulmonary veins into the left atrium.

Single-Ventricle Heart Defects

These lesions have many different varieties and involve some form of hypoplasia of either the right or left ventricle, and have a wide range of clinical severity. The hypoplastic left heart syndrome (HLHS), involving underdevelopment of the mitral valve, left ventricle, aortic valve, and aorta, is the prototypical single right ventricle lesion (Figure 30.3), while tricuspid atresia represents the prototypical single left

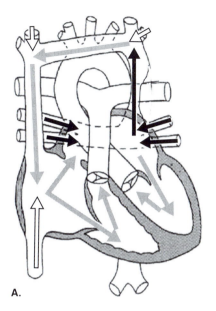 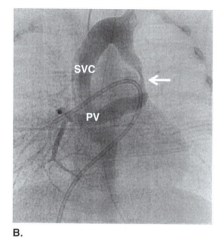

A. **B.**

FIGURE 30.2 • A. Supracardiac total anomalous pulmonary venous return with the pulmonary veins draining into a vertical vein that drains into the innominate vein. The white arrow with black border represent the course of desaturated blood, black arrows represent the course of completely saturated blood, and grey arrows represent the course of mixed saturated and desaturated blood. **B.** An angiogram from the right upper lung lobe demonstrates anomalous return of the pulmonary vein (PV) to an obstructed vertical vein (arrow) that drains to the innominate vein and then into the superior vena cava (SVC).

ventricle lesion. There are many other forms of single-ventricle lesions including the double inlet left ventricle spectrum of defects, double outlet right ventricle defects associated with mitral valve atresia, some forms of pulmonary atresia with an intact ventricular septum, and unbalanced atrioventricular canal defects. Single-ventricle physiology is characterized by complete mixing of systemic and pulmonary venous return most commonly with some form of obstruction to either pulmonary or systemic blood flow. Consequently, these are typically ductal-dependent lesions, and initial stabilization involves maintaining the patency of the ductus arteriosus with prostaglandins and ensuring that there is an effective means for mixing of desaturated and saturated blood (e.g., via an atrial septal defect). In single-ventricle physiology, excessive oxygen therapy can be harmful by encouraging pulmonary overcirculation. Thus some degree of cyanosis is tolerated, with goal oxygen saturations of 75–85% predicting an approximate even balance between pulmonary and systemic blood flow. The surgical approach for single-ventricle heart defects will vary depending on the lesion. When indicated, neonatal surgical intervention typically involves establishing a stable source of pulmonary blood flow (e.g., via a systemic to pulmonary shunt) and ensuring a stable source of systemic output. More definitive single ventricle palliation has evolved, typically involving a staged approach culminating in the Fontan operation.

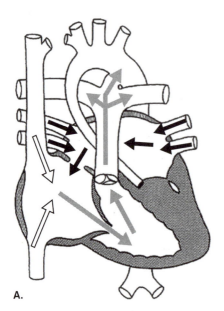
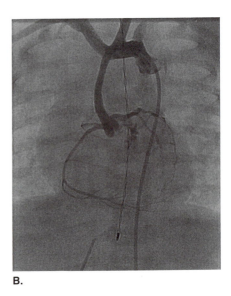

FIGURE 30.3 • A. Hypoplastic left heart syndrome features underdevelopment of the left-sided structures including the mitral and aortic valves and aorta. The white arrow with black border represent the course of desaturated blood, black arrows represent the course of completely saturated blood, and grey arrows represent the course of mixed saturated and desaturated blood. **B.** An aortic angiogram demonstrates the diminutive ascending aorta and coronary arteries in a neonate with hypoplastic left heart syndrome.

Ebstein's Anomaly

Ebstein's anomaly is a malformation of the tricuspid valve such that the leaflets are abnormal and the point of valve coaptation is displaced apically into the right ventricle, effectively "atrializing" a portion of the right ventricle. Severity of the defect is highly variable depending on the degree of displacement and the associated severity of tricuspid regurgitation. The most severe cases present in the neonatal period with severe cyanosis caused by an obligatory atrial level right to left shunt. The atrial level shunt is needed because severe tricuspid valve regurgitation limits antegrade pulmonary blood flow. In less severe forms, children can be completely asymptomatic. Physical examination, aside from cyanosis, can demonstrate a systolic regurgitant murmur that increases in intensity with inspiration, widely split S1 and S2 due to right bundle branch block, and venous distention in the form of hepatomegaly. CXR in neonates presenting with cyanosis often shows extreme cardiomegaly. ECG can be diagnostic with changes including PR prolongation, right bundle branch block, pre-excitation, and deep Q waves in leads V1–4 and inferior leads, as well as atrial and supraventricular tachycardias. Neonates presenting with cyanosis will sometimes improve as their pulmonary vascular resistance drops, thereby encouraging antegrade pulmonary blood flow. Neonatal surgical intervention is indicated for severe and unremitting cyanosis but is associated with a much poorer prognosis.

Pulmonary Atresia with or without a Ventricular Septal Defect

Pulmonary atresia with a ventricular septal defect (PA/VSD) and pulmonary atresia with intact ventricular septum (PA/IVS) are commonly classified together because both involve complete obstruction of antegrade pulmonary blood flow. However, in many respects these represent two physiologically and anatomically distinct lesions.

PA/VSD is characterized by a normally developed right ventricle with hypoplastic or sometimes nonexistent central pulmonary arteries (Figure 30.4). In this lesion, pulmonary blood flow is often dependent on multiple aortopulmonary collateral arteries (MAPCAs). In contrast, in PA/IVS the central pulmonary arteries are typically well formed but there may be tricuspid valve and/or right ventricular hypoplasia, and coronary artery development may be abnormal due to sinusoidal communications between the right ventricle and the coronary arteries. In both lesions cyanosis is evident due to complete mixing of saturated and desaturated blood in the heart (via an ASD or VSD). Worsening cyanosis often develops coincident with closure of

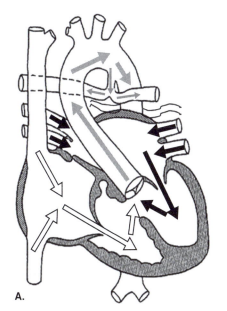
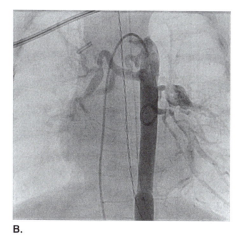

A.   B.

FIGURE 30.4 • **A.** Pulmonary atresia with a ventricular septal defect with blood flow to the native, hypoplastic pulmonary arteries from a patent ductus arteriosus. Also seen are several aortopulmonary collateral vessels supplying pulmonary blood flow. The white arrow with black border represent the course of desaturated blood, black arrows represent the course of completely saturated blood, and grey arrows represent the course of mixed saturated and desaturated blood. **B.** A descending aortic angiogram demonstrates several major aortopulmonary collaterals (MAPCAs). Not shown in this image are the native pulmonary arteries which originated more superiorly in this child from a reverse oriented ductus arteriosus. In PA/VSD pulmonary blood flow can be supplied entirely by native pulmonary arteries, entirely by MAPCAs or by some combination of the two.

the ductus arteriosus, although in the most severe forms of PA/VSD there may be no ductus arteriosus, with all pulmonary blood flow dependent upon MAPCAs. Physical examination findings include a normal or single first heart sound and a single second heart sound. A systolic murmur (louder with an intact ventricular septum) is often heard at the left lower sternal border secondary to tricuspid regurgitation in PA/IVS and from the VSD in PA/VSD. The CXR often shows decreased pulmonary vascular markings. A boot-shaped heart is often seen in PA/VSD, similar to TOF. The ECG in PA/IVS will show decreased right ventricular forces and right atrial enlargement with left axis deviation or left ventricular hypertrophy, while an ECG in PA/VSD, as a rule, shows right axis deviation with right ventricular hypertrophy. Infants diagnosed with PA with or without VSD typically require prostaglandin therapy for pulmonary blood flow. There are many variables in surgical decision-making with these heterogeneous anomalies.

In PA/IVS, cardiac catheterization is indicated, as coronary blood flow may be dependent upon sinusoidal coronary communications in the right ventricle. In the absence of right ventricle–dependent coronary circulation and/or right ventricular hypoplasia, the atretic pulmonary valve can sometimes be opened using transcatheter approaches, and neonatal surgery may not be needed. However, in cases with right ventricular hypoplasia or coronary involvement, single-ventricle palliation or heart transplant may be indicated. Management of PA/VSD is entirely dependent upon the presence or absence of central pulmonary arteries and delineation of all the potential sources of pulmonary blood flow. Management in the neonatal period can include a systemic to pulmonary artery shunt, complete repair, or in the most severe cases, no intervention may be feasible.

IMPLEMENTATION OF GUIDELINE

DESCRIPTION OF IMPLEMENTATION STRATEGY

Institutional and public health policies should be implemented to facilitate early identification of cyanotic congenital heart defects. Earlier diagnosis allows for stabilization before ductal closure, and transfer to a tertiary care center with expertise in the management of congenital heart disease. Prenatal evaluation with fetal echocardiography is optimal and should be performed in all high-risk pregnancies. Prenatal diagnosis allows planned delivery and immediate implementation of the appropriate postnatal medical, surgical, and transcatheter interventions. In the most severe cases where immediate intervention may be necessary, a prenatal diagnosis can facilitate availability and readiness of the appropriate care team.

In the absence of prenatal diagnosis, routine pulse oximetry screening is recommended for all term infants and should be performed after 24 hours of age but prior to hospital discharge. Transthoracic echocardiography should be performed in neonates that fail pulse oximetry screening or in those with other concerning clinical findings including unexplained clinical instability, abnormal cardiac findings on a prenatal ultrasound or fetal echocardiogram, and physical examination or other diagnostic findings (e.g., failed hyperoxia test, abnormal CXR, abnormal ECG) that suggest congenital heart disease. In the profoundly cyanotic infant, prostaglandins should be initiated if echocardiography is not immediately available. Once a diagnosis of cyanotic congenital heart disease is established, management and surgical intervention should be tailored to the specific cardiac lesion.

QUALITY METRICS

1. Frequency of pre- versus postnatal diagnosis of cyanotic congenital heart disease.
2. For postnatal diagnosis, time to diagnosis and implementation of appropriate therapy.
3. Mortality and major morbidity rates in children diagnosed with cyanotic congenital heart disease.

SUMMARY

Cyanotic congenital heart defects represent a heterogeneous collection of lesions characterized by obstruction to pulmonary blood flow and an associated intracardiac right-to-left shunt. Many of these lesions present with severe cyanosis in the neonatal period coincident with closure of the ductus arteriosus. Early diagnosis is critical for stabilization and to facilitate implementation of the appropriate treatment plan. Strategies to facilitate earlier diagnosis, including prenatal detection by fetal echocardiography or postnatal detection with pulse oximetry screening, have the potential to improve outcomes. Initial management includes stabilization and resuscitation by establishing a stable source of systemic and pulmonary blood flow. This is typically accomplished with prostaglandin therapy to maintain patency of the ductus arteriosus, although there are rare lesions where invasive intervention (surgical or transcatheter) is needed. Prostaglandin use should be considered in any cyanotic neonate if echocardiography is not immediately available. In most cases, transfer should be considered to a tertiary care center with expertise in management of congenital heart disease.

BIBLIOGRAPHIC SOURCE(S)

Al Habib HF, Jacobs JP, Mavroudis C, et al. Contemporary patterns of management of tetralogy of Fallot: data from the Society of Thoracic Surgeons Database. *Ann Thorac Surg.* 2010;90(3):813-9; discussion 819-20.

Alwi M. Management algorithm in pulmonary atresia with intact ventricular septum. *Catheter Cardiovasc Interv.* 2006;67(5):679-86.

Burroughs JT, Edwards JE. Total anomalous pulmonary venous connection. *Am Heart J.* 1960;59:913-31.

Cheung EW, Richmond ME, Turner ME, Bacha EA, Torres AJ. Pulmonary atresia/intact ventricular septum: influence of coronary anatomy on single-ventricle outcome. *Ann Thorac Surg.* 2014;98(4):1371-7.

Donofrio MT, Moon-Grady AJ, Hornberger LK, et al. Diagnosis and treatment of fetal cardiac disease: a scientific statement from the American Heart Association. *Circulation.* 2014;129(21): 2183-242.

Hoffman JI, Kaplan S. The incidence of congenital heart disease. *J Am Coll Cardiol.* 2002;39(12):1890-900.

Jones RW, Baumer JH, Joseph MC, Shinebourne EA. Arterial oxygen tension and response to oxygen breathing in differential diagnosis of congenital heart disease in infancy. *Arch Dis Child.* 1976;51(9):667-73.

Konstantinov IE, Karamlou T, Blackstone EH, et al. Truncus arteriosus associated with interrupted aortic arch in 50 neonates: a Congenital Heart Surgeons Society study. *Ann Thorac Surg.* 2006;81(1):214-22.

Lees MH. Cyanosis of the newborn infant. Recognition and clinical evaluation. *J Pediatr.* 1970;77(3):484-98.

Lim DS, Kulik TJ, Kim DW, Charpie JR, Crowley DC, Maher KO. Aminophylline for the prevention of apnea during prostaglandin E1 infusion. *Pediatrics.* 2003;112(1 Pt 1):e27-9.

Lundsgaard C. Studies on cyanosis: I. Primary causes of cyanosis. *J Exp Med*. 1919;30(3):259-69.

Mahle WT, Martin GR, Beekman RH 3rd, Morrow WR; Section on Cardiology and Cardiac Surgery Executive Committee. Endorsement of Health and Human Services recommendation for pulse oximetry screening for critical congenital heart disease. *Pediatrics*. 2012;129(1):190-2.

Mahle WT, Newburger JW, Matherne GP, et al. Role of pulse oximetry in examining newborns for congenital heart disease: a scientific statement from the American Heart Association and American Academy of Pediatrics. *Circulation*. 2009;120(5):447-58.

Malhotra SP, Hanley FL. Surgical management of pulmonary atresia with ventricular septal defect and major aortopulmonary collaterals: a protocol-based approach. *Semin Thorac Cardiovasc Surg Pediatr Card Surg Annu*. 2009:145-51.

Marcelletti C, McGoon DC, Danielson GK, Wallace RB, Mair DD. Early and late results of surgical repair of truncus arteriosus. *Circulation*. 1977;55(4):636-41.

Marino BS, Bird GL, Wernovsky G. Diagnosis and management of the newborn with suspected congenital heart disease. *Clin Perinatol*. 2001;28(1):91-136.

McElhinney DB, Driscoll DA, Emanuel BS, Goldmuntz E. Chromosome 22q11 deletion in patients with truncus arteriosus. *Pediatr Cardiol*. 2003;24(6):569-73.

Perloff JK, Marelli AJ. *Clinical Recognition of Congenital Heart Disease*. 6th ed. Philadelphia, PA: Elsevier/Saunders; 2012.

Quartermain MD, Pasquali SK, Hill KD, et al. Variation in prenatal diagnosis of congenital heart disease in infants. *Pediatrics*. 2015;136(2):378-85.

Reller MD, Strickland MJ, Riehle-Colarusso T, Mahle WT, Correa A. Prevalence of congenital heart defects in metropolitan Atlanta, 1998-2005. *J Pediatr*. 2008;153(6):807-13.

Seale AN, Uemura H, Webber SA, et al. Total anomalous pulmonary venous connection: morphology and outcome from an international population-based study. *Circulation*. 2010;122(25):2718-26.

Van Praagh R, Van Praagh S. The anatomy of common aorticopulmonary trunk (truncus arteriosus communis) and its embryologic implications. A study of 57 necropsy cases. *Am J Cardiol*. 1965;16(3):406-25.

Blood Pressure Management

Beau Batton, MD

SCOPE

DISEASE/CONDITION(S)

Cardiovascular support for extremely preterm infants in the first week after birth.

GUIDELINE OBJECTIVE(S)

1. Review evolving blood pressure (BP) parameters occurring immediately after birth.
2. Review the potential risks and benefits of commonly prescribed antihypotensive therapies.
3. Provide suggestions for early postnatal blood pressure management in extremely preterm infants.

BRIEF BACKGROUND

The intrinsically abnormal condition of extreme prematurity and the associated evolving complex physiology make it difficult to identify an acceptable range of BP values in the immediate postnatal period. Although BP is higher with increasing birth weight and gestational age (GA) at birth and increases spontaneously with advancing postnatal age similar to more mature infants, there is a wide range in observed BP values for extremely preterm infants during this time (Figure 31.1). These factors make it difficult to determine whether the BP for a given infant at a specific postnatal age is too high, too low, rising too quickly or not quickly enough. Multiple disease processes, unpredictable adaptation to extrauterine life, and difficulty assessing organ perfusion also make deciding when to institute therapy for perceived low BP challenging. Consequently, BP management is highly variable.

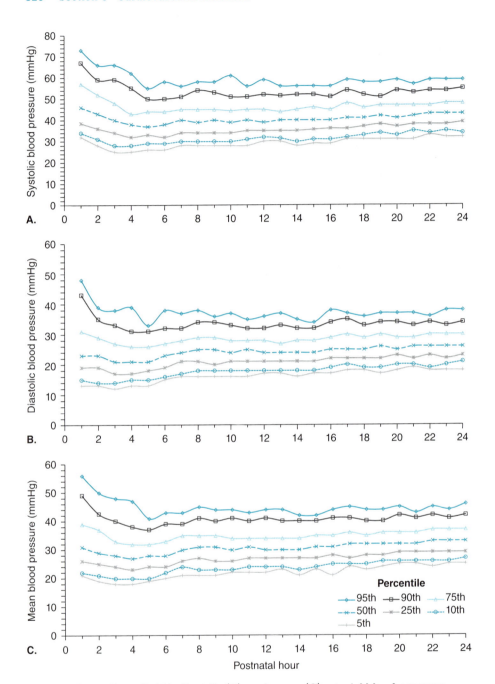

FIGURE 31.1 • Systolic (A), diastolic (B), and mean (C) arterial blood pressure curves for 367 extremely preterm infants. (From Batton B. *J Perinatol.* 2014;34:301-5; reprinted with permission.)

Numerous investigations over the last 25 years suggest preterm infants with perceived hypotension are at an increased risk for adverse outcomes. These observations have led many clinicians to administer therapies in an effort to raise BP and presumably improve an infant's chances of survival without major morbidity. No such improvement in outcomes has been demonstrated to date. More concerning is the possibility that commonly prescribed antihypotensive therapies such as isotonic fluid boluses, dopamine, dobutamine, epinephrine, and hydrocortisone may be harmful. Although these therapies may increase BP, it remains unclear whether these increases are distinct from the spontaneous rise in BP observed in the first postnatal week (Figure 31.2). Extremely preterm infants who receive antihypotensive therapies have higher mortality and morbidity rates versus untreated infants of a similar GA (Table 31.1). These risks persist even when considering confounding factors such as the frequency of low BP values, severity of illness, inclusion of infants in extremis who are likely to die irrespective of therapeutic interventions, and the underlying cause of perceived low BP (e.g., perinatal asphyxia, sepsis, hemorrhage).

RECOMMENDATIONS

MAJOR RECOMMENDATIONS

- Antihypotensive therapies should be used cautiously and reserved for infants in whom the perceived potential benefits outweigh the risks.
- A favorable risk-benefit ratio is unlikely unless there is strong clinical evidence of organ compromise or a condition associated with hemodynamic instability (e.g., shock due to sepsis, hypovolemia/hemorrhage, or myocardial dysfunction).
- There is currently insufficient data to support the routine use of echocardiography or indirect measures of end-organ perfusion/oxygen delivery to guide therapeutic decision-making.

PRACTICE OPTIONS

Practice Option #1

- Blood pressure values should not be the sole criteria to guide therapeutic decision-making.
- There is no numeric threshold defining hypotension for which outcomes have been shown to improve with antihypotensive therapy. A simple numeric cutoff for treating hypotension (e.g., a mean arterial BP < infant's GA in weeks) should not be used because it is not evidence based, will result in the overtreatment of hypotension, and exposes infants to unnecessary risks.
- A full physical examination to assess perfusion and a complete history to evaluate the likelihood of a condition which can lead to hypovolemic, cardiac, or septic shock should be incorporated into the decision to initiate therapy.
- Antihypotensive therapies are not indicated for infants with good perfusion (pink extremities, capillary refill ≤4 seconds, strong pulses) because these therapies have not been shown to benefit such infants and they may be harmful.

Practice Option #2

- Specific antihypotensive therapy treatment should be tailored to the individual patient and based on the suspected etiology.
- Isotonic fluids are only indicated if there is strong evidence of hypovolemia (hematocrit <35%, small cardiac silhouette on x-ray, history of fetal or neonatal hemorrhage, or umbilical cord complication).

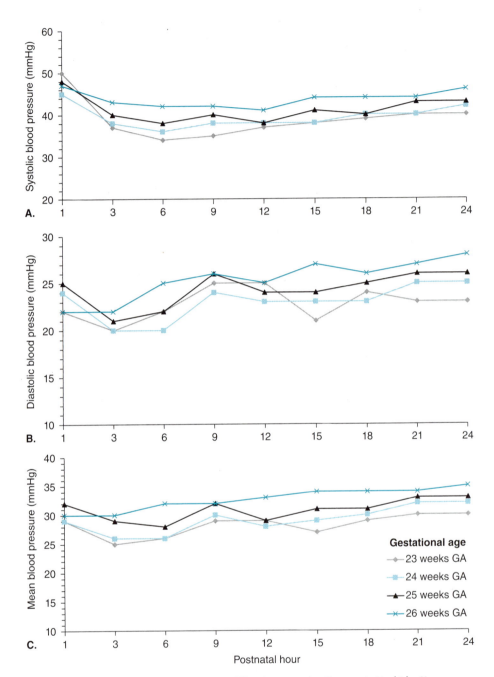

FIGURE 31.2 • Gestational age specific changes in the systolic (A), diastolic (B), and mean (C) arterial blood pressure 50th percentile curves for 367 extremely preterm infants. (From Batton B. *J Perinatol.* 2014;34:301-5; reprinted with permission.)

TABLE 31.1. Potential Risks and Benefits of Commonly Prescribed Antihypotensive Therapies

Antihypotensive Therapy	Potential Benefits	Potential Risks
Crystalloid	Restore intravascular volume	IVH, death, NDI
Inotropes*	Raise blood pressure	IVH, death, ROP, NDI
Dopamine	Raise blood pressure, increase cerebral blood flow, increase urine output	Pituitary gland suppression, IVH
Hydrocortisone	Raise blood pressure, improve lung function	Intestinal perforation, IVH, death

*Collectively refers to dopamine, dobutamine, or epinephrine.

IVH, intraventricular hemorrhage; NDI, neurodevelopmental impairment; ROP, retinopathy of prematurity.

- For infants with a high index of suspicion for septic shock, a vasopressor such as dopamine may be considered to increase systemic vascular resistance, and an isotonic fluid bolus may be considered to replace intravascular volume depletion through capillary leak.
- For infants with suspected myocardial dysfunction, especially those with a significant metabolic acidosis (base deficit ≥ 12 mEq/L), an inotrope such as dopamine, dobutamine, epinephrine, or hydrocortisone may be considered. There are insufficient data to recommend any specific inotrope.
- There are no data to support the routine use of milrinone for BP management in extremely preterm infants.

Practice Option #3

- Excessive or rapid infusion of fluid boluses are associated with increased rates of intraventricular hemorrhage and death and should be avoided unless there is an acute hemorrhage.
- Infusions of vasopressors or inotropes should be started at a low dose (2.5–5 µg/kg/min for dopamine and dobutamine; 0.1 µg/kg/min for epinephrine; 0.5–1 mg/kg/dose every 8 hours for hydrocortisone).
- The goal of antihypotensive therapy should be to increase BP at a physiologic rate (~5 mmHg/day) because more rapid rates of rise are not associated with clinical benefit and may be harmful.
- Titration of vasopressors or inotropes should be in a cautious stepwise manner at a slow rate (2.5 µg/kg/min every 30 minutes for dopamine and dobutamine and 0.1 µg/kg/min every 30 minutes for epinephrine).
- Clinical assessment of perfusion, BP values, and acid-base status should all be incorporated into the decision to titrate therapy.

IMPLEMENTATION OF GUIDELINE

QUALIFYING STATEMENTS

1. Blood pressure increases spontaneously with advancing postnatal age in preterm infants.
2. A wide range of BP values are observed at each postnatal hour for preterm infants.

3. There are no large randomized trials comparing any antihypotensive therapy to placebo in any population of preterm infants to guide decision-making.
4. Blood pressure correlates poorly with clinical measurements of perfusion or indices of end-organ oxygen delivery.
5. There is no evidence-based numeric threshold for defining hypotension or guiding therapeutic decision-making.

DESCRIPTION OF IMPLEMENTATION STRATEGY

Provide an algorithm for initiation of antihypotensive therapy treatment. Provide written guidelines for escalating, weaning, and discontinuing antihypotensive therapies. Guidelines should incorporate clinical markers of perfusion to guide treatment and a statement that therapy should be tailored to the individual patient based on the suspected etiology of perceived low BP. There is no "one size fits all" approach to BP management.

QUALITY METRICS

Monitor rates of antihypotensive therapy administration, in-hospital mortality rates, and incidence of intraventricular hemorrhage, retinopathy of prematurity, and necrotizing enterocolitis in both treated and untreated infants.

SUMMARY

Infants who receive an antihypotensive therapy are more likely to die or experience significant morbidity than untreated infants. Although numerous confounding variables preclude a direct correlation between treatment for perceived low BP and worse infant outcomes, this association is robust in the literature published over the last 30 years. As such, these therapies should be reserved for the most critically ill infants. When instituted, therapy should be directed to the suspected specific cause of low BP. A numeric threshold for deciding when to administer antihypotensive therapies is not evidence based, and this should not be the sole criterion for treatment.

BIBLIOGRAPHIC SOURCE(S)

Al-Aweel I, Pursley D, Rubin L, Shah B, Weisberger S, Richardson D. Variations in prevalence of hypotension, hypertension and vasopressor use in NICUs. *J Perinatol.* 2001;21:272-8.

Alderliesten T, Lemmers P, van Haastert I, et al. Hypotension in preterm neonates: low blood pressure alone does not affect neurodevelopmental outcome. *J Pediatr.* 2014;164:986-91.

Batton B, Batton D, Riggs T. Blood pressure in the first 7 days in premature infants born at postmenstrual age 23 to 25 weeks. *Am J Perinatol.* 2007;24:107-15.

Batton B, Li L, Newman N, et al. Early blood pressure, anti-hypotensive therapy and outcomes at 18 to 22 month corrected age in extremely preterm infants. *Arch Dis Child Fetal Neonat Ed.* 2016;101(3):F201-6.

Batton B, Li L, Newman N, et al. Evolving blood pressure dynamics for extremely preterm infants. *J Perinatol.* 2014;34:301-5.

Batton B, Li L, Newman N, et al. Prospective study of blood pressure management in extremely preterm infants. *Pediatrics.* 2013;131:e1865-73.

Batton B, Zhu X, Fanaroff J, et al. Blood pressure, anti-hypotensive therapy, and neurodevelopment in extremely preterm infants. *J Pediatr.* 2009;154:351-7.

Clark C, Clyman R, Roth R, et al. Risk factor analysis of intraventricular hemorrhage in low-birth-weight infants. *J Pediatr.* 1981;99:625-8.

Cordero L, Timan C, Waters H, Sachs L. Mean arterial pressures during the first 24 hours of life in ≤600-gram birth weight infants. *J Perinatol.* 2002;22:348-53.

Cunningham S, Symon A, Elton R, Changqing Z, McIntosh N. Intra-arterial blood pressure reference ranges, death and morbidity in very low birthweight infants during the first seven days of life. *Early Hum Dev.* 1999;56:151-65.

Dempsey E, Al Hazzani F, Barrington K. Permissive hypotension in the extremely low birthweight infant with signs of good perfusion. *Arch Dis Child Fetal Neonatal Ed.* 2009;94:F241-4.

Dempsey E, Barrington K. Diagnostic criteria and therapeutic interventions for the hypotensive very low birth weight infant. *J Perinatol.* 2006;26:677-81.

Dempsey E, Barrington K. Treating hypotension in the preterm infant: when and with what: a critical and systematic review. *J Perinatol.* 2007;27:469-78.

Evans N. Which inotrope for which baby? *Arch Dis Child Fetal Neonatal Ed.* 2006;91:F213-20.

Ewer A, Tyler W, Francis A, Drinkall D, Gardosi J. Excess volume expansion and neonatal death in preterm infants born at 2–28 weeks' gestation. *Paediatr Perinat Epidemiol.* 2003;17:180-6.

Fanaroff J, Wilson-Costello D, Newman N, et al. Symptomatic hypotension is associated with neonatal morbidity and hearing loss in extremely low birth weight infants. *Pediatrics.* 2006;117:1131-5.

Finer N, Powers R, Ou C, et al. Prospective evaluation of postnatal steroid administration: a 1-year experience from the California Perinatal Quality Care Collaborative. *Pediatrics.* 2006;117:704-13.

Goldstein R, Thompson R, Oehler J, et al. Influence of acidosis, hypoxemia, and hypotension on ND outcome in very low birth weight infants. *Pediatrics.* 1995;95:238243.

Hall R, Kronsberg S, Barton B, Kaiser J, Anand K. Morphine, hypotension, and adverse outcomes among preterm neonates: who's to blame? Secondary results from the NEOPAIN trial. *Pediatrics.* 2005;115:1351-9.

Laughon M, Bose C, Allred E, et al. Factors associated with treatment for hypotension in extremely low gestational age newborns during the first postnatal week. *Pediatrics.* 2007;119:273-80.

Lee J, Rafadurai V, Tan K. Blood pressure standards for very low birthweight infants during the first day of life. *Arch Dis Child.* 1999;81:F168-70.

Logan JW, O'Shea TM, Allred EB, et al. Early postnatal hypotension and developmental delay at 24 months of age among extremely low gestational age newborns. *Arch Dis Child Fetal Neonatal Ed.* 2011;96:F321-8.

Low J, Froese A, Egalbraith R, Smith J, Sauerbrei E, Derrick E. The association between preterm newborn hypotension and hypoxemia and outcome during the first year. *Acta Paediatr.* 1993;82:433-7.

Martens S, Rijken M, Stoelhorst G, et al. Is hypotension a major risk factor for neurological morbidity at term age in very preterm infants? *Early Hum Dev.* 2003;75:79-89.

Short B, Van Meurs K, Evans J. Summary proceedings from the cardiology group on cardiovascular instability in preterm infants. *Pediatrics.* 2006;117:S34-9.

Stranak Z, Semberova J, Barrington K, et al. International survey on diagnosis and management of hypotension in extremely preterm babies. *Eur J Pediatr.* 2014;173:793-8.

Watkins A, West C, Cooke R. Blood pressure and cerebral haemorrhage and ischaemia in very low birthweight infants. *Early Hum Dev.* 1989;19:103-10.

Shock

Sarah Mapp, MD • Wayne A. Price, MD

SCOPE

DISEASE/CONDITION(S)

Shock is a state of circulatory dysfunction that causes inadequate oxygen delivery to tissues. If left untreated, the mismatch in metabolic demand and supply of oxygen will cause organ damage and eventually death.

GUIDELINE OBJECTIVE(S)

To guide neonatologists, pediatricians, advanced practitioners, and nurses on the management of shock in the neonatal period.

BRIEF BACKGROUND

In the neonate, multiple factors can cause shock, such as myocardial dysfunction, sepsis, abnormal peripheral vasoregulation, hypovolemia, loss of vascular integrity, and adrenal insufficiency. The diagnosis of shock is based on indicators of inadequate perfusion such as tachycardia, respiratory distress (e.g., tachypnea, grunting, or retractions), temperature instability, delayed capillary refill time, cool extremities, poor color, oliguria, poor feeding or impaired feeding tolerance, low tone, and metabolic acidosis.

There are three phases of shock: compensated, uncompensated, and irreversible shock. During compensated shock, vital organ function is maintained by preserving blood flow to the heart, brain, and adrenal glands at the expense of the other organs such as the skin, kidneys and GI tract. During this phase, blood pressure (BP) is usually normal or near normal. Infants will likely have tachycardia, low urine output, increased respiratory rate, and delayed capillary refill time. If untreated or inadequately treated, the neonate's shock will progress to the uncompensated phase where compensatory mechanisms are no longer adequate to maintain perfusion to the vital organs. Decreased tissue and organ perfusion results in reduced oxygen delivery and subsequent anaerobic metabolism and production of lactic acid. Organ dysfunction may manifest as decreased myocardial contractility, kidney failure, liver failure, acute respiratory distress syndrome, pulmonary edema, pulmonary hypertension, adrenal insufficiency, capillary leak, or encephalopathy. The next step in rapidly progressing or untreated shock is an irreversible shock, with cellular damage and complete organ failure resulting in death.

RECOMMENDATIONS

MAJOR RECOMMENDATIONS

Clinicians should initiate treatment when there is evidence of systemic hypoperfusion (see above), even if the BP is in the normal range. General recommendations for management of neonatal shock are:

1. Assess respiratory function (airway and breathing) to assure adequate oxygen delivery. Infants may benefit from increased respiratory support and early intubation if apnea, increased work of breathing, or hypoxemia is present.
2. Assure adequate vascular access at the first signs of shock with venous access (preferably two sites) for the administration of fluids and medications.
3. Consider obtaining arterial access for continuous BP monitoring.
4. Carefully monitor blood pressure, perfusion, and urine output.
5. In addition to treating the underlying cause, provide supportive care such as maintenance of normothermia, avoidance of hypoglycemia, and correction of electrolyte abnormalities.
   a. Note that the use of sodium bicarbonate boluses to treat metabolic acidosis in neonates is controversial. Use of sodium bicarbonate as a bolus has not been shown to improve outcomes and may cause harm such as transient cardiac dysfunction.
6. Make infant NPO.
7. Correct fluid losses with the appropriate fluid. Use crystalloid boluses (normal saline or lactated Ringers, 10–20 mL/kg per bolus) for third-space losses or colloid (packed red blood cells, fresh frozen plasma, or platelets, 10–15 mL/kg) if anemia, disseminated intravascular coagulopathy (DIC), or thrombocytopenia are present. *Note:* Fluid boluses should be used cautiously in the preterm population early in life unless there is a history of volume loss. In extremely low birth weight (ELBW) infants, excess volume expansion ($\geq$ 30 mL/kg) in the first 48 hours of life has been associated with increased mortality.
8. If initial fluid resuscitation is ineffective, consider vasopressor treatment with dopamine, dobutamine, or epinephrine drips (see Chapter 31).
9. If hypotension is refractory (two vasopressors at maximum dosing), a trial of hydrocortisone may be indicated.
10. Look for other causes.
    a. A tension pneumothorax, pleural effusion, or cardiac tamponade may present as shock.
    b. Consider an echocardiogram to evaluate for myocardial dysfunction or congenital heart defects; consider starting prostaglandin if a ductal-dependent cardiac malformation is suspected.

PRACTICE OPTIONS

Practice Option #1: Septic Shock

Septic shock in neonates may present with peripheral vasodilation (warm shock) or peripheral vasoconstriction (cold shock). Vasodilation is characterized by increased or bounding pulses, a standard capillary refill time, and hypotension. Neonates with vasoconstriction initially are normotensive (due to increased vascular resistance) with delayed capillary refill time. Both types will have oliguria and lactic acidosis. Specific recommendations are as follows.

1. Assess respiratory function and assure adequate vascular access (see Major Recommendations).
2. Supportive care involves maintenance of normothermia and avoidance of hypoglycemia. Note comment above on the use of sodium bicarbonate boluses to treat metabolic acidosis in neonates.
3. Begin appropriate antibiotic therapy based on likely source and unit-specific antibiotic resistance patterns.
4. Initiate fluid resuscitation with crystalloid boluses or colloid transfusions. Clinicians may use aggressive initial volume expansion (20–60 mL/kg) for term or late preterm infants and premature infants after the first few days of life.
5. If shock is not reversed with initial fluid resuscitation as evidenced by reversal of the signs of shock, consider ongoing fluid resuscitation, watching for development of hepatomegaly or pulmonary edema from cardiac dysfunction or excess fluid administration; increased fluid requirements may continue for several days if profound capillary leak is present.
6. If cardiac dysfunction is suspected and vasopressor therapy is required, initiate dopamine as first-line agent for shock with vasodilation, followed by epinephrine then dobutamine; use dobutamine as the first-line agent for shock with peripheral vasoconstriction, followed by dopamine or epinephrine.
7. If there is significant hypoxemia and pulmonary hypertension is suspected, consider adding inhaled nitric oxide. The safety and efficacy of milrinone for the neonate with pulmonary hypertension is still under investigation.
8. Transfuse packed red blood cells, platelets, fresh frozen plasma, and/or cryoprecipitate as indicated if anemia, thrombocytopenia, or coagulopathy are present.

Practice Option #2: Hypovolemic Shock

Absolute hypovolemia can occur due to blood loss, loss of intravascular volume (e.g., necrotizing enterocolitis, sepsis, third spacing), loss of blood (e.g., pulmonary hemorrhage, intracranial hemorrhage, or subgaleal hemorrhage), excess transepidermal losses, or loss of other body fluids (polyuria, diarrhea, emesis). Relative hypovolemia can also occur secondary to vasodilation. Specific recommendations are as follows.

1. Assess respiratory function and assure adequate vascular access (see Major Recommendations).
2. Supportive care involves maintenance of normothermia and avoidance of hypoglycemia.
3. Initiate fluid resuscitation with crystalloid (normal saline or lactated Ringers) boluses of 10–20 mL/kg; replace measured losses with a fluid containing equivalent electrolyte concentrations.

4. Transfuse packed red blood cells (15 mL/kg) if there is known or suspected blood loss or anemia.
5. Monitor for improved perfusion and watch for development of hepatomegaly or pulmonary edema from excess fluid administration.
6. If hypotension or signs of inadequate perfusion persist after aggressive initial volume expansion (>40 mL/kg in term or >20 mL/kg in preterm), initiate vasopressor treatment with dopamine as first line, followed by dobutamine or epinephrine.

Practice Option #3: Asphyxia

Neonatal asphyxia can lead to multiorgan dysfunction due to hypoxic-ischemic injury. If myocardial injury occurs, cardiovascular dysfunction with decreased cardiac output and shock may result. Hypoxia and acidosis associated with asphyxia can increase the pulmonary vascular resistance and increase the risk for pulmonary hypertension. Therapeutic hypothermia for hypoxic-ischemic encephalopathy is associated with decreased cardiac output due to reduced heart rate and stroke volume. However, a meta-analysis of therapeutic hypothermia did not show any statistical difference in incidence of hypotension or pulmonary hypertension between the cooled or control groups. Specific recommendations to support cardiac output include the following:

1. Assess respiratory function and assure adequate vascular access (see Major Recommendations).
2. Avoid excessive volume resuscitation—give slowly only as indicated if there is evidence of hypovolemia.
3. Provide early vasopressor support for cardiac dysfunction; use dobutamine as the first line if there is evidence of myocardial dysfunction; other options are dopamine or epinephrine. Epinephrine may be preferable if pulmonary hypertension is present.
4. Assessment of and support for other end-organ damage.
5. If there is significant hypoxemia and pulmonary hypertension is suspected, consider adding inhaled nitric oxide. The safety and efficacy of milrinone for the neonate with pulmonary hypertension are currently under investigation.

Practice Option #4: Cardiogenic Shock

Major etiologies of cardiogenic shock in the neonatal period include cardiomyopathy, asphyxia (see above), arrhythmias, congenital heart defects with obstruction to blood flow, and metabolic disorders. Additional clinical findings with cardiogenic shock may be present including hepatomegaly, rales, peripheral edema, and a gallop rhythm. Management will differ based on the underlying cause; however, until identified, supportive management will be essential. Specific recommendations are as follows.

1. Assess respiratory function and assure adequate vascular access (see Major Recommendations).
2. Avoid excessive volume resuscitation—give volume slowly and only as indicated with evidence of hypovolemia.
3. Inotrope support as needed—recommend dobutamine as first line (inotropic effect with less heart rate effect). Depending on circumstances, may consider other inotropes (e.g., milrinone for postoperative cardiac patients).
4. Obtain chest radiograph to evaluate heart size and lung fields.
5. Obtain electrocardiogram and echocardiogram.
6. Consider infectious or metabolic workups, as indicated.

7. Consider starting prostaglandin if a ductal-dependent cardiac malformation is suspected.
8. Once the underlying cause has been identified, tailor treatment to the specific etiology (e.g., antiarrhythmics for dysrhythmias, surgical correction for congenital heart defects).

Practice Option #5: ELBW

Please see Chapter 31 for management of hypotension in the ELBW population.

CLINICAL ALGORITHM(S)

Initial resuscitative efforts should prioritize respiratory support, obtaining vascular access, and promoting normothermia. Once you accomplish these tasks, treat the patient's shock in accordance with the most likely etiology.

IMPLEMENTATION OF GUIDELINE

DESCRIPTION OF IMPLEMENTATION STRATEGY

Due to the heterogeneity of neonatal shock, specific treatments will vary based on underlying cause and severity. Written guidelines for basic early management of neonatal shock (see Major Recommendations) are recommended.

QUALITY METRICS

Monitor rates of death, organ dysfunction/failure (renal, cardiac, liver), and length of stay.

SUMMARY

The management of neonatal shock depends on the stage of shock as well as the underlying cause. Treatment will focus on supportive care and restoring adequate perfusion. Critical points of treatment are maintaining respiratory support, ensuring vascular access, replacing fluid/blood losses, and providing vasopressor/steroid treatment as indicated.

BIBLIOGRAPHIC SOURCE(S)

Aschner JL, Poland RL. Sodium bicarbonate: basically useless therapy. *Pediatrics.* 2008;122:831-5.

Brierley J, Carcillo JA, Choong K, et al. Clinical practice parameters for hemodynamic support of pediatric and neonatal septic shock: 2007 update from the American College of Critical Care Medicine. *Crit Care Med.* 2009;37(2):666-88.

Cheung P, Barrington KJ. The effects of dopamine and epinephrine on hemodynamics and oxygen metabolism in hypoxic anesthetized piglets. *Crit Care.* 2001;5:158-66.

Ewer AK, Tyler W, Francis A, Drinkall D, Gardosi JO. Excessive volume expansion and neonatal death in preterm infants born at 27-28 weeks gestation. *Paediatr Perinat Epidemiol.* 2003;17:180-6.

Fernandez E, Scrader R, Watterberg K. Prevalence of low cortisol values in term and near-term infants with vasopressor-resistant hypotension. *J Perinatol.* 2005;25:114-8.

Jacobs SE, Berg M, Hunt R, et al. Cooling for newborns with hypoxic ischaemic encephalopathy (Review). *Cochrane Database Syst Rev.* 2007;(4):CD003311.

Leone TA, Finer NN. Shock: a common consequence of neonatal asphyxia. *J Pediatr.* 2011;158(2S):e9-12.

Lokesh L, Kumar P, Murki S, et al. A randomized controlled trial of sodium bicarbonate in neonatal resuscitation: effect on immediate outcome. *Resuscitation.* 2004;60(2):219-23.

Ng PC, Lee CH, Bnur FL, et al. A double-blinded, randomized, controlled study of a "stress dose" of hydrocortisone for rescue treatment of refractory hypotension in preterm infants. *Pediatrics.* 2006;117:367-75.

Noori S, Friedlich P, Wong P, et al. Hemodynamic changes after low-dosage hydrocortisone administration in vasopressor treated preterm and term neonates. *Pediatrics.* 2006;118:1456-66.

Robel-Tillig E, Knupfer M, Pulzer F, et al. Cardiovascular impact of dobutamine in neonates with myocardial dysfunction. *Early Hum Dev.* 2007;83(5):307-12.

Samiee-Zafarghandy S, Raman SR, van den Anker JN, et al. Best Pharmaceuticals for Children Act—Pediatric Trials Network Administrative Core Committee. Safety of milrinone use in neonatal intensive care units. *Early Hum Dev.* 2015;91(1):31-5.

Seri BL, Tan R, Evans J. Cardiovascular effects of hydrocortisone in preterm infants with pressor-resistant hypotension. *Pediatrics.* 2001;107:1070-4.

Patent Ductus Arteriosus

Andrew Z. Heling, MD • Sofia R. Aliaga, MD, MPH, FAAP

SCOPE

DISEASE/CONDITION(S)

Patent ductus arteriosus (PDA) in preterm neonates.

GUIDELINE OBJECTIVE(S)

Review morbidities associated with a PDA; review risk factors for developing a PDA; identify PDA treatment options and their potential side effects and complications; identify a PDA treatment algorithm for preterm neonates.

BRIEF BACKGROUND

The ductus arteriosus is a fetal blood vessel that connects the main pulmonary artery to the aorta. In utero, the ductus arteriosus shunts blood away from the lungs and to the systemic circulation. Postnatally, blood flow typically reverses across the ductus arteriosus due to decreasing pulmonary vascular resistance and increasing systemic vascular resistance. When the ductus arteriosus fails to close after birth it is referred to as a patent ductus arteriosus (PDA).

Factors which increase the risk of having a PDA include low gestational age, low birth weight, and sepsis, among others. Approximately 60% of neonates delivered at <28 weeks' gestation are diagnosed with a PDA, with decreased rates observed with increased gestational age. Spontaneous PDA closure is ultimately likely to occur for preterm neonates of all gestational ages but is more likely to occur, and typically occurs sooner, with increased gestational age.

A physical examination is the first step in identifying a PDA. Examination findings consistent with a PDA include a systolic heart murmur, widened pulse pressure, bounding peripheral pulses, and a hyperdynamic precordium. A neonate may present with clinical signs or conditions that cannot otherwise be explained, including hypotension, pulmonary hemorrhage, and/or renal insufficiency. When a PDA is clinically suspected, an echocardiogram should be obtained to confirm clinical suspicion and to screen for ductal-dependent congenital cardiac lesions. In the setting where an echocardiogram cannot be obtained, one must use clinical judgment to weigh the risks and benefits of clinical diagnosis with empiric management versus transferring the preterm neonate to a referral hospital where subspecialty care is available.

A PDA is associated with, but has not been proven to be causative of, increased mortality and morbidity including chronic lung disease (CLD)/bronchopulmonary dysplasia (BPD), intraventricular hemorrhage (IVH), and necrotizing enterocolitis (NEC). It is pathophysiologically plausible that a sufficiently "hemodynamically significant" PDA may result in cardiopulmonary compromise, hypotension, and renal insufficiency due to increased pulmonary circulation and decreased systemic perfusion. However, there is no universally accepted and validated classification of PDA severity that correlates echocardiographic features or laboratory findings with clinical signs. The provider must determine to what extent, if any, a PDA is contributing to end-organ hypoperfusion and/or compromise. A "hemodynamically significant PDA" in this chapter is defined as a PDA with substantial left-to-right shunting of blood. In general, a ductus arteriosus diameter ≥ 1.5 mm, a left atrium/aortic root diameter ratio of $\geq 1.5:1$, and reversed diastolic blood flow in the descending aorta and/or renal arteries indicate greater hemodynamic significance.

RECOMMENDATIONS

MAJOR RECOMMENDATIONS

A PDA diagnosed before day 7 of life is likely to close spontaneously without treatment, particularly for neonates born at >28 weeks' gestation and with a birth weight of >1000 g. Clinical suspicion of a PDA should routinely be confirmed via echocardiogram to both confirm diagnosis and exclude additional etiologies. A conservative approach to therapy (Figure 33.1) is generally recommended over an aggressive approach due to a high spontaneous closure rate and insufficient data to support PDAs are causative of mortality and many morbidities. When treatment is initiated, pharmacotherapy should be used prior to surgical or catheterization therapy unless there are contraindications for pharmacotherapy (Figure 33.2).

PRACTICE OPTIONS

Practice Option #1: Conservative Therapy

The goal of conservative therapy is to limit shunt volume across the PDA and/or improve PDA tolerance. Data to support treatment efficacy utilizing conservative therapy is minimal. The risks of implementing conservative therapy are fewer than those for implementing pharmacotherapy. Implementation of conservative therapy should be

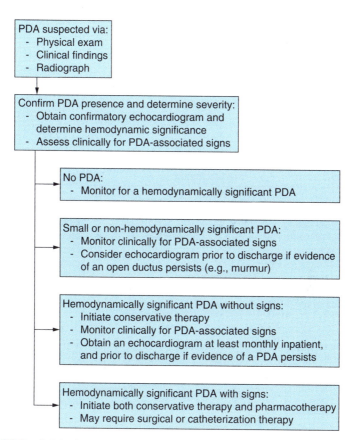

FIGURE 33.1 • Initial PDA workup and management algorithm for preterm neonates.

considered for any preterm neonate with a hemodynamically significant PDA. Conservative therapy consists of the following.

1. Modest fluid restriction. Maintain a maximum fluid intake of ≤130 mL/kg/day while maintaining hydration and optimizing caloric intake. In the setting of associated signs, such as renal insufficiency, fluid intake may need to be restricted further. Minimize energy expenditures by maintaining a neutral thermal environment.

2. Maintain a positive end-expiratory pressure (PEEP) that is at the higher limit of normal for the neonate's corrected age, if respiratory support is required. Maintain appropriate oxygenation and allow permissive hypercapnia.

3. Maintain the hematocrit ≥35%. Transfuse with packed red blood cells as needed.

4. For neonates with a hemodynamically significant PDA with worsening pulmonary overload and increased oxygenation and/or respiratory requirements, consider short courses of diuretic therapy. Administer hydrochlorothiazide (1–2 mg/kg/dose per os [PO] q12h) if a multiple-day course of diuretics is anticipated. Avoid furosemide as it may increase the risk of a PDA.

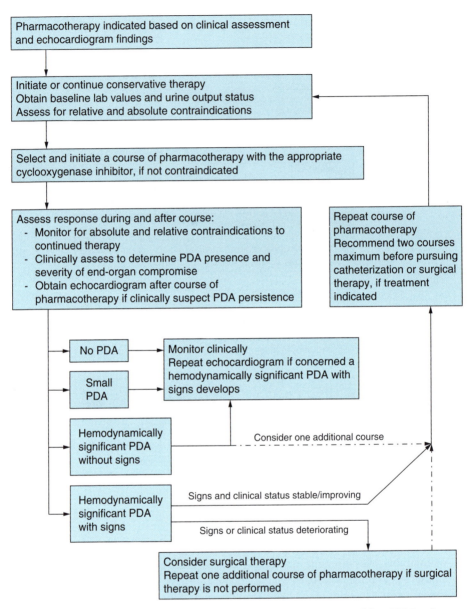

FIGURE 33.2 • Treatment algorithm for preterm neonates with a PDA when pharmacologic therapy is indicated.

Practice Option #2: Pharmacotherapy

The goal of pharmacotherapy is PDA closure. While neonates are likely to ultimately close their PDA without intervention, administration of particular pharmacologic medications make closure of the ductus more likely. Cyclooxygenase inhibitors, including ibuprofen and indomethacin, are acceptable pharmacotherapies to treat a

PDA. Acetaminophen is a promising alternative to cyclooxygenase inhibitors, but to date there are insufficient data to support its use. When pharmacotherapy is initiated:

1. Conservative therapy should be initiated or continued.
2. Low volume feedings (<20 mL/kg/day rate) should be considered while administering cyclooxygenase inhibitor therapy. Otherwise, feeds should be held at least 3 hours prior to the first dose and at least 6 hours after administering the last dose of cyclooxygenase inhibitor therapy. Administer the remainder of fluids and nutrition via total parental nutrition.
3. Obtain a baseline creatinine level and platelet count, determine urine output, and assess for active bleeding prior to initiating cyclooxygenase inhibitor therapy. A creatinine level of >1.8 mg/dL (or a level ≥200% from a previous trough level if previously obtained), a platelet count of <50,000/L, and urine output of ≤0.5 mL/kg/h are relative contraindications. Active bleeding and active or suspected NEC are contraindications. Concomitant or recent steroid exposure with cyclooxygenase inhibitor therapy is a contraindication due to increased risk for spontaneous intestinal perforation.
4. Select the appropriate cyclooxygenase inhibitor and administer as indicated. Ibuprofen and indomethacin are equally effective at closing a PDA. Both medications are most efficacious if used within the first week of postnatal life and have decreasing efficacy thereafter. Prophylactic use in selected patient populations has been shown to reduce the incidence of severe IVH but not reduce long-term neurodevelopmental impairment. Both medications have potential side effects including gastrointestinal bleeding, NEC, decreased platelet aggregation, oliguria, and renal insufficiency. Ibuprofen has a lower risk of NEC and renal insufficiency compared to indomethacin.
   a. Ibuprofen: In addition to side effects listed above, ibuprofen has additional potential side effects compared to indomethacin including hyperbilirubinemia and case reports of pulmonary hypertension. Each course of therapy consists of three doses of medication. The first dose of ibuprofen 10 mg/kg PO/IV is followed by two additional doses of ibuprofen 5 mg/kg PO/IV q24. Once a course is initiated, all three doses of medication should be administered per dosing recommendations unless contraindicated.
   b. Indomethacin: In addition to side effects listed above, indomethacin results in decreased mesenteric blood flow compared to ibuprofen. Each course of therapy consists of three doses of medication. The first dose of indomethacin 0.2 mg/kg IV/PO is to be followed by two additional doses of indomethacin 0.1–0.25 mg/kg IV/PO q12h–q24h, with dosing dependent on postnatal age. Intravenous administration should occur over 20–30 minutes. Once a course is initiated, all three doses of medication should be administered per dosing recommendations unless contraindicated.
5. Monitor for side effects throughout each course of medication, including:
   a. Oliguria: For the 24 hours following each dose of medication a urine output of ≤0.5 mL/kg/h is a relative contraindication to continuing cyclooxygenase inhibitor therapy. Urine output is expected to briefly drop following each dose of cyclooxygenase inhibitor but should promptly recover.
   b. Renal insufficiency: A creatinine level of >1.8 mg/dL or a level ≥200% from a previous trough level is a relative contraindication to continuing cyclooxygenase inhibitor therapy. Obtain daily creatinine levels while administering cyclooxygenase inhibitor therapy.

c. Bleeding: Active bleeding is a contraindication to continuing with pharmacotherapy. The platelet level needs only be checked prior to the initiation of each course of pharmacotherapy unless there is concern for bleeding and/or ongoing thrombocytopenia.

d. Spontaneous intestinal perforation and/or suspected or active NEC are contraindications to continuing pharmacotherapy.

6. Following each course of drug treatment, clinically assess for ductal closure and severity of end-organ compromise. Obtain a repeat echocardiogram if clinically uncertain of ductal patency, and then decide on the next course of action:

a. If the hemodynamically significant PDA closes, becomes small, or no longer has clinical consequences, monitor clinically for recurrence.

b. If the hemodynamically significant PDA persists but end-organ damage clinically resolves or is improving, consider conservative treatment or initiating an additional course of pharmacotherapy. Continue to monitor clinically for recurrence.

c. If the hemodynamically significant PDA persists and end-organ compromise is stable or is worsening, continue conservative therapy and/or initiate an additional course of pharmacotherapy. Cyclooxygenase inhibitors' effectiveness diminishes with increasing postnatal age, but late trials of pharmacotherapy may be considered, as some studies suggest pharmacotherapy efficacy may persist until 33–34 weeks postmenstrual age. While there are no limits to the total number of courses of pharmacotherapy that can administered, typically two courses are administered prior to performing surgical ligation if the hemodynamically significant PDA is persistent and end-organ compromise is not improving.

Practice Option #3: Surgical Ligation

The goal of surgical ligation is PDA closure. Surgical ligation is associated with worsened long-term outcomes and may result in significant short-term morbidities. Surgical ligation should be reserved for preterm neonates with a hemodynamically significant PDA with clinical signs who fail pharmacotherapy and are clinically worsening or are too clinically unstable for pharmacotherapy and who will likely die due to organ compromise secondary to the PDA. When surgical ligation is indicated:

1. Identify the appropriate procedure to be performed in consultation with the appropriate surgeons and specialists. Possible procedures include open thoracotomy and video-assisted thoracoscopic surgical (VATS) ligation. Procedure selection is dependent on procedure availability and patient characteristics. Open thoracotomy is the most commonly performed type of surgical PDA ligation. VATS ligation is less invasive, associated with fewer complications, and has a shorter healing time compared to open thoracotomy.

2. Provide routine postoperative care. Anticipate common potential complications and side effects, including cardiac and respiratory decompensation due to left ventricular systolic impairment. Hypotension is common postoperatively and is typically managed with vasopressors. Notably, surgical ligation carries considerable additional risks to the neonate including vocal cord paresis/paralysis, feeding difficulties, scoliosis, and an association with BPD and poor neurodevelopmental outcome.

Practice Option #4: Cardiac Catheterization

The goal of cardiac catheterization is PDA closure. Compared to surgical ligation, there are fewer and less severe complications associated with cardiac catheterization. This procedure should be considered for any neonate with a hemodynamically significant PDA with clinical signs who is large enough for the procedure. When cardiac catheterization is indicated:

1. Identify the appropriate procedure to be performed in consultation with the appropriate specialists. Possible procedures include coiling and occlusion devices. Procedure selection is dependent on procedure availability and patient characteristics. Transcatheter coiling is not effective in treating all PDAs, particularly those >2 mm in diameter or tubular in shape. Transcatheter occlusion devices have diminished efficacy, and increased side effects for neonates with a weight of <5 kg limits the availability for this patient population.
2. Provide routine postoperative care. Monitor for post-procedure bleeding and hematomas, and monitor extremity perfusion distal to the catheterization site.

CLINICAL ALGORITHM(S)

A society-sponsored treatment algorithm is not available, and consensus on treatment management does not exist. Figure 33.2 is a reasonable treatment algorithm to use when the provider determines pharmacologic therapy is indicated.

IMPLEMENTATION OF GUIDELINE

DESCRIPTION OF IMPLEMENTATION STRATEGY

Recommend written guidelines for PDA management; provide written materials for indications for treatment, contraindications to treatment, and potential side effects and complications of treatments.

QUALITY METRICS

Monitor for duration of and degree of respiratory support required, length of stay, and rates of CLD, IVH, NEC, ROP, hypotension, congestive heart failure, and renal insufficiency.

SUMMARY

A PDA is associated with, but has not been proven to be causative of, increased mortality and morbidity. A PDA has a higher incidence in preterm neonates with a lower gestational age and birth weight. Data increasingly supports treating only neonates who are symptomatic from their PDA and whose PDAs are unlikely to close spontaneously. Pharmacotherapy with cyclooxygenase inhibitors should be trialed prior to surgical therapy when treatment is indicated.

BIBLIOGRAPHIC SOURCE(S)

Benitz WE. Patent ductus arteriosus in preterm infants. *Pediatrics*. 2016;137:1-6.

Benitz WE. Patent ductus arteriosus: to treat or not to treat? *Arch Dis Child Fetal Neonatal Ed.* 2012;97:F80-2.

Benitz WE. Treatment of persistent patent ductus arteriosus in preterm infants: time to accept the null hypothesis? *J Perinatol*. 2010;30:241-52.

Bose CL, Laughon MM. Patent ductus arteriosus: lack of evidence for common treatments. *Arch Dis Child Fetal Neonatal Ed.* 2007;92:F498-502.

Clyman R, Cassady G, Kirklin JK, et al. The role of patent ductus arteriosus ligation in bronchopulmonary dysplasia: reexamining a randomized controlled trial. *J Pediatr.* 2009;154:873-6.

Clyman R, Wickremasinghe A, Jhaveri N, et al. Enteral feeding during indomethacin and ibuprofen treatment of a patent ductus arteriosus. *J Pediatr.* 2013;163:406–11.e4.

Clyman RI. The role of patent ductus arteriosus and its treatments in the development of bronchopulmonary dysplasia. *Semin Perinatol.* 2013;37:102-7.

Cordero L, Nankervis CA, DeLooze D, et al. Indomethacin prophylaxis or expectant treatment of patent ductus arteriosus in extremely low birth weight infants? *J Perinatol.* 2007;27:158-63.

Dang D, Wang D, Zhang C, et al. Comparison of oral paracetamol versus ibuprofen in premature infants with patent ductus arteriosus: a randomized controlled trial. *PloS ONE.* 2013;8:e77888.

Dani C, Bertini G, Corsini I, et al. The fate of ductus arteriosus in infants at 23–27 weeks of gestation: from spontaneous closure to ibuprofen resistance. *Acta Paediatr.* 2008;97:1176-80.

Dani C, Poggi C, Fontanelli G. Relationship between platelet count and volume and spontaneous and pharmacological closure of ductus arteriosus in preterm infants. *Am J Perinatol.* 2013;30:359-64.

Fowlie PW, Davis PG, McGuire W. Prophylactic intravenous indomethacin for preventing mortality and morbidity in preterm infants. *Cochrane Database Sys Rev.* 2010;7:CD000174.

Gokmen T, Erdeve O, Altug N, et al. Efficacy and safety of oral versus intravenous ibuprofen in very low birth weight preterm infants with patent ductus arteriosus. *J Pediatr.* 2011;158:549-54.

Hamrick SEG, Hansmann G. Patent ductus arteriosus of the preterm infant. *Pediatrics.* 2010;125:1020-30.

Jaillard S, Larrue B, Rakza T, et al. Consequences of delayed surgical closure of patent ductus arteriosus in very premature infants. *Ann Thorac Surg.* 2006;81:231-4.

Jensen EA, Dysart KC, Gantz MG, et al. Association between use of prophylactic indomethacin and the risk for bronchopulmonary dysplasia in extremely preterm infants. *J Pediatr.* 2017;186: 34-40.e2.

Johnston PG, Gillam-Krakauer M, Fuller MP, et al. Evidence-based use of indomethacin and ibuprofen in the neonatal intensive care unit. *Clin Perinatol.* 2012;39:111-36.

Kabra NS, Schmidt B, Roberts RS, et al. Neurosensory impairment after surgical closure of patent ductus arteriosus in extremely low birth weight infants: results from the trial of indomethacin prophylaxis in preterms. *J Pediatr.* 2007;150:229-34.

Kaempf JW, Wu YX, Kaempf AJ, et al. What happens when the patent ductus arteriosus is treated less aggressively in very low birth weight infants? *J Perinatol.* 2012;32:344-8.

Lee JH, Ro SK, Lee HJ, et al. Surgical ligation on significant patent ductus arteriosus in very low birth weight infants: comparison between early and late ligations. *Korean J Thorac Cardiovasc Surg.* 2014;47:444-50.

Malviya MN, Ohlsson A, Shah SS. Surgical versus medical treatment with cyclooxygenase inhibitors for symptomatic patent ductus arteriosus in preterm infants. *Cochrane Database Sys Rev.* 2013; 3:CD003951.

Mezu-Ndubuisi OJ, Agarwal G, Raghavan A, et al. Patent ductus arteriosus in premature neonates. *Drugs.* 2012;72:907-916.

Mosalli R, AlFaleh K. Prophylactic surgical ligation of patent ductus arteriosus for prevention of mortality and morbidity in extremely low birth weight infants. *Cochrane Database Sys Rev.* 2008;1:CD006181.

Naik-Mathuria B, Chang S, Fitch ME, et al. Patent ductus arteriosus ligation in neonates: preoperative predictors of poor postoperative outcomes. *J Pediatr Surg.* 2008;43:1100-5.

Nemerofsky SL, Parravicini E, Bateman D, et al. The ductus arteriosus rarely requires treatment in infants > 1000 grams. *Am J Perinatol.* 2008;25:661-6.

Ohlsson A, Walia R, Shah SS. Ibuprofen for the treatment of patent ductus arteriosus in preterm and/or low birth weight infants. *Cochrane Database Sys Rev.* 2013;4:CD003481.

Oncel MY, Yurttutan S, Erdeve O, et al. Oral paracetamol versus oral ibuprofen in the management of patent ductus arteriosus in preterm infants: a randomized controlled trial. *J Pediatr.* 2014;164:510-4.

Raval MV, Laughon MM, Bose CL, et al. Patent ductus arteriosus ligation in premature infants: who really benefits, and at what cost? *J Pediatr Surg.* 2007;42:69-75.

Sekar KC, Corff KE. Treatment of patent ductus arteriosus: indomethacin or ibuprofen? *J Perinatol.* 2008;28:S60-2.

Stephens BE, Gargus RA, Walden RV, et al. Fluid regimens in the first week of life may increase risk of patient ductus arteriosus in extremely low birth weight infants. *J Perinatol.* 2008;28:123-8.

Turck CJ, Marsh W, Stevenson JG, et al. Pharmacoeconomics of surgical interventions vs. cyclooxygenase inhibitors for the treatment of patent ductus arteriosus. *J Pediatr Pharmacol Ther.* 2007;12:183-93.

Vanhaesebrouck S, Zonnenberg I, Vandervoort P, et al. Conservative treatment for patent ductus arteriosus in the preterm. *Arch Dis Child Fetal Neonatal Ed.* 2007;92:F244-7.

Van Overmeire B, Smets K, Lecoutere D, et al. A comparison of ibuprofen and indomethacin for closure of patent ductus arteriosus. *N Engl J Med.* 2000;343:674-81.

Vida VL, Lago P, Salvatori S, et al. Is there an optimal timing for surgical ligation of patent ductus arteriosus in preterm infants? *Ann Thorac Surg.* 2009;87:1509-16.

Weisz DE, McNamara PJ. Patent ductus arteriosus ligation and adverse outcomes: causality or bias? *J Clin Neonatol.* 2014;3:67-75.

Blood Disorders

Anemia

Grant J. Shafer, MD, MA, FAAP • Vinayak Govande, MD, MS, MBA
• Gautham K. Suresh, MD, DM, MS, FAAP

SCOPE

DISEASE/CONDITION(S)

Neonatal anemia.

GUIDELINE OBJECTIVE(S)

Review the definition, risk factors, pathogenesis, clinical symptoms, diagnosis, outcomes, and clinical management of neonatal anemia.

BRIEF BACKGROUND

Neonatal anemia, a common condition in the neonatal intensive care unit (NICU) is defined as a hemoglobin (Hb) or hematocrit (Hct) concentration greater than two standard deviations below the mean for postnatal age and can be classified based on etiology into three categories: blood loss, inadequate red blood cell (RBC) production, and increased RBC destruction.

Blood loss due to significant bleeding can occur prior to, during, or after delivery. Fetomaternal hemorrhage is often small volume and clinically insignificant, but in severe cases can be catastrophic. External bleeding after delivery is usually obvious, but internal bleeding can be much more difficult to detect.

Inadequate RBC production is particularly common in the preterm neonate.

Erythropoiesis is in a constant state of evolution during the fetal and perinatal periods. Hb, Hct, and RBC counts vary throughout fetal life, and RBC indices and morphology at birth are different from pediatric or adult reference ranges. Compared to adult Hb, fetal Hb in the hypoxic fetal environment has a higher affinity for oxygen. As a newborn starts to breathe in the relatively high-oxygen environment at birth, Hb oxygen saturation increases rapidly. This induces a physiologic transition from fetal to adult Hb—which has a lower oxygen affinity—to facilitate increased delivery of Hb-bound oxygen to the tissues.

RBC production is stimulated by erythropoietin (EPO), which is downregulated by increased tissue oxygen delivery after birth. Erythropoiesis remains suppressed until tissue oxygen needs are greater than oxygen delivery. For term neonates, this nadir (Hb of 9.5–11 g/dL or Hct of 28.5–33%) is reached around 6–12 weeks of life, at which point EPO production increases and RBC production resumes. This is known as physiologic anemia of infancy.

For anemia of prematurity (AOP) in the preterm infant, this nadir is even more profound (typically ~Hb 8 g/dL or Hct 24% for infants 1000–1500 g and ~Hb 7 g/dL or Hct 21% for infants less than 100 g) and occurs earlier (4–8 weeks). One reason is the shorter lifespan—40–60 days—of RBCs in the premature neonate compared to 120 days in adults. In addition, EPO production in the preterm infant occurs in the liver, rather than the kidney, which is less responsive to anemia and hypoxia, leading to a blunted erythropoietic response. Finally, inadequate iron stores in the preterm infant further impair the ability of a preterm neonate to recover from anemia. Phlebotomy is a major iatrogenic contributor to AOP, and studies have demonstrated that phlebotomy volumes in the first 28 days of life represent up to 45% of total blood volume for preterm infants.

Increased RBC destruction (decreased RBC survival) is another important cause of neonatal anemia and can be caused by immune-mediated hemolysis (including allo-immune hemolytic anemia), non-immune hemolysis, hemoglobinopathies, erythrocyte membrane defects, and erythrocyte enzyme deficiencies (including glucose-6-phosphate dehydrogenase deficiency and pyruvate kinase deficiency).

Neonatal anemia leads to poor weight gain, tachycardia, greater supplemental oxygen requirement, or increased apnea or bradycardia. The clinical presentation is variable. Some term infants are relatively asymptomatic despite losing up to 33% of their circulating blood volume. Others manifest with shock—particularly with rapid and large-volume blood loss. Anemia is an independent risk factor for mortality in the neonate and has the potential to impair brain growth and development in both term and preterm infants.

RECOMMENDATIONS

MAJOR RECOMMENDATIONS

Management of neonatal anemia should aim to identify significant declines in Hb or Hct values early and restore them to sufficient levels to ensure adequate tissue oxygen delivery and support continued growth.

Diagnosis of neonatal anemia relies on Hb and Hct values adjusted for gestational age. There are currently no proven biomarkers that can predict which neonates will derive greater benefit than harm from treatment for anemia at various Hb or Hct levels. Therefore, clinical judgment is required in deciding about treatment.

When interpreting Hb and Hct values, the site where the blood was obtained should be considered, as capillary samples have a 5–10% higher Hb or Hct concentration than venous samples. This is due to sluggish circulation in the capillaries leading to transudation of plasma.

Identifying the etiology of neonatal anemia is essential to directing appropriate interventions. If the cause is high volume hemorrhage, emergent transfusion to re-expand the vascular space may be required. Occasionally, bleeding into internal organs may require surgical intervention. Congenital defects of the erythrocyte membranes or enzymes should prompt consultation with a pediatric hematologic specialist regarding further workup, management, and follow-up.

Anemia can be managed by expectant management, iron supplementation, or by RBC transfusion. The ideal threshold at which to transfuse remains elusive, despite multiple trials. Anemia can be prevented by alterations in clinical practices, while medications to prevent anemia are of less certain benefit.

PRACTICE OPTIONS

Practice Option #1: Investigation of Neonatal Anemia

History, physical examination, and a few laboratory tests should be sufficient to identify most causes for neonatal anemia.

History. A review of maternal history is important. Maternal Rh antigen status, treatment with Rh immune globulin if indicated, and ABO blood group status are important clues in mother's history. The clinician should also assess for a history of infections during pregnancy (such as parvovirus B19 infection) which might cause suppression of erythropoiesis in the neonate. Family history should be assessed for genetic diseases that cause anemia, and for a history of splenectomies.

Severe fetomaternal hemorrhage is a relatively rare (1 in 3000–10,000 births) but potentially life-threatening condition. Maternal history should be assessed for clues that the placental barrier may have been breached, including trauma during pregnancy, fetal interventions that breached the uterus, and velamentous cord insertion as well as history of maternal hemorrhage during pregnancy. Maternal history for many neonates with even severe fetomaternal hemorrhage may be normal.

Physical Examination. The physical examination is often normal, as neonates may not become symptomatic until 20–30% of total blood volume is lost. This is particularly true for chronic blood loss, which allows the patient time to compensate. Once this threshold is reached, however, patients will develop signs of shock such as tachycardia and hypotension. Masses in the abdomen may indicate bleeding into an internal organ such as the liver or adrenal gland (classically a flank mass with blueish hue). Anomalies of the thumb or radii, or café-au-lait spots are suggestive of Fanconi anemia.

Cranial bleeds may occur as a result of delivery—subarachnoid, subgaleal, or caput succedaneum—and the head should be examined for swelling, although enlargement may not occur until 72 hours after birth. If swelling is present, then serial head circumferences should be obtained. Subgaleal bleeds in particular can be life threatening, and every 1-cm increase in head circumference represents 38–40 mL of blood loss into the subgaleal space. Jaundice is another important clue, as significant jaundice with hyperbilirubinemia in a newborn with neonatal anemia suggests hemolysis, while the absence of jaundice with abrupt-onset signs or symptoms of anemia is more suggestive of internal bleeding.

Laboratory Studies. After the diagnosis of neonatal anemia is made, additional lab studies can help identify the etiology. The reticulocyte count indicates the bone marrow response to low RBC counts. Normal reticulocyte counts in a term infant at birth are ~5% and decrease to ~1% by 14 days of life. A decreased reticulocyte count in the setting of anemia should prompt consideration of a bone marrow deficiency, which may be infectious (e.g., due to parvo-19 virus), nutritional, or congenital (e.g., Diamond-Blackfan syndrome). Further workup, and in some cases a bone marrow biopsy, may be necessary in consultation with a pediatric hematologic specialist.

Immediately following an acute hemorrhage, the Hb and Hct are likely to be normal. This is because the RBC count and plasma volume are reduced proportionally. If rapid re-expansion of the intravascular space with fluid resuscitation occurs, then the Hb and Hct will drop as the vascular space is repleted. The reticulocyte count in these situations will be normal initially and may take several days to increase.

If fetomaternal hemorrhage is suspected, a Kleihauer-Betke count should be obtained on the mother's blood smear. An elevated reticulocyte count—particularly if accompanied by hyperbilirubinemia—is suggestive of increased RBC destruction, the commonest cause of which is hemolysis. Rh isoimmunization, ABO incompatibility, and minor blood group incompatibility are common causes of clinically significant hemolysis. If hemolysis is suspected, both the patient's and mother's Rh antigen status and ABO blood group should be obtained, followed by a direct antiglobulin test (DAT or Coombs) to evaluate for the presence of antibodies. A negative DAT does not completely exclude the presence of hemolytic disease, however, and an indirect antiglobulin test (IAT) should then be performed. Of note, for neonates with Rh-induced hemolysis who required intrauterine transfusions prior to delivery, the DAT is often negative but the IAT remains positive.

RBC indices can be helpful in identifying other causes of anemia. A low mean corpuscular volume (MCV) is suggestive of chronic fetal anemia or iron-deficiency anemia. A low MCV with a high mean corpuscular hemoglobin concentration (MCHC) should raise suspicion for hereditary spherocytosis. A review of the peripheral smear by a pathologist can reveal findings suggestive of congenital erythrocyte membrane (hereditary spherocytosis or elliptocytosis) or enzyme defects (glucose-6-phosphate dehydrogenase or pyruvate kinase deficiencies). Additional investigations for these congenital hematologic defects should be undertaken in consultation with a pediatric hematologic specialist.

Practice Option #2: Indications to Transfuse

The goal of RBC transfusion is to restore adequate oxygen delivery to the tissues. RBC transfusion inhibits native erythropoiesis and exposes the patient to the risks associated with RBC transfusions (e.g., infection, graft-versus-host disease, transfusion-associated lung injury, transfusion-associated circulatory overload, and reactions to the preservatives and anticoagulants used to store the RBCs).

When there is rapid, high-volume blood loss, the decision to transfuse is based on whether or not there are clinical signs of inadequate oxygen delivery (e.g., clinical cardiorespiratory distress or persistent lactic acidosis). For the acutely bleeding neonate with signs of instability, the intravascular volume should be restored with fluid resuscitation. This does not necessarily require RBC transfusion, however, as some infants will have adequate oxygen delivery following volume expansion with isotonic fluid, which can be administered more rapidly than RBCs. Indications for RBC transfusion in the setting of acute blood loss include greater than 20% blood loss, or 10–20% blood loss with evidence of ongoing inadequate oxygen delivery. External blood loss may be estimated by dividing the volume of blood loss (from difference in weight between blood-soaked and clean bandages, dressings, blankets, etc.) by the neonate's total blood volume (~85 mL/kg for term and 90 mL/kg for preterm infants, respectively). Internal blood loss is more difficult to quantify, although imaging may be helpful in select cases.

A special situation is a low Hb or Hct at delivery, which may represent either acute hemorrhage in the perinatal period or a chronic in utero process such a fetomaternal hemorrhage or twin-twin transfusion. Neonates with chronic hemorrhage while in utero may already have increased compensatory circulatory volume, and a simple transfusion may lead to heart failure. These neonates may instead require a partial exchange transfusion to improve oxygen-carrying capacity.

Similarly, many neonates with chronic anemia or AOP will require RBC transfusion. For example, up to 90% of extremely low birth weight (ELBW) infants (less than 1000 g) receive at least 1 RBC transfusion while in the NICU. However, while low versus high (an approximate Hct less than or greater than 40%, respectively) transfusion thresholds have been compared in multiple randomized control trials with the results pooled in meta-analyses, the optimal level at which to transfuse remains unclear.

An association between RBC transfusion and the development of necrotizing enterocolitis (NEC) has been noted in several observational studies, but a causal effect and methods of prevention have not been firmly established.

Selection and Administration of Transfusion Products. Once the decision to transfuse has been made, the clinician should ensure that the appropriate RBC product is chosen for the transfusion. NICU patients requiring RBC transfusion should receive leukoreduced, irradiated, and cytomegalovirus–safe RBC products if possible. Recent studies have not demonstrated a difference between RBC transfusions with fresh RBCs (within 7 days of donation) versus RBCs stored using standard blood bank practices. Often, an RBC unit can be split into multiple "satellite packs" for storage in the blood bank, which allows a neonate to receive multiple RBC transfusions while limiting exposure to the number of donors.

In emergency situations with life-threatening blood loss, particularly during resuscitation of the neonate in the delivery room, O-negative RBCs may be transfused.

Cord blood is sometimes used as a form of autologous blood donation. However, this capability is limited at most institutions. Similarly, family members may request to directly donate RBC products to a neonate, but the logistical issues and potential donation barriers limit the feasibility of direct donation in day-to-day practice.

Generally, RBC transfusions are given in 10–20 mL/kg aliquots and administered over several hours. Although some clinicians withhold enteral feeds during a packed RBC (PRBC) transfusion, it is uncertain whether this practice reduces the risk of transfusion-associated NEC, and it may have adverse nutritional consequences. If a specific rise in Hct is desired, the volume to transfuse can be calculated according to the formula:

$$\text{Volume to transfuse (mL)} = \text{weight (kg)} \times \text{blood volume per kg} \times [\text{desired Hct} - \text{observed Hct}]/\text{Hct of donor unit of RBCs}$$

Blood volume in the term newborn is ~85 mL/kg, and ~90 mL/kg in the preterm infant. The Hct of a standard donor unit RBCs is around 60%.

Practice Option #3: Strategies to Decrease Risk

There are multiple strategies to decrease the risk of neonatal anemia.

Delayed cord clamping (waiting 30–60 seconds after birth to clamp the umbilical cord) is supported by high-quality evidence and has been endorsed by both the

American Academy of Pediatrics and American College of Obstetricians and Gyne-cologists for both term and preterm neonates. For term infants, this practice increases the Hb and Hct and also improves iron stores for the first few months after birth. For preterm neonates, delayed cord clamping can decrease the need for blood transfusions and may reduce the risk of intraventricular hemorrhage. Polycythemia has been asso-ciated with delayed cord clamping, but this appears to be rare and without long-term consequences.

Umbilical cord milking—rapid transfer of umbilical cord blood to the neonate—as an alternative to delayed cord clamping is undergoing research and cannot be recom-mended at present.

While the current practice of neonatology requires serial lab monitoring, adherence to strict phlebotomy practices can reduce the volume of blood loss. This includes use of placental blood samples for admission laboratory studies, returning dead-space volume after sampling an arterial catheter, collection of the minimal blood volume requirements for lab draws, and recording the volume taken with each lab draw in the electronic med-ical record. Noninvasive and micro-sampling methods remain unproven and are not recommend for use in the NICU.

Preterm infants are at risk for iron-deficiency anemia, as their iron stores are often depleted by 2–3 months of age. All preterm infants receiving primarily breast-milk should receive iron supplementation for the first year of life. Term and preterm neonates receiving iron-containing formulas do not necessarily need additional iron supplementation.

As preterm neonates have impaired EPO production, the role of erythropoiesis-stimulating agents such as recombinant EPO have been widely studied. Both early and late (before and after 8 days of life, respectively) administration of recombinant EPO were analyzed in a recent Cochrane review. Early recombinant EPO reduced the risk of receiving one or more RBC transfusions but did not decrease exposure to total number of donors. Mortality was not decreased with questionable neuroprotective effect that was not well supported by evidence. Late recombinant EPO use showed minimal decrease in the number of RBC transfusions (by less than 1 RBC transfusion) and did not impact mortality or morbidity. Overall, there is not sufficient evidence to recommend routine recombinant EPO therapy for preterm neonates.

For premature infants whose parents decline RBC transfusion for religious reasons (e.g., Jehovah's Witnesses), use of EPO may be considered. Strict adherence to lab draw volumes and limitation of number of lab draws, however, is more likely to be successful in avoiding RBC transfusion in this population.

IMPLEMENTATION OF GUIDELINE

DESCRIPTION OF IMPLEMENTATION STRATEGY

All NICUs should develop standardized protocols for the volume of blood to collect for each lab study, as well as a system to record the volume taken with each lab draw. Units should work with their affiliated blood banks to determine which types of RBCs should be reserved for neonates, as well as methods to minimize exposure to multiple donors such as "satellite packs." Evidence-based institutional guidelines should be provided to the clinician with recommendations regarding at what Hb or Hct level to consider RBC transfusion, and how to best manage anemia in populations whose parents refuse RBC transfusions.

QUALITY METRICS

Potential metrics related to neonatal anemia are compliance, with unit guidelines for blood sampling practices, PRBC transfusion, and treatment with supplemental iron. Donor exposure can also be tracked.

SUMMARY

Neonatal anemia is a frequently-encountered problem in the NICU and is associated with increased mortality. The approach to neonatal anemia should consider the various etiologies of anemia in the term and preterm infant with thoughtful evaluation of a patient's clinical status prior to intervention. Expectant management or transfusion with RBCs are the mainstays of treatment, but the optimal transfusion threshold remains uncertain. Current evidence regarding therapy with erythropoiesis-stimulating agents is not sufficient to recommend their routine use.

BIBLIOGRAPHIC SOURCE(S)

Aher S, Malwatkar K, Kadam S. Neonatal anemia. *Semin Fetal Neonat Med.* 2008;13:239-47.

Aher SM, Ohlsson A. Early versus late erythropoietin for preventing red blood cell transfusion in preterm and/or low birth weight infants. *Cochrane Database Syst Rev.* 2012; 10:CD004865.

Andersen CC, Collins CL. Poor circulation, early brain injury, and the potential role of red cell transfusion in premature newborns. *Pediatrics.* 2006;117:1464.

Banerjee J, Aladangady N. Biomarkers to decide red blood cell transfusion in newborn infants. *Transfusion.* 2014;54:2574-82.

Calhoun D. Postnatal diagnosis and management of hemolytic disease of the fetus and newborn. In: Post TW, ed. Waltham, MA: UpToDate; 2018.

Colombatti R, Sainati L, Trevisanuto D. Anemia and transfusion in the neonate. *Semin Fetal Neonat Med.* 2016;21:2-9.

Dallman PR. Anemia of prematurity. *Ann Rev Med.* 1981;32:143.

Davis P, Herbert M, Davies DP, Jones ERV. Erythropoietin for anaemia in a preterm Jehovah's Witness baby. *Int J Gynecol Obstet.* 1992;39:366.

Del Vecchio A, Franco C, Petrillo F, D'Amato G. Neonatal transfusion practice: when do neonates need red blood cells or platelets? *Am J Perinatol.* 2016;33:1079-84.

Garcia-Prats J. Anemia of prematurity. In: Post TW, ed. Waltham, MA: UpToDate; 2017.

Hay S, Zupancic JA, Flannery DD, Kirpalani H, Dukhovny D. Should we believe in transfusion-associated enterocolitis? Applying a GRADE to the literature. *Semin Perinatol.* 2017;41:80-91.

Juul S. Erythropoiesis and the approach to anemia in premature infants. *J Matern Fetal Neonat Med.* 2012;25:97-9.

Kirpalani H, Whyte RK, Andersen C, et al. The premature infants in need of transfusion (pint) study: a randomized, controlled trial of a restrictive (LOW) versus liberal (HIGH) transfusion threshold for extremely low birth weight infants. *J Pediatr.* 2006;149:301-7.e3.

Kirpalani H, Zupancic JA. Do transfusions cause necrotizing enterocolitis? The complementary role of randomized trials and observational studies. *Semin Perinatol.* 2012;36:269-76.

Maier JT, Schalinski E, Schneider W, Gottschalk U, Hellmeyer L. Fetomaternal hemorrhage (FMH), an update: review of literature and an illustrative case. *Arch Gynecol Obstet*. 2015; 292:595-602.

Mohamed A, Shah PS. Transfusion associated necrotizing enterocolitis: a meta-analysis of observational data. *Pediatrics*. 2012;129:529.

Ohis R. Red blood cell transfusions in the newborn. In: Post TW, ed. Waltham, MA: UpToDate; 2018.

Ohlsson A, Aher SM. Early erythropoietin for preventing red blood cell transfusion in preterm and/or low birth weight infants. *Cochrane Database Syst Rev*. 2014:CD004863.

Strauss RG. Anaemia of prematurity: Pathophysiology and treatment. *Blood Rev*. 2010;24:221-5.

Bleeding Disorders and Thrombosis in Neonates

Renee M. Madden, MS, MD • Michael D. Tarantino, MD

SCOPE

DISEASE/CONDITION(S)

Disseminated intravascular coagulation (DIC).

GUIDELINE OBJECTIVE(S)

Identification of DIC and distinguish DIC from other bleeding disorders, laboratory analysis, and blood product support.

BRIEF BACKGROUND

Disseminated intravascular coagulation is an acquired bleeding diathesis. It is observed as a secondary event due to an underlying severe primary disease such as neonatal sepsis, trauma, asphyxia, blood product transfusion reactions, and respiratory distress. The ill neonate appears to be at particularly high risk of coagulopathy, due to quantitatively low plasma levels of procoagulant and anticoagulant factors at birth. Infection, asphyxia, or trauma can result in rapid depletion of these plasma factors, particularly in the ill preterm infant.

Although neonatal hemostasis is finely balanced in the healthy newborn, due to physiologically low neonatal procoagulant, anticoagulant, and fibrinolytic levels, exogenous events such as infection can readily disrupt this finely balanced system with a resultant hemorrhagic or thrombotic state in the ill neonate. In the healthy newborn, most of the

TABLE 35.1. Neonatal Laboratory Changes Associated with Bleeding Disorders

Disorder	Platelet Count	PT/INR	aPTT	Fibrinogen
DIC	Decreased	Increased	Increased	Decreased
HDN	Normal	Increased	Normal	Normal
Liver coagulopathy	Normal/ Decreased	Increased	Increased	Normal/ Decreased
Hemophilia A or B	Normal	Normal	Increased	Normal
NAIT	Decreased	Normal	Normal	Normal

DIC, disseminated intravascular coagulation; HDN, hemolytic disease of the newborn; NAIT, neonatal alloimmune thrombocytopenia.

procoagulant factors (vitamin K factors, contact factors) reach adult levels by 6 months of age. Similar findings are noted for several anticoagulants (antithrombin III, heparin cofactor II, and protein C and protein S).

DIC is characterized by coagulation activation, fibrin deposition, and microangiopathic thrombi, resulting in secondary fibrinolysis. Due to the varied clinical spectrums observed in neonatal DIC, the differential diagnosis of a bleeding neonate may be difficult to establish, and additional laboratory studies characterizing the activation of coagulation and fibrinolysis may or may not aid in the diagnosis. Newborn laboratory analysis must be based on neonatal age–corrected ranges. Laboratory analysis in neonatal DIC includes a decreased platelet count, prolonged PT/INR, aPTT, and decreased fibrinogen (Table 35.1). Fibrinogen depletion is associated with increased bleeding. Peripheral blood smear findings are often notable for schistocytes, due to the underlying microangiopathic changes. Typical confirmatory laboratory tests for DIC (i.e., D-dimer) in the newborn are generally unreliable due to a lack of specificity from altered plasma clearance.

Abnormal bleeding, thrombotic complications, or hemorrhage can be observed in the ill neonate with DIC. In contrast, abnormal bleeding in an otherwise healthy infant is more concerning for a congenital hemorrhagic disorder. The clinical spectrum of DIC may vary from mild clinical symptoms and coagulopathy to a fulminant thrombohemorrhagic state. Abnormal bleeding from central and peripheral line sites, catheterized sites, skin, and/or mucosal surfaces may be observed. The DIC state in the critically ill newborn may exacerbate areas of recent hemorrhage (intracranial or intraventricular hemorrhage). Vigilant monitoring and judicious replacement of the consumed and degraded blood elements aids in bleeding management; however, treatment of the primary disease process is of paramount importance in the management of DIC.

RECOMMENDATIONS

MAJOR RECOMMENDATIONS

Most important in the treatment for DIC is to treat the primary cause inciting the DIC state. Management of DIC bleeding is based on clinical symptoms and laboratory results. Laboratory results must be reported based on neonatal reference ranges. Blood products used to replete consumed and degraded hemostatic proteins should be prescribed with caution. Consultation with a pediatric hematologist is strongly recommended for management of DIC.

PRACTICE OPTIONS

Practice Option #1

- Severe, life-threatening bleeding requires maintaining adequate blood volumes (see Chapter 32). With any abnormal bleeding, obtain STAT screening coagulation studies with CBC, PT/INR, aPTT, and fibrinogen. Coagulation studies should optimally be obtained from a nonheparinized central or peripheral access line or from direct venipuncture. Normal coagulation study results in the setting of bleeding warrant repeating, since initial normal findings do not exclude activation of coagulation in the ill newborn.
- In the presence of bleeding with laboratory confirmation of DIC, replacement with fresh frozen plasma (FFP) at 10–15 mL/kg facilitates replacement of the consumed and degraded procoagulant factors, protein C and S and antithrombin.
- Some repletion of fibrinogen will occur with FFP; however, cryoprecipitate contains higher concentrations of fibrinogen along with factor VIII, factor XIII, and von Willebrand factor. For hypofibrinogenemia, cautious replacement with cryoprecipitate at 5–10 mL/kg is often useful (with concomitant monitoring for thrombosis).
- With active bleeding, maintain the platelet count >50,000/μL, with platelet transfusions at 10–15 mL/kg. For intracranial hemorrhage (ICH) or intraventricular hemorrhage (IVH), consider maintaining a platelet count >100,000/μL.
- Imaging with head ultrasound is recommended in the term and particularly in the preterm infant with abnormal bleeding.

Practice Option #2

Rarely is concomitant anticoagulation needed in the neonate during periods of blood product replacement. For overt thrombotic DIC, if anticoagulation is necessary, the cautious use of unfractionated low dose heparin should be considered.

CLINICAL ALGORITHM(S)

STAT labs: CBC, PT/INR, aPTT, fibrinogen

Bleeding in an ill-appearing neonate → Head ultrasound

Blood product replacement

IMPLEMENTATION OF GUIDELINE

QUALIFYING STATEMENTS

1. There are no recent prospective randomized clinical trials (RCT) for DIC in neonates.
2. Study of developmental hemostasis on healthy preterm infants at 30–36 weeks' gestation by Andrew et al (1988). Current NICU preterm population is <30 weeks' gestation and often ill, limiting the establishment of a normal range for this population.

DESCRIPTION OF IMPLEMENTATION STRATEGY

Recommend each NICU implement standard-of-care guidelines for replacement of each blood product component. Recommend NICU standard-of-care guidelines for blood product replacement be based on laboratory results and clinical findings. Recommend all NICU laboratory-reported results be based on neonatal standard ranges. In addition, recommend all blood products be CMV-negative and cellular blood products to be irradiated and leuko-poor filtered.

QUALITY METRICS

Monitor for improvement in clinical findings: improvement in bleeding and hemorrhage-associated morbidity or mortality. Monitor for improvement in laboratory coagulopathy testing parameters.

SCOPE

DISEASE/CONDITION(S)

Hemorrhagic disease of the newborn (HDN).

GUIDELINE OBJECTIVE(S)

Identification of HDN (three classifications of HDN) noted with vitamin K deficiency in infancy, and management and supportive care for neonates with HDN.

BRIEF BACKGROUND

HDN is caused by a vitamin K deficiency in the neonate and is also referred to as vitamin K deficiency bleeding (VKDB) in infancy. Infants are at increased risk for hemorrhage due to vitamin K deficiency secondary to endogenously low levels of almost all of vitamin K–dependent procoagulant proteins at birth (factors II, VII, IX, X), resulting in PT prolongation (Table 35.1). In addition, contributing to low infant levels of vitamin K is the poor transfer of maternal vitamin K across the placenta, the low breast milk content of vitamin K, and the lack of endogenous lower gastrointestinal bacteria in the infant at birth. HDN is an acquired bleeding diatheses and is classified into three forms—early, classic, and late HDN, based on onset of bleeding symptoms and localization of bleeding (Table 35.2).

The onset of **early HDN** is within the first 24 hours of life and is usually due to maternal medications during pregnancy (anticonvulsants, warfarin, antimicrobials). These medications are thought to cross the placenta and interfere with newborn vitamin K activity. Infants with early HDN can present with cephalohematomas, excessive scalp bleeding to due scalp monitor, bleeding from the umbilicus, ICH, and gastrointestinal (GI) or intra-abdominal bleeding. Recognizing and adjusting the offending maternal medication in the weeks prior to delivery or additional oral vitamin K replacement (for at least 2 weeks prior to delivery) has been shown to reduce incidence of early HDN.

Classic HDN is noted to occur 1–7 days after delivery is attributed to lack of vitamin K prophylaxis at birth. Infants can present with ICH, GI bleeding, bleeding at the umbilical stump, epistaxis, prolonged bleeding at injection sites, and additionally, male infants can present with prolonged bleeding after circumcision. Unexpected bleeding was noted to occur in up to 1.5% of healthy newborns within the first 7 days of life prior to routine vitamin K prophylaxis.

Late HDN can present 2 weeks to 6 months after birth. The vitamin K deficiency is secondary to other causes that compromise the ongoing vitamin K supply in the neonate.

TABLE 35.2. Clinical Presentation and Management of Hemolytic Disease of the Newborn

HDN Classification	Age	Sites of Bleeding	Management
Early HDN	0–24 hours	Scalp monitor, cephalohematoma, ICH, umbilicus, gastrointestinal, intra-abdominal	Discontinue or substitute interfering maternal medications or maternal vitamin K prophylaxis for several weeks prior to delivery
Classic HDN	1–7 days	ICH, umbilicus, gastrointestinal, circumcision, injection sites, mucosa	Newborn vitamin K prophylaxis
Late HDN	2 weeks– 6 months	ICH, intrathoracic, gastrointestinal, genitourinary, injection sites, skin, mucosa	Additional IM or enteral vitamin K

Adapted from Sutor A, von Kries R, Marlies, Cornelissen EAM, McNinch AW, Andrew M. Vitamin K deficiency bleeding (VKDB) in infancy. ISTH Pediatric/Perinatal Subcommittee. International Society on Thrombosis and Haemostasis. *Thromb Haemost.* 1999;81:456.

These causes include malabsorption syndromes, diarrhea, cystic fibrosis, α_1-antitrypsin deficiency, and hepatitis. ICH is noted in >50% of patients (subdural hemorrhage noted more frequently in term infants); bleeding from the GI tract, skin, or mucosal surfaces are noted to occur. Often additional oral or intramuscular (IM) vitamin K is needed.

RECOMMENDATIONS

MAJOR RECOMMENDATIONS

Infants should be treated if vitamin K deficiency is suspected (while awaiting laboratory results). Management of bleeding in HDN is based on symptoms and laboratory results.

PRACTICE OPTIONS

Practice Option #1

- Severe, life-threatening bleeding requires maintaining adequate blood volumes (see Chapter 32). Obtain STAT screening coagulation laboratory studies with CBC, PT/INR, aPTT, and fibrinogen. Coagulation studies should optimally be obtained from nonheparinized line. Normal coagulation studies warrant repeating in the setting of bleeding, since initial normal findings do not exclude activation of coagulation in the ill newborn.
- Imaging by ultrasonography of the head is recommended in the term and particularly in the preterm infant with abnormal bleeding.
- Vitamin K deficiency is confirmed by specific testing for coagulation factors II, VII, IX, and X, or PIVKA testing (proteins induced by vitamin K agonists).

- In the presence of bleeding, replacement with FFP at 10–20 mL/kg facilitates replacement of the procoagulant vitamin K–dependent factors, and protein C and protein S.
- **Early HDN:** FFP for neonatal bleeding. Vitamin K should be administered IM, or if actively bleeding give IV (slow administration due to association with anaphylactoid reaction ± test dose of vitamin K) or subcutaneously. Consider genetics consult for radiographic or phenotypic abnormalities due to vitamin K deficiency embryopathy. Re-evaluate need for additional maternal vitamin K for future pregnancies.
- **Classic HDN:** FFP for neonatal bleeding. Vitamin K should be administered IM or if actively bleeding give IV (slow administration due to association with anaphylactoid reaction ± test dose of vitamin K) or subcutaneously.
- **Late HDN:** FFP for neonatal bleeding. Additional oral vitamin K prophylaxis. If poor enteral vitamin K absorption, then IM or subcutaneously or IV (if actively bleeding, slow administration due to association with anaphylactoid reaction ± test dose of vitamin K) or subcutaneously.

Practice Option #2

In the presence of an isolated prolonged PT, also obtain hepatic function panel (AST, ALT, bilirubin) to evaluate for potential liver disorder. Early liver disease may result in initial isolated prolongation of PT. In addition, cholestasis with obstructive biliary tract disease may result in vitamin K deficiency due to impaired vitamin absorption.

CLINICAL ALGORITHM(S)

See prior algorithm for disseminated intravascular coagulation.

IMPLEMENTATION OF GUIDELINE

QUALIFYING STATEMENTS

Administer Vitamin K to all newborns as a single IM dose. Consultation with a pediatric hematologist is recommended to further evaluate the etiology of a bleeding diathesis in infancy.

DESCRIPTION OF IMPLEMENTATION STRATEGY

See prior recommendations.

QUALITY METRICS

See prior recommendations.

SCOPE

DISEASE/CONDITION(S)

Hemophilia A and hemophilia B.

GUIDELINE OBJECTIVE(S)

Identification, management, and blood product support guidelines for neonates with hemophilia A and B.

BRIEF BACKGROUND

Hemophilia is the most common inherited protein deficiency causing bleeding. The average incidence in the United States is estimated to be approximately 1 in 5000 live male births, with hemophilia A noted to be approximately 4–5 times more common than hemophilia B. Mutations or deletions in the genes synthesizing these specific coagulation proteins result in reduced or absent factor VIII or IX levels and can result in hemorrhagic symptoms in the neonatal period. Approximately 30% of newly diagnosed persons with hemophilia have no family history of hemophilia and it occurs due to a spontaneous mutation in the gene.

Hemophilia A is due to a deficiency in coagulation protein factor VIII (FVIII) and inherited in an X-linked recessive manner. The severity of disease is related to the degree of FVIII deficiency. Patients are considered to have mild hemophilia A with FVIII activity levels ranging from 6–49%, moderate hemophilia A patients have FVIII activity levels ranging from 1–5%, and patients with severe hemophilia A are noted to have FVIII activity levels of <1%. Approximately 60% of individuals with hemophilia A have severe disease. Males with severe hemophilia A usually present in the first year of life and may present at birth with ICH (1–4%) or prolonged bleeding after circumcision (50%) or phlebotomy.

Hemophilia B is an X-linked bleeding disorder, due to a hereditary deficiency of factor IX. The clinical presentation of neonates with hemophilia B is phenotypically similar to that observed in the neonatal period in males with hemophilia A. Severity of this bleeding disorder also correlates with the factor IX activity levels (mild: 6–49% activity level, moderate: 1–5% activity level, severe: <1% activity level). Identification of the specific missing factor is crucial to guiding treatment.

Coagulation laboratory studies for hemophilia A or B are notable for a prolonged aPTT, and normal PT/INR, platelet count, and fibrinogen (Table 35.1). Due to the prolongation of the aPTT, additional laboratory analysis with aPTT mixing studies would demonstrate a correction of the aPTT, supporting a plasma factor deficiency. Specific testing for FVIII or factor IX activity is needed to diagnose and distinguish between these bleeding disorders. Recommended treatment for bleeding episodes requires specific FVIII or factor IX replacement, with the goal to replace the missing factor and achieve normal hemostasis.

RECOMMENDATIONS

MAJOR RECOMMENDATIONS

Availability of factor VIII or factor IX concentrates vary from hospital to hospital. In addition, factor concentrate treatment may be thrombophilic and guidelines for dosing of factor IX products varies based on product type. We, therefore, recommend contact with the nearest hemophilia treatment center (HTC) for management guidelines prior to administration of either factor VIII or IX concentrates.

PRACTICE OPTIONS

Practice Option #1

- Consideration to cesarean delivery if: 1) the mother is a known carrier of hemophilia, 2) there is any morphometric disproportion that would predict a physically difficult delivery. No use of forceps or vacuum at delivery (both vaginal or cesarean delivery). STAT cord blood testing for factor VIII or factor IX activity and aPTT.

- Severe, life-threatening bleeding requires maintaining adequate blood volumes (see Chapter 32).
- Hemophilia A: Recombinant or high potency plasma-derived FVIII concentrate to raise factor VIII activity to 100%. Although FVIII is recovered in the cryoprecipitate fraction of blood and is often readily available for emergent bleeding episodes, preference is given to recombinant FVIII products (virtually no risk of blood born pathogen transmission) replacement in neonates with hemophilia A.
  - Factor VIII concentrate 50–80 U/kg as bolus for severe bleeding
  - Factor VIII concentrate at 25–50 U/kg every 8–12 hours based on factor VIII activity monitoring.
- Hemophilia B: Recombinant FIX or high purity plasma-derived FIX concentrate to raise factor IX activity to at least 100%. Although fresh frozen plasma is a source of factor IX, preference is for recombinant FIX replacement products; if emergent bleeding and no factor IX concentrate is available, replacement with FFP at 10–20 mL/kg.
  - Factor IX concentrate 100–120 U/kg as bolus for severe bleeding.
  - Factor IX concentrate at 20–40 U/kg every 12–24 hours based on factor VIII activity monitoring.

Practice Option #2

On occasion, additional von Willebrand testing may be needed to differentiate specific von Willebrand disease (type 2 Normandy variant) from patients with hemophilia A.

Practice Option #3

We strongly advocate that all neonates with hemophilia be referred to the nearest HTC soon after birth.

CLINICAL ALGORITHM(S)

See algorithm for disseminated intravascular coagulation.

IMPLEMENTATION OF GUIDELINE

QUALIFYING STATEMENTS

Contact with the nearest HTC is strongly recommended for guidelines prior to administration of either factor VIII or IX concentrates. Ideally, the delivery of a male infant to a mother known to carry the hemophilia gene mutation should be planned in consultation with a comprehensive HTC and pediatric hematologist. In addition, we strongly advocate that all neonates with hemophilia be referred to the nearest HTC soon after birth.

DESCRIPTION OF IMPLEMENTATION STRATEGY

See prior recommendations.

QUALITY METRICS

See prior recommendations.

SCOPE

DISEASE/CONDITION(S)

Liver disease coagulopathy.

GUIDELINE OBJECTIVE(S)

Identification, management, and supportive care for the neonate with coagulopathy-associated with liver disease.

BRIEF BACKGROUND

Newborn liver disease resulting in impaired hepatic synthetic function can result in significant coagulopathy. Neonatal liver diseases may be due to shock, viral hepatitis, disorders of cholestasis, or genetic or metabolic disorders. The diminished hepatic synthesis of procoagulants (factors II, V, VII, IX, X, XI, XII, and fibrinogen) and fibrinolytic proteins (plasminogen, tissue plasminogen activator, α_2-antiplasmin) due to liver disease, coupled with the endogenously low hemostatic proteins noted at birth, can result in significant bleeding. In addition, a secondary effect in neonatal liver coagulopathy is noted to be thrombocytopenia (Table 35.1), which may be attributed to hypersplenism and platelet sequestration, altered thrombopoietin production by the liver, immune-mediated. Infants with clinical bleeding require blood transfusion support with FFP and may also need additional blood product support (cryoprecipitate and/or platelets).

RECOMMENDATIONS

MAJOR RECOMMENDATIONS

Therapeutic success relies on recovery of hepatic function.

PRACTICE OPTION

Practice Option #1

- Severe, life-threatening bleeding requires maintaining adequate blood volumes (see Chapter 32). Obtain STAT laboratory screening coagulation studies with CBC, PT/INR, aPTT, and fibrinogen. Coagulation studies should optimally be obtained from nonheparinized line. Normal coagulation studies warrant repeating in the setting of bleeding, since initial normal findings do not exclude activation of coagulation in the ill newborn.
- Imaging with ultrasonography of the head is recommended in the term and particularly in the preterm infant with abnormal bleeding.
- In the presence of bleeding, replacement with FFP at 10–15 mL/kg facilitates replacement of the procoagulant factors.
- For hypofibrinogenemia, cautious replacement with cryoprecipitate at 5–10 mL/kg (with concomitant monitoring for thrombosis).
- With active bleeding, maintain the platelet count >50,000/μL, with platelet transfusions at 10–15 mL/kg. For ongoing ICH or IVH, consider maintaining a platelet count >100,000/μL.
- Additional administration of vitamin K (oral, IM, or subcutaneous) may be considered due to intestinal malabsorption and secondary vitamin K deficiency.

CLINICAL ALGORITHM(S)

See algorithm for disseminated intravascular coagulation.

IMPLEMENTATION OF GUIDELINE

QUALIFYING STATEMENTS

Consider pediatric gastrointestinal/hepatology consult; the therapeutic outcome of liver coagulopathy is heavily dependent upon liver function recovery and accurate diagnosis of etiology of newborn liver disease.

DESCRIPTION OF IMPLEMENTATION STRATEGY

See prior recommendations.

QUALITY METRICS

See prior recommendations.

SCOPE

DISEASE/CONDITION(S)

Neonatal alloimmune thrombocytopenia (NAIT).

GUIDELINE OBJECTIVE(S)

Identification, management, and supportive care for neonates with neonatal alloimmune thrombocytopenia.

BRIEF BACKGROUND

NAIT is noted to be the most common cause of immune-mediated thrombocytopenia. The incidence in Caucasians is 1 in 1000–2000 births. NAIT is to be considered in the well-appearing infant presenting with petechiae and bruising. It is the most common cause of ICH in full-term infants (10–20% of infants with symptoms). NAIT is a transient thrombocytopenia and noted to resolve in 2 weeks to several months.

Considered the platelet equivalent of Rh-mediated hemolytic disease of the newborn, NAIT is due to maternal alloantibodies in response to fetal antigens (fetal platelet antigens are paternally inherited and lacking in the mother). Not all cases of maternal alloantibody production result in neonatal thrombocytopenia. The most common alloantigen involved is HPA-1a (human platelet antigen 1a), the platelet alloantigen previously known as PL^{A1}. To date, HPA-1, -2, -3, -5, and -15 are noted in >95% of NAIT cases in Caucasians and HPA-4b, -6b, and -21b are noted to be more common in Asian populations.

RECOMMENDATIONS

MAJOR RECOMMENDATIONS

NAIT can be seen in first pregnancy (40–50%), and risk of NAIT is noted to increase with subsequent pregnancies (80–90%). Close monitoring of maternal HPA antibody titers with subsequent pregnancies is recommended, with intervention of maternal administration of IVIg and/or prednisone during subsequent pregnancies when indicated.

PRACTICE OPTIONS

Practice Option #1

- Severe, life-threatening bleeding requires maintaining adequate blood volumes (see Chapter 32).
- Imaging with ultrasonography of the head is recommended in the term and particularly in the preterm infant with abnormal bleeding.
- IVIg at 1 g/kg/day for 1–2 consecutive days is given (alternatively 0.4 g/kg/day may be given over a 5-day course).
- Methylprednisolone at 1 mg/kg/day given prior to each dose of the 1- to 2-day course of IVIg (or 1 mg methylprednisolone IV every 8 hours with IVIg).
- Transfusion with platelets at 10–15 mL/kg, for bleeding or for platelet count <30,000/µL.
- Transfuse with HPA-1a negative platelets if available, otherwise random donor platelets may be used, but with less and less durable platelet count recovery. Maternal washed platelets may be collected and transfused if bleeding and refractory to random donor or HPA1a negative transfusions.

Practice Option #2

NAIT is a transient thrombocytopenia and resolution is observed as the inciting maternal antibody is cleared from the neonate, usually over the course of one to several weeks.

CLINICAL ALGORITHM(S)

See algorithm for disseminated intravascular coagulation.

IMPLEMENTATION OF GUIDELINE

QUALIFYING STATEMENTS

NAIT is to be considered for thrombocytopenia not caused by infection, DIC, liver disease, congenital thrombocytopenia, or maternal immune-mediated autoimmune thrombocytopenia.

DESCRIPTION OF IMPLEMENTATION STRATEGY

See prior recommendations.

QUALITY METRICS

See prior recommendations.

SUMMARY FOR NEONATAL BLEEDING DISORDERS

The neonatal hemostatic system is a uniquely balanced system and differs quantitatively and qualitatively from the adult hemostatic system. Age-related physiologic changes occur in the hemostatic system from neonate to child to adult, and these differences often prevent direct comparison of newborn laboratory results based on the adult normal reference range. In the newborn, it is important to differentiate congenital bleeding disorders from acquired conditions and we strongly recommend involvement of a pediatric hematologist(s) to aid in diagnosis, management, and follow-up of the affected newborn.

SCOPE

DISEASE/CONDITION(S)

Venous thrombosis.

GUIDELINE OBJECTIVE(S)

Identification and management guidelines for venous thrombosis in the neonate.

BRIEF BACKGROUND

Neonatal venous thrombosis is an infrequent isolated occurrence. More often venous thrombosis is a secondary thrombotic event in critically ill infants, associated with sepsis, asphyxia, indwelling catheters, or congenital cardiac disease. Homozygous prothrombotic disorders are rare, and in infants with two of the congenital homozygous disorders (protein C and protein S deficiency), identification early in the newborn period is of paramount importance. In contrast, neonates with heterozygous prothrombotic disorders are not routinely diagnosed in the newborn period unless thrombosis develops as a secondary event.

Nevertheless, neonates may be at greater risk for thrombotic events due to decreased levels of endogenous anticoagulants (protein C and S, antithrombin III), excess procoagulant activity from factor V Leiden, prothrombin G20210A, hyperhomocysteinemia, and due to use of intravascular lines in small caliber vessels. In a prospective German survey, the reported incidence of symptomatic thrombosis (venous or arterial thrombus) was 5.1 per 100,000 live births with venous thrombosis making up approximately three quarters of these thrombotic events. An early report from Schmidt and Andrew in 1995 noted catheter-related venous thrombosis in 89% of neonates, after excluding infants with renal vein thrombosis.

Catheter-related venous thrombosis may be associated with limb edema, pain, and/or skin color changes (hyperemic to cyanotic in color). Use of umbilical venous catheters (UVCs) has been associated with portal vein thrombosis, and infants may have signs of hepatomegaly, splenomegaly, and liver dysfunction. Thrombosis of the inferior vena cava (IVC) has also been associated with use of UVCs, and lower limb swelling and signs of renal vein obstruction may also be noted. Often noninvasive methodology with Doppler ultrasound imaging is sufficient to confirm thrombotic affected vasculature (Table 35.3). Prompt central line removal after short-term use often minimizes thrombotic risk.

TABLE 35.3. **Neonatal Thrombus Imaging Modality**

Vasculature	Thrombus Location	Imaging
Arterial	CNS	MRI and MRA
	Extremity	Doppler ultrasound
	Aorta	ECHO (proximal lesions), Doppler ultrasound, angiography
Venous	CNS	MRI and MRV
	Renal vein	Doppler ultrasound
	Extremity	Doppler ultrasound
	IVC, portal vein, abdominal vein	Doppler ultrasound
	Cardiac, proximal IVC	ECHO, Doppler ultrasound

Adapted from Veldman A, Nold MF, Michel-Behnke I. Thrombosis in the critically ill neonate: incidence, diagnosis, and management. *Vasc Health Risk Manag.* 2008;4(6)1337 and Saxonhouse MA. Management of neonatal thrombosis. *Clin Perinatol.* 2012;39:191.

A common non-catheter–related venous thrombosis is renal vein thrombosis (RVT). Clinical signs and symptoms include gross hematuria, thrombocytopenia, renal dysfunction, and retroperitoneal or abdominal mass. Complications associated with RVT include renal failure, hypertension, adrenal hemorrhage, and thrombosis extension into the IVC.

The incidence of cerebral sinus thrombosis is approximately 0.67 cases per 100,000 children, and is observed more frequently in neonates. Infants may present with seizures and lethargy, while focal (hemiparesis, cranial nerve involvement) or diffuse neurologic signs are less frequently observed. deVeber et al described the thrombus in the neonate to be more frequently located in the superior sagittal sinus or the lateral sinus.

RECOMMENDATIONS

MAJOR RECOMMENDATIONS

Obtain appropriate imaging (consider consultation with a qualified radiologist) to determine extent of thrombus and evaluate for hemorrhagic component (Table 35.3). We often try to obtain the least invasive imaging modality to minimize radiation exposure when possible; however, CT scanning may be required in some infants.

Therapeutic options vary, and involvement of a pediatric hematologist is recommended. **Use of anticoagulation or thrombolytic therapy will increase risk of bleeding.** Depending on the neonate's clinical status and degree and location of thrombosis, therapeutic options include close monitoring and supportive care, anticoagulant therapy, thrombolytic therapy, and thrombectomy. Heparin-induced thrombocytopenia (which is extremely rare in the neonatal period) or hemorrhages are contraindications for heparin therapy.

Unfractionated heparin (UFH) is recommended in the infant at high risk for bleeding or if rapid anticoagulation reversal will be needed (perioperative period). UFH requires secure IV access and repeated blood monitoring. Maintaining UFH within the therapeutic goal range and monitoring with anti-Xa activity (target range: 0.35–0.7 U/mL) or aPTT at 2–3 times the baseline aPTT (if baseline aPTT is within normal age range) or aPTT 60–85 seconds (if this aPTT range correlates with anti-Xa activity range of 0.35–7) is typical (see Table 35.4).

Low-molecular-weight heparin (LMWH) has the advantage of a longer half-life and ease of administration, with every 12-hour subcutaneous injections. Adjusting the LMWH dose to maintain the anti-Xa activity between 0.5 U/mL and 1 U/mL is recommended (Table 35.4).

PRACTICE OPTIONS

Practice Option #1

- Obtain screening coagulation studies with CBC, PT/INR, aPTT, fibrinogen, and D-dimer prior to initiating anticoagulation or thrombolysis. Coagulation studies should optimally be obtained from nonheparinized line.
- Initial imaging with head ultrasound for neonatal central nervous system (CNS) thrombosis and then MRI/MRV for more definitive imaging.
- Ultrasonography of the head prior to therapeutic intervention with anticoagulation or thrombolysis, and at least daily during initiation phase of therapy.
- Maintain fibrinogen >100 mg/dL and platelet count at ≥50,000/μL during course of therapeutic intervention.
- Monitor aPTT or anti-Xa activity at 4 hours after changes to UFH dose and then every 12–24 hours and PRN new bleeding.

TABLE 35.4. Neonatal Heparin Dosing Guidelines

Heparin	Dosing Guidelines (Weeks' Gestation)
UFH	< 28 weeks: bolus dose 25 U/kg followed by maintenance: 15 U/kg/h
	28–37 weeks: bolus dose 50 U/kg followed by maintenance: 15 U/kg/h
	> 37 weeks: bolus dose 100 U/kg followed by maintenance: 28 U/kg/h
LMWH (Enoxaparin)	Preterm: 2 mg/kg/12 h
	Term: 1.7 mg/kg/12 h
	<2 months: 1.5 mg/kg/12 h
	>2 months: 1 mg/kg/12 h

Adapted from Manco-Johnson, MJ, Grabowski EF, Hellgreen M, et al. Recommendations for tPA thrombolysis in children. On behalf of the Scientific Subcommittee on Perinatal and Pediatric Thrombosis of the Scientific and Standardization Committee of the International Society of Thrombosis and Haemostasis. *Thromb Haemost.* 2002;88:157; Saxonhouse MA. Management of neonatal thrombosis. *Clin Perinatol.* 2012;39:191; Saxonhouse MA, Burchfield DJ. The evaluation and management of postnatal thrombosis. *J Perinatol.* 2009;29:467; Monagle P, Chan AKC, Goldenberg NA, et al. Antithrombotic therapy in neonates and children: Antithrombotic Therapy and Prevention of Thrombosis, 9th ed. American College of Chest Physicians Evidence-Based Clinical Practice Guidelines. *Chest.* 2012;141(2):737S.

- Monitor anti-Xa activity at 4–6 hours after LMWH injection.
- Non-life–threatening or non-limb–threatening thrombosis may be treated with UFH, LMWH, or supportive care, with vigilant monitoring of thrombus and intervention with heparin if extension of thrombosis observed. See Table 35.4.
- Thrombosis associated with central venous line: Line may be removed after 3–5 days of therapeutic anticoagulation with repeat imaging after line removal.
- Cerebral sinus venous thrombosis (without large intracerebral ischemic or hemorrhagic areas) should be treated with UFH or LMWH.
  - If unable to start heparin, repeat imaging in 5–7 days; begin heparin if thrombus extension noted.
- Life- or limb-threatening non-CNS thrombosis: Tissue plasminogen activator (t-PA) at 0.06 mg/kg/h with concomitant low-dose UFH at 10 U/kg/h. Dose escalation of t-PA can be done; however, this should be under the guidance of an experienced pediatric hematologist. At least daily fibrinogen monitoring is recommended and replacement with FFP as needed. Vigilant imaging (repeat imaging at least 4–6 hours after start of fibrinolysis) during t-PA administration.
  - **For major bleeding**: Stop t-PA infusion and administer cryoprecipitate (and FFP if indicated).
- Thrombolysis contraindications:
  - Major surgery within prior 10 days
  - Invasive procedure within prior 3 days
  - Major hemorrhage within prior 10 days
  - Active bleeding
  - Severe asphyxia within prior 7 days

- Seizures within prior 48 hours
- Systemic septicemia
- Inability to maintain platelet count 50,000–100,000/µL or fibrinogen >100 mg/dL
- <32 weeks' gestation (case reports/series of t-PA to <32-week infants and risk/benefit based on individual assessment)

Practice Option #2

- Thrombophilia evaluation: Factor V Leiden and prothrombin 20210A gene studies, protein C activity, protein S activity, antithrombin III activity, fasting homocysteine. We also obtain additional thrombophilia testing with antiphospholipid antibody panel, anti-beta-2 glycoprotein antibody panel and lupus anticoagulant, testing may be indicated in certain infants with neonatal stroke.
- Duration of anticoagulation as per consulting pediatric hematology recommendations.

Practice Option #3

- Prophylaxis with UFH at 0.5 U/kg/h in neonates with central venous lines.

SCOPE

DISEASE/CONDITION(S)

Arterial thrombosis.

GUIDELINE OBJECTIVE(S)

Identification and management guidelines for neonatal arterial thrombosis.

BRIEF BACKGROUND

(See also venous thrombosis background.) Occurrence of neonatal arterial thrombosis is reported less frequently than venous thrombosis (Nowak-Gottl et al noted 19 cases of arterial thrombosis in the 79 neonatal thrombotic events reported). Spontaneous arterial thrombotic events occurring in the absence of a central line is rare. Complications associated with thrombosis-associated umbilical arterial catheters (UACs) include ischemic limb damage (cold, pulseless, dusky- to pale-appearing extremity), mesenteric ischemia, organ dysfunction (renal failure, necrotizing enterocolitis, congestive heart failure), and blood pressure instability. American College of Clinical Pharmacy (ACCP) guidelines recommend high UAC placement and prophylactic UFH infusion for neonates with UACs.

Perinatal stroke is estimated to occur in 1 in 4000 births and often presents in the first week of life. Seizures are the most common presentation, although some neonates present with abnormal tone or a change in the level of consciousness. Noted to occur more in the left hemisphere. Evaluation for cardioembolic source is of paramount importance and will further guide anticoagulant recommendations.

RECOMMENDATIONS

MAJOR RECOMMENDATIONS

See venous thrombosis recommendations. In addition, echocardiogram is needed to evaluate for cardioembolic source.

PRACTICE OPTIONS

Practice Option #1

See venous thrombosis recommendations, with the following exceptions:

- Initial imaging with head ultrasound for neonatal CNS thrombosis and then MRI/MRA for more definitive imaging.
- For non-life–threatening or non-limb–threatening acute femoral artery thrombosis, begin UFH with transition to LMWH at later date.
- Immediate removal of the catheter is recommended for peripheral arterial catheter thrombosis.
- Anticoagulation with UFH or LMWH is recommended for new-onset neonatal arterial ischemic stroke due to a cardioembolic source.
- Life- or limb-threatening non-CNS thrombosis: Tissue plasminogen activator (t-PA) at 0.06 mg/kg/h with concomitant low dose UFH at 10 U/kg/h. Dose escalation of t-PA can be done; however, this should be under the guidance of an experienced pediatric hematologist. At least daily fibrinogen monitoring is recommended and replacement with FFP as needed. Vigilant imaging (repeat imaging at least 4–6 hours after start of fibrinolysis) during t-PA administration.
- If the risk of catastrophic embolism from chemical thrombolysis contraindicates its use (i.e., in the case of intracardiac or ascending aortic thrombosis), surgical thrombectomy should be considered by an experienced cardiovascular surgeon.

Practice Option #2

See venous thrombosis recommendations.

Practice Option #3

- Prophylaxis with UFH at 0.5 U/mL at 1 mL/h in neonates with peripheral arterial catheters.
- Prophylaxis with UFH at 0.25–1 U/mL (total dose 25–200 U/kg/day) for UACs.

IMPLEMENTATION OF GUIDELINE

QUALIFYING STATEMENTS

Recommend multidisciplinary approach with pediatric radiology, pediatric hematology, and pediatric neurology and neurosurgery (for neonates with CNS involvement).

SUMMARY FOR NEONATAL THROMBOSIS

There is a lack of prospective randomized clinical trials for the management of neonatal thrombosis, and management in infants is often based on retrospective studies, case series, individual pediatric hematologist team experience, and extrapolation of guidelines from adults. Evidence-based medicine for neonatal thrombosis management is a slowly emerging field. Consultation with pediatric hematology team is recommended with initiation of therapeutic anticoagulation or thrombolytic therapy.

BIBLIOGRAPHIC SOURCE(S)

Acharya SS. Rare bleeding disorders in children: identification and primary care management. *Pediatrics*. 2013;132(5):882.

Agrawal N, Johnston C, Wu YW, Sidney S, Fullerton HJ. Imaging data reveal a higher pediatric stroke incidence that prior US estimates. *Stroke*. 2009;40:3415.

American Academy of Pediatrics Committee on Fetus and Newborn. Controversies concerning vitamin K and the newborn. American Academy of Pediatrics Committee on Fetus and Newborn. *Pediatrics.* 2003;112(1):191.

Andrew M, Paes B, Milner R, et al. Development of the human coagulation system in the full-term infant. *Blood.* 1987;70(1):165.

Andrew M, Paes B, Milner R, et al. Development of the human coagulation system in the healthy premature infant. *Blood.* 1988;72(5):1651-7.

Aronis-Vournas S. The bleeding neonate. *Haematol Rep.* 2006;2(10):668.

Blumberg RW, Forbes GB, Fraser D, et al; Committee on Nutrition. Vitamin K compounds and the water-soluble analogues. *Pediatrics.* 1961;28:501.

Bussel J. Diagnosis and management of the fetus and neonate with alloimmune thrombocytopenia. *J Thromb Haemost.* 2009;7(S1):253.

Bussel JB, Sola-Visner M. Current approaches to the evaluation and management of the fetus and neonate with immune thrombocytopenia. *Semin Perinatol.* 2009;33(1):35.

Chalmers EA. Neonatal coagulation problems. *Arch Dis Child Fetal Neonatal Ed.* 2004;89:F475.

Chalmers EA. Perinatal stroke—risk factors and management. *Br J Haematol.* 2005;130:333.

Chalmers E, Williams M, Brennand J, Liesner R, Collins P, Richards M. Guideline on the management of haemophilia in the fetus and neonate. *Br J Haematol.* 2011;154:208.

D'Agata ID, Balistreri WF. Evaluation of liver disease in the pediatric patient. *Pediatr Rev.* 1999;20(11):376.

deVeber G, Andrew M, Adams C, et al. Cerebral sinovenous thrombosis in children. *N Engl J Med.* 2001;345(6):417.

Dhawan A, Mieli-Vergani G. Acute liver failure in neonates. *Early Hum Devel.* 2005;81:1005.

Hartmann J, Hussein A, Trowitzsch E, Becker J, Hennecke KH. Treatment of neonatal thrombus formation with recombinant tissue plasminogen activator: six years' experience and review of the literature. *Arch Dis Child Ed.* 2001;85(1):F18.

James AH, Hoots K. The optimal mode of delivery for the haemophilia carrier expecting an affected infant is caesarean delivery. *Haemophilia.* 2010;16(3):420.

Kenet G, Chan KC, Soucie JM, Kulkarni R. Bleeding disorders in neonates. *Haemophilia.* 2010;16(5):168.

Kirton A, Armstrong-Wells J, Chang T, et al. Symptomatic neonatal arterial ischemic stroke: The International Pediatric Stroke Study. *Pediatrics.* 2011;128(6):1402.

Loughnan PM, McDougall PN. Epidemiology of late onset haemorrhagic disease: a pooled data analysis. *J Pediatr Child Health.* 1993;29:177.

Lynch JK, Nelson KB. Epidemiology of perinatal stroke. *Curr Opin Pediatr.* 2001;13(6):499.

Manco-Johnson MJ. How I treat venous thrombosis in children. *Blood.* 2006;107(1):219.

Manco-Johnson MJ, Goldenberg NA. Use of fresh frozen plasma and plasma proteins in newborn infants. *Haematol Rep.* 2006;2(10):71.

Manco-Johnson MJ, Grabowski EF, Hellgreen M, et al. Recommendations for tPA thrombolysis in children. On behalf of the Scientific Subcommittee on Perinatal and Pediatric Thrombosis of the Scientific and Standardization Committee of the International Society of Thrombosis and Haemostasis. *Thromb Haemost.* 2002;88:157.

McMillan DD, Wu J. Approach to the bleeding newborn. *Paediatr Child Health.* 1998;3(6):399.

Medical and Scientific Advisory Board (MASAC). MASAC recommendations concerning products licensed for the treatment of hemophilia and other bleeding disorders. 2018; MASAC, Recommendation #253.

Monagle P, Chan AKC, Goldenberg NA, et al. Antithrombotic therapy in neonates and children: Antithrombotic Therapy and Prevention of Thrombosis, 9th ed. American College of Chest Physicians Evidence-Based Clinical Practice Guidelines. *Chest.* 2012;141(2):737S.

Motta M, Del Vecchio A, Radicioni M. Clinical use of fresh-frozen plasma and cryoprecipitate in neonatal intensive care unit. *J Matern Fetal Neonatal Med.* 2011;24S(1):129.

Nelson KB, Lynch JK. Stroke in newborn infants. *Lancet Neurol.* 2004;3(3):2004.

Nowak-Gottl U, von Kries R, Gobel U. Neonatal symptomatic thromboembolism in Germany: two-year study. *Arch Dis Child Ed.* 1997;76:F163.

Peterson JA, McFarland JG, Curtis BR, Aster RH. Neonatal alloimmune thrombocytopenia: pathogenesis, diagnosis and management. *Br J Haematol.* 2013;161(1):3.

Puckett RM, Offringa M. Prophylactic vitamin K for vitamin K deficiency bleeding in neonates. *Cochran Database Syst Rev.* 2000;4:CD002776.

Roach ES, Golomb MR, Adams R, et al. Management of stroke in infants and children: a scientific statement from a special writing group of the American Heart Association Stroke Council and the Council on cardiovascular disease in the young. *Stroke.* 2008;39:2644.

Saracco P, Parodi E, Fabris C, Cencinati V, Molinari AC, Giordano P. Management and investigation of neonatal thromboembolic events: genetic and acquired risk factors. *Thromb Res.* 2009;123:805.

Saxonhouse MA. Management of neonatal thrombosis. *Clin Perinatol.* 2012;39:191.

Saxonhouse MA, Burchfield DJ. The evaluation and management of postnatal thrombosis. *J Perinatol.* 2009;29:467.

Schmidt B, Andrew M. Neonatal thrombosis: report of a prospective Canadian and international registry. *Pediatrics.* 1995;96(5):939.

Soucie JM, Evatt B, Jackson D, et al. Occurrence of hemophilia in the United States. *Am J Hematol.* 1998;59:288.

Sutor A, von Kries R, Marlies, Cornelissen EAM, McNinch AW, Andrew M. Vitamin K deficiency bleeding (VKDB) in infancy. ISTH Pediatric/Perinatal Subcommittee. International Society on Thrombosis and Haemostasis. *Thromb Haemost.* 1999;81:456.

Veldman A, Fischer D, Nold MF, Wong FY. Disseminated intravascular coagulation in term and preterm neonates. *Semin Thromb Hemost.* 2010;36:419.

Veldman A, Nold MF, Michel-Behnke I. Thrombosis in the critically ill neonate: incidence, diagnosis, and management. *Vasc Health Risk Manag.* 2008;4(6)1337.

Wang M, Hays T, Balasa V, et al. Low-dose tissue plasminogen activator thrombolysis in children. *J Pediatr Hematol Oncol.* 2003;25(5):379.

Wicklund BM. Bleeding and clotting disorders in pediatric liver disease. *Hematology Am Soc Hematol Educ Program.* 2011;2011:170.

Williams MD, Chalmers EA, Gibson BE; Haemostasis and Thrombosis Task Force, British Committee for Standards in Haematology. The investigation and management of neonatal haemostasis and thrombosis. *Br J Haematol.* 2001;119:295.

Zidan AS, Abdel-Hady H. Surgical evacuation of neonatal intracranial hemorrhage due to vitamin K deficiency bleeding. *J Neurosurg Pediatr.* 2011;7:295.

Gut Disorders

Necrotizing Enterocolitis

Jonathan R. Swanson, MD, MSc • Phillip V. Gordon, MD, PhD

SCOPE

DISEASE/CONDITION(S)

Necrotizing enterocolitis (NEC) requiring medical and/or surgical treatment.

GUIDELINE OBJECTIVE(S)

Review risk factors and basic mechanisms of necrotizing enterocolitis; provide rationale for defining necrotizing enterocolitis; recommendations for the treatment of both medical and surgical necrotizing enterocolitis; identify areas for quality improvement.

BRIEF BACKGROUND

NEC is an acute acquired intestinal disease of neonates, the most common condition requiring surgical treatment and a leading cause of death in infants requiring care in a neonatal intensive care unit (NICU). The pathophysiology of NEC continues to be elucidated. In preterm infants, NEC is likely acquired through a series of steps. Preterm infants are born in a relative passive immune deficit without active transport of immunoglobulins in the third trimester. Secondly, the premature intestine undergoes excessive stimulation of the innate immune system. Specifically, toll-like receptor-4 is abundant and highly active in cell death–signaling pathways. Repeated exposure of bacterial lipopolysaccharide ramps up these pathways increasing the likelihood of apoptosis-induced necrosis. Finally, in the setting of passive immune deficit and innate immune priming, there is a window of vulnerability. During this window, infants may be exposed to one or more triggers that ultimately precipitate or permit NEC. These triggers may include anemia (transfusion-associated NEC), bacterial or viral pathogens, a hypoxic/ischemic event, cow's milk formula, or commercial thickening agents.

RECOMMENDATIONS

MAJOR RECOMMENDATIONS

Delineating between medical and surgical NEC requires both clinical and radiographic signs. Surgical treatment of NEC is suggested when there is free intraperitoneal air on radiograph or ultrasound, persistent ileus pattern that is unresponsive to medical management, and deteriorating clinical symptoms (persistent hypotension) or laboratory values (recalcitrant thrombocytopenia).

PRACTICE OPTIONS

Practice Option #1: Management of Medical NEC

Infants with a diagnosis of medical NEC require bowel rest and decompression. Bowel rest should continue for 3 days after radiographic evidence of NEC is absent. Abdominal radiographs, including anteroposterior and left lateral decubitus, should be monitored every 12 hours or until evidence of disease progression is absent. Laboratory studies including white blood cell count and differential, hematocrit, and platelet count should be monitored for disease progression and may aid in diagnosis and prognosis. Blood cultures should be obtained, and consideration should be made for viral cultures of stool. Antibiotics, including coverage of both gram-negative and gram-positive bacteria, should be instituted and continued for 5–7 days, depending on the severity of illness. It is unknown if there are specific antibiotic choices that could best optimize outcomes. When a cluster of NEC cases occur in a given NICU, consideration should be given to quarantining individual cases.

Practice Option #2: Management of Surgical NEC

Infants with a diagnosis of surgical NEC require bowel rest and decompression. Bowel rest should continue until radiographic evidence of NEC is absent and there is return of bowel function. Radiographs, including anteroposterior and left lateral decubitus, should be monitored every 12 hours or until evidence of disease progression is absent. Laboratory studies including white blood cell count and differential, hematocrit, and platelet count should be monitored for disease progression and may aid in diagnosis and prognosis. Blood cultures should be obtained, and consideration should be made for viral cultures of stool. Peritoneal fluid cultures should be obtained. Antibiotics, including coverage of both gram-negative and gram-positive bacteria, should be instituted and continued for 7–10 days. Use of anaerobic antimicrobial therapy may be considered. Surgical management should consider the clinical stability of the infant. If clinically stable, infants should be managed with laparotomy. Primary peritoneal drainage should be limited to infants too unstable for transfer to an operating room for laparotomy. Drain placement should not be used for definitive treatment in the majority of infants.

Practice Option #3: Practices for the Prevention of NEC

Prevention of medical and surgical NEC can be accomplished through several evidence-based practices. 1) Institution of human milk feeding programs, including the use of pasteurized human milk for infants without access to maternal breast milk. 2)

Implementation of unit-specific written feeding guidelines delineating volumes to be fed and when milk fortifiers are to be added. Advancement of feeding volumes can generally be tolerated up to 25–30 mL/kg/day. 3) Avoidance of unnecessary antibiotic exposure and implementation of antibiotic stewardship programs. 4) Removal of central venous lines expeditiously. 5) Limitation of elective transfusions of packed red blood cells but also avoidance of severe anemia. 6) Avoidance of acid inhibition. 7) Consideration of the use of probiotics.

IMPLEMENTATION OF GUIDELINE

QUALIFYING STATEMENTS

In order to accurately track and monitor NEC incidence, an appropriate diagnosis must be made. Recent reviews have suggested that the use of modified Bell's Staging criteria is out of date and fails to accurately capture NEC diagnosis. NEC can more accurately be diagnosed by the finding of at least two of the following:

1. Intestinal pneumatosis (on abdominal radiograph or ultrasound)
2. Platelet consumption (requirement of daily platelet transfusions or decreasing platelet count less than 150,000/μL over 72 hours)
3. Onset of acquired neonatal intestinal disease that corresponds to an appropriate gestational window (Figure 36.1)

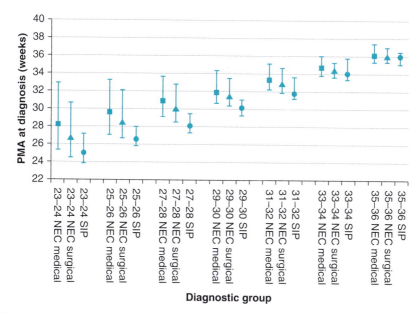

FIGURE 36.1 • Graph of postmenstrual age at diagnosis versus gestational groupings for medical and surgical NEC as well as SIP from a refined national dataset, excluding congenital anomalies and dual diagnoses. Shapes represent medians; bars represent 10th–90th percentiles. (Used with permission from Gordon PV, Clark R, Swanson JR, Spitzer A. Can a national dataset generate a nomogram for necrotizing enterocolitis onset? *J Perinatol.* 2014;34:732.)

Infants should be excluded from a traditional NEC diagnosis if they have major congenital anomalies or suspected NEC (traditionally Bell's Stage I). A more refined diagnosis of NEC improves classification and subtyping of NEC cases, which allows for improved ability to initiate quality improvement programs.

DESCRIPTION OF IMPLEMENTATION STRATEGY

New Disease

The response to a patient with a new diagnosis of NEC should be immediate and with highest priority. Intestinal decompression, initiation of antibiotics, and a switch from enteral to IV nutrition should be a universal response. Additional supports for physiologic stability depend on the severity of presentation and the baseline of illness prior to acquiring NEC. This is a disease that has the potential to progress rapidly. Infants can die in hours. For this reason, two additional things should always occur. 1) An experienced neonatologist should examine an infant with suspected NEC at the time of diagnosis to assess for severity of disease. 2) Parents should always be called and informed of this ominous status change at the time of diagnosis (regardless of the time of day).

Disease Prevention

Because NEC occurs in runs and clusters, it is a challenging outcome for quality improvement. Fortunately, comprehensive multipronged approaches have been shown to improve NEC rates, and these should be implemented universally. All NICUs should seek to increase human milk feedings, to standardize their feeding advances, to eradicate the use of acid inhibitors, and to minimize unnecessary antibiotic exposure in culture-negative infants. Evidence is less strong for how to combat NEC associated with blood transfusions but most agree that limiting unnecessary transfusions, avoiding severe anemia, and limiting or holding feeds in infants at highest risk are the approaches that seem sound. Center-to-center variation in practice and product use likely accounts for much of the remaining regional variation in NEC rates. Centers with high rates should subtype their NEC into clinical groupings that help identify these practice variations, thus providing targets for additional quality improvement. Data analyses of this type require commitment and a solid knowledge base. Individuals should be immersed in the NEC literature and have a basic understanding of statistics before attempting a more detailed NEC quality improvement assessment.

QUALITY METRICS

Neonatal intensive care units should tailor quality improvement strategies to their own data and incidence of NEC subsets. Other metrics that should be monitored include use of human milk at initiation of feeds, use of human milk at discharge, surgical NEC rates, and time to "full" feeds (150–160 mL/kg/day). Useful tools for tracking NEC include run charts, NEC per 1000 patient days (as a means of quantifying clusters), and quarterly incidence stratified by gestational age groups.

SUMMARY

The clinical management of NEC today consists of two parts: 1) acute management of the infant with NEC and 2) prevention of disease through system-wide quality improvement efforts. Both aspects are essential to providing the standard of care.

BIBLIOGRAPHIC SOURCE(S)

Alexander VN, Northrup V, Bizzarro MJ. Antibiotic exposure in the newborn intensive care unit and the risk of necrotizing enterocolitis. *J Pediatr.* 2011;159(3):392-7.

AlFaleh K, Anabrees J. Probiotics for prevention of necrotizing enterocolitis in preterm infants. *Cochrane Database Syst Rev.* 2014;(4):CD005496.

Autmizguine J, Hornik CP, Benjamin DK Jr, et al. Anaerobic antimicrobial therapy after necrotizing enterocolitis in VLBW infants. *Pediatrics.* 2015;135(1):e117-25.

Bailey SM, Hendricks-Muñoz KD, Mally PV. Variability in splanchnic tissue oxygenation during preterm red blood cell transfusion given for symptomatic anaemia may reveal a potential mechanism of transfusion-related acute gut injury. *Blood Transfus.* 2015;13(3):429-34.

Beal J, Silverman B, Bellant J, Young TE, Klontz K. Late onset necrotizing enterocolitis in infants following use of a xanthan gum-containing thickening agent. *J Pediatr.* 2012;161(2):354-6.

Berdon WE, Grossman H, Baker DH, Mizrahi A, Barlow O, Blanc WA. Necrotizing enterocolitis in the premature infant. *Radiology.* 1964;83:879-87.

Bohnhorst B, Muller S, Dordelmann M, Peter CS, Petersen C, Poets CF. Early feeding after necrotizing enterocolitis in preterm infants. *J Pediatr.* 2003;143(4):484-7.

Christensen RD, Gordon PV, Besner GE. Can we cut the incidence of necrotizing enterocolitis in half—today? *Fetal Pediatr Pathol.* 2010;29(4):185-98.

Christensen RD, Lambert DK, Henry E, et al. Is "transfusion-associated necrotizing enterocolitis" an authentic pathogenic entity? *Transfusion.* 2010;50(5):1106-12.

Cotten CM, Taylor S, Stoll B, et al; NICHD Neonatal Research Network. Prolonged duration of initial empirical antibiotic treatment is associated with increased rates of necrotizing enterocolitis and death for extremely low birth weight infants. *Pediatrics.* 2009;123(1):58-66.

Egan CE, Sodhi CP, Good M, et al. Toll-like receptor 4-mediated lymphocyte influx induces neonatal necrotizing enterocolitis. *J Clin Invest.* 2015;126(2):495-508.

Elgin TG, Kern SL, McElroy SJ. Development of the neonatal intestinal microbiome and its association with necrotizing enterocolitis. *Clin Ther.* 2016;38(4):706-15.

Ellsbury DL, Clark RH, Ursprung R, Handler DL, Dodd ED, Spitzer AR. A multifaceted approach to improving outcomes in the NICU: the Pediatrix 100000 babies campaign. *Pediatrics.* 2016;137(4):e20150389.

Gordon P, Christensen R, Weitkamp JH, Maheshwari A. Mapping the new world of necrotizing enterocolitis (NEC): review and opinion. *EJ Neonatol Res.* 2012;2(4):145-72.

Gordon PV. Necrotizing enterocolitis (NEC) and Darwinism (reviewing the evolutionary basis for NEC). *EJ Neonatol Res.* 2013; 3(1):23-30.

Gordon PV, Clark R, Swanson JR, Spitzer A. Can a national dataset generate a nomogram for necrotizing enterocolitis onset? *J Perinatol.* 2014;34(10):732-5.

Gordon PV, Swanson JR. Necrotizing enterocolitis is one disease with many origins and potential means of prevention. *Pathophysiology.* 2014;21(1):13-9.

Gordon PV, Swanson JR, Attridge JT, Clark R. Emerging trends in acquired neonatal intestinal disease: is it time to abandon Bell's criteria? *J Perinatol.* 2007;27(11):661-71.

Gordon PV, Swanson JR, Clark R, Spitzer A. The complete blood cell count in a refined cohort of preterm NEC: the importance of gestational age and day of diagnosis when using the CBC to estimate mortality. *J Perinatol.* 2016;36(2):121-5.

Guillet R, Stoll BJ, Cotton CM, et al. Association of H2-blocker therapy and higher incidence of necrotizing enterocolitis in very low birth weight infants. *Pediatrics.* 2006;117(2):e137-42.

Henderson G, Anthony MY, McGuire W. Formula milk versus maternal breast milk for feeding preterm or low birth weight infants. *Cochrane Database Syst Rev.* 2007;(4):CD002972.

Leaphart CL, Cavallo J, Gribar SC, et al. A critical role for TLR4 in the pathogenesis of necrotizing enterocolitis by modulating intestinal injury and repair. *J Immunol.* 2007;179(7):4808-20.

Lee HC, Kurtin PS, Wight NE, et al. A quality improvement project to increase breast milk use in very low birth weight infants. *Pediatrics.* 2012;130(6):e1679-87.

Meinzen-Derr J, Morrow AL, Hornung RW, Donovan EF, Dietrich KN, Succop PA. Epidemiology of necrotizing enterocolitis temporal clustering in two neonatology practices. *J Pediatr.* 2009;154(5):656-61.

Morgan J, Young L, McGuire W. Slow advancement of enteral feed volumes to prevent necrotizing enterocolitis in very low birth weight infants. *Cochrane Database Syst Rev.* 2015;(10):CD001241.

Patel AL, Trivedi S, Bhandari NP, et al. Reducing necrotizing enterocolitis in very low birth weight infants using quality-improvement methods. *J Perinatol.* 2014;34(11):850-7.

Patel RM, Knezevic A, Shenvi N, et al. Association of red blood cell transfusion, anemia, and necrotizing enterocolitis in very low-birth-weight infants. *JAMA.* 2016;315(9):889-97.

Quigley M, McGuire W. Formula versus donor breast milk for feeding preterm or low birth weight infants. *Cochrane Database Syst Rev.* 2014;(4):CD002971.

Remon J, Kampanatkosol R, Kaul RR, Muraskas JK, Christensen RD, Maheshwari A. Acute drop in blood monocyte count differentiates NEC from other causes of feeding intolerance. *J Perinatol.* 2014;34(7):549-54.

Shah D, Sinn JK. Antibiotic regimens for the empirical treatment of newborn infants with necrotizing enterocolitis. *Cochrane Database Syst Rev.* 2012;(8):CD007448.

Sharma R, Garrison RD, Tepas JJ 3rd, et al. Rotavirus-associated necrotizing enterocolitis: an insight into a potentially preventable disease? *J Pediatr Surg.* 2004;39(3):453-7.

Soliman A, Michelsen KS, Karahashi H, et al. Platelet-activating factor induces TLR4 expression in intestinal epithelial cells: implication for the pathogenesis of necrotizing enterocolitis. *PLoS One.* 2010;5(10):e15044.

Swanson JR, Jilling T, Lu J, Landseadel JB, Marcinkiewicz M, Gordon PV. Ileal immunoglobulin binding by the neonatal Fc receptor: a previously unrecognized mechanism of protection in the neonatal rat model of necrotizing enterocolitis? *EJ Neonatol Res.* 2011;1(1):12-22.

Walsh MC, Kliegman RM. Necrotizing enterocolitis: treatment based on staging criteria. *Pediatr Clin North Am.* 1986;33:179-201.

Woods CW, Oliver T, Lewis K, Yang Q. Development of necrotizing enterocolitis in premature infants receiving thickened feeds using SimplyThick®. *J Perinatol.* 2012;32(2):150-2.

Intestinal Perforation

Kendall R. Johnson, MD • James E. Moore, MD, PhD

SCOPE

DISEASE/CONDITION(S)

Management of intestinal and gastric perforations.

GUIDELINE OBJECTIVE(S)

Review spontaneous intestinal and gastric perforations; recommendations for initial management, surgical involvement, and postoperative care.

DISEASE/CONDITION(S)

Spontaneous intestinal perforation

GUIDELINE OBJECTIVE(S)

Review and identify recommendations for the medical management of spontaneous intestinal perforations.

BRIEF BACKGROUND

Spontaneous Intestinal Perforation

Spontaneous intestinal perforation (SIP), also known as isolated or focal intestinal perforation, commonly presents in very low birth weight (VLBW) infants. It is characterized as isolated bowel perforation, particularly in the distal small intestines, without clinical or radiographic evidence of necrotizing enterocolitis (NEC). Presentation is typically within the first week of life and does not have a close association with enteral feedings.

An association has been found between SIP and exposure to indomethacin and corticosteroids. Typically, infants with SIP lack evidence of significant intestinal or systemic inflammation. A common radiographic finding is pneumoperitoneum without pneumatosis intestinalis. Though differences exist between SIP and NEC, it can be difficult to distinguish the two entities prior to laparotomy.

RECOMMENDATIONS

MAJOR RECOMMENDATIONS

1. An increased risk of developing SIP has been associated with administration of both a nonsteroidal anti-inflammatory agent and corticosteroids. As such, concomitant administration of these medications should be avoided if possible, particularly in VLBW infants.
2. As soon as a diagnosis of SIP is suspected, initial medical management should include bowel rest, abdominal decompression with a gastric tube, blood culture, administration of broad-spectrum antibiotics, and initiation of intravenous fluids.
3. Surgical consultation should be obtained for all infants with suspected SIP.
4. Preoperatively, it can be difficult to distinguish NEC from SIP, particularly when the only radiographic finding is pneumoperitoneum. As such, the initial management of SIP is similar to NEC and requires urgent surgical evaluation.
5. A commonly used broad-spectrum antibiotic regimen is ampicillin and gentamicin, however other antimicrobial agents such as piperacillin with tazobactam, cephalosporins, or other aminoglycosides may be used depending on local resistance patterns, renal function, or allergies. A Cochrane review demonstrated insufficient evidence from two randomized controlled trials to recommend a particular antibiotic regimen. If known, local antimicrobial resistance patterns should be taken into consideration when initiating treatment. Duration of antibiotic treatment has not been well studied, but typical practices are 7–14 days of treatment.

PRACTICE OPTIONS

Practice Option #1: Initial Management

1. Initiate bowel rest (cessation of feedings and enteral medications), abdominal decompression with gastric tube on suction, broad-spectrum antibiotics, and intravenous fluids.
2. Consult general surgery.
3. The following laboratory studies should be obtained: CBC, blood culture, electrolytes, and blood gas.
4. Initiate antibiotic regimen, commonly ampicillin and gentamicin, though other regimens may be considered based on local resistance patterns and patient characteristics. Alternative regimens include piperacillin with tazobactam or ampicillin with cefotaxime. Anaerobic coverage with metronidazole or clindamycin should be added for infants requiring surgical intervention.
5. Based on clinical status, further medical management may include intravenous fluid resuscitation, blood product transfusion, pressor initiation, increased respiratory support, correction of electrolyte imbalances, and pain control, with the focus on stabilizing the infant prior to surgical intervention.

6. Infants with deterioration of respiratory status or frequent apneic episodes may require intubation.
7. If peritoneal fluid is obtained, send for Gram stain and culture.

Practice Option #2: If Surgery is Required

Postoperative care:

1. Closely monitor intravascular fluid status via serum electrolytes, monitoring of net fluid balance, daily weights and strict intake and urinary output assessment. Postoperative third spacing may result in infants requiring 1.5 maintenance fluids or more to maintain adequate intravascular volume. In addition, gastric output should be replaced with an isotonic intravenous fluid with potassium chloride, such as lactated ringer's or normal saline with potassium chloride.
2. Regular interval monitoring for and correction of anemia, thrombocytopenia, coagulopathy, or metabolic acidosis is essential postoperatively. Persistence of these abnormalities after surgical intervention, despite optimized medical management, may indicate residual necrotic bowel requiring further surgical exploration.
3. Continue broad-spectrum antibiotics for 7–14 days, adjusting treatment regimen based on culture results if available. Duration of antibiotic treatment has not been well studied, except in the setting of bacteremia for which treatment should continue for 14 days.
4. Attention to pain control is needed, especially during the early postoperative period, with the use of intermittent or continuous intravenous analgesics to achieve adequate pain control.
5. To ensure a positive nitrogen balance and allow injured tissues to repair, parenteral nutrition with 3.5–4 g/kg/day of protein should be initiated early.
6. Maintain bowel rest and decompression with gastric tube until there is evidence of bowel function. Initiate small tube feeds, with close attention to stoma/stool output. If large segments of bowel were resected, the remaining intestine may be unable to absorb adequate nutrition, therefore requiring long-term parenteral nutrition. Due to the risk of intestinal failure in these patients, many centers have multidisciplinary bowel rehabilitation programs to assist with long-term management.

IMPLEMENTATION OF GUIDELINE

DESCRIPTION OF IMPLEMENTATION STRATEGY

Recommend written guidelines for initial approach to SIP, including surgical evaluation, medical stabilization, laboratory studies, and antibiotic therapy.

QUALITY METRICS

TPN duration, length of stay, mortality rates.

SCOPE

DISEASE/CONDITION(S)

Perforation secondary to intestinal obstruction.

GUIDELINE OBJECTIVE(S)

Review the common causes of neonatal obstruction complicated by perforation. Review and identify recommendations for the medical management of perforations secondary to intestinal obstructions.

BRIEF BACKGROUND

Intestinal obstruction should be suspected in infants with a history of maternal polyhydramnios, bilious emesis, failure to pass meconium within 24 hours of life, or abdominal distension. Incidence of neonatal obstruction is estimated to be approximately 1 in 2000 live births. A potential complication of intestinal obstruction is visceral perforation. Etiologies of obstruction most commonly associated with perforation include midgut malrotation with volvulus, meconium ileus (MI), Hirschsprung disease (HD), and anorectal malformations. More detailed specifics on these obstructive conditions are discussed in Chapter 38.

Malrotation results from abnormal rotation of the gut as it returns to the abdominal cavity during early development. Midgut volvulus occurs when the abnormally narrow mesenteric base twists resulting in intestinal obstruction and vascular compromise. Late presentation resulting in significant ischemia and necrosis of the bowel can result in perforation, leading to peritonitis, sepsis, shock, and possibly death.

MI is caused by thick, tenacious meconium which is high in protein and low in water, pancreatic enzymes, lactase, and sucrase. Complex MI has a varied clinical presentation, ranging from an incidental finding of calcifications to frank peritonitis. Radiographic findings in complex MI include calcifications, free air, air–fluid levels, pseudocysts, ascites, and distended small bowel. While most symptoms develop from sterile chemical irritation, pseudocysts are at risk of developing infection.

HD has a male predominance and is the cause of 15–20% of all neonatal intestinal obstructions. HD is a functional obstruction of the intestines due to lack of peristalsis in an abnormally innervated distal colon. Perforation presents in less than 2% of infants with HD.

Anorectal malformations (ARM) occur in approximately 1 in 5000 live births. Perforation occurs in approximately 2–9% of infants with ARM, resulting in increased risk of mortality. Though diagnostic or therapeutic delay has been implicated in the development of perforations, there have been reports of perforations occurring within the first 24 hours or in utero.

RECOMMENDATIONS

MAJOR RECOMMENDATIONS

1. Upon suspicion of bowel obstruction, initial medical management should include bowel rest, abdominal decompression with a gastric tube on low suction, and initiation of intravenous fluids. Fluid removed via gastric tube should be replaced with isotonic IV fluids, such as lactated ringer's or normal saline, with potassium chloride if losses are more than 20–30 mL/kg/day.
2. Obtain two view abdominal radiographs, supine and left lateral decubitus, to confirm presence of free air.

3. Infants with perforated bowel are at increased risk for acidosis and shock. As such, fluid resuscitation with normal saline in 10–20 mL/kg aliquots may be indicated.

4. Electrolytes should be sent to evaluate for abnormalities that may require correction. In addition, a CBC and coagulation studies should be sent to evaluate for signs of infection, anemia, thrombocytopenia, or coagulopathy, which may require treatment with blood products prior to or during surgery.

5. Particularly if perforation is present, a blood culture should be obtained and broad-spectrum antibiotics initiated.

6. Surgical evaluation is indicated for bowel obstruction to determine operative plan as well as ongoing management. In the setting of an obstruction with bowel perforation, surgical consultation should be obtained urgently.

PRACTICE OPTIONS

Practice Option #1: Malrotation with Midgut Volvulus

1. The gold standard for diagnosis is an upper GI contrast study, but if the infant is unstable or clinical suspicion of the diagnosis is high then surgical treatment should not be delayed.

2. Abdominal x-rays may be normal. There are no radiographic plain film findings that rule out malrotation with volvulus.

3. Along with preoperative bowel rest, abdominal decompression with gastric tube, fluid resuscitation, and blood cultures should be obtained in addition to broad-spectrum antibiotic initiation.

Practice Option #2: Meconium Ileus

1. After consultation with surgery, simple MI can be initially treated with hyperosmolar enemas, but the presence of bowel perforation requires immediate surgical evaluation and treatment.

2. All infants with MI should be tested for cystic fibrosis.

Practice Option #3: Hirschsprung Disease

1. Contrast enema is the standard approach for diagnosis. A positive study demonstrates a transition zone between the smaller rectum and proximally dilated bowel. Definitive diagnosis requires rectal suction biopsy demonstrating absent ganglion cells in the submucosal and myenteric plexus and increased acetylcholinesterase in parasympathetic nerve fibers.

2. Management of HD requires surgical involvement. If a bowel perforation is present, then a surgical consult should be obtained urgently, as operative management may be needed immediately.

3. The most serious complication of HD is enterocolitis, which presents as diarrhea, shock, and dehydration. It can occur early at any time, before or after surgical repair. Bacterial overgrowth and mucosal ischemia develops secondary to stasis of fluid and stool within the colon. Enemas should be avoided during enterocolitis as there is a high risk of perforation.

Practice Option #4: Anorectal Malformations

1. Clinical signs of perforation are often absent, so abdominal radiographs including a left lateral decubitus view should be obtained to evaluate for pneumoperitoneum.
2. Operative repair is urgently needed for ARM complicated by perforation, particularly in unstable infants.
3. Given the high risk of associated anomalies, infants with ARM should be evaluated with an echocardiogram, renal and bladder ultrasound, spinal ultrasound, and plain radiographs of the abdomen and lower spine.

IMPLEMENTATION OF GUIDELINE

DESCRIPTION OF IMPLEMENTATION STRATEGY

Recommend written guidelines for initial approach to intestinal obstruction.

QUALITY METRICS

Rates of intestinal perforation from obstruction, mortality rates, length of stay.

SCOPE

DISEASE/CONDITION(S)

Gastric perforations.

GUIDELINE OBJECTIVE(S)

Review potential etiology of neonatal gastric perforation. Review and identify recommendations for initial management of gastric perforations.

BRIEF BACKGROUND

Neonatal gastric perforation is a rare, serious, and life-threatening problem. The etiology and pathogenesis remain unknown. Historically, these perforations were thought to be spontaneous, though many potential risk factors have been identified, including prematurity, NEC, asphyxia, postnatal corticosteroid administration, nasal ventilation, and gastric trauma. Potential explanations include mechanical pneumatic rupture from severely increased gastric pressure, congenital defects of the gastric muscle wall, stress ulceration, and ischemia secondary to vascular shunting. Gastric perforation typically occurs between the second to seventh day of life. The most common site of perforation is the greater curvature of the stomach. Mortality rates are high, ranging from 25% to 83% in case reports. Potential poor prognostic indicators may include metabolic acidosis, hyponatremia, male gender, and low birth weight. Early diagnosis and urgent surgical intervention are essential for improved survival.

RECOMMENDATIONS

MAJOR RECOMMENDATIONS

1. As a preventative measure, all infants receiving nasal ventilation or clinically demonstrating abdominal distension should be decompressed with a gastric tube.

2. Particularly for infants with potential risk factors for gastric perforation, such as low birth weight, prematurity or asphyxia, enteral feeds should be initiated slowly, and tolerance of feeding monitored closely.

3. Urgent surgical intervention is necessary for all infants suspected of gastric perforation. Delayed surgical involvement is a poor prognostic indicator.

4. Initial stabilization should include bowel rest, initiation of IV fluids, and abdominal radiograph to confirm presence of perforation.

5. Obtain a blood gas and electrolytes to evaluate for metabolic acidosis or electrolyte abnormalities that require correction. If stable, obtain blood culture prior to initiation of broad-spectrum antibiotics.

IMPLEMENTATION OF GUIDELINE

DESCRIPTION OF IMPLEMENTATION STRATEGY

Recommend written guidelines for initial management of gastric perforations.

QUALITY METRICS

Rates of gastric perforations, mortality rates, time to surgical involvement.

SUMMARY

Intestinal and gastric perforation can occur in neonates due to variety of diseases including necrotizing enterocolitis, spontaneous intestinal perforation, and intestinal obstruction. Gastric perforation is a rare but life-threatening problem that may also result in pneumoperitoneum. Abdominal radiographs, both supine and left lateral decubitus views, should verify the presence of abdominal free air. Initial medical management should focus on stabilization of the infant through bowel rest, abdominal decompression via gastric tube, and initiation of intravenous fluids and broad-spectrum antibiotics. Hemodynamically unstable infants may require further management with increased respiratory support, pressor initiation, isotonic fluid boluses, or blood product transfusion. Laboratory studies should be obtained to evaluate for acidosis, electrolyte abnormalities, infection, coagulopathy, anemia, thrombocytopenia, and systemic inflammation. Surgery consultation is indicated for further management of perforated viscera and should be obtained urgently for unstable patients.

BIBLIOGRAPHIC SOURCE(S)

Berman L, Moss RL. Necrotizing enterocolitis: an update. *Semin Fetal Neonatal Med.* 2011;16:145-50.

Dominquez KM, Moss RL. Necrotizing enterocolitis. *Clin Perinatol.* 2012;39:387-401.

Duran R, Inan M, Vatansever U, Aladag N, Acunas D. Etiology of neonatal gastric perforations: review of 10 years' experience. *Pediatr Int.* 2007;49:626-30.

Gordon PV, Young ML, Marshall DD. Focal small bowel perforation: an adverse effect of early postnatal dexamethasone therapy in extremely low birth weight infants. *J Perinatol.* 2001;21:156-60.

Juang D, Snyder CL. Neonatal bowel obstruction. *Surg Clin N Am.* 2012;92:685-711.

Khope S, Vivekanand S. Neonatal colonic perforation with low anorectal anomaly: a case report. *J Postgrad Med.* 1989;35:226-7.

Lin C, Lee H, Kao H, et al. Neonatal gastric perforation: report of 15 cases and review of the literature. *Pediatr Neonatol.* 2008;49:65-70.

Neu J, Walker WA. Necrotizing enterocolitis. *N Engl J Med.* 2011;364(3):255-64.

Raveenthiran V. Spontaneous perforation of the colon and rectum complicating anorectal malformations in neonates. *J Pediatr Surg.* 2012;47:720-6.

Shah D, Sinn JKH. Antibiotic regimens for the empirical treatment of newborn infants with necrotising enterocolitis. *Cochrane Database Syst Rev.* 2012;(8):CD007448.

Sharma R, Hudak ML. A clinical perspective of necrotizing enterocolitis: past, present and future. *Clin Perinatol.* 2013;40(1):27-51.

Sharma R, Hudak ML, Tepas JJ 3rd, et al. Prenatal or postnatal indomethacin exposure and neonatal gut injury associated with isolated intestinal perforation and necrotizing enterocolitis. *J Perinatol.* 2010;30(12):786-93.

Stark AR, Carlo WA, Tyson JE, et al. Adverse effects of early dexamethasone in extremely-low-birth-weight infants. *N Engl J Med.* 2001; 344:95–101.

Terui K, Iwai J, Yamada S, et al. Etiology of neonatal gastric perforation: a review of 20 years' experience. *Pediatr Surg Int.* 2012;28:9-14.

Tongsong T, Chanprapaph P. Prenatal diagnosis of isolated anorectal atresia with colonic perforation. *J Obstet Gynaecol Res.* 2001;27:241-4.

Gastrointestinal Obstruction

Jennifer M. Trzaski, MD • James E. Moore, MD, PhD

SCOPE

DISEASE/CONDITION(S)

Diagnosis and treatment of neonates with symptoms of gastrointestinal obstruction.

GUIDELINE OBJECTIVE(S)

The objectives of this chapter are to review the symptoms of neonatal gastrointestinal obstruction, describe diagnostic approaches to the neonate with symptoms of gastrointestinal obstruction, and identify treatment options for infants with gastrointestinal obstruction.

BRIEF BACKGROUND

Gastrointestinal obstruction is a common reason for neonatal intensive care. The overall incidence of gastrointestinal obstruction is approximately 1:2000. Early symptoms of gastrointestinal obstruction include nonbilious or bilious emesis, abdominal distention, and failure to pass meconium. Left unrecognized, the sequelae of gastrointestinal obstruction can be life threatening and include sepsis, shock, and necrosis of significant portions of bowel. Early recognition and treatment can prevent lifelong complications and death.

SCOPE

DISEASE/CONDITION(S)

Pyloric stenosis.

GUIDELINE OBJECTIVE(S)

To identify and review diagnostic approaches to and pre- and postoperative management of pyloric stenosis.

BRIEF BACKGROUND

Epidemiology

The incidence of pyloric stenosis varies based on geographic location with rates of 2–5/1000 live births in the Western world and decreased incidence in Asian and African populations. There is a male predominance with a male:female ratio of 4–5:1.

Pathophysiology

The etiology of pyloric stenosis is poorly understood and considered to be multifactorial, with a combination of environmental and genetic factors playing a role.

There appears to be abnormal innervation of the pylorus making the muscle unable to relax, leading to increased synthesis of growth factors and hypertrophy of the muscle.

Bottle-fed infants have an increased risk of developing pyloric stenosis compared to breastfed infants, with the theory that breast milk contains vasoactive intestinal peptide which serves to relax the pylorus.

Macrolide antibiotics, specifically erythromycin, have been associated with the development of pyloric stenosis by serving as motilin agonists.

The genetic etiology behind the development of pyloric stenosis is poorly understood but may involve single-nucleotide polymorphisms (SNPs) regulating the production of nitric oxide, as well as other SNPs which have been identified in genome-wide association studies.

Presentation

Infants usually present between 3 weeks and 3 months of age with non-bilious, projectile vomiting.

Because the hypertrophied pylorus will prevent bile reflux into the stomach, bilious emesis should prompt urgent evaluation for other intestinal obstruction.

Pathognomonic acid-base and electrolyte abnormalities include a hypochloremic, hypokalemic metabolic alkalosis; however, many infants may present with normal laboratory values.

RECOMMENDATIONS

MAJOR RECOMMENDATIONS

Diagnosis

History of vomiting and physical examination finding of the hypertrophied pyloric muscle or "olive" is considered diagnostic of pyloric stenosis with a positive predictive value of 99%.

However, successful palpation of the hypertrophied muscle or "olive" is difficult and requires an experienced examiner. Sensitivity and specificity of physical examination to diagnose pyloric stenosis ranged from 31% to 100% across various studies.

Ultrasound is the preferred imaging modality for diagnosis of pyloric stenosis due to the rapid, noninvasive nature of the test and lack of radiation exposure.

Ultrasound diagnosis demonstrating the hypertrophied pyloric canal, length >15 mm and muscle thickness >3 mm, has near 100% sensitivity and specificity.

When performed at referral centers, upper GI has high sensitivity (96%) and specificity (100%) for diagnosing pyloric stenosis, but is more invasive than ultrasound, exposes infants to radiation, and due to potential for vomiting during the study, increases the risk of aspiration.

Preoperative Fluid Resuscitation

Evaluation of the degree of dehydration, identification and correction of electrolyte abnormalities, and fluid resuscitation are essential prior to surgical intervention.

IV access should be obtained promptly.

Fluid resuscitation is recommended with 5% dextrose with 0.45% normal saline at 1.25–2 times maintenance until adequate rehydration and urine output are achieved and electrolytes and acid-base status normalize.

10–20 mEg/L potassium chloride can be added to IV fluids either initially or once urine output is established.

Potassium chloride concentration can be increased too but should not exceed 30 mEq/L depending on the degree of hypokalemia.

Electrolytes should be obtained with initial clinical evaluation and followed serially until levels normalize.

Chloride levels >100 and HCO_3 levels <30 are felt to be acceptable levels at which the metabolic alkalosis is corrected sufficiently to ensure safe anesthesia and prevent post-operative apnea related to carbon dioxide retention as compensatory mechanism for the metabolic alkalosis.

Cl and HCO_3 normal, but K abnormal, then 20 mL/kg normal saline bolus and repeat electrolytes.

If Cl ≤97 or HCO_3 ≥33, then 20 mL/kg normal saline × 2 boluses and repeat electrolytes.

If Cl <85 or HCO_3 ≥40, then 20 mL/kg normal saline × 3 boluses and repeat electrolytes.

Postoperative Management

Ad libitum feeding significantly decreases length of stay following pyloromyotomy versus a structured feeding regimen.

Therefore, ad libitum and early feeding following pyloromyotomy is recommended.

Upon awakening from general anesthesia, infants may be fed full-strength formula or breast milk ad libitum and IV fluids weaned off.

Discharge may occur once tolerating feeds and off IV fluids.

While postoperative emesis has been shown to be increased in infants fed early and often, this has no negative impact or increase in postoperative complications.

Significant emesis may necessitate use of a structured feeding regimen.

IMPLEMENTATION OF GUIDELINE

DESCRIPTION OF IMPLEMENTATION STRATEGY

- Recommend written guidelines for diagnosis of pyloric stenosis using ultrasonography.
- Recommend written guidelines for fluid resuscitation and electrolyte monitoring.
- Recommend written guidelines for postoperative feeding protocol.

QUALITY METRICS

- Monitor time to correction of electrolyte abnormalities, rehydration, and time to surgical repair.
- Monitor quantity and frequency of emesis following postoperative initiation of feeds.
- Monitor length of stay.

SUMMARY

Pyloric stenosis is a common surgical condition in the infant. Rapid identification of the condition and the degree of dehydration and electrolyte abnormalities can lead to appropriate fluid resuscitation and optimal timing for surgical repair. A postoperative feeding protocol employing early, ad libitum feeds leads to shortened length of stay following pyloromyotomy.

SCOPE

DISEASE/CONDITION(S)

Malrotation and volvulus.

GUIDELINE OBJECTIVE(S)

To identify and review diagnostic approaches to and management of infants with malrotation and volvulus.

BRIEF BACKGROUND

Epidemiology

Incidence of malrotation varies with estimates ranging from approximately 1:500 to 1:6000 live births.

Extra-intestinal associations are common, occurring in approximately 30–60% of cases of malrotation, and include congenital heart disease, specifically heterotaxy syndrome, duodenal, jejunoileal and colonic atresia, anorectal malformations, Hirschsprung disease, and abdominal wall defects.

Pathophysiology

Disorders of rotation occur early in development, with failure of normal rotation and fixation of the intestine during embryogenesis.

Genetics

Malrotation with volvulus is usually not associated with genetic or syndromic causes. However, recent gene analysis has demonstrated that in some cases malrotation has been associated with FOXF1 mutations.

Presentation

Malrotation may be asymptomatic, chronic, or present acutely.

Approximately 50% of cases present within the first week of life, 75% within the first month, and approximately 90% of cases within the first year.

Infants present with bilious emesis with or without abdominal tenderness and distention.

If diagnosis is delayed, symptoms of sepsis and shock develop, including abdominal wall erythema, hematemesis, leukocytosis or leukopenia, thrombocytopenia, metabolic acidosis, and electrolyte abnormalities.

RECOMMENDATIONS

MAJOR RECOMMENDATIONS

Diagnosis

Infants who are clinically stable should have abdominal radiographs, including a lateral view to evaluate for obstruction; however, there are no findings on plain x-rays that can effectively rule out malrotation and volvulus.

The gold standard for diagnosis is the upper GI series, which looks to evaluate the position of the ligament of Treitz and the duodenojejunal junction.

Malrotation with obstruction or volvulus may result in the corkscrew appearance of the duodenum.

If the upper GI study is equivocal, small bowel follow-through or barium enema may be considered to document the position of the cecum.

Preoperative Management

Infants should be made NPO and have a nasogastric tube placed for gastric decompression.

IV access should be secured, and infants should receive IV fluid resuscitation.

Infants should have complete blood counts and chemistries obtained along with blood cultures and consideration of coagulation factors.

Broad-spectrum antibiotic therapy should be administered.

Acutely ill infants may need urgent surgical intervention with the Ladd procedure.

Postoperative Management

Infants will return from the operating room intubated and ventilated. Ventilator management should be optimized and the infant extubated when appropriate.

Central venous line (CVL) may be placed intraoperatively depending on the extent of disease and bowel resection.

Nasogastric tube remains in place and volume and quality of output is closely monitored. Consider isotonic fluid, either normal saline or lactated Ringer's replacement with KCL supplementation if output is excessive.

Total parenteral nutrition (TPN) should be initiated early if initiation of enteral feeds is expected to be delayed.

Traditionally, the nasogastric tube is removed and enteral feeds are started when nasogastric tube output decreases in volume, is no longer bilious, and the infant is stooling.

IMPLEMENTATION OF GUIDELINE

DESCRIPTION OF IMPLEMENTATION STRATEGY

- Recommend written guidelines for diagnostic approach for infants with suspected malrotation and volvulus.
- Recommend written guidelines for preoperative management of infants diagnosed with malrotation and volvulus.
- Recommend written guidelines for postoperative management of infants diagnosed malrotation and volvulus.

QUALITY METRICS

- Monitor time from diagnosis to surgical repair.
- Monitor number of infants requiring bowel resection.
- Monitor development of short gut syndrome for infants requiring more extensive bowel resection.
- Monitor time to initiation of and time to full enteral feedings.
- Monitor CVL days and line infections.
- Monitor TPN days.
- Monitor length of stay following surgical repair.
- Monitor for postoperative complications including infection, postoperative ileus, and obstruction due to development of adhesions.

SUMMARY

Bilious emesis in the newborn can be an ominous sign of intestinal obstruction from malrotation with volvulus. Malrotation alone may be asymptomatic, but the majority of infants present within the first month of life. Upper GI is considered the gold standard for evaluation and diagnosis of malrotation. Acutely ill infants or infants with evidence of malrotation with volvulus require urgent surgical intervention. Time for normal bowel function to return may be prolonged in some infants depending on the extent of bowel involved and resected.

SCOPE

DISEASE/CONDITION(S)

Duodenal obstruction: atresia, webs.

GUIDELINE OBJECTIVE(S)

To identify and review diagnostic approaches to and management of infants with duodenal atresia.

BRIEF BACKGROUND

Epidemiology

The incidence of duodenal atresia ranges from 1:5000 to 1:10,000 live births with a male predominance.

More than 50% of infants with duodenal obstruction have other associated congenital anomalies, including congenital heart disease, esophageal atresia, imperforate anus, renal anomalies, and skeletal and central nervous system (CNS) anomalies.

Approximately 25% of infants with duodenal obstruction have other associated GI anomalies.

Between 25% and 30% of infants with duodenal atresia have Down syndrome.

Other anomalies may be related to the VACTERL association.

Studies have shown duodenal obstruction to be associated with prematurity and small for gestational age; however, incidence varies and appears to be higher when duodenal obstruction is caused by an annular pancreas.

Pathophysiology

The etiology of duodenal obstruction is felt to be related to abnormal foregut development, possibly related to lack of recanalization of the intestine at the solid cord stage of development during the 8th–10th weeks of gestation versus errors in cellular signaling and migration early in development. Anatomic pancreatic abnormalities such as annular pancreas can also cause duodenal obstruction.

Duodenal obstructions are classified into three types: type 1 defect is a mucosal web with a normal muscular wall, type 2 defects are described as two atretic ends of the duodenum connected by a short fibrous cord, and type 3 defects have complete separation of the atretic ends of the duodenum.

In the majority of cases, the ampulla of Vater is located proximal to the obstruction.

Presentation

Cardinal signs of duodenal obstruction in the fetus include polyhydramnios and a double bubble resulting from a dilated stomach and proximal duodenum. Other associated congenital anomalies may be diagnosed on prenatal ultrasound.

For infants undiagnosed prenatally, age at diagnosis is earlier for infants with duodenal atresia (1–10 days, mean 5.5 days) or annular pancreas (1–30 days, mean 15.5 days). Infants with a duodenal web causing the obstruction present later (3–90 days, mean 46.5 days).

Eighty to ninety percent of infants present with bilious emesis within a few hours of birth. Clinical examination may detect subtle distention of the stomach; however, the abdomen is generally described as being scaphoid. For a small number (10–15%) of infants in which the ampulla of Vater is distal to the obstruction, emesis may be non-bilious.

RECOMMENDATIONS

MAJOR RECOMMENDATIONS

Diagnosis

Approximately half of mothers with polyhydramnios will have fetuses with a double bubble suggestive of duodenal atresia.

Antenatal suspicion of duodenal obstruction should prompt investigation for other associated congenital anomalies.

Postnatal acquisition of an abdominal radiograph demonstrating the double bubble appearance of the dilated stomach and proximal duodenum and a paucity of distal bowel gas is diagnostic of duodenal obstruction.

Upper GI may be diagnostic for cases of partial duodenal obstruction due to stenosis or duodenal web, in which case the windsock appearance is pathognomonic.

Careful physical examination should be performed, looking for other congenital anomalies. Cardiac echocardiogram and renal ultrasound should be considered.

Preoperative Management

Infants should be made NPO and nasogastric tube placed to suction.

IV fluids should be started with the goal of achieving fluid resuscitation, maintaining appropriate hydration status, and restoring any electrolyte abnormalities.

Surgical correction is non-urgent and should be performed only once the infant is clinically stable.

Postoperative Management

Infants will return from the operating room intubated and ventilated. Ventilator management should be optimized with expected extubation within 1–4 days postoperatively.

Central venous line may be placed intraoperatively, and parenteral nutrition provided until enteral feeds are established postoperatively.

Nasogastric tube is placed, and volume and quality of output is closely monitored.

Traditionally, the nasogastric tube is removed and enteral feeds are started when nasogastric tube output decreases in volume and is no longer bilious.

While some infants may be managed without parenteral nutrition when feedings are started early, delayed initiation of parenteral nutrition has been shown to compromise infants' growth.

Parenteral nutrition can be stopped when the volume of enteral feeds reaches 100–120 mL/kg/day.

More recent evidence has demonstrated success with earlier initiation of enteral feeds, regardless of the quantity and quality of gastric output.

Consideration may be given to performing an upper GI study between postoperative days 5–7. If the study demonstrates no anastomotic leak or stricture, the nasogastric tube can be removed and enteral feeds started and advanced.

An alternative approach to postoperative enteral feedings is to place a transanastomotic feeding tube and initiate continuous enteral feeds within 24–48 hours postoperatively. This approach may decrease the time to full enteral feeds and the need for CVL and parenteral nutrition. However, other studies have demonstrated longer time to full enteral feeds or longer length of stay with this approach.

IMPLEMENTATION OF GUIDELINE

DESCRIPTION OF IMPLEMENTATION STRATEGY

- Recommend written guidelines for diagnostic approach for infants with suspected duodenal obstruction.
- Recommend written guidelines for preoperative management of infants diagnosed with duodenal obstruction.
- Recommend written guidelines for postoperative management of infants diagnosed with duodenal obstruction.

QUALITY METRICS

- Monitor time to initiation of feeds and time to full enteral feeds postoperatively.
- Monitor CVL days and line infections.
- Monitor TPN days.
- Monitor length of stay following surgical repair.
- Monitor for postoperative complications including infection due to bowel bacterial translocation, stricture formation and anastomotic leak.

SUMMARY

Duodenal obstruction may be diagnosed antenatally in mothers with polyhydramnios whose fetuses are found to have a double-bubble appearance of the stomach and proximal duodenum on ultrasound. Postnatally, infants present shortly after birth with bilious emesis and a non-distended, scaphoid abdomen. Abdominal x-ray demonstrating a double bubble is diagnostic of duodenal obstruction.

Infants with duodenal obstruction should be made NPO, a nasogastric tube should be placed to suction, and IV fluid resuscitation should commence with correction of any electrolyte abnormalities. Infants should undergo surgical repair once clinically stable. A CVL may be placed intraoperatively.

Postoperative management includes ventilator management, maintaining the nasogastric tube while monitoring quantity and quality of output, and administration of parenteral nutrition. Enteral feeds may be started at the recommendation of the surgical team when the quantity of gastric output has decreased and is non-bilious in quality.

SCOPE

DISEASE/CONDITION(S)

Jejunoileal atresia.

GUIDELINE OBJECTIVE(S)

To identify and review diagnostic approaches to and management of infants with jejunoileal atresia.

BRIEF BACKGROUND

Epidemiology

The incidence of jejunoileal atresia (JIA) is approximately 1:5000 and it affects both genders equally.

Approximately one-third of infants with JIA are premature, with a higher incidence of prematurity occurring in type IIIb apple-peel deformity JIA.

Most cases of JIA are sporadic.

There is a low incidence of associated congenital anomalies; however, cystic fibrosis, gastroschisis, and malrotation are associated with JIA in approximately 10% of cases. Other studies have documented a higher incidence of associated anomalies.

Pathophysiology

JIA is thought to occur due to vascular disruption and ischemic insult to the midgut during fetal life resulting in ischemic necrosis of a segment or segments of bowel.

There has been some association between maternal cigarette smoking, use of vasoconstrictive medications, or cocaine and subsequent development of JIA.

There are four types of JIA: type I is a stenosis or diaphragm; type II is an atresia with a gap in the lumen of the intestine, but mesenteric continuity; type III is further subdivided into two groups, IIIa being a gap defect in the intestine and mesentery and type IIIb is the apple-peel deformity; type IV is multiple atresias.

The type IIIb apple-peel deformity JIA consists of a proximal jejunal atresia with a foreshortened small bowel. The ileocolic or right colic artery supplies the distal small bowel.

Atresia of the small intestine usually results in dilation and dysfunction of the bowel proximal to the atresia and a microcolon distal to the atresia.

Presentation

Polyhydramnios, dilated loops, and echogenic bowel may be present antenatally.

Postnatal presentation varies depending on the location of the obstruction.

Proximal obstruction presents with bilious emesis usually within the first 24 hours of life, while more distal obstruction presents slightly later within 48 hours of life with abdominal distention and visible bowel loops.

Failure to pass meconium may occur with more distal obstruction, but this is not diagnostic, as infants with more proximal obstruction may pass meconium.

RECOMMENDATIONS

MAJOR RECOMMENDATIONS

Diagnosis

Approximately one-third of cases can be diagnosed prenatally when polyhydramnios, dilated bowel loops, and echogenic bowel are found on ultrasound.

Infants with bilious emesis or abdominal distention should have an abdominal radiograph.

Abdominal radiograph demonstrates dilated loops of bowel, sometimes with a triple bubble indicative of dilated stomach, duodenum, and proximal jejunum, and air–fluid levels.

Upper GI is usually not indicated unless there is concern for intestinal stenosis or malrotation with volvulus.

Contrast enema can be useful to confirm the diagnosis of atresia, distinguish from other obstructive etiologies, evaluate rotation of the intestine, and evaluate the caliber of the colon.

If peritoneal calcifications are seen on abdominal films, intrauterine perforation with meconium peritonitis should be suspected and raise concern for a diagnosis of cystic fibrosis.

Sweat testing and genetic testing should be considered to evaluate for cystic fibrosis.

Preoperative Management

Infants should be made NPO and nasogastric tube placed to suction to decompress the stomach.

IV fluids should be started with the goal of achieving fluid resuscitation, maintaining appropriate hydration status, and restoring any electrolyte abnormalities.

Broad-spectrum antibiotics should be administered.

Surgical correction should be performed once the infant is clinically stable, unless there is concern for associated malrotation with volvulus necessitating more urgent repair or gastroschisis, in which case delayed repair may take place after recovery from gastroschisis closure.

Postoperative Management

Infants will return from the operating room intubated and ventilated. Ventilator management should be optimized and the infant extubated when appropriate.

Central venous line should be placed intraoperatively.

Nasogastric tube remains in place and volume and quality of output is closely monitored.

Total parenteral nutrition should be initiated early.

Traditionally, the nasogastric tube is removed and enteral feeds are started when nasogastric tube output decreases in volume, is no longer bilious, and the infant is stooling.

Parenteral nutrition can be stopped when the volume of enteral feeds reaches 100–120 mL/kg/day.

A multidisciplinary team consisting of neonatologists, gastroenterologists, pediatric surgeons, and dieticians has been shown to optimize outcomes in infants at highest risk for intestinal failure.

Short Bowel Syndrome

Infants with jejunoileal atresia are at high risk for development of short bowel syndrome depending on both quantity of bowel remaining following resection and function of the remaining bowel, which is often abnormal due to dysmotility, and dysfunction of the remaining segments of bowel.

The goal of surgical repair of JIA focuses on resecting necessary sections of bowel while preserving the maximum amount of bowel possible.

Infants with short bowel syndrome will have prolonged TPN dependence while adaptation to enteral feeding takes place over months to years.

IMPLEMENTATION OF GUIDELINE

DESCRIPTION OF IMPLEMENTATION STRATEGY

- Recommend written guidelines for diagnostic approach for infants with suspected JIA.
- Recommend written guidelines for preoperative management of infants diagnosed with JIA.
- Recommend written guidelines for postoperative management of infants diagnosed with JIA.
- Consider development of a multidisciplinary team of neonatologists, gastroenterologists, pediatric surgeons, and dieticians to manage infants at highest risk for intestinal maladaptation and failure.

QUALITY METRICS

- Monitor time to initiation of feeds and time to full enteral feeds postoperatively.
- Monitor CVL days and line infections.
- Monitor TPN days.
- Monitor length of stay following surgical repair.
- Monitor for postoperative complications including infection due to bowel bacterial translocation, stricture formation, anastomotic leak, functional obstruction or dysmotility.
- Monitor incidence of short bowel syndrome.

SUMMARY

JIA may be suspected antenatally in mothers with polyhydramnios whose fetuses are found to have echogenic bowel. Postnatally, infants may present within 24–48 hours with bilious emesis. Infants with more distal obstruction present with marked abdominal distention. Abdominal x-ray demonstrating dilated loops of bowel with air fluid levels, possibly a triple bubble, with a paucity of distal bowel gas is concerning for JIA. Contrast enema can differentiate distal atresia from other forms of obstruction, evaluate for intestinal rotation and microcolon.

Infants with JIA should be made NPO, a nasogastric tube should be placed to suction, IV fluid resuscitation should commence with correction of any electrolyte abnormalities, and broad-spectrum antibiotic administered.

Infants should undergo surgical repair once clinically stable unless there is concern for malrotation with volvulus or gastroschisis is present. A CVL may be placed intraoperatively. Postoperative management includes ventilator management, maintaining the nasogastric tube while monitoring quantity and quality of output, and administration of parenteral nutrition. Enteral feeds may be started at the recommendation of the surgical team when the quantity of gastric output has decreased, is non-bilious in quality, and the infant is stooling.

Infants with JIA are at high risk for development of short bowel syndrome. A multidisciplinary team may help optimize outcomes in this group of high-risk infants.

SCOPE

DISEASE/CONDITION(S)

Meconium disease.

GUIDELINE OBJECTIVE(S)

To identify and review diagnostic approaches to and management of infants with meconium ileus (MI) and meconium plug syndrome (MPS).

BRIEF BACKGROUND

Epidemiology

Meconium Ileus. The incidence of MI is approximately 1:3000–3500 and is believed to account for between 10% and 30% of bowel obstruction in the neonate.

MI is one of the earliest manifestations of cystic fibrosis (CF). Between 80% and 95% of infants with MI have CF; conversely, between 10% and 20% of infants with CF have MI.

The majority of infants who present with simple MI have CF, while presentation with complex MI is less likely to be associated with CF.

MI associated with prematurity is less likely to be associated with CF and more likely to be related to poor intestinal motility, slow peristalsis causing failure of meconium to move through the intestine, and increased absorption of water from meconium leaving thick, inspissated meconium in the bowel.

Meconium Plug Syndrome. MPS occurs in approximately 1 in 500 liveborn infants.

Some have questioned the association of MPS with Hirschsprung disease, cystic fibrosis, in utero exposure to magnesium, and small left colon syndrome, but more recent reports discount these associations.

Pathophysiology

Meconium Ileus. MI is classified as simple MI or complex MI. Simple MI presents with failure to pass meconium, and abdominal distention, while with complex MI, obstruction is associated with other pathology including bowel atresia, necrosis, perforation, meconium peritonitis, or pseudocyst formation.

Infants who present with complex MI who also have CF are most likely to be homozygous for the delta F08 mutation, while those with simple MI have other mutations.

Mutations in the delta-F508 and G542X genes are associated with an increased incidence of MI disease, while mutations in G551D and R117H are associated with a decreased incidence of MI disease in infants with CF.

In addition, modifier genes have been discovered that may influence the development of MI in infants with CF.

No genetic factors have been identified in infants with MI who do not have CF.

Meconium peritonitis is broken down into four types: adhesive, pseudocyst, ascites, or infected pseudocyst.

In situations where MI is associated with CF, the underlying pathology is felt to be caused by thick, adhesive, desiccated meconium that obstructs the lumen of the ileum.

Mutations in the CF transmembrane conductance regulator (CFTR) chloride channels of CF patients create an abnormal electrolyte balance in the lumen of the bowel that results in thick, dehydrated meconium.

In cases where MI is not associated with CF, the proposed etiology for MI is immaturity of the myenteric plexus and interstitial cells of Cajal leading to hypomotility of the intestine. Gastrointestinal malformations may also play a causative role, creating an anatomic obstruction that leads to impaction of meconium proximal to the site of obstruction.

Meconium Plug. MPS is a benign intestinal obstruction caused by colonic obstruction from inspissated meconium.

Presentation

Meconium Ileus. Simple MI often presents within 24–48 hours of birth with delayed passage of meconium, abdominal distention, and bilious emesis. Examination may be significant for palpable loops of bowel, but abdominal tenderness and respiratory embarrassment are uncommon.

Presentation of complex MI is variable. Infants who perforate in utero earlier in gestation may be asymptomatic at delivery with an incidental finding of calcifications on abdominal radiograph.

Infants with an in utero perforation that occurs later in gestation often present soon after delivery with signs and symptoms of acute peritonitis and possibly shock.

Meconium Plug. MPS presents with failure to pass meconium within 24–48 hours of birth, abdominal distention, and emesis.

RECOMMENDATIONS

MAJOR RECOMMENDATIONS

Meconium Ileus

Diagnosis. Antenatal ultrasound features suggestive of MI are hyperechoic masses possibly representing inspissated meconium, dilated bowel loops, and inability to visualize the gallbladder.

All women of childbearing age should be offered preconception or prenatal screening for CF. Pregnancies are considered low risk if ultrasound features of MI are suspected in a fetus with a mother with negative CF carrier status, and high risk if features of MI are suspected in a fetus with parents who are known CF carriers or have had a previous child with CF.

Following delivery or with onset of symptoms, abdominal radiograph should be obtained.

In simple MI, abdominal radiographs demonstrate dilated loops of proximal bowel, and the distal bowel may have a ground glass appearance due to the presence of inspissated meconium.

With complex MI, abdominal radiographs may show dilated loops of bowel, calcifications, free air, air–fluid levels, pseudocyst formation, or ascites.

Water-soluble hyperosmolar contrast enema may be both diagnostic and therapeutic if it demonstrates inspissated meconium pellets and a microcolon.

Preoperative Management. Infant should be made NPO and nasogastric tube should be placed for gastric decompression.

Infants should receive IV fluid resuscitation.

Broad-spectrum antibiotic therapy should be administered.

For simple MI, rectal washouts with a water-soluble hyperosmotic enema should be tried before proceeding with operative management.

If washouts are successful in producing meconium stools, they are continued until the infant stools spontaneously.

Serial radiographs may be considered to confirm evacuation of the bowel and to rule out perforation related to the washouts.

If rectal washouts fail to result in passage of meconium or the infant presents with complex MI, the infant requires operative management.

Postoperative Management. Intestinal lavage of the bowel via nasogastric tube or enterostomy may help flush out residual meconium.

Initial postoperative management focuses on fluid resuscitation to replace preoperative losses from hyperosmolar enemas inducing diarrhea, intraoperative fluid losses, and nasogastric or enterostomy drainage.

Total parenteral nutrition should be used in the early postoperative period.

Enteral feeds may be started once the infant passes stool.

If the infant required a large resection of bowel, continuous feeds may be considered with partially hydrolyzed or elemental formulas.

Management of MI in the Face of CF. All infants with MI should have genetic and sweat testing to rule out CF.

If infants are confirmed to have CF, pancreatic insufficiency should be presumed and infants started on pancreatic enzyme replacement therapy.

Growth trends, electrolytes, and nutritional status should be followed closely, particularly if infants require enterostomy placement.

Meconium Plug Syndrome

Diagnosis. Abdominal radiograph should be obtained.

Contrast enema is performed and is both diagnostic and therapeutic for MPS.

Treatment. Infants with suspected MPS may respond to rectal stimulation.

If rectal stimulation alone does not result in passage of meconium, contrast enema should be performed.

MPS usually resolves following the contrast enema, however on occasion infants who fail to respond to nonoperative management require surgery.

If infants continue to have an abnormal stooling pattern following contrast enema, further evaluation should be pursued, including rectal suction biopsy to evaluate for Hirschsprung disease.

PRACTICE OPTIONS

Meconium Ileus

Consider attempt to solubilize inspissated meconium with water-soluble hyperosmotic contrast enemas.

Simple MI may require enterotomy with intraoperative intestinal washout.

MI may require enterostomy placement versus primary anastomotic repair depending on complexity and extent of disease and infant's illness severity.

Controversy exists as to duration of enterostomy placement—early versus late takedown depending on infant's nutritional and electrolyte status.

IMPLEMENTATION OF GUIDELINE

DESCRIPTION OF IMPLEMENTATION STRATEGY

- Recommend written guidelines for diagnostic approach for infants with MI.
- Recommend written guidelines for preoperative management of infants diagnosed with MI.
- Recommend written guidelines for postoperative management of infants diagnosed with MI.
- Recommend written guidelines for diagnostic and therapeutic management of infants with suspected MPS.

QUALITY METRICS

Meconium Ileus

- Monitor success of treatment of simple MI with water-soluble hyperosmolar contrast enemas.
- Monitor for perforation, inflammation, enterocolitis, or shock following treatment with enemas.
- Monitor outcomes of infants who undergo enterotomy with bowel irrigation, resection with primary anastomosis, or resection with enterostomy placement for management of MI including development of post-anastomotic leak, stoma prolapse, development of adhesions and secondary bowel obstruction, development of peritonitis, growth and nutritional status, serum electrolytes, duration of TPN, time to commencement of enteral feeds, time to full enteral feeds, length of hospital stay.

Meconium Plug Syndrome

- Successful treatment of obstruction with nonoperative measures.
- Number of infants requiring further evaluation for other etiologies of obstruction, including Hirschsprung disease.

SUMMARY

Meconium Ileus

MI is caused by impaction of thick inspissated meconium in the terminal ileum leading to bowel obstruction in the neonate. MI is often associated with CF, and all infants with MI should have genetic and sweat testing for CF.

Water-soluble hyperosmolar contrast enemas can be both diagnostic and therapeutic for infants with simple MI. Rectal washouts may be efficacious in relieving the obstruction and avoiding surgery. If rectal washouts are unsuccessful or the infant has complex MI, the infant may require surgery including enterotomy with intraoperative bowel irrigation or resection with either enterostomy or primary anastomosis. Postoperative fluid, electrolyte, and nutritional management is imperative, especially for infants diagnosed with CF.

Meconium Plug Syndrome

MPS is a benign bowel obstruction caused by inspissated meconium in the colon. MPS is successfully treated in a nonoperative manner with either rectal stimulation or contrast enema. On occasion, abnormal stooling patterns persist and the infant may require further evaluation or other etiologies of obstruction, specifically Hirschsprung disease.

SCOPE

DISEASE/CONDITION(S)

Colonic atresia.

GUIDELINE OBJECTIVE(S)

To identify and review diagnostic approaches to and management of infants with colonic atresia.

BRIEF BACKGROUND

Epidemiology

Colonic atresia is very rare, with an incidence of approximately 1:20,000, and comprises between 2% and 15% of intestinal atresias.

Colonic atresia has been shown to be associated with Hirschsprung disease, gastroschisis, and multiple small intestinal atresias as well as urologic and skeletal anomalies.

Pathophysiology

Colonic atresia is felt to be caused by a vascular injury during fetal life.

There are three types of colonic atresia: type 1, where there is a mucosal atresia with an intact bowel wall and mesentery; type 2, when a fibrous cord separates atretic ends of bowel; and type 3, where a V-shaped mesenteric gap separates the atretic ends of bowel.

Genetics

No genetic association or predisposition has been linked to development of colonic atresia.

Presentation

Infants with colonic atresia usually present within 1–5 days after birth with abdominal distention, bilious emesis, and failure to pass meconium.

RECOMMENDATIONS

MAJOR RECOMMENDATIONS

Diagnosis

Diagnosis of colonic atresia may be suspected prenatally if the diameter of the colon is larger than expected for gestational age, but in general findings are nonspecific and other forms of bowel obstruction or intestinal atresia cannot be ruled out.

Infants with bilious emesis or abdominal distention should have an abdominal radiograph.

Abdominal radiograph demonstrates dilated loops of bowel with air-fluid levels indicative of bowel obstruction. A large, dilated loop of colon proximal to the atresia may be seen.

Contrast enema can be useful to confirm the diagnosis of atresia, distinguish from other obstructive etiologies, and evaluate the caliber of the colon.

Evaluation for Hirschsprung disease is recommended.

Preoperative Management

Infants should be made NPO and nasogastric tube placed to suction to decompress the stomach.

IV fluids should be started with the goal of achieving fluid resuscitation, maintaining appropriate hydration status, and restoring any electrolyte abnormalities.

Broad-spectrum antibiotics should be administered.

Surgical correction should be performed as soon as possible, ideally after clinical stabilization, fluid resuscitation has occurred, and electrolyte abnormalities corrected. However, correction is relatively urgent due to the presence of the ileocecal valve preventing colonic decompression, which can create massive proximal colonic dilation with risk of bowel necrosis and perforation.

Infants operated on 72 hours after birth had an increased mortality rate in comparison to infants who underwent surgical repair within 72 hours of birth.

Postoperative Management

Infants will return from the operating room intubated and ventilated. Ventilator management should be optimized and the infant extubated when appropriate.

Central venous line should be placed intraoperatively.

Nasogastric tube remains in place and volume and quality of output is closely monitored.

Total parenteral nutrition should be initiated early.

Traditionally, the nasogastric tube is removed and enteral feeds are started when nasogastric tube output decreases in volume, is no longer bilious, and the infant is stooling.

Parenteral nutrition can be stopped when the volume of enteral feeds reaches 100–120 mL/kg/day. It has been demonstrated that most infants with colonic atresia transition from TPN to full enteral feeds in approximately 1 week.

IMPLEMENTATION OF GUIDELINE

DESCRIPTION OF IMPLEMENTATION STRATEGY

- Recommend written guidelines for diagnostic approach for infants with suspected colonic atresia.
- Recommend written guidelines for preoperative management of infants diagnosed with colonic atresia.
- Recommend written guidelines for postoperative management of infants diagnosed with colonic atresia.

QUALITY METRICS

- Monitor time to initiation of feeds and time to full enteral feeds postoperatively.
- Monitor CVL days and line infections.
- Monitor TPN days.
- Monitor length of stay following surgical repair.
- Monitor for postoperative complications including infection, postoperative ileus, prolapse of stoma, and obstruction due to development of adhesions.

SUMMARY

Colonic may be suspected antenatally; however, ultrasound findings are generally non-specific. Postnatally, infants may present with bilious emesis, marked abdominal distention, and failure to pass meconium. Abdominal x-ray demonstrating dilated loops of bowel with air-fluid levels or a massively dilated loop of colon suggests distal bowel obstruction. Contrast enema can differentiate distal atresia from other forms of obstruction and can evaluate for microcolon.

Infants with colonic atresia should be made NPO, a nasogastric tube should be placed to suction, IV fluid resuscitation should commence with correction of any electrolyte abnormalities, and broad-spectrum antibiotic administered.

Infants should undergo surgical repair once fluid resuscitation has occurred and electrolyte abnormalities corrected, ideally within 72 hours of birth as the ileocecal valve creates a closed loop obstruction increasing risk of perforation. A CVL may be placed intraoperatively. Postoperative management includes ventilator management, maintaining the nasogastric tube while monitoring quantity and quality of output, and administration of parenteral nutrition. Enteral feeds may be started at the recommendation of the surgical team when the quantity of gastric output has decreased, is non-bilious in quality, and the infant is stooling.

SCOPE

DISEASE/CONDITION(S)

Hirschsprung disease.

GUIDELINE OBJECTIVE(S)

To identify and review diagnostic approaches to and management of infants with Hirschsprung disease.

BRIEF BACKGROUND

Epidemiology

The incidence of Hirschsprung disease is approximately 1 in 5000 live births. There is a male predominance, particularly in rectosigmoid disease, where the male:female ratio is 4:1; male:female ratio for long-segment disease is estimated to be 1:1–2:1.

Pathophysiology

Hirschsprung disease is characterized as a functional obstruction caused by absence of enteric nervous system parasympathetic ganglion cells.

Inability of the aganglionic segment to relax leads to spasm of the affected section of bowel and causes functional distal obstruction.

The transition zone is identified as the segment of bowel between the aganglionic and normal segments where ganglion cells are present, but enteric nervous system abnormalities lead to impaired motility.

The bowel proximal to the transition zone is dilated.

"Classic-segment disease" comprises the majority of cases, where disease is limited to the rectum and sigmoid.

In approximately 10% of cases, longer segments are affected, including total colonic aganglionosis.

Genetics

Underlying genetic factors associated with Hirschsprung disease are complex with mutations identified in 10 different genes including mutations in the RET gene, EDNRB gene, and END3 gene.

Hirschsprung disease is associated with other congenital anomalies, including cardiac, gastrointestinal, central nervous system, and genitourinary anomalies, and genetic syndromes—specifically, trisomy 21, congenital hypoventilation syndrome, multiple endocrine neoplasia type 2, neurofibromatosis, and Waardenburg syndrome.

Presentation

The typical presentation is described as delayed passage or lack of meconium within the first 24–48 hours after birth in association with abdominal distention, feeding intolerance, and bilious emesis.

Abdominal x-ray demonstrates dilated loops of bowel.

On occasion, infants may present with Hirschsprung-associated enterocolitis (HAEC), but early recognition, diagnosis, and improved medical management has decreased the number of infants presenting with HAEC.

Delayed diagnosis may increase the risk of initial presentation with HAEC.

One study found a delay in passage of meconium (53 vs 44 hours) and delay in diagnosis (16.6 vs 4.6 days) to be associated with development of HAEC, and another demonstrated risk of developing HAEC increased from 11% to 24% when diagnosis was delayed beyond the first week of life.

Other risk factors associated with development of HAEC include a family history of Hirschsprung disease, trisomy 21, long-segment disease, and previous episodes of HAEC.

Symptoms of HAEC include explosive, foul-smelling diarrhea, fever, and abdominal distention.

RECOMMENDATIONS

MAJOR RECOMMENDATIONS

Diagnosis

Full thickness rectal biopsy is considered to be the gold standard for diagnosing Hirschsprung disease; however, this approach requires exposure to general anesthesia and suturing of the biopsy site, and carries the risk of bleeding, perforation, and infection.

Other tests used to diagnose Hirschsprung disease include contrast enema (CE), anorectal manometry (AM), and rectal suction biopsy (RSB).

Systematic review analyzing these alternative diagnostic approaches demonstrates that rectal suction biopsy stained for acetylcholinesterase activity (RSB-AChE) has the highest sensitivity (93%) and specificity (97%) in comparison to AM and CE.

The sensitivity of AM was comparable to RSB at 91%, however specificity was found to be significantly lower at 94%.

CE has the lowest sensitivity (70%) and specificity (83%) and the highest false negative rate.

When limited to studies evaluating these diagnostic approaches in neonates, RSB had the highest sensitivity and specificity. RSB with hematoxylin and eosin (RSB-H&E) stain had sensitivity ranging from 97% to 100% and specificity ranging from 99% to 100%, RSB-AChE had sensitivity ranging from 91% to 100% and specificity from 97% to 100%, while AM had slightly lower and variable sensitivity and specificity ranging from 75% to 100% and 85% to 97%, respectively. CE had the lowest sensitivity, ranging 65% to 80% and specificity from 66% to 100% and has also been demonstrated to have a high rate of inconclusive results.

Rectal suction biopsy is felt to be the optimal diagnostic test for Hirschsprung disease as it is a simple, low-risk procedure.

While it is a noninvasive test, AM requires the availability of expensive equipment and extensive experience in performing the procedure, especially in infants under 1 year of age.

Preoperative Management

Infants suspected of having Hirschsprung disease should be made NPO and have a nasogastric tube placed for decompression.

Maintenance IV fluids should be administered.

Rectal washouts three times daily are recommended.

Broad-spectrum antibiotics can be considered until washouts have decompressed the distal bowel.

Enteral feeds may be started and advanced to full volume, monitoring for emesis, abdominal distention, and stooling.

Rectal washouts can be reduced to once daily when full enteral feeds are tolerated.

Caregivers should be instructed in the rectal washout technique and the infant may be discharged home to grow prior to definitive repair.

Postoperative Management

Following definitive repair with a primary pull-through procedure, enteral feeds are usually started 2 days postoperatively.

Length of stay following a primary pull-through procedure is reported to be between 3 and 7 days.

There is controversy surrounding postoperative management to HAEC.

Some institutions recommend routine daily anal dilations to prevent stricture formation following pull-through. One study showed a significant decrease in development of postoperative HAEC when patients had daily anal dilations.

More recent evidence has questioned the need for daily dilations, demonstrating that weekly dilations by the surgical team leads to similar rates of HAEC while decreasing the negative psychosocial effects experienced by families performing daily dilations.

Other studies demonstrate that postoperative prophylactic rectal washouts with 10–20 mL/kg warm saline 1–2 times daily beginning 1–2 weeks postoperatively and continued for 6 months decrease the incidence and severity of HAEC.

Some authors have suggested a less invasive technique with application of topical nitrates, either isosorbide dinitrate or nitroglycerine, to relax the smooth muscle of the anal canal.

Hirschsprung-Associated Enterocolitis

Radiographic findings associated with HAEC include the "cutoff" sign in the rectosigmoid colon with absent distal air, dilated loops of bowel, air-fluid levels, pneumatosis intestinalis, the "sawtooth" appearance with irregular intestinal lining, and free air due to perforation.

Ultrasound was used in case reports to identify ascites or septations consistent with peritonitis or intestinal inflammation.

Contrast enema is not recommended due to risk of perforation, and CT is not recommended due to radiation exposure.

Management of HAEC includes prompt initiation of antibiotics, usually metronidazole for mild cases, and broad-spectrum therapy with ampicillin, gentamicin, and metronidazole in severe cases.

Vancomycin may be added if *Clostridium difficile* is isolated in stool cultures.

Stool studies should be sent to evaluate for microbes involved in HAEC and to guide appropriate antimicrobial treatment.

Fluid resuscitation is necessary with 20 mL/kg isotonic boluses and initiation of IV fluids at 1.5 times maintenance.

Rectal washouts with 10–20 mL/kg warm saline using a large-bore rubber catheter should be performed 2–4 times daily.

Severe cases of HAEC requiring prolonged periods of NPO will require initiation of TPN.

Diverting enterostomy may be considered for patients presenting with sepsis and severe HAEC.

There is no evidence to support prophylactic antibiotic therapy for prevention of HAEC.

IMPLEMENTATION OF GUIDELINE

DESCRIPTION OF IMPLEMENTATION STRATEGY

- Recommend written guidelines for diagnostic approach to suspected cases of Hirschsprung disease.
- Recommend written guidelines for preoperative management of infants diagnosed with Hirschsprung disease.
- Recommend written guidelines for postoperative management, focusing on strategies to prevent HAEC.
- Recommend written guidelines for diagnosis and management of HAEC.

QUALITY METRICS

- Monitor incidence of preoperative development of HAEC.
- Monitor incidence of postoperative development of HAEC.
- Monitor length of stay following definitive surgical repair.

SUMMARY

Diagnosis of Hirschsprung disease should be made by RSB with contrast enema used to determine the extent of colonic disease.

Preoperative management should include rectal washouts, ensuring infants can tolerate full enteral feeds and monitoring for development of HAEC. Postoperative management options include daily anal dilations beginning within the first month postoperatively and prevention of HAEC with rectal washouts.

All infants should be closely followed for development of HAEC. If symptoms concerning for HAEC develop, patients should be treated with antibiotic therapy and rectal washouts.

SCOPE

DISEASE/CONDITION(S)

Anorectal malformation, focusing on imperforate anus.

GUIDELINE OBJECTIVE(S)

To identify and review diagnostic approaches to and management of infants with anorectal malformations (ARM), specifically imperforate anus.

BRIEF BACKGROUND

Epidemiology

The incidence of ARM is approximately 1:4000–5000 with a slight male predominance. One-third is isolated, and the remaining two-thirds of cases are associated with other congenital anomalies.

Pathophysiology

Current thinking is that imperforate anus develops during the 9th week of gestation and is caused by failure of the anal opening of the hindgut to recanalize after the cloaca is separated into the urogenital sinus and anus during the 7th week of gestation.

Genetics

ARMs are associated with many genetic syndromes, most frequently trisomy 21 and microdeletion of chromosome 22q11.2.

There also appears to be a familial inheritance pattern, with almost 15% of patients with ARM having a positive family history.

Approximately 50–70% of ARMs are associated with other congenital anomalies, especially vertebral, cardiac, trachea/esophageal, renal, and limb anomalies (VACTERL association).

Presentation

ARMs are difficult to diagnose prenatally, as the observation of a dilated colon is nonspecific. However, ARM may be suspected prenatally when other congenital anomalies are found on prenatal ultrasound; specifically, dilated or calcified bowel, lack of meconium at the expected level, renal anomalies, neural tube defects, tethered cord, hydrocolpos, vertebral anomalies, limb anomalies, and omphalocele with absent bladder.

Postnatally, the majority of ARMs should be diagnosed on the initial newborn examination with special attention focused on the perineum and location of any fistulae, and on the urethral and vaginal openings. Given the high likelihood of other anomalies, a thorough examination for additional congenital anomalies should ensue.

Presence of meconium in the urine or at the urethral meatus suggests a rectourethral fistula.

In female infants, the presence of a single perineal opening is indicative of a cloacal malformation.

RECOMMENDATIONS

MAJOR RECOMMENDATIONS

Diagnosis

Diagnosis of ARM is made based on physical examination findings on the initial newborn examination.

Inversion radiographs or prone cross-table radiographs at 24 hours of life can be used to distinguish high from low malformations. Visualization of air below the level of the coccyx is indicative of a low lesion, while air terminating above the level of the coccyx is consistent with a high lesion. Studies done prior to 24 hours may falsely identify lesions as high due to air having not completely traversed through the distal rectum.

Prone cross-table radiographs are used most commonly to determine the level of the rectal pouch when there is no obvious fistula on examination.

Ultrasound may also be used to determine distance from the rectal pouch to the perineal skin, and to determine presence and type of fistula.

CT scan can be used to demonstrate the level of the rectal pouch, however this is not recommended due to radiation exposure to the newborn.

Use of MRI in the neonate with ARM is limited due to the small size of the area and inability to discern structure. It can be used to demonstrate the level of the rectal pouch and pelvic musculature; however, fistulae can be visualized in only 20% of cases.

All radiologic studies for diagnosis and assessment of ARM are considered to be relatively inaccurate. Diagnosis is best made with careful and thorough physical examination, completely probing all external orifices to look for fistulae. Radiologic studies can be most helpful to plan the surgical approach.

For infants with an imperforate anus with rectoperineal fistula, physical examination is diagnostic and no other imaging modalities are necessary.

Infants diagnosed with ARM should have a comprehensive evaluation for other anomalies beginning with a thorough physical examination. Workup should include cardiac echocardiography, radiographic evaluation for vertebral anomalies, spinal ultrasound to evaluate for tethered cord, renal ultrasound, voiding cystourethrogram (VCUG) if renal anomalies are noted on ultrasound, evaluation for esophageal atresia with chest radiograph following attempt to pass a nasogastric tube to the stomach, and pelvic ultrasound to evaluate for hydrocolpos or other uterine and vaginal anomalies.

VCUG may be used to detect rectourethral fistulae in male infants, however there is no evidence to support this practice.

Preoperative Management

Maintenance IV fluids should be administered.

A Foley catheter is placed in the operating room.

For premature infants or those infants with associated defects preventing early repair, the fistula may be dilated and repair delayed, with close attention paid to ensure that the infant is stooling appropriately from the fistula.

Postoperative Management

Following primary anorectal repair without a diverting colostomy, feeding is usually started after the first bowel movement. Some surgeons begin feeds later on the day of surgery, while others wait 2–3 days postoperatively.

In males undergoing repair of rectourethral fistula, the Foley catheter is removed within the first postoperative week, otherwise the catheter may be removed after 24 hours.

For females with rectovestibular fistulae who undergo primary repair in the newborn period, the recommendation is to remain NPO, receiving TPN for 5 days postoperatively. For repair of a perineal fistula or delayed repair of a rectovestibular fistula, the recommendation is for preoperative bowel irrigation followed postoperatively by 7–10 days NPO, receiving TPN.

Postoperative antibiotic administration varies among centers, with the majority of surgeons continuing postoperative antibiotic therapy for 2–7 days. Antibiotic ointment may be applied to the perineum for 7 days.

Postoperative anal dilations are used to prevent anal stenosis. Daily dilations usually begin approximately 2 weeks postoperatively and continue for 2 weeks to 6 months at the discretion of the surgical team.

More recent evidence has questioned the need for daily dilations, demonstrating that weekly dilations by the surgical team leads to comparable outcomes while decreasing the negative psychosocial effects experienced by families performing daily dilations.

IMPLEMENTATION OF GUIDELINE

DESCRIPTION OF IMPLEMENTATION STRATEGY

- Recommend written guidelines for diagnostic approach for infants with anorectal malformations.
- Recommend written guidelines for preoperative management of infants diagnosed with anorectal malformations.
- Recommend written guidelines for postoperative management of infants diagnosed with anorectal malformations.

QUALITY METRICS

- Monitor length of stay following surgical repair.
- Monitor the incidence of the development of postoperative complications, including wound dehiscence, anal stenosis, rectal stenosis, and urethral diverticulum.
- Monitor the incidence of long-term outcomes, including continence and constipation.

SUMMARY

Diagnosis of anorectal malformations is primarily clinical based on thorough newborn examination. Radiography can be useful to guide the surgical approach when the anatomy is unclear based on clinical examination. Comprehensive evaluation for associated congenital anomalies is essential, including echocardiogram, radiography of the spine, ultrasound of the spine, kidneys, and pelvis, evaluation for esophageal atresia/TEF, and VCUG.

Preoperative management should include the above evaluations and initiation of IVF.

Postoperative management of feedings is dependent upon the classification of the anorectal malformation and type of operative repair. Postoperative management options include anal dilations beginning 2 weeks postoperatively.

BIBLIOGRAPHIC SOURCE(S)

ACOG Committee Opinion No. 486: Update on carrier screening for cystic fibrosis. *Obstet Gynecol.* 2011;117(4):1028-31.

Adibe OO, Iqbal CW, Sharp SW, et al. Protocol versus ad libitum feeds after laparoscopic pyloromyotomy: a prospective randomized trial. *J Pediatr Surg.* 2014;49(1):129-32; discussion 132.

Adibe OO, Nichol PF, Lim FY, Mattei P. Ad libitum feeds after laparoscopic pyloromyotomy: a retrospective comparison with a standardized feeding regimen in 227 infants. *J Laparoendosc Adv Surg Tech A.* 2007;17(2):235-7.

Amiel J, Sproat-Emison E, Garcia-Barcelo M, et al. Hirschsprung disease, associated syndromes and genetics: a review. *J Med Genet.* 2008;45(1):1-14.

Anderson N, Malpas T, Robertson R. Prenatal diagnosis of colon atresia. *Pediatr Radiol.* 1993;23(1):63-4.

Applebaum H, Lee S, Puapong D. Duodenal atresia and stenosis-annular pancreas. In: Grosfeld JL, O'Neill JA, Fronkalsrud EW, et al, eds. *Pediatric Surgery.* 6th ed. Philadelphia: Mosby; 2006: 1260-8.

Applegate KE, Anderson JM, Klatte EC. Intestinal malrotation in children: a problem-solving approach to the upper gastrointestinal series. *Radiographics.* 2006;26(5):1485-500.

Arnbjornsson E, Larsson M, Finkel Y, Karpe B. Transanastomotic feeding tube after an operation for duodenal atresia. *Eur J Pediatr Surg.* 2002;12(3):159-62.

Aspelund G, Langer JC. Current management of hypertrophic pyloric stenosis. *Semin Pediatr Surg.* 2007;16(1):27-33.

Baglaj M, Carachi R, MacCormack B. Colonic atresia: a clinicopathological insight into its etiology. *Eur J Pediatr Surg.* 2010;20(2):102-5.

Bagwell CE, Langham MR Jr, Mahaffey SM, Talbert JL, Shandling B. Pseudomembranous colitis following resection for Hirschsprung's disease. *J Pediatr Surg.* 1992;27(10):1261-4.

Bekhit E, Murphy F, Puri P, Hutson J. The clinical features and diagnostic guidelines for identification of anorectal malformations. In: AM H, Hutson J, eds. *Anorectal Malformations in Children.* Berlin: Springer; 2006:185-200.

Benson CD, Lotfi MW, Brogh AJ. Congenital atresia and stenosis of the colon. *J Pediatr Surg.* 1968;3(2):253-7.

Best KE, Tennant PW, Addor MC, et al. Epidemiology of small intestinal atresia in Europe: a register-based study. *Arch Dis Child Fetal Neonatal Ed.* 2012;97(5):F353-8.

Bischoff A, Levitt MA, Lim FY, Guimaraes C, Pena A. Prenatal diagnosis of cloacal malformations. *Pediatr Surg Int.* 2010;26(11):1071-5.

Bischoff A, Levitt MA, Pena A. Update on the management of anorectal malformations. *Pediatr Surg Int.* 2013;29(9):899-904.

Bishay M, Lakshminarayanan B, Arnaud A, et al. The role of parenteral nutrition following surgery for duodenal atresia or stenosis. *Pediatr Surg Int.* 2013;29(2):191-5.

Bittencourt DG, Barini R, Marba S, Sbragia L. Congenital duodenal obstruction: does prenatal diagnosis improve the outcome? *Pediatr Surg Int.* 2004;20(8):582-5.

Blackman SM, Deering-Brose R, McWilliams R, et al. Relative contribution of genetic and nongenetic modifiers to intestinal obstruction in cystic fibrosis. *Gastroenterology.* 2006;131(4):1030-9.

Blumhagen JD, Maclin L, Krauter D, Rosenbaum DM, Weinberger E. Sonographic diagnosis of hypertrophic pyloric stenosis. *AJR Am J Roentgenol* 1988;150(6):1367-70.

Boczar M, Sawicka E, Zybert K. Meconium ileus in newborns with cystic fibrosis - results of treatment in the group of patients operated on in the years 2000-2014. *Dev Period Med.* 2015;19(1):32-40.

Bonham JR, Dale G, Scott DJ, Wagget J. A 7-year study of the diagnostic value of rectal mucosal acetylcholinesterase measurement in Hirschsprung's disease. *J Pediatr Surg.* 1987;22(2):150-2.

Boles ET Jr, Vassy LE, Ralston M. Atresia of the colon. *J Pediatr Surg.* 1976;11(1):69-75.

Burjonrappa SC, Crete E, Bouchard S. Prognostic factors in jejuno-ileal atresia. *Pediatr Surg Int.* 2009;25(9):795-8.

Calvo-Garcia MA, Kline-Fath BM, Levitt MA, et al. Fetal MRI clues to diagnose cloacal malformations. *Pediatr Radiol.* 2011;41(9):1117-28.

Carlyle BE, Borowitz DS, Glick PL. A review of pathophysiology and management of fetuses and neonates with meconium ileus for the pediatric surgeon. *J Pediatr Surg.* 2012;47(4):772-81.

Carpenter RO, Schaffer RL, Maeso CE, et al. Postoperative ad lib feeding for hypertrophic pyloric stenosis. *J Pediatr Surg.* 1999;34(6):959-61.

Clatworthy HW Jr, Howard WH, Lloyd J. The meconium plug syndrome. *Surgery.* 1956;39(1):131-42.

Choudhry MS, Rahman N, Boyd P, Lakhoo K. Duodenal atresia: associated anomalies, prenatal diagnosis and outcome. *Pediatr Surg Int.* 2009;25(8):727-30.

Cooper WO, Ray WA, Griffin MR. Prenatal prescription of macrolide antibiotics and infantile hypertrophic pyloric stenosis. *Obstet Gynecol.* 2002;100(1):101-6.

Coran AG, Caldamone A, Adzick NS, et al. Hypertrophic pyloric stenosis. In: *Pediatric Surgery.* Philadelphia: Elsevier Saunders; 2012:1021-8.

Cox SG, Numanoglu A, Millar AJ, Rode H. Colonic atresia: spectrum of presentation and pitfalls in management. A review of 14 cases. *Pediatr Surg Int.* 2005;21(10):813-8.

Cuenca AG, Ali AS, Kays DW, Islam S. "Pulling the plug"–management of meconium plug syndrome in neonates. *J Surg Res.* 2012;175(2):e43-6.

Cuschieri A, Group EW. Descriptive epidemiology of isolated anal anomalies: a survey of 4.6 million births in Europe. *Am J Med Genet.* 2001;103(3):207-15.

Cystic Fibrosis Genotype-Phenotype Consortium. Correlation between genotype and phenotype in patients with cystic fibrosis. *N Engl J Med.* 1993;329(18):1308-13.

Dagli TE. Neonatal gastrointestinal obstruction. In: Burge DM, Griffiths DM, Steinbrecher HA, et al, eds. *Paediatric Surgery.* 2nd ed. London: Hodder Arnold; 2010:135-45.

Dalla Vecchia LK, Grosfeld JL, West KW, Rescorla FJ, Scherer LR, Engum SA. Intestinal atresia and stenosis: a 25-year experience with 277 cases. *Arch Surg.* 1998;133(5):490-6; discussion 6-7.

Dalton BG, Gonzalez KW, Boda SR, Thomas PG, Sherman AK, St Peter SD. Optimizing fluid resuscitation in hypertrophic pyloric stenosis. *J Pediatr Surg.* 2016; 51(8):1279-82.

Dassinger M, Jackson R, Smith S. Management of colonic atresia with primary resection and anastomosis. *Pediatr Surg Int.* 2009;25(7):579-82.

Davenport M. Intestinal atresia. In: Davenport M, Pierro A, eds. *Oxford Handbook of Paediatric Surgery.* Oxford: Oxford University Press; 2009:146-9.

Davenport M, Bianchi A, Doig CM, Gough DC. Colonic atresia: current results of treatment. *J R Coll Surg Edinb.* 1990;35(1):25-8.

de Lorijn F, Kremer LC, Reitsma JB, Benninga MA. Diagnostic tests in Hirschsprung disease: a systematic review. *J Pediatr Gastroenterol Nutr.* 2006;42(5):496-505.

De Lorijn F, Reitsma JB, Voskuijl WP, et al. Diagnosis of Hirschsprung's disease: a prospective, comparative accuracy study of common tests. *J Pediatr.* 2005;146(6):787-92.

Draus JM Jr, Maxfield CM, Bond SJ. Hirschsprung's disease in an infant with colonic atresia and normal fixation of the distal colon. *J Pediatr Surg.* 2007;42(2):e5-8.

Drewett M, Johal N, Keys C, J Hall N, Burge D. The burden of excluding malrotation in term neonates with bile stained vomiting. *Pediatr Surg Int.* 2016;32(5):483-6.

Elhalaby EA, Coran AG, Blane CE, Hirschl RB, Teitelbaum DH. Enterocolitis associated with Hirschsprung's disease: a clinical-radiological characterization based on 168 patients. *J Pediatr Surg.* 1995;30(1):76-83.

Emir H, Akman M, Sarimurat N, Kilic N, Erdogan E, Soylet Y. Anorectal manometry during the neonatal period: its specificity in the diagnosis of Hirschsprung's disease. *Eur J Pediatr Surg.* 1999;9(2):101-3.

Escobar MA, Grosfeld JL, Burdick JJ, et al. Surgical considerations in cystic fibrosis: a 32-year evaluation of outcomes. *Surgery.* 2005;138(4):560-71; discussion 571-2.

Escobar MA, Ladd AP, Grosfeld JL, et al. Duodenal atresia and stenosis: long-term follow-up over 30 years. *J Pediatr Surg.* 2004;39(6):867-71; discussion -71.

Etensel B, Temir G, Karkiner A, et al. Atresia of the colon. *J Pediatr Surg.* 2005;40(8):1258-68.

Fakhoury K, Durie PR, Levison H, Canny GJ. Meconium ileus in the absence of cystic fibrosis. *Arch Dis Child.* 1992;67(10 Spec No):1204-6.

Feenstra B, Geller F, Carstensen L, et al. Plasma lipids, genetic variants near APOA1, and the risk of infantile hypertrophic pyloric stenosis. *JAMA.* 2013;310(7):714-21.

Feenstra B, Geller F, Krogh C, et al. Common variants near MBNL1 and NKX2-5 are associated with infantile hypertrophic pyloric stenosis. *Nat Genet.* 2012;44(3):334-7.

Feingold J, Guilloud-Bataille M. Genetic comparisons of patients with cystic fibrosis with or without meconium ileus. Clinical Centers of the French CF Registry. *Ann Genet.* 1999;42(3):147-50.

Fishman SJ, Islam S, Buonomo C, Nurko S. Nonfixation of an atretic colon predicts Hirschsprung's disease. *J Pediatr Surg.* 2001;36(1):202-4.

Frischer JS, Azizkhan RG. Jejunoileal atresia and stenosis. In: Coran AG, ed. *Pediatric Surgery.* 7th ed. Philadelphia: Elsevier Saunders; 2012.

Frongia G, Gunther P, Schenk JP, et al. Contrast enema for Hirschsprung disease investigation: diagnostic accuracy and validity for subsequent diagnostic and surgical planning. *Eur J Pediatr Surg.* 2016;26(2):207-14.

Frykman PK, Short SS. Hirschsprung-associated enterocolitis: prevention and therapy. *Semin Pediatr Surg.* 2012;21(4):328-35.

Gao Y, Li G, Zhang X, et al. Primary transanal rectosigmoidectomy for Hirschsprung's disease: preliminary results in the initial 33 cases. *J Pediatr Surg.* 2001;36(12):1816-9.

Garza JJ, Morash D, Dzakovic A, Mondschein JK, Jaksic T. Ad libitum feeding decreases hospital stay for neonates after pyloromyotomy. *J Pediatr Surg.* 2002;37(3):493-5.

Georgeson KE, Robertson DJ. Laparoscopic-assisted approaches for the definitive surgery for Hirschsprung's disease. *Semin Pediatr Surg.* 2004;13(4):256-62.

Gorter RR, Karimi A, Sleeboom C, Kneepkens CM, Heij HA. Clinical and genetic characteristics of meconium ileus in newborns with and without cystic fibrosis. *J Pediatr Gastroenterol Nutr.* 2010;50(5):569-72.

Gray S, Skandalakis J. *Embryology for Surgeons.* Philadelphia, PA: WB Saunders; 1972.

Grosfeld JL, Ballantine TV, Shoemaker R. Operative management of intestinal atresia and stenosis based on pathologic findings. *J Pediatr Surg*. 1979;14(3):368-75.

Hall NJ, Drewett M, Wheeler RA, Griffiths DM, Kitteringham LJ, Burge DM. Trans-anastomotic tubes reduce the need for central venous access and parenteral nutrition in infants with congenital duodenal obstruction. *Pediatr Surg Int*. 2011;27(8):851-5.

Han TI, Kim IO, Kim WS. Imperforate anus: US determination of the type with infracoccygeal approach. *Radiology*. 2003;228(1):226-9.

Haricharan RN, Georgeson KE. Hirschsprung disease. *Semin Pediatr Surg*. 2008;17(4):266-75.

Haxhija EQ, Schalamon J, Hollwarth ME. Management of isolated and associated colonic atresia. *Pediatr Surg Int*. 2011;27(4):411-6.

Herman RS, Teitelbaum DH. Anorectal malformations. *Clin Perinatol*. 2012;39(2):403-22.

Hernanz-Schulman M, Sells LL, Ambrosino MM, Heller RM, Stein SM, Neblett WW 3rd. Hypertrophic pyloric stenosis in the infant without a palpable olive: accuracy of sonographic diagnosis. *Radiology*. 1994;193(3):771-6.

Ikawa H, Yokoyama J, Sanbonmatsu T, et al. The use of computerized tomography to evaluate anorectal anomalies. *J Pediatr Surg*. 1985;20(6):640-4.

Ikeda K, Goto S. Diagnosis and treatment of Hirschsprung's disease in Japan. An analysis of 1628 patients. *Ann Surg*. 1984;199(4):400-5.

Irish MS. Surgical aspects of cystic fibrosis and meconium ileus. *Medscape*. 2011.

Jawaheer J, Khalil B, Plummer T, et al. Primary resection and anastomosis for complicated meconium ileus: a safe procedure? *Pediatr Surg Int*. 2007;23(11):1091-3.

Jensen AR, Short SS, Anselmo DM, et al. Laparoscopic versus open treatment of congenital duodenal obstruction: multicenter short-term outcomes analysis. *J Laparoendosc Adv Surg Tech A*. 2013;23(10):876-80.

Juang D, Snyder CL. Neonatal bowel obstruction. *Surg Clin North Am*. 2012;92(3):685-711, ix-x.

Karimi A, Gorter RR, Sleeboom C, Kneepkens CM, Heij HA. Issues in the management of simple and complex meconium ileus. *Pediatr Surg Int*. 2011;27(9):963-8.

Karnak I, Ciftci AO, Senocak ME, Tanyel FC, Buyukpamukcu N. Colonic atresia: surgical management and outcome. *Pediatr Surg Int*. 2001;17(8):631-5.

Keckler SJ, St Peter SD, Spilde TL, et al. Current significance of meconium plug syndrome. *J Pediatr Surg*. 2008;43(5):896-8.

Kenny SE, Tam PK, Garcia-Barcelo M. Hirschsprung's disease. *Semin Pediatr Surg*. 2010;19(3): 194-200.

Kim IO, Han TI, Kim WS, Yeon KM. Transperineal ultrasonography in imperforate anus: identification of the internal fistula. *J Ultrasound Med*. 2000;19(3):211-6.

Kimura K, Loening-Baucke V. Bilious vomiting in the newborn: rapid diagnosis of intestinal obstruction. *Am Fam Physician*. 2000;61(9):2791-8.

Kimura K, Mukohara N, Nishijima E, Muraji T, Tsugawa C, Matsumoto Y. Diamond-shaped anastomosis for duodenal atresia: an experience with 44 patients over 15 years. *J Pediatr Surg*. 1990;25(9):977-9.

Kohda E, Fujioka M, Ikawa H, Yokoyama J. Congenital anorectal anomaly: CT evaluation. *Radiology*. 1985;157(2):349-52.

Krogh C, Biggar RJ, Fischer TK, Lindholm M, Wohlfahrt J, Melbye M. Bottle-feeding and the risk of pyloric stenosis. *Pediatrics*. 2012;130(4):e943-9.

Kucinska-Chahwan A, Posiewka A, Bijok J, Jakiel G, Roszkowski T. Clinical significance of the prenatal double bubble sign - single institution experience. *Prenat Diagn*. 2015;35(11):1093-6.

Kulkarni M. Duodenal and small intestinal atresia. *Surgery (Oxford)*. Elsevier; 2010;28(1): 33-7.

Kumaran N, Shankar KR, Lloyd DA, Losty PD. Trends in the management and outcome of jejuno-ileal atresia. *Eur J Pediatr Surg*. 2002;12(3):163-7.

Kurer MH, Lawson JO, Pambakian H. Suction biopsy in Hirschsprung's disease. *Arch Dis Child*. 1986;61(1):83-4.

Levitt M, Pena A. Management in the newborn period. In: Holschneider AM, Hutson J, eds. *Anorectal Malformations in Children*. Berlin: Springer; 2006:289-93.

Levitt M, Pena A. Operative management of anomalies in males. In: Holschneider AM, Hutson J, eds. *Anorectal Malformations in Children*. Berlin: Springer; 2006:295-302.

Livingston JC, Elicevik M, Breech L, Crombleholme TM, Pena A, Levitt MA. Persistent cloaca: a 10-year review of prenatal diagnosis. *J Ultrasound Med*. 2012;31(3):403-7.

Loening-Baucke V, Pringle KC, Ekwo EE. Anorectal manometry for the exclusion of Hirschsprung's disease in neonates. *J Pediatr Gastroenterol Nutr*. 1985;4(4):596-603.

Louw JH, Barnard CN. Congenital intestinal atresia; observations on its origin. *Lancet*. 1955;269(6899):1065-7.

Macdessi J, Oates RK. Clinical diagnosis of pyloric stenosis: a declining art. *BMJ*. 1993; 306(6877):553-5.

MacMahon B. The continuing enigma of pyloric stenosis of infancy: a review. *Epidemiology*. 2006;17(2):195-201.

Martin V, Shaw-Smith C. Review of genetic factors in intestinal malrotation. *Pediatr Surg Int*. 2010;26(8):769-81.

Marty TL, Seo T, Sullivan JJ, Matlak ME, Black RE, Johnson DG. Rectal irrigations for the prevention of postoperative enterocolitis in Hirschsprung's disease. *J Pediatr Surg*. 1995;30(5):652-4.

Materne R. The duodenal wind sock sign. *Radiology*. 2001;218(3):749-50.

Melendez E, Goldstein AM, Sagar P, Badizadegan K. Case records of the Massachusetts General Hospital. Case 3-2012. A newborn boy with vomiting, diarrhea, and abdominal distention. *N Engl J Med*. 2012;366(4):361-72.

McAteer JP, Ledbetter DJ, Goldin AB. Role of bottle feeding in the etiology of hypertrophic pyloric stenosis. *JAMA Pediatr*. 2013;167(12):1143-9.

McHugh K, Dudley NE, Tam P. Pre-operative MRI of anorectal anomalies in the newborn period. *Pediatr Radiol*. 1995;25(Suppl 1):S33-6.

Millar AJW, Rode H, Cwyes S. Intestinal atresia and stenosis. In: Ashcraft KW, Holcomb GW, Murphy JP, eds. *Pediatric Surgery*. Philadelphia: Elsevier Saunders; 2005:416-34.

Mirza B, Iqbal S, Ijaz L. Colonic atresia and stenosis: our experience. *J Neonat Surg*. 2012;1(1):4.

Moore KL, Persaud TV. *The Developing Human*. 8th ed. Philadelphia: Saunders; 2008.

Moore SW. Congenital anomalies and genetic associations in Hirschsprung's disease. In: Holschneider AM, Puri P, eds. *Hirschsprung's Disease and Allied Disorders*. 3rd ed. New York, NY: Springer; 2008:115-31.

Morandi A, Ure B, Leva E, Lacher M. Survey on the management of anorectal malformations (ARM) in European pediatric surgical centers of excellence. *Pediatr Surg Int*. 2015;31(6):543-50.

Morris G, Kennedy A Jr, Cochran W. Small bowel congenital anomalies: a review and update. *Curr Gastroenterol Rep*. 2016;18(4):16.

Mundt E, Bates MD. Genetics of Hirschsprung disease and anorectal malformations. *Semin Pediatr Surg*. 2010;19(2):107-17.

Mustafawi AR, Hassan ME. Congenital duodenal obstruction in children: a decade's experience. *Eur J Pediatr Surg*. 2008;18(2):93-7.

Nakao M, Suita S, Taguchi T, Hirose R, Shima Y. Fourteen-year experience of acetylcholinesterase staining for rectal mucosal biopsy in neonatal Hirschsprung's disease. *J Pediatr Surg*. 2001;36(9):1357-63.

Narasimharao KL, Prasad GR, Katariya S, Yadav K, Mitra SK, Pathak IC. Prone cross-table lateral view: an alternative to the invertogram in imperforate anus. *AJR Am J Roentgenol* 1983;140(2):227-9.

Nixon HH, Tawes R. Etiology and treatment of small intestinal atresia: analysis of a series of 127 jejunoileal atresias and comparison with 62 duodenal atresias. *Surgery*. 1971;69(1):41-51.

Noblett HR. Treatment of uncomplicated meconium ileus by Gastrografin enema: a preliminary report. *J Pediatr Surg*. 1969;4(2):190-7.

Nunez R, Torres A, Agulla E, Moreno C, Marin D, Santamaria JI. Rectal irrigation and bowel decontamination for the prevention of postoperative enterocolitis in Hirschsprung's disease. *Cir Pediatr.* 2007;20(2):96-100.

O'Donovan AN, Habra G, Somers S, Malone DE, Rees A, Winthrop AL. Diagnosis of Hirschsprung's disease. *AJR Am J Roentgenol.* 1996;167(2):517-20.

Oldham KT, Arca MJ. Atresia, stenosis, and other obstructions of the colon. In: Grosfeld JL, O'Neil JA, Fonkalsrud EW, eds. *Pediatric Surgery.* 2. Philadelphia: Mosby; 2006:1493-500.

O'Keeffe FN, Stansberry SD, Swischuk LE, Hayden CK Jr. Antropyloric muscle thickness at US in infants: what is normal? *Radiology.* 1991;178(3):827-30.

Oppenheimer DA, Carroll BA, Shochat SJ. Sonography of imperforate anus. *Radiology.* 1983;148(1):127-8.

Oue T, Puri P. Smooth muscle cell hypertrophy versus hyperplasia in infantile hypertrophic pyloric stenosis. *Pediatr Res.* 1999;45(6):853-7.

Parmentier B, Peycelon M, Muller CO, El Ghoneimi A, Bonnard A. Laparoscopic management of congenital duodenal atresia or stenosis: a single-center early experience. *J Pediatr Surg.* 2015;50(11):1833-6.

Pastor AC, Osman F, Teitelbaum DH, Caty MG, Langer JC. Development of a standardized definition for Hirschsprung's-associated enterocolitis: a Delphi analysis. *J Pediatr Surg.* 2009;44(1):251-6.

Pearl RH, Irish MS, Caty MG, Glick PL. The approach to common abdominal diagnoses in infants and children. Part II. *Pediatr Clin North Am.* 1998;45(6):1287-326, vii.

Peters B, Oomen MW, Bakx R, Benninga MA. Advances in infantile hypertrophic pyloric stenosis. *Expert Rev Gastroenterol Hepatol.* 2014;8(5):533-41.

Piper HG, Alesbury J, Waterford SD, Zurakowski D, Jaksic T. Intestinal atresias: factors affecting clinical outcomes. *J Pediatr Surg.* 2008;43(7):1244-8.

Powell RW, Raffensperger JG. Congenital colonic atresia. *J Pediatr Surg.* 1982;17(2):166-70.

Puapong D, Kahng D, Ko A, Applebaum H. Ad libitum feeding: safely improving the cost-effectiveness of pyloromyotomy. *J Pediatr Surg.* 2002;37(12):1667-8.

Putnam LR, John SD, Greenfield SA, et al. The utility of the contrast enema in neonates with suspected Hirschsprung disease. *J Pediatr Surg.* 2015;50(6):963-6.

Rice HE, Caty MG, Glick PL. Fluid therapy for the pediatric surgical patient. *Pediatr Clin North Am.* 1998;45(4):719-27.

Ruangtrakool R, Mungnirandr A, Laohapensang M, Sathornkich C. Surgical treatment for congenital duodenal obstruction. *J Med Assoc Thai.* 2001;84(6):842-9.

Rudolph CD. Meconium diseases of infancy. In: Rudolph CD, Rudolph AM, Hostetter MK, et al, eds. *Rudolph's Pediatrics.* 21st ed. New York: McGraw-Hill; 2001:1407-9.

Ryan ET, Ecker JL, Christakis NA, Folkman J. Hirschsprung's disease: associated abnormalities and demography. *J Pediatr Surg.* 1992;27(1):76-81.

Sato S, Nishijima E, Muraji T, Tsugawa C, Kimura K. Jejunoileal atresia: a 27-year experience. *J Pediatr Surg.* 1998;33(11):1633-5.

Saur D, Vanderwinden JM, Seidler B, Schmid RM, De Laet MH, Allescher HD. Single-nucleotide promoter polymorphism alters transcription of neuronal nitric oxide synthase exon 1c in infantile hypertrophic pyloric stenosis. *Proc Natl Acad Sci U S A.* 2004;101(6):1662-7.

Sencan A, Mir E, Gunsar C, Akcora B. Symptomatic annular pancreas in newborns. *Med Science Mon.* 2002;8(6):Cr434-7.

Seo T, Ando H, Watanabe Y, et al. Colonic atresia and Hirschsprung's disease: importance of histologic examination of the distal bowel. *J Pediatr Surg.* 2002;37(8):E19.

Schramm C, Draaken M, Tewes G, et al. Autosomal-dominant non-syndromic anal atresia: sequencing of candidate genes, array-based molecular karyotyping, and review of the literature. *Eur J Pediatr.* 2011;170(6):741-6.

Schuster SR, Teele RL. An analysis of ultrasound scanning as a guide in determination of "high" or "low" imperforate anus. *J Pediatr Surg.* 1979;14(6):798-800.

Shawis R, Antao B. Prenatal bowel dilatation and the subsequent postnatal management. *Early Hum Dev.* 2006;82(5):297-303.

Shuman FI, Darling DB, Fisher JH. The radiographic diagnosis of congenital hypertrophic pyloric stenosis. *J Pediatr.* 1967;71(1):70-4.

Sizemore AW, Rabbani KZ, Ladd A, Applegate KE. Diagnostic performance of the upper gastrointestinal series in the evaluation of children with clinically suspected malrotation. *Pediatr Radiol.* 2008;38(5):518-28.

Smith G, Cass D. Infantile Hirschsprung's disease: is a barium enema useful? *Pediatr Surg Int.* 1991;6:318-21.

Smith S. Disorders of intestinal rotation and fixation. In: Grosfeld JL, O'Neil JA, Fronkalsrud EW, et al, eds. *Pediatric Surgery.* 6th ed. Philadelphia: Mosby Elsevier; 2006:1342-57.

Snyder CL, Miller KA, Sharp RJ, et al. Management of intestinal atresia in patients with gastroschisis. *J Pediatr Surg.* 2001;36(10):1542-5.

Somme S, Langer JC. Primary versus staged pull-through for the treatment of Hirschsprung disease. *Semin Pediatr Surg.* 2004;13(4):249-55.

Spilde TL, St Peter SD, Keckler SJ, Holcomb GW 3rd, Snyder CL, Ostlie DJ. Open vs laparoscopic repair of congenital duodenal obstructions: a concurrent series. *J Pediatr Surg.* 2008;43(6):1002-5.

Spouge D, Baird PA. Hirschsprung disease in a large birth cohort. *Teratology.* 1985;32(2):171-7.

Stoll C, Alembik Y, Dott B, Roth MP. Associated malformations in patients with anorectal anomalies. *Eur J Med Genet.* 2007;50(4):281-90.

Stollman TH, de Blaauw I, Wijnen MH, et al. Decreased mortality but increased morbidity in neonates with jejunoileal atresia; a study of 114 cases over a 34-year period. *J Pediatr Surg.* 2009;44(1):217-21.

Strouse PJ. Disorders of intestinal rotation and fixation ("malrotation"). *Pediatr Radiol.* 2004;34(11):837-51.

Stunden RJ, LeQuesne GW, Little KE. The improved ultrasound diagnosis of hypertrophic pyloric stenosis. *Pediatr Radiol.* 1986;16(3):200-5.

Sullivan KJ, Chan E, Vincent J, Iqbal M, Wayne C, Nasr A. Feeding post-pyloromyotomy: a meta-analysis. *Pediatrics.* 2016;137(1):1-11.

Surana R, Quinn FM, Puri P. Evaluation of risk factors in the development of enterocolitis complicating Hirschsprung's disease. *Pediatr Surg Int.* 1994;9:234-6.

Sutcliffe J, Sugarman I, Levitt M. Anorectal anomalies and Hirschsprung disease (including stomas). *Surgery - Oxford International Edition.* 2013;31(12):631-8.

Tam PK, Garcia-Barcelo M. Molecular genetics of Hirschsprung's disease. *Semin Pediatr Surg.* 2004;13(4):236-48.

Taxman TL, Yulish BS, Rothstein FC. How useful is the barium enema in the diagnosis of infantile Hirschsprung's disease? *Am J Dis Child.* 1986;140(9):881-4.

Teitelbaum DH, Qualman SJ, Caniano DA. Hirschsprung's disease. Identification of risk factors for enterocolitis. *Ann Surg.* 1988;207(3):240-4.

Temple SJ, Shawyer A, Langer JC. Is daily dilatation by parents necessary after surgery for Hirschsprung disease and anorectal malformations? *J Pediatr Surg.* 2012;47(1):209-12.

Tiryaki T, Demirbag S, Atayurt H, Cetinkursun S. Topical nitric oxide treatment after pull through operations for Hirschsprung disease. *J Pediatr Gastroenterol Nutr.* 2005;40(3):390-2.

Torres AM, Ziegler MM. Malrotation of the intestine. *World J Surg.* 1993;17(3):326-31.

Toyosaka A, Tomimoto Y, Nose K, Seki Y, Okamoto E. Immaturity of the myenteric plexus is the aetiology of meconium ileus without mucoviscidosis: a histopathologic study. *Clin Auton Res.* 1994;4(4):175-84.

Upadhyay V, Sakalkale R, Parashar K, et al. Duodenal atresia: a comparison of three modes of treatment. *Eur J Pediatr Surg.* 1996;6(2):75-7.

van Rooij IA, Wijers CH, Rieu PN, et al. Maternal and paternal risk factors for anorectal malformations: a Dutch case-control study. *Birth Defects Res A Clin Mol Teratol.* 2010;88(3):152-8.

Vieten D, Spicer R. Enterocolitis complicating Hirschsprung's disease. *Semin Pediatr Surg.* 2004;13(4):263-72.

Vinocur DN, Lee EY, Eisenberg RL. Neonatal intestinal obstruction. *AJR Am J Roentgenol.* 2012;198(1):W1-10.

Waldhausen JH, Sawin RS. Improved long-term outcome for patients with jejunoileal apple peel atresia. *J Pediatr Surg.* 1997;32(9):1307-9.

Wangensteen OH, Rice CO. Imperforate anus: a method of determining the surgical approach. *Ann Surg.* 1930;92(1):77-81.

Werler MM, Sheehan JE, Mitchell AA. Association of vasoconstrictive exposures with risks of gastroschisis and small intestinal atresia. *Epidemiology.* 2003;14(3):349-54.

Werner H, Koch Y, Fridkin M, Fahrenkrug J, Gozes I. High levels of vasoactive intestinal peptide in human milk. *Biochem Biophys Res Commun.* 1985;133(1):228-32.

Wetherill C, Sutcliffe J. Hirschsprung disease and anorectal malformation. *Early Hum Dev.* 2014;90(12):927-32.

White MC, Langer JC, Don S, DeBaun MR. Sensitivity and cost minimization analysis of radiology versus olive palpation for the diagnosis of hypertrophic pyloric stenosis. *J Pediatr Surg.* 1998;33(6):913-7.

Willital GH. Advances in the diagnosis of anal and rectal atresia by ultrasonic-echo examination. *J Pediatr Surg.* 1971;6(4):454-7.

Wilmott RW, Tyson SL, Dinwiddie R, Matthew DJ. Survival rates in cystic fibrosis. *Arch Dis Child.* 1983;58(10):835-6.

Wyllie R. Intestinal atresia, stenosis and malrotation. In: Kliegmann RM, Behrman RE, Jenson HB, et al, eds. *Nelson Textbook of Pediatrics.* 18th ed. Philadelphia: Saunders Elsevier; 2007:1559-62.

Yoo SY, Jung SH, Eom M, Kim IH, Han A. Delayed maturation of interstitial cells of Cajal in meconium obstruction. *J Pediatr Surg.* 2002;37(12):1758-61.

Ziegler M. Meconium ileus. In: Grosfeld JL, O'Neil JA, Fonkalsrud EW, et al, eds. *Pediatric Surgery.* Philadelphia: Mosby Elsevier; 2006:1289-303.

Abdominal Wall Defects

Saleem Islam, MD, MPH

SCOPE

DISEASE/CONDITION(S)

Congenital abdominal wall defects.

GUIDELINE OBJECTIVE(S)

The objectives of this chapter are to review the resuscitation and perinatal management of neonates with abdominal wall defects.

BRIEF BACKGROUND

Congenital abdominal wall defects (AWD), with an increasing incidence over the last several decades, represent one of the more commonly encountered neonatal surgical conditions. While often considered together, they can be divided into two distinct clinical entities; namely omphalocele and gastroschisis. AWD in gastroschisis is typically <4 cm in size, located to the right of the umbilical cord, and lacks a covering sac. Consequently, the exteriorized abdominal contents, most frequently midgut derivatives (rarely part of the liver, gonads, and bladder), are exposed to amniotic fluid during gestation. In contrast, an omphalocele is characterized by a defect typically >4 cm in size, located at the base of the umbilical cord, and the exteriorized intra-abdominal contents are typically covered by a sac made by the layers of the umbilical cord. Multiple additional congenital anomalies can be associated with AWD. Up to half of neonates with omphalocele may have an associated cardiac anomaly; other associations include chromosomal anomalies and musculoskeletal and neural tube defects. In contrast, gastroschisis is most commonly associated with intestinal atresias (5% incidence), while other extra-intestinal malformations are encountered relatively less frequently. As a result, despite numerous advances in neonatal and surgical care, considerable morbidity and mortality remains associated with AWD. Moreover, certain aspects of management, such as the timing and mode of delivery, utility of fetal interventions, and the timing and type of repair performed for AWD remain controversial.

RECOMMENDATIONS

MAJOR RECOMMENDATIONS

1. Optimal timing of and mode of delivery for both types of AWD are controversial and have been debated considerably. In patients with gastroschisis, exposure of the exteriorized bowel to the amniotic fluid is thought to lead to the development of an inflammatory peel, which in turn causes bowel dysmotility and delayed transition to full enteral nutrition. However, multiple studies and a Cochrane review failed to demonstrate any significant advantage of elective preterm delivery. Similarly, the perceived risk of injury to the viscera in the birth canal during vaginal delivery led to an interest in performing routine cesarean sections. However, multiple studies as well as a systematic review of the literature do not demonstrate any advantage to cesarean section for AWD in the absence of obstetrical indications. In patients with omphalocele, the timing and mode of delivery is a little less controversial; in the absence of obstetrical indications, term vaginal deliveries are more universally advocated. Cesarean deliveries, however, may be considered in the case of giant omphaloceles with liver in the sac, ruptured omphaloceles, ectopia cordis, and cloacal exstrophy. Therefore, the recommendation is a term vaginal delivery in the absence of any fetal issues, with close monitoring.

2. Studies from the UK and Australia have not demonstrated improved outcomes with prenatal referral to a tertiary care center as measured by time to discharge or time to attain enteral feeds. Despite these results, most experts favor referral of patients with prenatal diagnosis of AWD to tertiary care center for delivery and postnatal care, which may allow for expeditious surgical care.

3. Immediate versus delayed repair with a silo is another controversial topic in the management of gastroschisis. A recent meta-analysis of 20 studies comparing these two approaches concluded that delayed silo closure was associated with slightly better clinical outcomes, particularly in the studies with the least selection bias. The improved outcomes with some neonates after immediate closure is most likely related to the diminished "matting" or inflammatory peel over the intestines that allowed for easier closure in the first place. However, given the significant variations in the designs of the studies included at present, either technique would work well in appropriately selected patients, with silo closure preferred in cases in which there is a large amount of bowel extruded.

4. Gastroschisis is divided into either a "simple" or "complex" category, depending on the presence of an atresia, ischemic bowel, or perforation. Simple gastroschisis carries a more favorable prognosis and will have shorter NICU stay as well as a more rapid attainment of enteral feedings.

5. Omphalocele management is individualized based on the status of the patient and the relative size of the defect. Thus, patients with a major congenital heart defect or a large/giant omphalocele will mostly be managed using techniques that will allow for eschar formation (scarification treatment) and gradual epithelialization, with delay

of final repair to early childhood. Neonates with no cardiac defect or small to moderate sized defects may have a primary repair performed, while others can have a staged repair using mesh.

PRACTICE OPTIONS

Practice Option #1: Fluid Resuscitation

Fluid losses in children with gastroschisis are extremely high compared to a healthy newborn. Recognition of these needs and appropriate replacement are essential to reduce the perioperative morbidity and mortality. However, it is important to note that over-resuscitation can lead to increased edema and bowel ischemia and should be avoided. Lactated ringer's solution is usually used initially with a 10-cc/kg bolus followed by 150 mL/kg/day of maintenance fluids with close monitoring of urine output. Most neonates require parenteral nutrition, which may be required for several weeks following the repair until complete enteral autonomy is achieved. This degree of resuscitation is not generally required with an intact omphalocele.

Practice Option #2: Hypothermia

The neonate with gastroschisis is at risk for insensible heat and fluid losses from exposure of the eviscerated bowel. This is best avoided by covering the exposed bowel with silo or bowel bag.

Practice Option #3: Antibiotic Prophylaxis

The role of antibiotics is somewhat controversial in the management of neonates with gastroschisis. Broad-spectrum antimicrobials are frequently used at birth and during the silo; however, there is no evidence to support the duration or specific type of antibiotic, which is dictated by the unit policies. Antibiotics should not be used in intact omphaloceles other than a topical application.

CLINICAL ALGORITHM(S)

See Figure 39.1.

IMPLEMENTATION OF GUIDELINE

DESCRIPTION OF IMPLEMENTATION STRATEGY

Consensus-based management guidelines for patients with AWD need to be developed and implemented.

QUALITY METRICS

There are no specific quality metrics that apply to AWDs. However, the typical outcome measures that have been used consist of length of stay and time to attaining full enteral feeds. When implementing a clinical algorithm, patients with simple gastroschisis can be compared using these two outcome measures.

SUMMARY

Congenital AWDs represent one of the more commonly encountered neonatal surgical conditions. They represent two distinct clinical entities; namely gastroschisis and omphaloceles, and are frequently associated with other malformations. The management of AWD is guided

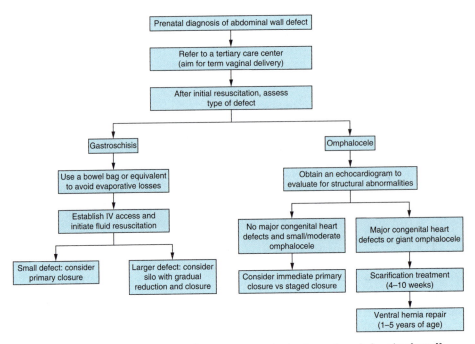

FIGURE 39.1 • Flow diagram of management strategy for abdominal wall defects.

by the nature of the defect and the overall condition of the neonate. Given the significant heterogeneity seen in the clinical course, these patients, after initial stabilization, are best suited for an early referral to a tertiary care center for expeditious pediatric surgical evaluation.

BIBLIOGRAPHIC SOURCE(S)

Brantberg A, Blass HG, Haugen SE, Eik-Nes SH. Characteristics and outcome of 90 cases of fetal omphalocele. *Ultrasound Obstet Gynecol.* 2005;26:527-37.

Islam S. Abdomen: congenital abdominal wall defects. In: Holcomb GW, Murphy P, Ostlie D, eds. *Ashcraft's Pediatric Surgery.* 6th ed. London: Saunders Elsevier; 2014:660-72.

Islam S. Clinical care outcomes in abdominal wall defects. *Curr Opin Pediatr.* 2008;20(3):305-10.

Keys C, Drewett M, Burge DM. Gastroschisis: the cost of an epidemic. *J Pediatr Surg.* 2008;43(4):654-7.

Klein M. Congenital defects of the abdominal wall. In: Coran AG, Adzick NS, eds. *Pediatric Surgery.* Philadelphia: Elsevier Saunders; 2012:973-84.

Kronfli R, Bradnock TJ, Sabharwal A. Intestinal atresia in association with gastroschisis: a 26-year review. *Pediatr Surg Int.* 2010;26(9):891-4.

Kunz SN, Tieder JS, Whitlock K, Jackson JC, Avansino JR. Primary fascial closure versus staged closure with silo in patients with gastroschisis: a meta-analysis. *J Pediatr Surg.* 2013;48(4):845-57.

Mayer TH, Black RI, Matlak ME, Johnson DG. Gastroschisis and omphalocele. An eight-year review. *Ann Surg.* 1980;192(6):783.

Mollitt DL, Ballantine TV, Grosfeld JL, Quinter P. A critical assessment of fluid requirements in gastroschisis. *J Pediatr Surg.* 1978;13(3):217-9.

Segel SY, Marder SJ, Parry S, Macones GA. Fetal abdominal wall defects and mode of delivery: a systematic review. *Obstet Gynecol.* 2001;98:867-73.

Direct Hyperbilirubinemia

Maria Estefania Barbian, MD • Vani V. Gopalareddy, MD

SCOPE

GUIDELINE OBJECTIVE(S)

The objectives of this chapter are to review the causes of direct hyperbilirubinemia/neonatal cholestasis as well as to provide a step-wise approach to the evaluation and management of neonates with conjugated hyperbilirubinemia.

BRIEF BACKGROUND

Jaundice is a common finding in neonates, with as many as 50% of infants having transient jaundice in the first 5 days of life. Neonatal jaundice lasting greater than 2–3 weeks requires additional evaluation as it may suggest cholestasis, a condition that is not normal at any age.

Conjugated hyperbilirubinemia is defined as direct bilirubin level greater than 2 mg/dL or 20% of the total bilirubin. Conjugated hyperbilirubinemia is caused by cholestasis—the pathologic reduction in bile formation or flow. Cholestasis may be caused by hepatocellular injury, obstruction to bile flow, or the presence of bile canalicular transport defects. Newborns are particularly prone to developing cholestasis because of the liver's immature excretory capacity.

Many disease processes can cause neonatal cholestasis and often these diseases lack specific diagnostic testing, making the evaluation of neonatal cholestasis complex. Table 40.1 provides a complete list of differential diagnoses to consider in infants with neonatal cholestasis and the diagnostic evaluation for each diagnosis. However, a few conditions account for most cases of neonatal cholestasis. In term infants, over 70% of the cases of cholestasis are caused by neonatal hepatitis and biliary atresia (BA), while α_1-antitrypsin (A1AT)

TABLE 40.1. Causes of Neonatal Cholestasis and Diagnostic Approach

	Disease	Key Diagnostic Strategy
Anatomic	BA	Delayed or absent excretion on hepatobiliary scan, biliary obstruction on histology
	Choledochal cyst	Ultrasound
	Inspissated bile syndrome	Ultrasound
	Neonatal sclerosing cholangitis	Cholangiogram
	Spontaneous perforation of bile duct	Ultrasound, paracentesis
Infectious	*Congenital*	
	Cytomegalovirus	Urine, blood, or CSF for viral culture or PCR within 2–4 weeks of birth, hearing test
	Toxoplasmosis	IgM-specific antibodies
	Rubella	IgM-specific antibodies
	Herpes simplex virus	HSV PCR
	Syphilis	STS, VDRL, FTA-ABS
	HIV	Anti-HIV immunoglobulins, CD4 count
	HHV-6, herpes zoster	Serology, PCR
	Hepatitis B	HBV panel, HBV DNA
	Hepatitis C	HCV RNA PCR
	Parvovirus B19	IgM-specific antibodies
	Enteric viral sepsis (echoviruses, Coxsackie A and B viruses, adenoviruses)	Serologies, CSF for viral studies
	Acquired	
	Urinary tract infection	Urine culture
	Bacteremia/sepsis	Blood culture
Metabolic	*Disorders of carbohydrate metabolism*	
	Galactosemia	Galactose-1-6-phosphate uridyl transferase
	Fructosemia	Liver biopsy: EM, enzyme activity
	Type IV glycogen storage disease	Liver biopsy
	Disorders of amino acid metabolism	
	Tyrosinemia	Serum tyrosine, methionine, alpha-fetoprotein, urine succinylacetone
	Disorders of lipid metabolism	
	Niemann-Pick, type A	Sphingomyelinase, BM aspirate
	Niemann-Pick, type C	Storage cells in BM aspirate, liver, rectal biopsy
	Wolman disease	Abdominal x-ray of adrenal glands

(Continued)

TABLE 40.1. Causes of Neonatal Cholestasis and Diagnostic Approach (Continued)

	Disease	Key Diagnostic Strategy
	Disorders of bile acid synthesis	Urinary bile acid intermediates by fast-atom bombardment-mass spectroscopy
	Zellweger syndrome	Very-long-chain fatty acid studies
	Other metabolic defects α_1-Antitrypsin deficiency	Serum AAT concentration, Pi type
	Cystic fibrosis	Sweat chloride test
Cholestatic syndromes	Alagille syndrome	Echocardiogram, chest x-ray, genetic testing
	PFIC	GGTP, genetic testing
	Trisomy 18	Karyotype
	Trisomy 21	Karyotype
Endocrinopathies	Hypothyroidism	High TSH, low T4, T3, free T4
	Hypopituitarism	Low cortisol, TSH, and T4
Drug/toxin	Parenteral nutrition	Feeding history
	Drugs	Medication history
Systemic disorder	Congenital heart disease/failure	Echocardiogram
	Idiopathic neonatal hepatitis	Liver biopsy
	Shock	
Immune	Neonatal lupus erythematosus	Anti-Ro and anti-La antibodies (in infant and mother)
	Autoimmune hemolytic anemia with giant-cell hepatitis	Coombs test, giant cell hepatitis on liver biopsy

BA, biliary atresia; BM, bone marrow; PFIC, progressive familial intrahepatic cholestasis.
Adapted from Roberts EA. The jaundiced baby. In: *Disease of the Liver and the Biliary System in Children.* 2nd ed. Malden, MA: Blackwell;2004:35-64.

deficiency accounts for 5–15% of the cases. In contrast, cholestasis in premature infants is often caused by prolonged parenteral nutrition or sepsis. Refer to Table 40.2 for a list of the most common causes of neonatal cholestasis in term infants.

INITIAL ASSESSMENT

An infant with jaundice lasting longer than 2–3 weeks requires evaluation for cholestasis. The differential for neonatal cholestasis is broad and requires a thorough evaluation. The evaluation should begin with a detailed history, including prenatal and family histories. Next, growth parameters should be assessed, followed by a complete physical examination evaluating for hepatosplenomegaly, cephalohematoma, ascites, heart failure, dysmorphic features, petechiae, and/or bruising. Infants with Alagille syndrome, metabolic liver disease, and intrauterine infection may be small for gestational age (SGA) or have evidence of intrauterine growth restriction (IUGR). Infants that are ill appearing should

TABLE 40.2. Most Common Causes of Neonatal Cholestasis

α_1-Antitrypsin deficiency
Idiopathic neonatal hepatitis
Hepatitis secondary to infection (i.e., cytomegalovirus, sepsis)
Parenteral nutrition
Biliary atresia
Metabolic disease (i.e., galactosemia)
Alagille syndrome
Progressive familial intrahepatic cholestasis

Gottesman LE, Del Vecchio MT, Aronoff SC. Etiologies of conjugated hyperbilirubinemia in infancy: a systematic review of 1692 subjects. *BMC Pediatr.* 2015;15:192.

be evaluated for infection or metabolic disease, whereas infants with BA are typically well appearing but may have hepatomegaly. Splenomegaly is suggestive of a storage or hematologic disease. Dysmorphic features may be noted in trisomy 18, trisomy 21, Alagille syndrome, Zellweger syndrome, and with certain congenital infections. Ascites may be noted in metabolic liver disease. Observation of stool color and urine color is also helpful, as acholic stools and dark urine indicate significant cholestasis.

DIAGNOSTIC EVALUATION

Laboratory evaluation should begin with measurement of total and direct serum bilirubin levels since unconjugated hyperbilirubinemia is indistinguishable from conjugated hyperbilirubinemia. Refer to Table 40.3 for a complete list of diagnostic tests to consider upon diagnosing direct hyperbilirubinemia. Table 40.4 provides further diagnostic recommendations for these infants. Once conjugated hyperbilirubinemia is confirmed, serious conditions such as sepsis, hypothyroidism, panhypopituitarism, and inborn errors of metabolism should be considered early on to avoid devastating sequelae. Conjugated hyperbilirubinemia that presents in the first 24 hours of life is highly suggestive of infection. BA should also be considered early on, as diagnosing BA before 60 days of life leads to earlier surgical intervention and improved outcome for the infant.

Next, serum aspartate aminotransferase (AST), alanine aminotransferase (ALT), alkaline phosphatase (AP), and gamma-glutamyl transpeptidase (GGTP) should be obtained. Elevation in AST and ALT do not provide specific information regarding the etiology. In infectious processes, aminotransferases may be more than 4 times the normal levels. Significantly elevated serum AP levels may indicate BA or rickets. GGTP is usually elevated in cholestasis; however, reference values change during the first 3 months of life, with neonates having higher levels of GGTP than older children. Very elevated GGTP is typically noted in Alagille syndrome and progressive familial intrahepatic cholestasis type 3 (PFIC-3). Normal or low GGTP in infants with cholestasis has been associated with hypopituitarism, PFIC-1, PFIC-2, and bile salt synthetic defects.

Hepatic function should be evaluated. This includes coagulation testing (prothrombin [PT] and international normalized ratio [INR]), albumin, ammonia, lactate, and glucose levels. Hypoglycemia is present in metabolic liver disease, hypopituitarism, or severe liver disease. Prolonged prothrombin times (PT and INR) are associated with vitamin K deficiency or severe liver disease. If there is impaired hepatic function, evidenced by prolonged PT and INR values, elevated ammonia level, low serum albumin, or hypoglycemia, the infant should be transferred immediately to a tertiary care facility.

TABLE 40.3. Initial Diagnostic Evaluation of the Persistently Jaundiced Infant

Blood	Total bilirubin
	Direct bilirubin
	AST
	ALT
	AP
	GGTP
	Albumin
	Glucose
	Ammonia
	Lactate
	PT/INR
	TSH
	T4
	CPK
	α_1-Antitrypsin phenotype (Pi typing)
	CBC with differential
	Blood culture
	Verify newborn screen results
Urine	Urinalysis
	Urine culture
	Urine reducing substances
Imaging	Fasting abdominal ultrasound

TABLE 40.4. Secondary Diagnostic Evaluation of the Persistently Jaundiced Infant

Blood	Serum bile acids
	Random cortisol level
	Cholesterol
	Red blood cell galactose-1-phosphate uridyl transferase
	Gene panels or exome sequencing
Urine	Succinylacetone
	Organic acids
	Bile salts profiling
Special testing	PCR for CMV, HSV, *Listeria*
	Sweat chloride test
	Liver biopsy
Imaging	Chest x-ray to evaluate for lung and heart disease
	Plain film of spine to assess for butterfly vertebrae
	Echocardiogram
	HIDA scan (phenobarbital primed)
Consultation	Consider:
	GI/Hepatology
	Metabolic/Genetic
	Ophthalmology
	Cardiology
	Nutrition

Severe coagulopathy unresponsive to vitamin K administration may be secondary to gestational alloimmune liver disease, metabolic disease, or sepsis.

Evaluation for infection, particularly urinary tract infection, and sepsis should be considered. A complete blood count with differential, urinalysis, urine culture, and blood culture should be obtained. If the urine is noted to have reducing substances, this suggests galactosemia.

The newborn screen should be reviewed for cystic fibrosis, hypothyroidism, galactosemia, and tyrosinemia. Screening for A1AT deficiency should also be obtained.

Finally, a fasting abdominal ultrasound should be performed. If the abdominal ultrasound reveals abnormal bile ducts or abnormal gallbladder, then a phenobarbital-primed hepatobiliary scintigraphy scan with technetium-labeled iminodiacetic acid (HIDA scan) should be performed. If the scan indicates no definite excretion even after 24 hours, liver biopsy should be obtained to determine the diagnosis. If the liver biopsy reveals bile duct paucity, gene testing for Alagille syndrome should be obtained. If the liver biopsy is indicative of BA, then an operative cholangiogram and surgical intervention should be pursued.

MANAGEMENT

Infants with chronic cholestasis often have failure to thrive. The cause is multifactorial; however, reduced bile flow to the intestine results in fat malabsorption and steatorrhea. Medium-chain triglycerides (MCT) do not require bile for intestinal absorption and are the preferred fats for infants with cholestasis. There are formulas with high levels of MCT, and MCT supplements that can be administered as well. These infants often need high-calorie diets, careful monitoring of serum vitamin levels, and use of oral fat-soluble vitamin supplements.

Ursodeoxycholic acid, a hydrophilic bile acid, can be useful in cholestasis by stimulating bile flow and reducing cholestasis. Ursodeoxycholic acid may also be beneficial in displacing toxic bile acids from the hepatocyte, potentially minimizing the hepatocyte injury associated with cholestasis. For pruritus secondary to bile acid deposition in the skin, ursodeoxycholic acid can be helpful. For refractory pruritus, oral rifampin is another therapeutic option.

SCOPE

DISEASE/CONDITION(S)

Biliary atresia (BA).

GUIDELINE OBJECTIVE(S)

To review the etiology and clinical features of BA as well as the recommendations for the evaluation and treatment of BA.

BRIEF BACKGROUND

BA is the most common cause of neonatal cholestasis. There are two forms of BA: congenital and acquired. The acquired form is the most prevalent (~80%). The congenital form is seen with other congenital anomalies, such as heterotaxy and polysplenia.

Etiology

The etiology of acquired BA is unclear. It is thought to be due to an inflammatory response involving the intra- and extrahepatic bile ducts. This causes destruction of the ducts and formation of fibrous scar tissue. The lumen of the bile duct becomes obliter-ated and bile flow is impaired, causing cholestasis. Acquired BA presents in the first few weeks of life, and the infant is usually asymptomatic at birth.

Clinical Features

Infants present with progressive jaundice and are usually well appearing. As the infant's jaundice worsens, the stools will transition from a normal color to acholic. Hepatomeg-aly is always present. Splenomegaly is a late finding, suggesting hepatic fibrosis.

RECOMMENDATIONS

PRACTICE OPTION

Practice Option #1

Evaluation. Total and direct bilirubin levels, serum aminotransferases, serum AP, GGTP, serum albumin, PT/INR, and serum glucose level. An abdominal ultrasound is required to rule out other obstructive etiologies such as choledochal cyst, choledocholithiasis, and spontaneous perforation of the common bile duct. A phenobarbital primed HIDA scan may needed. A liver biopsy is often performed. The gold standard for diagnosis of BA is intraoperative cholangiogram, showing obstruction of flow within a segment of the extrahepatic bile duct.

Treatment. Kasai procedure—excision of fibrous bile duct followed by hepatoportoenterostomy. This operation is done to reestablish bile flow to the intestine. If this procedure is done before 60 days of life it leads to biliary flow in up to 80% of the patients. If the procedure is performed after 90 days of life, the rate of biliary drainage decreases significantly. Despite a successful Kasai procedure, BA is a progressive disease in most patients. The inflammatory injury progresses, causing fibrosis, portal hypertension, and eventually cirrhosis. BA is the most common reason for liver transplant in pediatric patients.

SCOPE

DISEASE/CONDITION(S)

Idiopathic neonatal hepatitis.

GUIDELINE OBJECTIVE(S)

To review idiopathic neonatal hepatitis, including the clinical features, evaluation, and treatment of idiopathic neonatal hepatitis.

BRIEF BACKGROUND

In up to 25% of neonates with cholestasis, an etiology is not determined. It may be diffi-cult to distinguish idiopathic neonatal hepatitis from BA. Infants with idiopathic neonatal hepatitis are more likely to be premature or SGA than those with BA. Prognosis is gen-erally good. Poor prognostic factors include jaundice longer than 6 months, acholic stools, family history of idiopathic neonatal cholestasis, and severe inflammation on biopsy.

Clinical Features

Jaundice, hepatosplenomegaly may be present; if liver biopsy is performed, giant-cell transformation of hepatocytes with inflammation is noted, while bile ducts are normal.

RECOMMENDATIONS

PRACTICE OPTION

Practice Option #1

Evaluation. Total and direct bilirubin levels, serum aminotransferases, serum AP, GGTP, serum albumin, PT/INR, and blood glucose level. Abdominal ultrasound, followed by HIDA scan and/or liver biopsy, may be performed to rule out BA. An intraoperative cholangiogram may be necessary to distinguish from BA.

Treatment. Nutritional support, fat-soluble vitamin supplementation, and ursodeoxycholic acid (15–30 mg/kg/day) to promote bile flow and improve cholestasis.

SCOPE

DISEASE/CONDITION(S)

Neonatal cholestasis secondary to congenital cytomegalovirus (CMV) infection.

GUIDELINE OBJECTIVE(S)

To review congenital CMV infection, including the clinical features, evaluation, and treatment of neonatal cholestasis secondary to congenital CMV infection.

BRIEF BACKGROUND

CMV is the most common congenital infectious cause of neonatal cholestasis. It may be associated with extrahepatic BA. CMV can cause a late presentation of extrahepatic BA from infecting the bile duct epithelial cells.

Clinical Features

Most term infants are asymptomatic as congenital CMV rarely causes acute liver failure in term infants. Preterm infants are more likely to be symptomatic. Infants affected may be growth restricted. Clinical findings include petechial rash, hepatosplenomegaly, jaundice, microcephaly, intracranial calcifications, hearing loss, and chorioretinitis.

RECOMMENDATIONS

PRACTICE OPTION

Practice Option #1

Evaluation. Urine for CMV culture or CMV-DNA by PCR.

Treatment. Ganciclovir (infectious disease consultation).

SCOPE

DISEASE/CONDITION(S)

Neonatal cholestasis secondary to bacterial infection.

GUIDELINE OBJECTIVE(S)

To review the clinical features, evaluation, and treatment of neonatal cholestasis secondary to bacterial infection.

BRIEF BACKGROUND

Neonatal cholestasis may present with sepsis or localized extrahepatic infection that may not be apparent, such as a urinary tract infection. Streptococcal, staphylococcal, and gram-negative bacterial sepsis may cause cholestasis. If there is high suspicion for infection or infection has been confirmed, especially with gram-negative bacteria, the infant should be evaluated for galactosemia. Infants with galactosemia may present with jaundice and gram-negative sepsis.

Clinical Features

Jaundice; infant is likely ill appearing and may be hemodynamically unstable.

Evaluation

CBC with differential, blood culture, urinalysis and urine culture. If available, review metabolic screen from birth. If suspicion for galactosemia is high, obtain urine-reducing substances, erythrocyte galactose-1-phosphate uridyl transferase.

RECOMMENDATIONS

PRACTICE OPTION

Practice Option #1

Treatment. Antibiotics.

SCOPE

DISEASE/CONDITION(S)

Neonatal cholestasis secondary to parenteral nutrition.

GUIDELINE OBJECTIVE(S)

To review the clinical features, evaluation, and treatment of neonatal cholestasis secondary to parenteral nutrition.

BRIEF BACKGROUND

Total parenteral nutrition (TPN)-associated cholestasis is more likely to develop in premature infants or infants that require TPN for prolonged periods of time with limited enteral nutrition. Fasting interrupts enterohepatic circulation, which decreases the secretion of gut hormones needed for normal hepatobiliary function. This may lead to bacterial small bowel overgrowth, leading to production of endotoxins or modification of endogenous bile acids to toxic chemicals. All of these factors are heightened by hypoxia, hypoperfusion, infection, and medications commonly used in the preterm population. The more premature an infant is, the less mature their hepatocellular mechanisms of bile formation, only increasing the risk of TPN-associated cholestasis.

Clinical Presentation

Jaundice, hepatomegaly, and acholic stools may be present. There is usually an elevation in AST, ALT, AP, and GGTP. Albumin and PT/INR are usually normal.

RECOMMENDATIONS

PRACTICE OPTION

Practice Option #1

Evaluation. Feeding history, medication history, and history of intercurrent illnesses. Total and direct bilirubin levels, serum aminotransferases, serum AP, GGTP, serum albumin, PT/INR, and blood glucose level.

Treatment. If possible, begin enteral nutrition. If parenteral nutrition is needed, use a lipid emulsion containing a mixture of soybean oil, olive oil, medium-chain fatty triglycerides and fish oil (SMOF lipids). Content of amino acids in TPN should not exceed required levels and trace elements should be adjusted. Once enteral feeds are initiated, ursodeoxycholic acid (20 mg/kg/day) can be initiated to promote bile flow and improve cholestasis.

SCOPE

DISEASE/CONDITION(S)

Galactosemia.

GUIDELINE OBJECTIVE(S)

To review the clinical features, evaluation, and treatment of neonatal cholestasis secondary to galactosemia.

BRIEF BACKGROUND

Galactosemia is the elevation of blood galactose concentration which is caused by the impaired metabolism of galactose. Galactose is produced from the breakdown of lactose into glucose and galactose. Impaired galactose metabolism may be caused by enzyme deficiencies or liver dysfunction. Infants will have signs of liver dysfunction including cholestasis, abnormal liver function tests, coagulopathy, elevated plasma amino acid levels, renal tubular dysfunction causing metabolic acidosis, galactosuria (urine-reducing substances), and hemolytic anemia.

Clinical Features

Signs and symptoms present within a few days of birth for infants who are breastfeeding or consuming cow's milk-based formula. These infants present with jaundice, vomiting, hepatomegaly, failure to thrive, poor feeding, lethargy, and hypotonia. In addition, they may present with ascites, edema, bleeding/bruising, encephalopathy, cataracts, and gram-negative sepsis.

RECOMMENDATIONS

PRACTICE OPTION

Practice Option #1

Evaluation. Total and direct bilirubin levels, serum aminotransferases, serum AP, GGTP, serum albumin, PT/INR, and blood glucose level. Urinalysis for reducing substances, serum erythrocyte galactose-1-phosphate uridyl transferase.

Treatment. Discontinuation of breast milk or cow's milk-based formula and initiation of soy formula. Lactose-free formulas should not be used in place of soy formula.

SCOPE

DISEASE/CONDITION(S)

α_1-Antitrypsin (A1AT) deficiency.

GUIDELINE OBJECTIVE(S)

To review the clinical features, evaluation, and treatment of neonatal cholestasis secondary to A1AT deficiency.

BRIEF BACKGROUND

A1AT deficiency is an autosomal recessive condition with more than 75 variants. It is caused by a mutation in the gene at the Pi locus on chromosome 14. This gene mutation produces a variant A1AT which accumulates within hepatocytes, causing abnormal bile formation and secretion. This deficiency affects the lungs, liver, and skin (rare). It is the most common inherited cause of neonatal cholestasis. Infants with A1AT deficiency who develop liver disease may have severe cholestasis, and it may be difficult to distinguish their disease from BA.

Clinical Features

Jaundice, acholic stools, hepatomegaly, IUGR. Approximately 2% of infants present with coagulopathy responsive to vitamin K.

RECOMMENDATIONS

PRACTICE OPTION

Practice Option #1

Evaluation. Total and direct bilirubin levels, serum aminotransferases, serum AP, GGTP, serum albumin, PT/INR, and blood glucose level. Ultrasound may reveal intrahepatic cholestasis with a contracted gallbladder. The impaired secretion of the variant gene product is seen on liver biopsy as periodic acid-Schiff (PAS)-positive diastase-resistant granules. Diagnosis is confirmed with low serum A1AT levels (<100 mg/dL) and confirmation of the phenotype Pi by isoelectric focusing. Of note, A1AT is an acute-phase reactant and may be elevated from hepatic inflammation.

Treatment. Nutritional support, fat-soluble vitamin supplementation, treatment of cholestasis and pruritus. Family should be counseled not to smoke due to development of emphysema from the effects of this defect on the lungs.

SCOPE

DISEASE/CONDITION(S)

Alagille syndrome.

GUIDELINE OBJECTIVE(S)

To review the clinical features, evaluation, and treatment of neonatal cholestasis secondary to Alagille syndrome.

BRIEF BACKGROUND

Alagille syndrome is an autosomal dominant multisystem disorder with variable penetrance. It is characterized by abnormalities of the liver, heart, skeletal system, kidneys, and eyes. Cholestasis is secondary to a paucity of interlobular ducts. It is the most common form of familial intrahepatic cholestasis.

Clinical Features

Acholic stools, dysmorphic facies (broad forehead, triangular facies, deep-set eyes), butterfly vertebrae, posterior embryotoxon, renal disease, cardiac defects (peripheral pulmonic stenosis or tetralogy of Fallot). Infant may be SGA. Cholestasis varies, with some experiencing gradual improvement and others requiring liver transplantation in childhood.

RECOMMENDATIONS

PRACTICE OPTION

Practice Option #1

Evaluation. Total and direct bilirubin levels, serum aminotransferases, serum AP, GGTP, serum albumin, PT/INR, and blood glucose level. Cholesterol and triglyceride levels should be evaluated, as they may be three times the upper limit of normal. Diagnosis is confirmed by sequencing JAG1 and NOTCH2 genes. Liver biopsy shows a paucity of bile ducts.

Treatment. Dependent on distribution and severity of disease. Nutritional support, fat-soluble vitamin supplementation is recommended in patients with cholestasis.

SCOPE

DISEASE/CONDITION(S)

Progressive familial intrahepatic cholestasis (PFIC).

GUIDELINE OBJECTIVE(S)

To review the clinical features, evaluation, and treatment of neonatal cholestasis secondary to PFIC.

BRIEF BACKGROUND

PFIC is a disorder caused by defects in transporter proteins along the apical surface of hepatocytes that are responsible for transport of bile components into the bile canaliculus. These defects cause progressive cholestasis and liver injury. There are three types of PFIC. An autosomal recessive mutation produces phenotypes PFIC-1 and 2 which may cause liver failure early in life.

Clinical Features

PFIC-1, in addition to causing cholestasis, may also present with diarrhea and growth failure. With PFIC-3, GGTP levels are usually elevated, and presentation occurs later when compared to PFIC-1 and 2. With PFIC-1 and 2, GGTP levels are low or normal.

RECOMMENDATIONS

PRACTICE OPTION

Practice Option #1

Evaluation. Total and direct bilirubin levels, serum aminotransferases, serum AP, GGTP, serum albumin, PT/INR, and blood glucose level. Genetic evaluation needs to be pursued.

Treatment. Nutritional support, correction of fat-soluble vitamin deficiencies, and ursodeoxycholic acid.

BIBLIOGRAPHIC SOURCE(S)

Balistreri WF. Neonatal cholestasis. *J Pediatr*. 1985;106(2):171.

Balistreri WF, Grand R, Hoofhagle JH, et al. Biliary atresia: current concepts and research directions. *Hepatology*. 1996;23:1682-92.

Brumbaugh D, Mack C. Conjugated hyperbilirubinemia in children. *Pediatr Rev*. 2012;33(7): 291-301.

Davis AR, Rosenthal P, Escobar GJ, Newman TB. Interpreting conjugated bilirubin levels in newborns. *J Pediatr*. 2011;158(4):562-5.

El-Youssef M, Whitington PF. Diagnostic approach to the child with hepatobiliary disease. *Semin Liver Dis*. 1998;18(3)3:195-202.

Hartley JL, Davenport M, Kelly DA. Biliary atresia. *Lancet*. 2009;374(9702):1704-13.

Moyer V, Freese DK, et al. Guideline for the evaluation of cholestatic jaundice in infants: recommendations of the North American Society for Pediatric Gastroenterology, Hepatology and Nutrition. *J Pediatr Gastroenterol Nutr*. 2004;39(2):115-28.

Roberts EA. The jaundiced baby. In: *Disease of the Liver and the Biliary System in Children*. 2nd ed. Malden, MA: Blackwell; 2004:35-64.

Waggoner DD, Buist NR, Donnell GN. Long-term prognosis in galactosaemia: results of a survey of 350 cases. *J Inherit Metab Dis*. 1990;13(6):802.

Infections

Neonatal Sepsis

Kamlesh V. Athavale, MD • C. Michael Cotten, MD, MHS

SCOPE

DISEASE/CONDITION(S)

Neonatal sepsis.

GUIDELINE OBJECTIVE(S)

Review risk factors, clinical presentation, evaluation, and treatment options for sepsis in neonates.

BRIEF BACKGROUND

Introduction

Sepsis is a clinical syndrome caused by invasion of a microbial pathogen into the bloodstream. Early-onset neonatal sepsis (EOS) is defined as onset of symptoms before 7 days of age, while late-onset neonatal sepsis (LOS) refers to the onset of symptoms after 7 days and up to 3 months of age. Suspected sepsis, presumed sepsis, and "rule-out" sepsis are common diagnoses in neonatal intensive care units (NICUs).

Incidence

The overall incidence of neonatal sepsis ranges from 1 to 10 cases/1000 live births, with higher incidence observed in lower-birth-weight infants, and in lower-income versus higher-resourced countries. The incidence of EOS has decreased in developed countries with the use of intrapartum Group B *Streptococcus* (GBS) prophylaxis. In the United States, while the incidence of EOS is less than 1 per 1000 live births, about 35% of extremely low birth weight (ELBW) (<1000 g birth weight) infants in the NICU develop LOS. In low-income countries, the burden of EOS and LOS remains high.

Etiology

Pathogens vary across geographic regions. GBS and *Escherichia coli* are the most common causes of EOS in the United States. *Listeria monocytogenes* is a rare cause of EOS. In the developing world, *Klebsiella*, *E. coli*, staphylococci, and streptococci are prevalent. In term infants, LOS is usually caused by GBS, *E. coli*, or other gram-negative organisms. In low birth weight infants in the NICU, about 50% cases of LOS are caused by coagulase-negative *Staphylococcus* (CONS) species, about 25% caused by other gram-positive organisms (*S. aureus*, *Enterococcus*, or GBS), 20% by gram-negative organisms (*E. coli*, *Klebsiella*, *Serratia*, *Pseudomonas*, *Acinetobacter*, *Enterobacter*) and about 10% by *Candida*. The common pathogens causing EOS or LOS are listed in Table 41.1. Mortality is highest with gram-negative bacterial and fungal infections.

Pathophysiology

EOS is believed to result from ascending bacterial infection of the amniotic membranes (intra-amniotic infection [IAI]) from the vaginal flora. Risk factors that predispose an infant for EOS may be classified into maternal, intrapartum, and neonatal factors, and are summarized in Table 41.2. In preterm infants with EOS, the primary associated risk factor

TABLE 41.1. Microbial Agents Associated With Early- and Late-Onset Neonatal Sepsis

Microbial Agent	Comment
Group B *Streptococcus*	EOS/LOS up to 3 months of age
Listeria monocytogenes	EOS; contaminated unprocessed food ingestion (especially raw milk products) by mother; LOS rare
Staphylococcus aureus (methicillin sensitive and methicillin resistant)	LOS; associated with skin infections, osteomyelitis or arthritis, central line infections; rarely EOS
Enterococcus	LOS/EOS; seen in preterm, UTI common
Coagulase-negative *Staphylococcus* (CONS)	LOS; preterm, indwelling catheters, biofilm production
Escherichia coli	EOS/LOS
Klebsiella, *Haemophilus*	EOS/LOS; *Haemophilus* rare, but affects preterm
Enterobacter, *Citrobacter*, *Pseudomonas*, *Acinetobacter*, *Serratia*	Usually LOS, cause nosocomial infections in NICUs
Rare organisms: *Streptococcus viridans*, other *Streptococcus* species, anaerobes (*B. fragilis*, *Peptostreptococcus*)	EOS/LOS
Candida species	EOS/LOS in ELBW infants with history of prolonged antibiotic therapy, central lines
Virus: herpes simplex, enteroviruses, respiratory viruses, cytomegalovirus	Sepsis-like syndrome of early or late onset

ELBW, extremely low birth weight; EOS, early-onset sepsis; LOS, late-onset sepsis; UTI, urinary tract infection.

TABLE 41.2. **Risk Factors for Early-Onset Neonatal Sepsis**

Maternal
1. GBS colonization, GBS bacteriuria, previous infant affected with GBS illness, inadequate GBS prophylaxis
2. Multiple UTIs in pregnancy
3. History of multiple STD
4. Bacterial vaginosis

Intrapartum
1. Chorioamnionitis (intra-amniotic infection [IAI]) (intrapartum fever, lower abdominal tenderness, foul-smelling amniotic fluid, maternal leukocytosis, fetal tachycardia)
2. Intrapartum fever >38°C
3. Prolonged rupture of membranes (>18 hours)
4. Prolonged labor
5. Instrumentation in labor
6. Multiple vaginal examinations
7. Fetal distress

Neonatal
1. Prematurity
2. Low birth weight
3. Low Apgar score with need for resuscitation
4. Congenital anomalies (e.g., open neural tube defects)

is IAI. Risk factors for LOS include low birth weight, mechanical ventilation, prolonged hospitalization in NICU, presence of central lines, delayed enteral feeds, prolonged total parenteral nutrition (TPN), postoperative status, and other complications of prematurity such as patent ductus arteriosus, bronchopulmonary dysplasia, and necrotizing enterocolitis. Besides being exposed to the above risk factors, newborn infants also have relative immunodeficiency compared to adults, with more reliance on innate immune system response and transfer of maternal antibody and less contribution from cell-mediated, adaptive immunity. Within their innate immune function, infants are faced with a reduced neutrophil (polymorphonuclear [PMN]) pool, limited PMN migration, decreased cytokine production, and reduced complement levels compared to older children or adults. In addition, premature infants have immature skin and mucosal barriers and lack adequate maternal humoral protection. Once bacteria enter the bloodstream, it is common in newborn infants, and particularly in premature infants, to have dissemination of bacteria via hematogenous route to other organs such as the meninges, kidneys, and bone.

Pathogenesis

Even with antibiotic treatment, bacterial toxins, enzymes, or cell wall constituents activate macrophages, triggering the systemic inflammatory response. Various cytokines such as interleukin (IL)-6, IL-8, and tumor necrosis factor-α (TNF-α) are released. These cytokines can alter vascular tone and vascular permeability, decrease myocardial contractility, activate clotting systems, increase pulmonary vascular resistance, and activate other phagocytic cells, such as PMNs.

Signs and Symptoms

For EOS, in some cases the diagnosis is made on an asymptomatic infant in whom a blood culture was done as part of an evaluation based on antenatal risk factors.

Other cases of EOS present with poor feeding and respiratory distress (mild to severe) and some with respiratory failure. Other common signs include lethargy or irritability, vomiting, abdominal distension, paralytic ileus. Temperature instability is frequently seen, with hypothermia being more common in sepsis than hyperthermia. Neonatal *Listeria, Candida,* or herpes simplex virus (HSV) infections may be associated with a skin rash. Decrease in heart rate variability is another early physiologic marker of neonatal sepsis. Other cardiovascular signs include mottling, pulmonary hypertension, or systemic hypotension progressing to distributive shock. In severe cases, disseminated intravascular coagulation and thrombocytopenia may be seen. Apnea or seizures can occur in the presence or in the absence of meningitis. Renal and liver dysfunction may occur. For EOS, differential diagnoses include other respiratory conditions of the newborn such as RDS or meconium aspiration syndrome, congenital heart disease, congenital anomalies, metabolic disorders, or systemic viral infections. LOS can also present with any of the symptoms listed in EOS above. Focal findings such as pneumonia can be seen with EOS, while meningitis, urinary tract infection, cellulitis, omphalitis, and osteomyelitis are more commonly seen with LOS.

RECOMMENDATIONS

MAJOR RECOMMENDATIONS

A positive blood culture remains the gold standard for making the diagnosis of sepsis. Testing body fluids for molecular biomarkers has also been used recently but has not reached the level of standard practice. Indirect evidence for inflammation can be detected by ancillary tests such as changes in WBC count or elevations in biomarkers, but these are not conclusive, especially for the presence of infection. For EOS in term and near-term infants, current guidelines emphasize risk factors (prematurity, maternal fever, duration of ruptured membranes, intrapartum antibiotics for GBS prophylaxis) and clinical signs (temperature, respiratory, and cardiovascular signs) rather than laboratory values in decision-making regarding initiation of empirical antibiotics.

The mainstay for treatment of neonatal sepsis, both EOS and LOS, is antimicrobial therapy. When bacterial sepsis is suspected based on clinical signs and basic laboratory data, but culture results are awaited, empiric antibiotics that target common pathogens effectively should be initiated. If an organism is identified by Gram stain, the laboratory should be contacted to provide specific identification of the species and its antibiotic sensitivity. Treatment then is directed based on these sensitivity results for a total duration of 10 days (or 10 days from the first negative blood culture), for isolated bloodstream infections.

PRACTICE OPTIONS

Practice Option #1: What Diagnostic Tests Should We Choose?

Blood Culture. At least 1 mL of peripheral blood should always be collected prior to starting antimicrobial therapy. Modern culture systems can detect from 1 to 10 colony-forming units per mL if a volume of 1 mL is inoculated. It is unnecessary to collect a separate specimen for fungal culture. If the blood culture is positive, it should be repeated every 24–48 hours until clearance from the blood. For LOS in the NICU, if an organism is identified on the initial collection, a repeat blood culture should be sent prior to changing to the specific antimicrobial agent. This practice is usually helpful to detect for contaminants; for example, in cases of CONS, if the repeat blood culture is negative prior to initiating vancomycin, and the infant is stable clinically, therapy may be discontinued.

Lumbar Puncture. The incidence of meningitis is higher in LOS than in EOS and is also higher in premature infants than in term infants. A small but significant portion of infants with positive cerebrospinal fluid cultures will have a negative blood culture. If the infant presents with obvious signs of sepsis, a lumbar puncture (LP) is recommended. Ideally a LP should be performed prior to initiating antibiotics, since these can negatively affect cerebrospinal fluid (CSF) culture results, and CSF cell counts may not always be elevated in meningitis. However, treatment should not be delayed awaiting the LP. The LP can be delayed if the procedure itself could compromise the infant's cardiorespiratory status. An LP is also recommended for infants exhibiting central nervous system signs, and in any infant with a positive blood culture.

Urine Culture. The incidence of urinary tract infection (UTI) is low (<2%) in the first few days of life even in infants who are bacteremic. However, a urine culture plus sensitivity testing of any identified organism is recommended in screening an infant with signs of LOS. Gram-negative bacteremia is often associated with a UTI. Urine may be sterilely obtained by urinary bladder catheterization or a suprapubic bladder tap.

Chest Radiograph. In the presence of respiratory symptoms, a chest radiograph should be obtained to evaluate for possible findings suggestive of a pneumonic process.

White Blood Cell Count. For EOS, if a clinician is using white blood cell (WBC) counts to assess likelihood of infection of asymptomatic infants as one factor in a risk factor–based approach to decide on empirical treatment, the initial WBC should be delayed for at least 4–6 hours after birth to avoid falsely low WBC at birth. Elevations or reductions in WBC counts may be attributed to several factors other than infection. A low WBC count is more predictive of EOS than a high WBC count. Very high and very low WBC counts, high absolute neutrophil counts, high immature-to-total neutrophil ratios may be observed with LOS; however, a normal WBC count can also be seen in LOS.

Other Cultures. In EOS from chorioamnionitis or IAI, a placental culture may provide diagnostic clues to the etiologic agent. In freshly intubated patients with radiologic findings of pneumonia, an endotracheal culture may provide clues to diagnostic agent. However, in older intubated patients, it can be difficult to interpret since colonization is frequent and difficult to distinguish from infection. Superficial or deep collections of pus should be drained and cultured.

Molecular-Based Tests. Conventional polymerase chain reaction (PCR) and real-time PCR (qPCR) can be used on culture specimens or directly on body fluids. They can identify microbial DNA within hours of sampling. These tests may be useful in low-density bacteremia, or where pretreatment with antibiotics has occurred, and to test for viruses. The tests can be oversensitive, and contamination concerns can increase false positive results. Multiplex PCR involves testing for multiple organisms from a single specimen, and various laboratory panels are available for testing for blood, CSF, and respiratory secretions. Unexpected or unusual pathogens may be missed if qPCR or multiplex primers target only one bacterial species/family.

Viral Studies. If HSV is suspected, viral cultures/PCR of conjunctiva, oropharynx, skin, and anus as well as CSF DNA PCR for HSV should be obtained. Enterovirus, respiratory syncytial virus (RSV), and rhinovirus are common in the NICU and should be suspected during the specific seasons. CMV may also mimic EOS or LOS; therefore obtaining urine, saliva, and blood samples for CMV should be considered, particularly in infants with gastrointestinal signs such as heme-positive stools with distension.

Biomarkers. Elevations in biomarkers such as nCD64, interleukins (soluble IL-2 receptor, IL-6, IL-8), TNF-α, procalcitonin (PCT), or C-reactive protein (CRP) have been described in association with neonatal sepsis. The latter two are used by some in practice. They are nonspecific tests with a low positive predictive value, and levels can be elevated due to other conditions such as perinatal asphyxia as well as bacterial sepsis and meningitis, and also with viral infections. CRP and PCT both naturally rise in the first 24 postnatal hours. CRP peaks at about 48 hours after infection, while PCT peaks at about 24 hours. Serially normal values might reliably exclude sepsis and can guide discontinuation of antibiotics.

Future Trends. There is future potential for proteomics and metabolomics to assess host response in sepsis, as well as transcriptomics to monitor gene expression changes during sepsis. Newer molecular diagnostic platforms such as MALDI-TOF mass spectrometry and broad range 16S rDNA PCR are exciting and available, but their use is not widespread and still experimental.

Practice Option #2: Which Antibiotics to Initiate
See Table 41.3.

EOS. In EOS for the United States, the empiric choice of antibiotic is usually ampicillin or penicillin and an aminoglycoside, such as gentamicin. This combination covers GBS, *Listeria*, and most *E. coli* effectively. If meningitis is strongly suspected, only then cefotaxime, which has excellent CSF penetration, can be used for gram-negative coverage.

LOS. For LOS, if an infant is admitted from the community, the initial empiric choice remains ampicillin and gentamicin. For infants in the NICU, the choice for empiric antibiotic is based on site of infection, the possible sources of infection, and the local microbiogram. Generally, an agent that covers gram-positive organisms (such as oxacillin or nafcillin) is selected along with an agent that covers gram-negative organisms (such as gentamicin). In sites where methicillin-resistant *S. aureus* (MRSA) infections are endemic, consideration should be given to use of empirical vancomycin.

Meningitis. If meningitis is diagnosed, then an agent with good penetration into CSF such as third- (cefotaxime) or fourth-generation cephalosporin (cefepime) should be selected. If a shunt or ventricular reservoir is present, coverage for *Staphylococcus* is recommended. The duration of treatment is a minimum of 14 days for gram-positive and 21 days for gram-negative meningitis. Repeat LP is indicated to confirm sterility of CSF in cases where uncommon or drug-resistant organisms are identified. In such cases, treatment is recommended for minimum of 21 days, with at least 2 weeks of therapy after sterilization of CSF.

TABLE 41.3. **Antimicrobial Agents in Neonatal Sepsis**

Organism in Blood	Initial Agent(s) Choice	Comment
GBS	Penicillin G	May use ampicillin; use gentamicin initially for synergistic effect
L. monocytogenes	Ampicillin	May need 14 days, and 14–21 days for meningitis; use gentamicin initially for synergistic effect
E. coli	Ampicillin + AG	If sensitive to ampicillin, use ampicillin alone; use piperacillin-tazobactam or cephalosporin if resistant to ampicillin
Enterococcus	Ampicillin + AG	Vancomycin if resistant to ampicillin; linezolid or daptomycin* if resistant to vancomycin; cephalosporins not effective
S. aureus	Nafcillin or oxacillin	If blood or superficial infection only, can use cefazolin (not good CNS penetration); cefepime also effective If methicillin-resistant species, use vancomycin or linezolid Clindamycin for localized infections or isolated bacteremia (poor CSF penetration)
Coagulase negative *Staphylococcus*	Vancomycin	Common contaminant; alternatively, use teicoplanin*
Pseudomonas	Ceftazidime ± AG	Alternatively, use piperacillin-tazobactam ± AG
Enterobacteriaceae	Based on sensitivity	Piperacillin-tazobactam ± AG, *or* cefepime ± AG, *or* meropenem
Anaerobes	Metronidazole	Alternatively, clindamycin, ampicillin-sulbactam, piperacillin-tazobactam, or meropenem Metronidazole has good CNS coverage *Peptostreptococcus*: penicillin G
Candida	Amphotericin	Alternatively, use fluconazole or micafungin Liposomal amphotericin does not penetrate well into urine

*Not adequately studied in neonates/children.
AG, aminoglycoside.

General Principles of Therapy

1. If culture is positive and probability of contaminants is low (contaminants usually grow late, beyond 36 hours of collection time, except fungus that can grow up to 72 hours), antibiotics are continued to complete a 10-day course. In the case of resistant organisms or *Staphylococcus*, some have recommended a 10-day course from the first sterile culture.

2. If mild clinical signs persist, discontinuation of antibiotics in presence of sterile cultures may be safe; however, clinical judgment should be exercised. In this situation, biomarkers may be used to aid decision-making, but their positive predictive value when used in cohorts with and without positive cultures is not infallibly high. Whatever the decision, to go long or short with the antibiotic course in the absence of positive cultures, the infant should be monitored in the hospital setting until clinical symptoms abate.
3. If the infant is critically ill from suspected sepsis but cultures are sterile, continuation of antibiotics beyond 48 hours, up to 5–7 days may be appropriate but may not, in the long run, be helpful.

Anaerobic Infections. Suspected intra-abdominal infections, bowel perforation, and abscesses within internal organs must be covered with agents that cover for anaerobes such as *Bacteroides* and *Peptostreptococcus*.

Fungal Sepsis. Empiric antifungal coverage may be appropriate to initiate in a symptomatic extremely premature infant with signs of LOS, especially if known to be colonized with fungus, has new onset of thrombocytopenia, or has received third-generation cephalosporin in the past 7 days. CSF and urine should be cultured if fungemic, and amphotericin B deoxycholate or fluconazole therapy initiated. It is necessary to screen the internal organs for fungal involvement. Liposomal amphotericin is less toxic, however has lesser penetration into the urine and meninges. Treatment for fungal sepsis should be continued for 21 days, and much longer (4–6 weeks) for meningitis or end-organ involvement.

Monitoring on Antimicrobial Therapy. Aminoglycoside and vancomycin levels are necessary while subjecting infants to courses greater than 48 hours, due to their toxicity potential. Other antibiotics do not routinely require drug levels. Renal function should be monitored on patients receiving aminoglycoside or vancomycin. Liver function should be monitored in patients on prolonged antimicrobial therapy. Neonatal physiology is quite different than adults; also disease states can affect pharmacodynamics, resulting in differences in the efficacy or toxicity of antibiotics. Therefore caution is to be exercised while using antimicrobials that have not been adequately tested in neonates.

Failure of Therapy. Sometimes the blood culture may remain positive and the infant may deteriorate despite treatment. The most common reasons for this include inadequate antibiotic levels or regimens, resistant organisms, colonization of indwelling catheters or other objects (such as surgical meshes, etc.), or focal infection as seen in abscess formation, osteomyelitis, meningitis, or endocarditis.

Multidrug-Resistant Organisms (MDRO). Ampicillin resistance is increasingly reported for *E. coli*, as is resistance of *Enterococcus* and even CONS to vancomycin. A large number of other gram-negative bacteria are becoming resistant to cephalosporins. Many bacteria are now resistant to multiple agents. This type of antibiotic resistance can be due to extended-spectrum beta lactamases (ESBL) which are plasmid-mediated enzymes that are rapidly evolving. The plasmids can carry other resistant genes as well. Usually *E. coli* and *Klebsiella* are the most common, but *Enterobacter, Haemophilus*, and *Serratia* can also produce ESBL. Such organisms can be resistant to penicillin or cephalosporins. For all of the above, fourth-generation cephalosporins or carbapenems are effective options. However, resistance of *Acinetobacter, Klebsiella*, and *Stenotrophomonas* to carbapenems is also increasing. Note that ESBL are rare in EOS. In the case of aminoglycoside resistance, which is rare, the available options are amikacin or netilmicin. These agents are resistant to the enzyme-modifying bacteria. When MDRO are isolated, the patients should be isolated from other patients to limit spread within the unit.

Antibiotic Stewardship. While antimicrobials are highly beneficial in the presence of true infection, continuing antibiotics in the absence of a positive culture is not, and in fact may be harmful. Increased risks of fungal colonization and infection, NEC, LOS, and death have been demonstrated. Overuse of broad-spectrum antibiotics raises the probability of introducing MDRO into the NICU. Long-term health effects have also been reported. When initiating antibiotics, it is important to use antibiotics with the narrowest spectrum of coverage. Once an organism is identified by the laboratory, antimicrobial coverage should be narrowed further based on antibiotic sensitivity. Antibiotics should be used for minimal duration. Prolonged early courses of antibiotics longer than 5–7 days may be associated with NEC and subsequent LOS. Third-generation cephalosporins should be used with caution due to the association with invasive candidiasis in ELBW infants. Routine use of these agents can also result in emergence of cephalosporin-resistant gram-negative bacteria. Their use should be restricted to gram-negative meningitis. Broad-spectrum antibiotics should be avoided, especially for prolonged durations, and should be either discontinued or de-escalated to narrower spectrum after 48–72 hours, based on culture results. Empiric usage of antibiotics, especially vancomycin or very broad-spectrum antibiotics such as carbapenems or extended-spectrum penicillins such as piperacillin-tazobactam, should be avoided beyond 48 hours if all cultures are sterile. Use of vancomycin as first-line antibiotics for nosocomial infection should be avoided, unless MRSA is a common local NICU pathogen. Vancomycin should be only used if bacteria are only susceptible to vancomycin, or in MRSA-colonized infants with clinical deterioration. Targeting empiric use of vancomycin to only those infants with the highest risk of complicated CONS infections would greatly minimize their exposure in the neonatal unit. Use of carbapenems and fourth-generation cephalosporins should be reserved for MDRO.

Antibiotic stewardship for early- and late-onset neonatal infection should also include consideration of drug dosing and schedules based on pharmacokinetic data obtained from an appropriate, similar gestational and chronologic age cohort, if available.

Practice Option #3: What Other Interventions Should Be Considered?

Central Line Removal. This is recommended for all gram-negative infections and fungal infections. In the case of a gram-positive infection, central lines should be removed if the peripheral blood culture is repeatedly positive in the presence of the line. Once a line is removed, antibiotics are continued and a new central line can be placed after about 48 hours of therapy, if the condition allows, and ideally only if the repeat blood culture is negative. In cases of fungal sepsis, clearance can be reliably achieved only after removal of any central lines.

Immunotherapy. Infusion of IV immunoglobulin, which can help boost passive immunity and recombinant granulocyte and granulocyte macrophage colony-stimulating factor (G-CSF and GM-CSF) have been used in cases of severe neutropenia and overwhelming sepsis. Others have used pentoxifylline to improve microcirculation. All these therapies have limited evidence to support their routine use.

Consultation. Failure to clear infection from blood, or presence of MDROs usually warrant expert opinion from pediatric infectious disease specialists.

Practice Option #4: Other Supportive Care

The infant should be thoroughly examined, including type of breathing, tone, activity, posture, capillary refill, organomegaly, and presence of rashes. Vital signs with BP should be monitored closely, and urine output as well as serum electrolytes measured. Neonates with apnea or respiratory distress could need mechanical ventilation. Feeds should be withheld, and intravenous fluids or TPN initiated. Infants should be monitored and treated for hypoglycemia, hyperglycemia, and jaundice. Clotting function should be evaluated if concerned, and any bleeding diathesis should be corrected with the help of Vitamin K and fresh-frozen plasma infusion. Platelets should be transfused if bleeding and thrombocytopenic. Optimal acid–base balance should be achieved using adjustments to TPN. Endotoxic shock is treated with continuous infusion of vasopressors such as epinephrine or dopamine. Volume expansion may be used—however, with caution in ELBW infants—during the first week of life. Infants should be evaluated for adrenal insufficiency by measuring serum cortisol levels and treated with mineralocorticoids, if indicated. If in multi-organ failure, fluid restriction is helpful.

IMPLEMENTATION OF GUIDELINE

DESCRIPTION OF IMPLEMENTATION STRATEGY

Well-baby nurseries should develop local algorithms for EOS risk assessment and clinical management of symptomatic and asymptomatic newborn infants either using categorical algorithms or by following recommendations of validated multivariate risk tools such as the online Neonatal Sepsis Calculator (https://neonatalsepsiscalculator. kaiserpermanente.org/). For NICUs, guidelines for evaluation and management of sepsis and other infectious conditions should be developed, and a single leader should be appointed. A team consisting of the neonatology provider, unit pharmacist, pediatric ID specialist, laboratory microbiologist, and nursing leadership are essential in decision-making.

QUALITY METRICS

It is important to monitor the incidence of early- and late-onset sepsis in any NICU. For central line infections, the number of central line infections per 1000 line-days can be tracked, as should central lines that are not discontinued, despite infant being on full feeds. From an antibiotic stewardship perspective, the following metrics can be used: tracking microbial antibiotic resistance patterns for EOS and LOS organisms, days of antibiotic therapy per 1000 patient days, number of patients on antibiotics per 1000 patient days, percentage of infants started on antibiotics at admission, antibiotic usage beyond 48 hours in the absence of positive cultures, utilization of vancomycin and other broad-spectrum agents in the NICU as well as percentage of patients discharged without receiving any antibiotics.

SUMMARY

Neonatal sepsis continues to be an important cause of mortality and morbidity in newborn infants. Although the incidence of EOS is falling in the United States, the number of infants affected by LOS has not changed much. Prompt and thorough evaluation of symptomatic infections coupled with early initiation of antibiotic therapy are highly beneficial and generally associated with good outcomes. Identifying true bacterial infection in a symptomatic patient in the absence of positive cultures continues to remain a diagnostic challenge. Antimicrobials, although life-saving, also have short-term and long-term side effects, along with risk of development of MDRO; therefore judicious use of antimicrobials is to be highly encouraged.

BIBLIOGRAPHIC SOURCE(S)

Benitz WE. Adjunct laboratory tests in the diagnosis of early-onset neonatal sepsis. *Clin Perinatol.* 2010;37(2):421-38.

Benjamin DK, Stoll B, Goldberg R; National Institute for Child Health and Human Development Neonatal Research Network. Neonatal candidiasis: epidemiology, risk factors, and clinical judgment. *Pediatrics.* 2010;126(4):e865-73.

Bradley JS, Nelson DJ, eds. *Nelson's Pediatric Antimicrobial Therapy.* 24th ed. Elk Grove Village, IL: American Academy of Pediatrics; 2018.

Cantey JB, Baird SD. Ending the culture of culture-negative sepsis in the neonatal ICU. *Pediatrics.* 2017;140(4). pii: e20170044.

Cantey JB, Wozniak PS, Pruszynski JE, Sánchez PJ. Reducing unnecessary antibiotic use in the neonatal intensive care unit (SCOUT): a prospective interrupted time-series study. *Lancet Infect Dis.* 2016;16(10):1178-84.

Chiesa C, Natale F, Pascone R, et al. C reactive protein and procalcitonin: reference intervals for preterm and term newborns during the early neonatal period. *Clin Chim Acta.* 2011;412(11-12):1053-9.

Clark RH, Bloom BT, Spitzer AR, et al. Empiric use of ampicillin and cefotaxime, compared with ampicillin and gentamicin, for neonates at risk for sepsis is associated with an increased risk of neonatal death. *Pediatrics.* 2006;117:67-74.

Cotten CM, McDonald S, Stoll B, et al; National Institute for Child Health and Human Development Neonatal Research Network. The association of third-generation cephalosporin use and invasive candidiasis in extremely low birth-weight infants. *Pediatrics* 2006;118:717-22.

Cotten CM, Taylor S, Stoll B, et al. Prolonged duration of initial empirical antibiotic treatment is associated with increased rates of necrotizing enterocolitis and death for extremely low birth weight infants. *Pediatrics.* 2009;123:58–66.

Hofer N, Zacharias E, Muller W, Resch B. An update on the use of C-reactive protein in early-onset neonatal sepsis: current insights and new tasks. *Neonatology.* 2012;102:25-36.

Hornik CP, Benjamin DK, Becker KC, et al. Use of the complete blood cell count in late-onset neonatal sepsis. *Pediatr Infect Dis J.* 2012;31(8):803-7.

Kimberlin DW, Brady MT, Jackson MA, Long SS, eds. *Red Book 2018: Report of the Committee on Infectious Diseases.* 31st ed. Itasca, IL: American Academy of Pediatrics; 2018.

Ku LC, Boggess KA, Cohen-Wolkowiez M. Bacterial meningitis in infants. *Clin Perinatol.* 2015;42(1):29-45.

Kuzniewicz MW, Puopolo KM, Fischer A, et al. A quantitative, risk-based approach to the management of neonatal early-onset sepsis. *JAMA Pediatr.* 2017;171(4):365-71.

Muller-Pebody B, Johnson AP, Heath PT, et al; iCAP Group (Improving Antibiotic Prescribing in Primary Care). Empirical treatment of neonatal sepsis: are the current guidelines adequate? *Arch Dis Child Fetal Neonatal Ed.* 2011;96(1):F4-8.

Newman TB, Puopolo KM, Wi S, Draper D, Escobar GJ. Interpreting complete blood counts soon after birth in newborns at risk for sepsis. *Pediatrics.* 2010;126(5):903-9.

Ng S, Strunk T, Jiang P, Muk T, Sangild PT, Currie A. Precision medicine for neonatal sepsis. *Front Mol Biosci.* 2018;5:70.

Pammi M, Brocklehurst P. Granulocyte transfusions for neonates with confirmed or suspected sepsis and neutropenia. *Cochrane Database Syst Rev.* 2011;(10):CD003956.

Polin R; Committee on Fetus and Newborn. Management of neonates with proven early onset bacterial sepsis. *Pediatrics*. 2012;129(5):1006-16.

Puopolo KM, Benitz WE, Zaoutis TE; AAP Committee on Fetus and Newborn, AAP Committee on Infectious Diseases. Management of neonates born at ≤34 6/7 weeks' gestation with suspected or proven early-onset bacterial sepsis. *Pediatrics*. 2018;142(6):e20182896.

Puopolo KM, Benitz WE, Zaoutis TE; Committee on Fetus and Newborn, AAP Committee on Infectious Diseases. Management of neonates born at ≥35 0/7 weeks' gestation with suspected or proven early-onset bacterial sepsis. *Pediatrics*. 2018;142(6):e20182894.

Rawat D, Nair D. Extended-spectrum β-lactamases in gram negative bacteria. *J Glob Infect Dis*. 2010;2(3):263-74.

Ronchi A, Michelow IC, Chapin KC, et al. Viral respiratory tract infections in the neonatal intensive care unit: the VIRIoN-I study. *J Pediatr*. 2014;165(4):690-6.

Russell AB, Sharland M, Heath PT. Improving antibiotic prescribing in neonatal units: time to act. *Arch Dis Child Fetal Neonatal Ed*. 2012;97(2):F141-6.

Schelonka RL, Chai MK, Yoder BA, Hensley D, Brockett RM, Ascher DP. Volume of blood required to detect common neonatal pathogens. *J Pediatr*. 1996;129(2):275-8.

Stoll BJ, Hansen NI, Bell EF, et al. Neonatal outcomes of extremely preterm infants from the NICHD Neonatal Research Network. *Pediatrics*. 2010;126(3):443-56.

Stoll BJ, Hansen N, Fanaroff AA, et al. Late-onset sepsis in very low birth weight neonates: the experience of the NICHD Neonatal Research Network. *Pediatrics*. 2002;110(2 Pt 1):285-9.

Stoll BJ, Hansen N, Fanaroff AA, et al; National Institute for Child Health and Human Development Neonatal Research Network. Changes in pathogens causing early-onset sepsis in very-low-birth-weight infants. *N Engl J Med*. 2002;347(4):240-7.

Stoll BJ, Hansen NI, Sánchez PJ, et al; Eunice Kennedy Shriver National Institute of Child Health and Human Development Neonatal Research Network. Early onset neonatal sepsis: the burden of group B *Streptococcal* and *E. coli* disease continues. *Pediatrics*. 2011;127(5):817-26.

Wortham JM, Hansen NI, Schrag SJ, et al; Eunice Kennedy Shriver NICHD Neonatal Research Network. Chorioamnionitis and culture-confirmed, early-onset neonatal infections. *Pediatrics*. 2016;137(1).

Zaidi AK, Thaver D, Ali SA, Khan TA. Pathogens associated with sepsis in newborns and young infants in developing countries. *Pediatr Infect Dis J*. 2009;28(1 Suppl):S10-8.

Candida Infections

Kanecia Zimmerman, MD, MPH • Daniel K. Benjamin Jr, MD, PhD, MPH

SCOPE

DISEASE/CONDITION(S)

Evaluation and management of neonatal candidiasis.

GUIDELINE OBJECTIVE(S)

Review morbidity and mortality associated with invasive candidiasis; provide recommendations for prevention, diagnosis, empirical therapy, and treatment of neonatal candidiasis.

BRIEF BACKGROUND

Invasive candidiasis (IC) is common in premature infants, occurring in up to 6% of infants <1000 g birth weight. IC in premature infants is associated with significant mortality and morbidity. Death occurs in up to 34% of affected infants and neurodevelopmental impairment occurs in up to 63% of survivors. IC is also associated with increased hospital stay, hospital costs, severe retinopathy of prematurity, and bronchopulmonary dysplasia. Although the overall incidence of invasive candidiasis has recently decreased, prevention and appropriate management of this disease leads to reduced morbidity and mortality.

RECOMMENDATIONS

MAJOR RECOMMENDATIONS: PREVENTION

Prevention of IC is paramount. Methods to prevent IC are centered around minimization of risk factors that promote colonization of mucosal surfaces, disrupt anatomic barriers, or weaken the host immune response. Preventive efforts should focus on the judicious use of broad-spectrum antibiotics, early removal of central venous catheters, early initiation of enteral feeds, and infection control practices to prevent horizontal transmission. In addition, fluconazole prophylaxis is safe and effective, and should be used at moderate- to high-incidence centers and in high-risk infants <1000 g birth weight.

PRACTICE OPTION

Practice Option #1

Several randomized controlled trials have demonstrated safety and efficacy of fluconazole prophylaxis for the prevention of IC in premature infants. However, in the largest trial of infants <750 g birth weight, there was no difference in death or IC for those who received 6 mg/kg of fluconazole twice weekly for 42 days compared to those who received placebo (odds ratio [OR]: 0.73; 95% CI 0.43–1.23). Centers included in this trial had low incidence of IC compared to previous trials conducted in high-incidence centers. Based on available evidence, we recommend fluconazole prophylaxis (6 mg/kg twice weekly for 42 days) in infants who are <1000 g birth weight and admitted to moderate- or high-incidence centers (>5–10% incidence of IC).

IMPLEMENTATION OF GUIDELINE

DESCRIPTION OF IMPLEMENTATION STRATEGY

Recommend written guidelines for prevention of IC and implementation of prophylactic therapy; written guidelines for prevention should include identification of triggers for central line removal and protocols for attainment of oral feeds. Guidance on antibiotic stewardship should also be included.

QUALITY METRICS

Adherence to guidelines; incidence of IC; need for replacement of central lines after early removal.

RECOMMENDATIONS

MAJOR RECOMMENDATIONS: DIAGNOSIS AND EMPIRICAL THERAPY

Isolation of *Candida* from sterile body fluid is the current gold standard for diagnosis of IC. Once IC is identified, providers should initiate evaluation for disseminated infection. Empirical therapy may be helpful but has not been evaluated in well-powered, randomized trials of infants.

PRACTICE OPTIONS

Practice Option #1

Large-volume blood cultures may be positive in as few as 29% of cases of IC in adults. The smaller volume (0.5–1 mL) of cultures obtained from infants is likely to have even lower sensitivity. Further, diagnosis of IC by culture is time intensive, often requiring days for growth of the organism, speciation, and sensitivity testing. New techniques,

TABLE 42.1. Routine Workup for Dissemination of IC

Organ	Evaluation
Bloodstream	Blood culture (1 mL)
Urinary tract	Urinalysis, urine culture
CNS	Lumbar puncture for cerebral spinal fluid (cells, white blood cell differential, glucose, protein, culture); head ultrasound
Kidneys/liver/spleen	Abdominal ultrasound
Eyes	Examination by ophthalmology
Heart	Transthoracic echocardiogram

including detection of *Candida* DNA by polymerase chain reaction, matrix-assisted laser desorption/ionization time of flight mass spectrometry (MALDI-TOF MS), and mannan, D-arabinitol/L-arabinitol, and 1,3-β-D-glucan antigen assays, are promising methods that may improve sensitivity and decrease time to diagnosis and speciation. However, these methods have not been systematically validated in infants.

Practice Option #2

IC can affect any organ system, most commonly the kidneys and central nervous system (CNS). Up to 40% of infants have kidney involvement, and CNS infection is common in extremely low birth weight infants. In a meta-analysis of 21 studies, the median prevalence of other end-organ effects in infants included endophthalmitis (3%), endocarditis (5%), and hepatosplenic abscesses (1%). Providers should routinely perform investigation to identify IC dissemination (Table 42.1).

Practice Option #3

Given the significant morbidity and mortality associated with IC, clinicians may consider empirical antifungal therapy in high-risk infants. According to a clinical predictive model for IC in preterm infants, infants with the following characteristics are at high risk for IC: 1) gestational age <25 weeks, 2) thrombocytopenia at the time of blood culture, or 3) 25–27 weeks gestational age with exposure to cephalosporins or carbapenems in the preceding 7 days before blood culture. Use of a clinical model that incorporated *Candida*-like dermatitis, central venous catheter, mode of infant delivery, absence of enteral feeding, gestational age, glucose, platelets, and antibiotic therapy proved superior to clinical judgment ($p = 0.0022$) in predicting IC in premature infants.

Importantly, well-designed randomized trials are needed to assess the risks and benefits of empirical antifungal therapy in high-risk infants. Existing observational studies have evaluated the efficacy of this strategy with mixed results. In a cohort of 295 infants with IC, antifungal therapy on or before the day of first positive culture did not decrease mortality compared to no receipt of empirical therapy (34/104, 33% with empirical therapy and 53/191, 28% without empirical therapy). In contrast, a multicenter cohort study of 136 infants <1000 g birth weight demonstrated a reduced composite endpoint of mortality and neurodevelopmental impairment with initiation of systemic antifungal therapy on the day of or before culture (OR, 0.27; 95% CI, 0.08–0.86).

IMPLEMENTATION OF GUIDELINE

DESCRIPTION OF IMPLEMENTATION STRATEGY

Guidelines for routine workup for IC dissemination.

QUALITY METRICS

Adherence to complete workup for IC dissemination.

RECOMMENDATIONS

MAJOR RECOMMENDATIONS: TREATMENT

Initial choice of antifungal therapy should consider the presence of routine fluconazole prophylaxis and organism predominance in the intensive care unit. With notable exceptions, appropriately dosed amphotericin B deoxycholate, micafungin, or fluconazole should be used as first-line therapy because of penetration into the CNS. In addition, prompt removal of central venous catheters should occur after IC diagnosis. Infants should receive a total of 21 days of antifungal therapy from the time of first negative culture.

PRACTICE OPTIONS

Practice Option #1: Polyenes

Amphotericin B deoxycholate, liposomal amphotericin B, amphotericin B colloidal dispersion, and amphotericin B lipid complex are the available polyene compounds. Amphotericin B deoxycholate, typically dosed at 1 mg/kg/day, is the oldest and preferred amphotericin compound because of penetration into the CNS and kidneys. Lipid amphotericin compounds do not have reliable penetration into the kidneys but have demonstrated efficacy for eradication of IC in settings where amphotericin B has failed.

Practice Option #2: Triazoles

Fluconazole, dosed at 25 mg/kg/day on day 1, then 12 mg/kg/day, achieves rapid target serum concentrations and penetrates both the urine and CNS. Despite appropriate dosing, *C. krusei* and *C. glabrata* are intrinsically resistant to fluconazole, and in adult populations, there is concern for emerging *C. albicans* and *C. parapsilosis* species resistance to fluconazole.

Practice Option #3: Echinocandins

Micafungin, anidulafungin, and caspofungin have efficacy against all *Candida* species. In general, echinocandins do not have good penetration into the CNS; however, adequate systemic exposures of micafungin (AUC0–24, >170 µg•h/mL) have been associated with 90% decreased fungal burden in rabbit brain tissue. Although pharmacokinetics of micafungin have been well described in infants and support dosing of 10 mg/kg/day, limited data exist for caspofungin and anidulafungin. With rare exceptions, anidulafungin use should be avoided in the neonatal intensive care unit.

Practice Option #4: Central Venous Catheter Removal

In addition to administration of antifungal therapy for 21 days from negative culture and evaluation for disseminated disease, providers should promptly remove central venous catheters. Prompt removal of central venous catheters after IC diagnosis has been associated with decreased mortality compared to delayed removal. In addition, delayed removal has been linked to worse neurodevelopmental outcomes. Providers should document clearance of infection within 1 week of antifungal initiation. In the event that clearance does not occur, providers should consider addition of a second antifungal agent.

IMPLEMENTATION OF GUIDELINE

DESCRIPTION OF IMPLEMENTATION STRATEGY

Develop guidelines for antifungal therapy in the setting of IC diagnosis.

QUALITY METRICS

Adherence to guidelines; emergence of antifungal resistance.

SUMMARY

IC is a significant cause of morbidity and mortality in premature infants. Potential methods to prevent IC include early removal of central venous catheters, prevention of *Candida* colonization, and prophylactic therapy. Because of its safety profile and demonstrated efficacy, we recommend fluconazole prophylaxis for up to 6 weeks in infants <1000 g birth weight who are admitted to moderate- or high-incidence centers (>5–10%). Diagnosis remains difficult due to the low sensitivity of blood cultures; however, emerging therapies may improve the sensitivity and speed of diagnosis. Once a diagnosis of IC is made, appropriate antifungal therapy is imperative as is evaluation for the presence of IC dissemination.

BIBLIOGRAPHIC SOURCE(S)

Adams-Chapman I, Bann CM, Das A, et al. Neurodevelopmental outcome of extremely low birth weight infants with Candida infection. *J Pediatr.* 2013;163(4):961-7.e3.

Ahmad S, Khan Z. Invasive candidiasis: a review of nonculture-based laboratory diagnostic methods. *Indian J Med Microbiol.* 2012;30(3):264-9.

Aliaga S, Clark RH, Laughon M, et al. Changes in the incidence of candidiasis in neonatal intensive care units. *Pediatrics.* 2014;133(2):236-42.

Ascher SB, Smith PB, Watt K, et al. Antifungal therapy and outcomes in infants with invasive Candida infections. *Pediatr Infect Dis J.* 2012;31(5):439-43.

Austin N, McGuire W. Prophylactic systemic antifungal agents to prevent mortality and morbidity in very low birth weight infants. *Cochrane Database Syst Rev.* 2013;4:CD003850.

Benjamin DK Jr, DeLong ER, Steinbach WJ, Cotton CM, Walsh TJ, Clark RH. Empirical therapy for neonatal candidemia in very low birth weight infants. *Pediatrics.* 2003;112(3 Pt 1):543-7.

Benjamin DK Jr, Hudak ML, Duara S, et al. Effect of fluconazole prophylaxis on candidiasis and mortality in premature infants: a randomized clinical trial. *JAMA.* 2014;311(17):1742-9.

Benjamin DK Jr, Poole C, Steinbach WJ, Rowen JL, Walsh TJ. Neonatal candidemia and end-organ damage: a critical appraisal of the literature using meta-analytic techniques. *Pediatrics.* 2003;112(3 Pt 1):634-40.

Benjamin DK Jr, Smith PB, Arrieta A, et al. Safety and pharmacokinetics of repeat-dose micafungin in young infants. *Clin Pharmacol Ther.* 2010;87(1):93-9.

Benjamin DK Jr, Stoll BJ, Fanaroff AA, et al. Neonatal candidiasis among extremely low birth weight infants: risk factors, mortality rates, and neurodevelopmental outcomes at 18 to 22 months. *Pediatrics.* 2006;117(1):84-92.

Benjamin DK Jr, Stoll BJ, Gantz MG, et al. Neonatal candidiasis: epidemiology, risk factors, and clinical judgment. *Pediatrics.* 2010;126(4):e865-73.

Berenguer J, Buck M, Witebsky F, Stock F, Pizzo PA, Walsh TJ. Lysis-centrifugation blood cultures in the detection of tissue-proven invasive candidiasis. Disseminated versus single-organ infection. *Diagn Microbiol Infect Dis.* 1993;17(2):103-9.

Chapman RL, Faix RG. Invasive neonatal candidiasis: an overview. *Semin Perinatol.* 2003;27(5):352-6.

Fridkin SK, Kaufman D, Edwards JR, Shetty S, Horan T. Changing incidence of Candida bloodstream infections among NICU patients in the United States: 1995-2004. *Pediatrics.* 2006;117(5):1680-7.

Goudjil S, Kongolo G, Dusol L, et al. (1-3)-Beta-D-glucan levels in candidiasis infections in the critically ill neonate. *J Matern Fetal Neonat Med.* 2013;26(1):44-8.

Greenberg RG, Benjamin DK Jr, Gantz MG, et al. Empiric antifungal therapy and outcomes in extremely low birth weight infants with invasive candidiasis. *J Pediatr.* 2012;161(2):264-9.e2.

Hope WW, Smith PB, Arrieta A, et al. Population pharmacokinetics of micafungin in neonates and young infants. *Antimicrob Agents Chemother.* 2010;54(6):2633-7.

Hsieh E, Smith PB, Jacqz-Aigrain E, et al. Neonatal fungal infections: when to treat? *Early Hum Dev.* 2012;88(Suppl 2):S6-S10.

Juster-Reicher A, Leibovitz E, Linder N, et al. Liposomal amphotericin B (AmBisome) in the treatment of neonatal candidiasis in very low birth weight infants. *Infection.* 2000;28(4):223-6.

Kaufman D, Boyle R, Hazen KC, Patrie JT, Robinson M, Donowitz LG. Fluconazole prophylaxis against fungal colonization and infection in preterm infants. *N Engl J Med.* 2001;345(23):1660-6.

Lehmann LE, Hunfeld KP, Emrich T, et al. A multiplex real-time PCR assay for rapid detection and differentiation of 25 bacterial and fungal pathogens from whole blood samples. *Med Microbiol Immunol.* 2008;197(3):313-24.

Maenza JR, Keruly JC, Moore RD, Chaisson RE, Merz WG, Gallant JE. Risk factors for fluconazole-resistant candidiasis in human immunodeficiency virus-infected patients. J Infect Dis. 1996;173(1):219-25.

Manzoni P, Stolfi I, Pugni L, et al. A multicenter, randomized trial of prophylactic fluconazole in preterm neonates. *N Engl J Med.* 2007;356(24):2483-95.

Morace G, Pagano L, Sanguinetti M, et al. PCR-restriction enzyme analysis for detection of Candida DNA in blood from febrile patients with hematological malignancies. *J Clin Microbiol.* 1999;37(6):1871-5.

Oliveri S, Trovato L, Betta P, Romeo MG, Nicoletti G. Experience with the Platelia Candida ELISA for the diagnosis of invasive candidosis in neonatal patients. *Clin Microbiol Infect.* 2008;14(4):391-3.

Pfaller MA, Diekema DJ, Boyken L, et al. Effectiveness of anidulafungin in eradicating Candida species in invasive candidiasis. *Antimicrob Agents Chemother.* 2005;49(11):4795-7.

Piper L, Smith PB, Hornik CP, et al. Fluconazole loading dose pharmacokinetics and safety in infants. *Pediatr Infect Dis J.* 2011;30(5):375-8.

Rowen JL, Tate JM. Management of neonatal candidiasis. Neonatal Candidiasis Study Group. *Pediatr Infect Dis J.* 1998;17(11):1007-11.

Schelonka RL, Chai MK, Yoder BA, Hensley D, Brockett RM, Ascher DP. Volume of blood required to detect common neonatal pathogens. *J Pediatr.* 1996;129(2):275-8.

Smith PB, Morgan J, Benjamin JD, et al. Excess costs of hospital care associated with neonatal candidemia. *Pediatr Infect Dis J.* 2007;26(3):197-200.

Smith PB, Walsh TJ, Hope W, et al. Pharmacokinetics of an elevated dosage of micafungin in premature neonates. *Pediatr Infect Dis J.* 2009;28(5):412-5.

Stoll BJ, Hansen N, Fanaroff AA, et al. Late-onset sepsis in very low birth weight neonates: the experience of the NICHD Neonatal Research Network. *Pediatrics.* 2002;110(2 Pt 1):285-91.

Tan KE, Ellis BC, Lee R, Stamper PD, Zhang SX, Carroll KC. Prospective evaluation of a matrix-assisted laser desorption ionization-time of flight mass spectrometry system in a hospital clinical microbiology laboratory for identification of bacteria and yeasts: a bench-by-bench study for assessing the impact on time to identification and cost-effectiveness. *J Clin Microbiol.* 2012;50(10):3301-8.

Trovato L, Betta P, Romeo MG, Oliveri S. Detection of fungal DNA in lysis-centrifugation blood culture for the diagnosis of invasive candidiasis in neonatal patients. *Clin Microbiol Infect.* 2012;18(3):E63-5.

Wurthwein G, Groll AH, Hempel G, Adler-Shohet FC, Lieberman JM, Walsh TJ. Population pharmacokinetics of amphotericin B lipid complex in neonates. *Antimicrob Agents Chemother.* 2005;49(12):5092-8.

Zaoutis TE, Argon J, Chu J, Berlin JA, Walsh TJ, Feudtner C. The epidemiology and attributable outcomes of candidemia in adults and children hospitalized in the United States: a propensity analysis. *Clin Infect Dis.* 2005;41(9):1232-9.

TORCH Infections

Kelly C. Wade, MD, PhD, MSCE

SCOPE

DISEASE/CONDITION(S)

Congenital infections secondary to toxoplasmosis, other (varicella zoster virus [VZV], parvovirus, and enterovirus), rubella, and cytomegalovirus (CMV); herpes simplex virus (HSV) and syphilis reviewed in Chapter 44.

GUIDELINE OBJECTIVE(S)

Review clinical features that are useful in identifying infants with congenital infections; outline diagnostic tests to confirm or refute congenital infections; outline treatments for congenital infections.

BRIEF BACKGROUND

The TORCH acronym (*Toxoplasma*, other, rubella, CMV, and HSV) was originally designated to group congenital infections with similar clinical features in newborns that included intrauterine growth restriction (IUGR), microcephaly, hepatosplenomegaly, rashes, and eye findings or in utero fetal demise. Congenital rubella syndrome has declined with improved immunizations; however, the "other" category has expanded to include viral pathogens such as VZV, parvovirus, and enterovirus. Serologic testing of mothers and infants along with polymerase chain reaction (PCR)-based diagnostic tests have improved the ability to identify the specific pathogens responsible for congenital infections.

RECOMMENDATIONS

MAJOR RECOMMENDATIONS

Recognition of clinical features of congenital infections is important to facilitate early diagnosis and treatment. Infants with congenital infections often present with IUGR, hepatosplenomegaly, eye findings, and skin rashes. Alternatively, they can be asymptomatic, hydropic, or suffer in utero demise. Careful review of maternal history and serologies for infections during pregnancy is critical. Further evaluation of infant characteristics may help distinguish different pathogens. Congenital infection is confirmed by pathogen-specific IgM in infant and PCR-based detection of microbe in the amniotic fluid, neonatal skin lesions, or body fluids (blood, urine, CSF, and nasopharyngeal secretions). Treatment targets the specific pathogen.

PRACTICE OPTIONS

Practice Option #1

Identify infants at risk for congenital infections using two triggers: 1) infants born to women who had serious infections in pregnancy and 2) newborns with common clinical features of congenital infection (IUGR, microcephaly, hepatosplenomegaly, skin rashes, and eye findings or nonimmune hydrops). Newborns with positive trigger may benefit from further evaluation, including complete blood count, liver function tests, hearing test, eye examination (cataracts, glaucoma, or chorioretinitis), and neuroimaging (calcifications or CNS abnormalities).

Practice Option #2

Maternal history and clinical features of the newborn direct the pathogen-specific workup. Diagnostic evaluation includes maternal and neonatal pathogen-specific serologic evaluation and PCR test of amniotic fluid or infant body fluids (Table 43.1).

Practice Option #3

Infants with confirmed infection require treatment (Table 43.1) and follow-up surveillance for long-term sequelae tailored to the specific pathogen. Consultation with infectious disease specialist is often recommended.

IMPLEMENTATION OF GUIDELINE

QUALIFYING STATEMENTS

1. Some serologic assays are not approved for diagnostic use in infants by the US Food and Drug Administration and may not be commercially available. False negative, false positive, and equivocal tests have been reported. Specific laboratories and infectious disease specialist may be required.
2. The optimal drugs, doses, and duration of therapy are not established definitively. Consultation with infectious disease specialist is often warranted.
3. Clinical features of congenital infections can also be seen in inborn errors of metabolism and genetic syndromes.

TABLE 43.1. Clinical Features and Evaluation of Congenital Infections

Clinical features	Specific clinical features
General	• Diffuse CNS calcifications—*Toxoplasma*
IUGR	• Periventricular calcifications—CMV
Microcephaly	• Hearing loss—CMV, rubella, *Toxoplasma*; onset at
Liver disease	birth or during infancy
Thrombocytopenia	• Limb hypoplasia—VZV
Skin rash	• Cataracts—VZV, rubella
Eye chorioretinitis	• Congenital heart disease—rubella
Hearing impairment	• Radiolucent bone disease—rubella
	• Nonimmune hydrops or myocarditis—parvovirus, enterovirus
	Severe congenital syndromes (rubella, CMV, VZV) occur most often when maternal primary infection occurs at <20 weeks' gestation
	Acute viral illness in newborns most often occurs when maternal illness, e.g., VZV or enterovirus, occurs near the time of delivery, prior to placental transfer of maternal IgG

Serology	Basic interpretation of serologic studies	IgG	IgM
	• No serologic evidence infection	–	–
	• New primary infection or false positive	–	+
	• Immunity from past infection or immunization	+	–
	• Recent primary infection *or*	+	+
	Immunity from past infection with new exposure or reactivation		
	Immunity from past infection with false positive IgM		

- **High-avidity IgG testing** can help determine timing of infection. Initial infection leads to low-avidity IgG, then after 2–4 months high-avidity IgG is produced. Low-avidity IgG suggests primary infection within the past 2–4 months, while high-avidity IgG suggests infection more than 2–4 months ago. High-avidity IgG in first trimester indicates infection prior to pregnancy.
- **False positive IgM** due to rheumatoid factor, heterophile Ab, or other viral IgM

Detection	Polymerase chain reaction (PCR)

- Most sensitive diagnostic test for microbes
- Performed on different body fluids including amniotic fluid, placenta, blood, urine, CSF, skin lesions, and respiratory/nasopharyngeal secretions
- Reverse transcriptase PCR for rubella, an RNA virus
- Rubella: high sensitivity for nasopharyngeal specimen
- CMV: high sensitivity for urine
- VZV: high sensitivity for skin lesions

Direct fluorescent antibody (DFA) and viral culture

(Continued)

TABLE 43.1. Clinical Features and Evaluation of Congenital Infections (Continued)

Treatment	***Toxoplasma gondii:*** pyrimethamine, sulfadiazine, folinic acid, ± prednisone
	CMV: consider ganciclovir or valganciclovir for CNS disease based on improved hearing outcomes at 6 months age
	VZV: acyclovir for active neonatal infections
	Enterovirus: consider IVIG if myocarditis
	VZV post-exposure prophylaxis: VZ IG or if not available IVIG
	• Maternal infection <5 days prior to or 2 days after birth
	• Hospitalized, preterm infant <28 weeks' gestation
	• Hospitalized, preterm infant >28 weeks' gestation born to a non-immune mother

DESCRIPTION OF IMPLEMENTATION STRATEGY

Recommend written guidelines for evaluation of infants born to mothers with serious infections acquired in pregnancy or those with clinical features consistent with congenital infections.

QUALITY METRICS

Review specific diagnosis and outcome of infants born with clinical features consistent with congenital infections. Identify infants diagnosed with congenital infection after hospital discharge using reporting systems or feedback from infectious disease specialists to birth hospitals.

SUMMARY

The identification of infants with congenital infections requires a high index of suspicion, recognition of common clinical features, interpretation of maternal and neonatal serologies, and diagnostic tests for specific pathogens. Additional studies are needed to optimize drug treatments for congenital infections in infants.

BIBLIOGRAPHIC SOURCE(S)

AAP. *Red Book Online.* 2012. http://redbook.solutions.aap.org/. Accessed February 14, 2015.
Centers for Disease Control. http://www.cdc.gov/. Accessed February 14, 2015.

HIV and Sexually Transmitted Diseases

Matthew S. Kelly, MD, MPH • Ross McKinney Jr, MD

SCOPE

DISEASE/CONDITION(S)

Evaluation and antiretroviral (ARV) prophylaxis of HIV-exposed infants.

GUIDELINE OBJECTIVE(S)

Review routes of HIV transmission; evaluation of HIV-exposed infants; recommendations for infant ARV prophylaxis

BRIEF BACKGROUND

Mother-to-child transmission (MTCT) of HIV can occur during pregnancy (intrapartum), at the time of birth (perinatal), or through breastfeeding (postpartum). The risk of MTCT of HIV can be reduced from 25–30% to <1% with maternal combination ARV therapy during pregnancy, infant ARV prophylaxis, and avoidance of breastfeeding. Risk factors for perinatal HIV transmission include high maternal viral load, low maternal CD4 count, chorioamnionitis, other sexually transmitted infections, and vaginal delivery. Most infants with HIV infection are asymptomatic at birth, but approximately 25% of these infants progress rapidly to AIDS and death. Early diagnosis and treatment reduces mortality by at least 75% among HIV-infected infants.

RECOMMENDATIONS

MAJOR RECOMMENDATIONS

Strict avoidance of breastfeeding is recommended for all HIV-exposed infants in the United States. A blood HIV DNA polymerase chain reaction (PCR) or qualitative HIV RNA PCR should be drawn from all HIV-exposed newborns after a brief bath is performed (do not delay starting infant ARV prophylaxis). In addition, HIV DNA PCR or qualitative HIV RNA PCR should be performed at ages 2 weeks, 1–2 months, and 4 months. For very high-risk infants, virologic testing could also be considered at 6 months of age. Infants with positive virologic testing should have immediate confirmatory testing (repeat DNA PCR or qualitative HIV RNA PCR on a new blood specimen) and evaluation by a pediatric infectious diseases specialist for consideration of combination ARV therapy. The ARV regimen for infant prophylaxis is determined based on an assessment of the risk of MTCT.

PRACTICE OPTIONS

Practice Option #1

For low-risk infants born to HIV-infected mothers on combination ARV therapy with undetectable HIV viral loads during pregnancy, a 4–6-week course of zidovudine (AZT) (term infants: 4 mg/kg by mouth twice daily) is recommended (with first dose given as soon as possible after birth).

Practice Option #2

For high-risk infants born to HIV-infected mothers with a detectable viral load near delivery or who were not on combination ARV therapy prior to delivery, two-drug ARV prophylaxis is recommended. In addition to a 6-week course of AZT, three doses of nevirapine (NVP) (birth weight >2 kg: 12 mg per dose by mouth) should be given. The first dose is administered as soon as possible after birth, the second dose is given 48 hours after the first dose, and the third dose is given 96 hours after the second dose.

Practice Option #3

For very high-risk infants (e.g., mother had a high HIV viral load prior to delivery or has suspected or known ARV-resistant virus), a three-drug ARV prophylaxis regimen should be considered in consultation with a pediatric infectious disease specialist.

CLINICAL ALGORITHM(S)

Figure 44.1 presents an algorithm for risk stratification and ARV prophylaxis of HIV-exposed infants.

IMPLEMENTATION OF GUIDELINE

QUALIFYING STATEMENTS

1. The optimal duration of AZT for infant prophylaxis has not been established. For low-risk infants whose mothers were on combination ARV therapy during pregnancy, had serial undetectable HIV viral loads, and no concerns regarding adherence, a 4-week course of AZT can be considered.
2. No clinical trials demonstrate that a three-drug ARV prophylaxis regimen is superior to two-drug ARV prophylaxis in very high-risk infants.

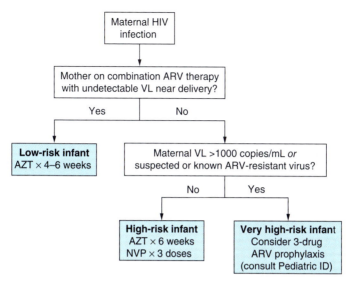

FIGURE 44.1 • Algorithm for risk stratification and ARV prophylaxis of HIV-exposed infants. ARV, antiretroviral; AZT, zidovudine; ID, infectious diseases; NVP, nevirapine; VL, viral load.

DESCRIPTION OF IMPLEMENTATION STRATEGY

All pregnant women should be tested routinely for HIV. Rapid HIV testing using a combined HIV antibody/antigen assay should be performed on women with unknown HIV status who present in labor or after delivery. All infants born to HIV-infected mothers should receive ARV prophylaxis as soon as possible after birth. For infants of mothers with unknown HIV status who have positive rapid HIV testing at the time of delivery, infant ARV prophylaxis should be started while awaiting testing to confirm maternal HIV infection.

QUALITY METRICS

ARV prophylaxis should be administered to all HIV-exposed infants by 6–12 hours of life, and ideally within the first hour after birth.

SUMMARY

MTCT of HIV can be effectively prevented through maternal combination ARV therapy during pregnancy, timely administration of ARV prophylaxis to HIV-exposed infants, and strict avoidance of breastfeeding. The choice of infant ARV prophylaxis regimen is based on an assessment of the risk of MTCT, taking into account the mother's history of ARV treatment, viral load, and HIV resistance testing. HIV-infected infants should be started on combination ARV therapy to prevent progression to AIDS and reduce mortality during infancy.

SCOPE

DISEASE/CONDITION(S)

Diagnosis and treatment of infants with congenital syphilis.

GUIDELINE OBJECTIVE(S)

Review the evaluation and treatment of infants born to mothers with syphilis.

BRIEF BACKGROUND

Congenital syphilis results from transmission of the spirochete *Treponema pallidum* from mother to fetus. Intrauterine infection results in stillbirth in 30–40% of cases. Among live born infants, clinical manifestations of congenital syphilis include lymphadenopathy, hepatosplenomegaly, profuse nasal discharge ("snuffles"), pneumonia, osteochondritis, and mucocutaneous lesions. Thrombocytopenia, hemolytic anemia, or hyperbilirubinemia are often identified on laboratory testing. However, two-thirds of infants with congenital syphilis are asymptomatic at birth. Without appropriate treatment, infants with congenital syphilis can develop late complications of the central nervous system (CNS), bones and joints, teeth, and eyes. Penicillin G is the only proven effective therapy for congenital syphilis.

RECOMMENDATIONS

MAJOR RECOMMENDATIONS

The American Academy of Pediatrics (AAP) Committee on Infectious Diseases published guidelines for the evaluation and treatment of infants born to mothers with syphilis. The decision to treat is based upon infant physical examination, adequacy of maternal syphilis treatment during pregnancy, and results of non-treponemal test (e.g., rapid plasma reagin [RPR] or venereal disease research laboratory [VDRL] testing) from the infant. Adequate treatment of pregnant women for syphilis is defined as:

- Receipt of penicillin G treatment >4 weeks prior to delivery
- *And* receipt of a treatment regimen that is appropriate for the stage of syphilis
- *And* documentation of serological response to treatment:
  - Early syphilis: ≥fourfold reduction in RPR or VDRL
  - Late syphilis: stable low titer (RPR<1:4 or VDRL<1:2)
- *And* no evidence of relapse or reinfection (≥fourfold increase in RPR or VDRL)

PRACTICE OPTIONS

Practice Option #1

Infants with perinatal exposure and examination findings consistent with congenital syphilis should have serum non-treponemal test (e.g., RPR or VDRL), complete blood count (CBC) with differential, and lumbar puncture for cerebrospinal fluid (CSF) cell count, protein, and CSF quantitative VDRL. Additional diagnostic testing (e.g., skeletal and chest radiographs, liver enzymes, ophthalmological examination) should be performed if clinically indicated. All infants should receive aqueous penicillin G 50,000 units/kg IV every 12 hours (if age <1 week) or every 8 hours (if age ≥1 week) for 10 days.

Practice Option #2

Evaluation and treatment of infants with normal physical examination whose mothers received inadequate treatment for syphilis during pregnancy:

- CBC with differential, lumbar puncture (CSF cell count, protein, CSF quantitative VDRL)
- Treat with aqueous penicillin G 50,000 units/kg IV every 12 hours (if age <1 week) or every 8 hours (if age ≥1 week) for 10 days

Practice Option #3

Infants with normal physical examination whose mothers received adequate treatment during pregnancy should have a serum non-treponemal test:

- Infant RPR or VDRL titer ≥fourfold the maternal titer (which is diagnostic for congenital infection):
  - CBC with differential, lumbar puncture (CSF cell count, protein, CSF quantitative VDRL)
  - Treat with aqueous penicillin G 50,000 units/kg IV every 12 hours (if age <1 week) or every 8 hours (if age ≥1 week) for 10 days
- Infant RPR or VDRL <fourfold the maternal titer:
  - No further evaluation
  - Treat with aqueous penicillin G 50,000 units/kg IV every 12 hours (if age <1 week) or every 8 hours (if age ≥1 week) for 10 days

Practice Option #4

Infants of mothers who were treated for syphilis before pregnancy do not require evaluation or treatment if all of the following criteria are met:

1. The mother received adequate treatment before pregnancy
2. *And* the mother had a non-treponemal test that remained stable and low (RPR<1:4, VDRL<1:2) during pregnancy and at delivery
3. *And* the infant has a normal physical examination
4. *And* the infant's RPR or VDRL is the same or lower than the maternal titer

Practice Option #5

Infants with neurosyphilis (CSF pleocytosis, elevated CSF protein, or positive CSF quantitative VDRL) should have repeat lumbar puncture at 6 months of age to document normalization of CSF cell count and other parameters; infants with continued abnormal CSF parameters or reactive CSF VDRL at 6 months should undergo retreatment with aqueous penicillin G IV.

CLINICAL ALGORITHM(S)

The recommended diagnostic evaluation and treatment of infants born to mothers with syphilis during pregnancy is summarized in Table 44.1.

IMPLEMENTATION OF GUIDELINE

QUALIFYING STATEMENTS

1. Procaine penicillin G 50,000 units/kg IM once daily for 10 days is an alternative to treatment with aqueous penicillin G IV. However, as the CSF levels achieved with procaine penicillin G are lower than those observed with aqueous penicillin G, it should not be used to treat neurosyphilis.
2. No randomized controlled trials examined the optimal treatment duration for congenital syphilis.

TABLE 44.1. Treatment of Infants Born to Mothers With Syphilis During Pregnancy

Infant Examination	Maternal Treatment	Infant RPR or VDRL	Diagnostic Evaluation	Treatment
Abnormal	–	–	CBC CSF cell count, protein, VDRL	Penicillin G IV 50,000 units/kg IV q8h (<1 week) or q12h (≥1 week) × 10 days
Normal	Inadequate	–		
Normal	Adequate	≥ Fourfold maternal titer		
Normal	Adequate	< Fourfold maternal titer	None	Penicillin G IV 50,000 units/kg IV q8h (<1 week) or q12h (≥1 week) × 10 days

DESCRIPTION OF IMPLEMENTATION STRATEGY

All women should be screened for syphilis using a non-treponemal test (e.g., RPR or VRDL) early in pregnancy. In high-prevalence settings or in high-risk patients, repeat testing should be performed during the third trimester and again at the time of delivery. Confirmation of maternal syphilis infection should be performed using a treponemal test (e.g., fluorescent treponemal antibody absorption [FTA-ABS] test, T. pallidum particle agglutination [TP-PA]). All pregnant women with syphilis should be tested for other sexually transmitted infections including HIV. Infants born to mothers with a history of syphilis infection during pregnancy should have a thorough physical examination as soon as possible after birth.

SUMMARY

As most infants with congenital syphilis are asymptomatic at birth, evaluation and treatment for congenital syphilis is based upon history of maternal infection during pregnancy and the adequacy of treatment. A conservative approach is warranted because congenital syphilis can occur despite adequate maternal treatment as a result of relapse or reinfection.

SCOPE

DISEASE/CONDITION(S)

Neonatal herpes simplex virus (HSV) infection.

GUIDELINE OBJECTIVE(S)

Discuss route and risk factors for transmission of HSV; review evaluation and treatment of neonatal HSV infection.

BRIEF BACKGROUND

Neonatal HSV infection most frequently results from exposure to infected maternal genital secretions at the time of delivery. Signs of neonatal HSV infection can develop from birth to 6 weeks of age, although most infants present during the first month of life. The risk of HSV transmission is higher from mothers with primary infection during pregnancy (particularly near delivery) than from women with a history of genital HSV preceding pregnancy. Neonatal HSV infection is associated with three clinical presentations: skin, eye, and mucous membrane (SEM) disease, CNS disease (meningoencephalitis), and disseminated infection. Infants with SEM disease have mucocutaneous vesicles that most frequently develop during the first 2 weeks of life. HSV meningoencephalitis occurs most commonly in the second or third week of life and may be associated with temperature instability, irritability, lethargy, poor feeding, or seizures. HSV meningoencephalitis may present similarly to serious bacterial infections (e.g., bacteremia, febrile urinary tract infection). Disseminated infection often presents in the first 2 weeks of life and is typically associated with hepatitis and liver failure, hematological abnormalities, shock physiology, and disseminated intravascular coagulation (DIC). There is substantial overlap in these clinical presentations, and infants with any manifestation of HSV infection may have disease at other sites.

RECOMMENDATIONS

PRACTICE OPTIONS

Practice Option #1

Infants with suspected HSV disease (regardless of clinical presentation) should be evaluated with surface cultures (conjunctivae, mouth, nasopharynx, and rectum), blood HSV PCR, and lumbar puncture for CSF cell counts, glucose, protein, and CSF HSV PCR. Any skin lesions should also be sent for HSV testing by PCR. Infants with suspected neonatal HSV disease should receive acyclovir 20 mg/kg IV every 8 hours immediately and while awaiting the results of this diagnostic evaluation.

Practice Option #2

For infants with confirmed neonatal HSV infection, the duration of treatment with acyclovir IV depends on the site(s) of disease. Infants with localized SEM disease (without CNS or disseminated infection) should be treated with acyclovir IV (20 mg/kg IV every 8 hours) for at least 14 days. Infants with CNS or disseminated disease require treatment with acyclovir IV (20 mg/kg IV every 8 hours) for a minimum of 21 days. For infants with CNS disease, repeat lumbar puncture should be performed near the end of the treatment course to ensure that CSF parameters have normalized and repeat CSF HSV PCR is negative. Once clinically stable, infants with CNS disease should also have neuroimaging (i.e., brain MRI or, if unavailable, CT) as this may provide useful prognostic information.

Practice Option #3

After completion of the treatment course of acyclovir IV, infants with CNS or disseminated disease should receive suppressive therapy (acyclovir 300–500 mg/m²/dose orally given thrice daily) for at least 6 months (improves neurodevelopmental outcomes). Some experts recommend suppressive therapy with acyclovir 500 mg/m²/dose orally given thrice daily for as long as 2 years.

Practice Option #4

Infants born to mothers with a history of genital HSV infection but no active lesions at the time of delivery require close monitoring only. The AAP developed guidelines for the management of asymptomatic infants born to mothers with active genital lesions at the time of delivery. Maternal genital lesions should be sent for HSV PCR and culture. The extent of the initial evaluation of the infant and the decision regarding empirical acyclovir treatment is guided by whether maternal infection is primary or a reactivation.

- For infants of mothers with a history of genital HSV preceding the pregnancy:
  - Surface cultures (conjunctivae, mouth, nasopharynx, and rectum)
  - Blood HSV PCR
  - No empirical acyclovir while awaiting results of the diagnostic evaluation provided that the infant displays no signs of infection
- For infants of mothers with *no* history of genital HSV preceding the pregnancy:
  - Send serum HSV-1/HSV-2 antibodies from mother
  - Surface cultures (conjunctivae, mouth, nasopharynx, and rectum)
  - Blood HSV PCR
  - Lumbar puncture for CSF cell counts, glucose, protein, and CSF HSV PCR
  - Liver enzymes
  - Start acyclovir 20 mg/kg IV every 8 hours while awaiting results of this diagnostic evaluation

The interpretation of maternal HSV serologies and decisions regarding definitive acyclovir treatment based on the results of the diagnostic evaluation are beyond the scope of this text but are discussed in detail in the AAP guidelines.

IMPLEMENTATION OF GUIDELINE

QUALIFYING STATEMENTS

1. Although CSF HSV PCR is very sensitive (>95%) for the diagnosis of CNS disease, false negatives do occur, particularly on samples obtained early in the disease course or after several days of treatment with acyclovir.
2. Neither the optimal duration nor the optimal acyclovir dose for oral suppressive therapy in infants with CNS disease or disseminated infection have been defined. Long-term oral suppressive therapy has not been shown to improve neurodevelopmental outcomes among infants with isolated SEM disease but does prevent skin recurrences.

DESCRIPTION OF IMPLEMENTATION STRATEGY

Pregnant women should be routinely asked whether they have a history of genital HSV infection or ulcerations and should undergo careful examination for the presence of genital lesions at the time of delivery. The American College of Obstetricians and Gynecologists recommends cesarean delivery for women with genital HSV lesions or prodromal symptoms at the onset of labor.

SUMMARY

Neonatal HSV infection is a potentially devastating condition that presents during the first 6 weeks of life. Acyclovir reduces morbidity and mortality of neonatal HSV disease and should be started immediately in infants with clinical suspicion for HSV infection. The risk of HSV transmission to infants depends on the timing of maternal infection. Infants born to mothers with primary infection during pregnancy are at highest risk and should receive empirical acyclovir while being evaluated for HSV infection.

SCOPE

DISEASE/CONDITION(S)

Neonatal gonococcal infections.

GUIDELINE OBJECTIVE(S)

Review the prevention, diagnosis, and treatment of neonatal gonococcal infections.

BRIEF BACKGROUND

Infants may become infected with *Neisseria gonorrhea* from exposure to infected maternal genital secretions during the birthing process. Infection most frequently causes conjunctivitis (ophthalmia neonatorum) developing within 2–5 days of birth, characterized by conjunctival erythema, profuse purulent exudate, and periorbital edema. Prompt antibiotic treatment is critical to preventing progression to corneal ulceration, scarring, and long-term visual impairment. Infants can also develop gonococcal scalp abscesses at the sites of electrodes for fetal monitoring or disseminated infections including bacteremia, septic arthritis, and meningitis.

RECOMMENDATIONS

MAJOR RECOMMENDATIONS

All infants should receive prophylaxis with 0.5% erythromycin ophthalmic ointment into both eyes as soon as possible after birth. Parenteral antibiotic therapy is required to treat gonococcal conjunctivitis, scalp abscess, or disseminated infection.

PRACTICE OPTIONS

Practice Option #1

Conjunctival exudate should be sent for Gram stain and culture (request modified Thayer-Martin media) if gonococcal conjunctivitis is suspected. Infants with presumed or confirmed gonococcal conjunctivitis should undergo evaluation for disseminated infection including a thorough joint examination, blood culture, and lumbar puncture (CSF cell counts, glucose, protein, Gram stain, and culture). If disseminated infection is excluded, infants with conjunctivitis should receive a single dose of ceftriaxone 25 mg/kg IV/IM (maximum dose: 125 mg). Eyes should be irrigated frequently with sterile saline until the purulent discharge has resolved.

Practice Option #2

Infants with scalp abscess, bacteremia, or septic arthritis should be treated with ceftriaxone 25–50 mg/kg IV/IM once daily for a minimum of 7 days. Cefotaxime 25 mg/kg IV/IM every 12 hours for 7 days is an alternative if the infant has hyperbilirubinemia. Duration of treatment for meningitis is 10–14 days.

TABLE 44.2. Treatment of Neonatal Gonococcal Infections

Infection Site	Antibiotic Regimen	Duration
Eye (conjunctivitis)	Ceftriaxone 25 mg/kg IV/IM (max dose: 125 mg)	× 1
Scalp abscess Bacteremia Septic arthritis	Ceftriaxone 25–50 mg/kg IV/IM q24h *or* Cefotaxime 25 mg/kg IV/IM q12h	7 days
Meningitis	Ceftriaxone 25–50 mg/kg IV/IM q24h *or* Cefotaxime 25 mg/kg IV/IM q12h	10–14 days

Practice Option #3

Asymptomatic infants born to mothers with untreated urogenital gonorrhea infection should receive prophylaxis with a single dose of ceftriaxone 25–50 mg/kg IV/IM (maximum dose: 125 mg).

CLINICAL ALGORITHM(S)

Antibiotic regimens and treatment durations for neonatal gonococcal infections by site are shown in Table 44.2.

IMPLEMENTATION OF GUIDELINE

QUALIFYING STATEMENTS

1. No randomized controlled trials identified the optimal duration of treatment for disseminated gonococcal infections among infants.
2. No randomized controlled trials evaluated the efficacy of single-dose ceftriaxone for prophylaxis of infants born to mothers with untreated gonococcal infections.

DESCRIPTION OF IMPLEMENTATION STRATEGY

All pregnant women should be tested for gonorrhea as part of standard prenatal care. Mothers with gonorrhea should be evaluated for other sexually transmitted infections including HIV. Hospitals should have a system in place to identify infants who do not receive erythromycin ophthalmic ointment in the delivery room.

QUALITY METRICS

Monitor rates of testing for gonorrhea among pregnant women, proportion of infants receiving erythromycin ophthalmic ointment in the delivery room.

SUMMARY

Neonatal gonococcal infections can be vision- or life-threatening, but the vast majority are preventable through routine screening of pregnant women and universal administration of erythromycin ophthalmic ointment to infants. Treatment of gonococcal infections in infants requires parenteral therapy, with the dosing and duration of antibiotic therapy determined based on the site of the infection.

SCOPE

DISEASE/CONDITION(S)

Chlamydial infections in young infants.

GUIDELINE OBJECTIVE(S)

Review diagnosis and treatment of chlamydial infections in infants.

BRIEF BACKGROUND

Chlamydia trachomatis is the most common sexually transmitted infection in the United States. Infection in young infants most frequently manifests as conjunctivitis or pneumonia. Chlamydial conjunctivitis typically occurs between 5 days and 2 weeks of life, with signs and symptoms that can range from mild conjunctival hyperemia with scant watery or mucoid discharge to severe chemosis, periorbital edema, and pseudomembrane formation. Chlamydial pneumonia occurs most frequently 2 weeks to 4 months after birth and is classically characterized by tachypnea and a staccato cough, with hyperinflation and bilateral infiltrates on chest radiograph; fever is generally absent.

RECOMMENDATIONS

MAJOR RECOMMENDATIONS

Routine screening and treatment of *C. trachomatis* infections in pregnant women can prevent chlamydia infections in infants. Erythromycin 0.5% ophthalmic ointment is ineffective in preventing chlamydial conjunctivitis but should be administered to prevent gonococcal ophthalmologic disease.

PRACTICE OPTIONS

Practice Option #1

Chlamydial infection should be considered in all infants with conjunctivitis during the first month of life. Infants with suspected chlamydial conjunctivitis should have a specimen collected from the everted eyelid using a Dacron-tipped swab. This specimen must include epithelial cells (not just exudate) and should be sent for chlamydial culture and PCR. Infants with chlamydial conjunctivitis should receive erythromycin 50 mg/kg/day PO in four divided doses for 14 days. Close follow-up is necessary, as up to 20% of infants will have continued symptoms and require a second course of treatment. Topical (ophthalmologic) therapy should not be used, as it is associated with a high treatment failure rate and does not eradicate nasopharyngeal infection.

Practice Option #2

Evaluation for chlamydial pneumonia should include chlamydial culture and PCR of a nasopharyngeal specimen obtained using a Dacron-tipped swab. Tracheal or bronchoalveolar lavage specimens should also be tested by culture and PCR when available. Infants with chlamydial pneumonia should be treated with erythromycin 50 mg/kg/day PO in four divided doses for 14 days. Close follow-up is necessary, as up to 20% of infants will require a second course of treatment for continued symptoms.

Practice Option #3

No effective prophylaxis regimen is available for infants born to mothers with untreated *C. trachomatis* urogenital infection. Approximately 50% of these infants will acquire chlamydia infection, with 25–50% of infected infants developing conjunctivitis and 5–20% developing pneumonia.

IMPLEMENTATION OF GUIDELINE

QUALIFYING STATEMENTS

1. Although PCR for chlamydia is likely more sensitive than culture, PCR-based assays have not been approved by the US Food and Drug Administration for detection of chlamydia from conjunctival swabs or respiratory specimens.
2. Azithromycin (20 mg/kg PO daily × 3 days) is often used as an alternative for the treatment of chlamydial conjunctivitis or pneumonia. However, there are limited data regarding the efficacy of azithromycin for treatment of chlamydial infections among infants, and both erythromycin and azithromycin are associated with an increased risk of infantile hypertrophic pyloric stenosis.
3. No randomized controlled trials identified the optimal duration of treatment for chlamydial conjunctivitis or pneumonia among infants.

DESCRIPTION OF IMPLEMENTATION STRATEGY

All pregnant women should be tested for chlamydia infection as part of standard prenatal care. Healthcare facilities should have Dacron-tipped swabs or commercial kits available for the collection of chlamydia culture and PCR.

SUMMARY

Prevention of neonatal chlamydia infections relies on screening of pregnant mothers because no effective infant prophylaxis is available. Chlamydia should be considered in young infants with conjunctivitis or pneumonia, particularly if the child's mother did not receive prenatal care or has a prior history of sexually transmitted infections. Close monitoring of infants with chlamydial conjunctivitis or pneumonia is warranted because retreatment is often necessary with current antibiotic regimens.

BIBLIOGRAPHIC SOURCE(S)

ACOG Practice Bulletin. Clinical management guidelines for obstetrician-gynecologists No. 82. Management of herpes in pregnancy. *Obstet Gynecol.* 2007;109(6):1489-98.

American Academy of Pediatrics. Chlamydia trachomatis. In: *Red Book: 2012 Report of the Committee on Infectious Diseases.* 29th ed. Elk Grove Village, IL: American Academy of Pediatrics; 2012.

American Academy of Pediatrics. Gonococcal infections. In: *Red Book: 2012 Report of the Committee on Infectious Diseases.* 29th ed. Elk Grove Village, IL: American Academy of Pediatrics; 2012.

American Academy of Pediatrics. Herpes simplex. In: *Red Book: 2012 Report of the Committee on Infectious Diseases.* 29th ed. Elk Grove Village, IL: American Academy of Pediatrics; 2012.

American Academy of Pediatrics. Syphilis. In: *Red Book: 2012 Report of the Committee on Infectious Diseases.* 29th ed. Elk Grove Village, IL: American Academy of Pediatrics; 2012.

Azimi PH, Janner D, Berne P, et al. Concentrations of procaine and aqueous penicillin in the cerebrospinal fluid of infants treated for congenital syphilis. *J Pediatr.* 1994;124(4):649.

Diaz C, Hanson C, Cooper ER, et al. Disease progression in a cohort of infants with vertically acquired HIV infection observed from birth: the Women and Infants Transmission Study (WITS). *J Acquir Immune Defic Syndr Hum Retrovirol.* 1998;18:221-8.

Eberly MD, Eide MB, Thompson JL, Nylund CM. Azithromycin in early infancy and pyloric stenosis. *Pediatrics.* 2015;135(3):483-8.

Hammerschlag MR, Cummings C, Roblin PM, Williams TH, Delke I. Efficacy of neonatal ocular prophylaxis for the prevention of chlamydial and gonococcal conjunctivitis. *N Eng J Med.* 2009;320:769-72.

Jensen HB. Congenital syphilis. *Semin Pediatr Infect Dis.* 1999;10:183-94.

Kimberlin DW, Baley J. Guidance on management of asymptomatic neonates born to women with active genital herpes lesions. *Pediatrics.* 2013;131:383-6.

Kimberlin DW, Whitley RJ, Wan W, et al. Oral acyclovir suppression and neurodevelopment after neonatal herpes. *N Engl J Med.* 2011;365:1284-92.

Siegfried N, van der Merwe L, Brocklehurst P, Sint TT. Antiretrovirals for reducing the risk of mother-to-child transmission of HIV infection. *Cochrane Database Syst Rev.* 2011; (7):CD003510.

The Working Group on MTCT of HIV. Rates of mother-to-child transmission of HIV-1 in Africa, America and Europe: results of 13 perinatal studies. *J Acquir Immune Defic Syndr.* 1995;8:506-10.

Tiffany KF, Benjamin DK Jr, Palasanthiran P, O'Donnell K, Gutman LT. Improved neurodevelopmental outcomes following long-term high-dose oral acyclovir therapy in infants with central nervous system and disseminated herpes simplex disease. *J Perinatol.* 2005;25:156-61.

U. S. Public Health Service Task Force. Recommendations for use of antiretroviral drugs in pregnant HIV-1-infected women for maternal health and interventions to reduce perinatal HIV-1 transmission in the United States. Available at http://AIDSinfo.nih.gov. Accessed January 24, 2015.

Violari A, Cotton MF, Gibb DM, et al. Early antiretroviral therapy and mortality among HIV-infected infants. *N Engl J Med.* 2008;359(21):2233-44.

Wolff T, Shelton E, Sessions C, Miller T. Screening for syphilis infection in pregnant women: evidence for the US Preventive Services Task Force reaffirmation recommendation statement. *Ann Intern Med.* 2009;150(10):710-6.

Woods CR. Gonococcal infections in neonates and young children. *Semin Pediatr Infect Dis.* 2005;16(4):258-70.

Workowski KA, Berman S, Centers for Disease Control and Prevention (CDC). Sexually transmitted diseases treatment guidelines, 2010. *MMWR Recomm Rep.* 2010;59(RR-12):1.

Endocrine and Metabolic Disorders

Hypothyroidism

Ari J. Wassner, MD

SCOPE

DISEASE/CONDITION(S)

Fetal and neonatal hypothyroidism.

GUIDELINE OBJECTIVE(S)

Review the clinical significance of fetal and neonatal hypothyroidism, review causes of fetal and neonatal hypothyroidism, and present recommendations for diagnosis and management of fetal and neonatal hypothyroidism.

BRIEF BACKGROUND

Thyroid hormone is essential for normal growth and development. Because thyroid hormone plays a critical role in brain development from fetal life through 2–3 years of age, hypothyroidism during this period can cause abnormal neurodevelopment. Worldwide, hypothyroidism in infancy is the most common cause of preventable mental retardation in children, but neurocognitive deficits can be avoided by prompt and adequate treatment. Since the 1970s, the implementation of universal newborn screening for hypothyroidism has essentially eliminated hypothyroidism as a cause of severe mental retardation in many parts of the world. Nevertheless, with an incidence of around 1:2000 births, congenital hypothyroidism poses a significant risk to many infants, and care is needed to ensure early diagnosis and initiation of therapy.

Preterm and low birth weight (LBW) infants are at increased risk of thyroid function abnormalities due to many factors, including immaturity of the hypothalamic–pituitary–thyroid (HPT) axis, systemic illness (e.g., cardiovascular disease, respiratory distress syndrome, sepsis), medications that affect thyroid function (e.g., dopamine, glucocorticoids), and iodine excess or deficiency. Very low birth weight (VLBW) infants have a much higher incidence of hypothyroidism (up to 1:250) than do normal weight infants, and low levels of thyroxine (T4) are observed in up to 50% of infants born prior to 28 weeks. Hypothyroxinemia is correlated with poor medical and developmental outcomes in preterm infants. While a randomized trial suggested a possible benefit of treatment on *short-term* neurodevelopment in infants born under 27 weeks, subsequent studies have failed to show a clear benefit on *long-term* developmental outcomes. Hypothyroidism in preterm/LBW infants may manifest later than in term infants, so repeat screening at 2–4 weeks of age is indicated in this population.

Nearly all T4 circulates bound to plasma proteins, primarily thyroxine-binding globulin (TBG), but only unbound free T4 (fT4) is able to exert biological effects. Therefore, direct measurement of fT4 is desirable when assessing for hypothyroidism. However, many current fT4 assays can be confounded by acute illness, medications, or abnormalities of binding proteins that are present in many hospitalized patients. In such cases, measurement of *total* T4 may be helpful but should always be accompanied by measurement of protein binding such as a thyroid hormone binding ratio or T3 resin uptake, which can be used calculate the free T4 index (an estimate of fT4).

RECOMMENDATIONS

MAJOR RECOMMENDATIONS

1. Maternal history of thyroid disease should be elicited in all cases to assess risk factors for fetal or neonatal thyroid dysfunction.
2. Fetal goiter may be assessed by ultrasound. If present and causing airway compression, and caused by fetal hypothyroidism, it should be treated by maternal administration of levothyroxine (LT4).
3. All newborns should be screened for hypothyroidism to facilitate early diagnosis and treatment, and prevention of poor neurocognitive outcomes. Repeat screening after 2–4 weeks is advisable in infants at high risk of hypothyroidism.
4. Infants with confirmed primary hypothyroidism (elevated TSH and low fT4) should be treated promptly with LT4. Infants with compensated hypothyroidism (elevated TSH and normal fT4) and no clinical findings of hypothyroidism may be observed without treatment, depending on the severity and persistence of TSH elevation.
5. In infants with hypothyroxinemia (normal TSH and low fT4), the possibility of hypopituitarism should be considered. In preterm or VLBW infants with hypothyroxinemia, treatment may be considered in those born under 27 weeks, although data do not show a clear benefit of treatment and risks are uncertain.
6. The goal of treatment is to achieve normal serum TSH and serum fT4 in the upper half of the normal range.
7. Enteral LT4 should be given in tablet form, which can be crushed and delivered in a small amount of liquid (e.g., breastmilk, formula). Although liquid LT4 formulations are available in some countries, data on their use are limited and tablets should be used if possible. Enteral absorption of LT4 is impaired by calcium, iron, and soy products/formulas; concurrent enteral administration of these substances with LT4 should be avoided. For patients requiring intravenous (IV) administration of LT4, 70–80% of the enteral dose should be used.
8. A pediatric endocrinologist should participate in the management and ongoing care of all patients with confirmed thyroid abnormalities, particularly those in whom treatment is considered or initiated.

PRACTICE OPTIONS

Practice Option #1: Assessment of Maternal History

All pregnant women should be evaluated for a history of conditions that may place the fetus or neonate at risk of hypothyroidism:

1. Maternal thyrotoxicosis, most commonly due to Graves' disease, can result in neonatal central hypothyroidism that is usually transient (see Practice Option #6). More commonly, treatment of maternal hyperthyroidism with antithyroid drugs (e.g., methimazole, propylthiouracil) can result in fetal or transient neonatal hypothyroidism.
2. Maternal autoimmune thyroid disease—including autoimmune (Hashimoto) thyroiditis and Graves' disease—can cause transient primary hypothyroidism due to transplacental passage of maternal TSH receptor–blocking antibodies (see Practice Option #4).
3. Maternal iodine deficiency or excess can cause congenital hypothyroidism.

Practice Option #2: Assessment for Fetal Hypothyroidism

Fetal goiter is most often caused by fetal hypothyroidism due to maternal administration of antithyroid drugs, intrinsic defects in fetal thyroid hormone synthesis, or maternal iodine deficiency. Severe fetal goiter can compress the trachea, which may cause prenatal pulmonary hypoplasia or postnatal airway obstruction.

1. Fetal goiter can be assessed by ultrasound.
2. Severe fetal goiter due to fetal hypothyroidism that is causing tracheal compression should be treated with administration of LT4 to the mother to reduce goiter size.

Practice Option #3: Newborn Screening for Hypothyroidism

1. All newborns should be screened for hypothyroidism prior to hospital discharge, following local newborn screening protocols (if applicable).
2. Ideally, newborns should be screened at 48–72 hours of life. Because of the normal, transient surge in TSH that occurs in the first 24–48 hours of life, a sample obtained prior to 48 hours may result in a false-positive screen based on elevated TSH levels. Therefore, if screening must be performed earlier than 48 hours (e.g., prior to early hospital discharge or prior to a blood transfusion), results should be interpreted in light of this normal physiology.
3. Any thyroid abnormality detected by newborn screening of a whole blood sample (e.g., heel prick blood spot) should be confirmed by laboratory measurement of serum TSH and fT4. Results should be interpreted based on gestational age- and postnatal age-specific reference ranges (Table 45.1). Attention should be paid to whether the patient is receiving medications that may interfere with thyroid hormone assays, such as heparin, furosemide, fatty acids, or biotin.
4. Patients at high risk of thyroid function abnormalities should be rescreened at 2–4 weeks of age, even if the initial newborn screen was normal. Such infants include those with any of the following (Table 45.2): preterm birth, LBW, trisomy 21, acute illness, excess iodine exposure (e.g., cardiac catheterization, surgical wounds dressed in iodine-containing antiseptic), dependence on total parenteral nutrition (low iodine intake), history of maternal thyroid dysfunction, or clinical signs of hypothyroidism (Table 45.3). Monozygotic twins also require re-screening, because a twin with normal thyroid function may compensate in utero for congenital

TABLE 45.1. Gestational Age- and Postnatal Age-Specific Normal Ranges for Neonatal Thyroid Function Tests

Gestational Age (Weeks)	Postnatal Age			
	Cord	7 Days	14 Days	28 Days
TSH (mIU/L)				
23–27	6.8 ± 2.9	3.5 ± 2.6	3.9 ± 2.7	3.8 ± 4.7
28–30	7.0 ± 3.7	3.6 ± 2.5	4.9 ± 11.2	3.6 ± 2.5
31–34	7.9 ± 5.2	3.6 ± 4.8	3.8 ± 9.3	3.5 ± 3.4
≥37	6.7 ± 4.8	2.6 ± 1.8	2.5 ± 2.0	1.8 ± 0.9
Free T4 (ng/dL)				
23–27	1.3 ± 0.4	1.5 ± 0.6	1.4 ± 0.5	1.5 ± 0.4
28–30	1.4 ± 0.4	1.8 ± 0.7	1.6 ± 0.4	1.7 ± 0.4
31–34	1.5 ± 0.3	2.1 ± 0.6	2.0 ± 0.4	1.9 ± 0.5
≥37	1.4 ± 0.4	2.7 ± 0.6	2.0 ± 0.3	1.6 ± 0.3
Total T4 (μg/dL)				
23–27	5.4 ± 2.0	4.0 ± 1.8	4.7 ± 2.6	6.1 ± 2.3
28–30	6.3 ± 2.0	6.3 ± 2.1	6.6 ± 2.3	7.5 ± 2.3
31–34	7.6 ± 2.3	9.4 ± 3.4	9.1 ± 3.6	8.9 ± 3.0
≥37	9.2 ± 1.9	12.7 ± 2.9	10.7 ± 1.4	9.7 ± 2.2
TBG (mg/L)				
23–27	18.8 ± 5.7	17.1 ± 4.0	18.9 ± 5.2	22.8 ± 6.0
28–30	19.6 ± 5.1	20.2 ± 4.9	21.1 ± 5.2	22.0 ± 6.1
31–34	24.0 ± 8.2	24.4 ± 7.9	23.4 ± 7.9	23.1 ± 7.6
≥37	29.2 ± 5.6	33.5 ± 10.7	27.5 ± 3.8	27.3 ± 6.7

Adapted from Williams FL, Simpson J, Delahunty C, et al. Developmental trends in cord and postpartum serum thyroid hormones in preterm infants. *J Clin Endocrinol Metab.* 2004;89(11):5314-20.

hypothyroidism in the other twin via shared placental circulation, potentially leading to a false-negative initial screen. Protocols regarding rescreening (including timing and which patients are rescreened) may vary among newborn screening programs.

TABLE 45.2. Neonates Requiring Repeat Newborn Screening

Preterm birth (<37 weeks)
Low birth weight (<2500 g)
Monozygotic twins
Trisomy 21
Acute illness
Excess iodine exposure
　　Cardiac catheterization
　　Open wounds exposed to iodine-containing antiseptic
Dependence on total parenteral nutrition (low iodine intake)
History of maternal thyroid dysfunction
Clinical signs of hypothyroidism (Table 45.3)

TABLE 45.3. Clinical Manifestations of Neonatal Hypothyroidism

Macroglossia
Enlarged posterior fontanelle
Umbilical hernia
Dry skin
Hypothermia
Bradycardia
Lethargy
Poor feeding
Constipation
Decreased muscle tone
Prolonged jaundice (unconjugated hyperbilirubinemia)

Practice Option #4: Infants with Primary Hypothyroidism (Elevated TSH and Low fT4)

1. These infants have been clearly shown to benefit from early initiation of LT4 therapy. Therefore, infants confirmed to have elevated TSH and low fT4 should be treated for hypothyroidism. Patients with a screening TSH above 40 mIU/mL should begin treatment immediately after having confirmatory serum tests drawn, without awaiting their results. LT4 should be started at a dose of 10–15 µg/kg daily. The highest dose in this range should be used for infants with severe disease (very high TSH or very low fT4), while lower doses may be used for those with less severe disease.

2. Serum TSH and fT4 should be checked 1–2 weeks after starting treatment, with a shorter interval preferred in acutely ill or hospitalized patients. TSH and fT4 should be checked at least every 2 weeks until TSH has normalized, and every 1–3 months thereafter for the first year of life.

3. For diagnosis of the underlying etiology of hypothyroidism, consider performing the following tests. However, obtaining one of these tests should never delay initiation of LT4 therapy.

    a. *Thyroid imaging using ultrasound and/or scintigraphy.* Ultrasound can assess the presence and size of the thyroid gland. Scintigraphy can evaluate the size of the thyroid and its ability to take up iodine, as well as locate ectopic thyroid tissue.

    b. *Measurement of serum thyroglobulin concentration,* which correlates with the volume of thyroid tissue present. If performed, thyroglobulin concentration should be measured while TSH remains elevated.

    c. *Measurement of TSH receptor antibodies,* which can cause transient hypothyroidism that resolves within the first 3–4 months of life in infants with a maternal history of autoimmune thyroid disease.

4. For infants with a history of maternal Graves' disease, primary hypothyroidism may be caused by maternal treatment with antithyroid drugs (e.g., methimazole, propylthiouracil) or, less commonly, by transplacental passage of maternal TSH receptor-blocking antibodies. These forms of hypothyroidism resolve after the etiologic agent is cleared from the newborn circulation, which occurs within 7–10 days for antithyroid drugs and 3–4 months for TSH receptor antibodies. After resolution of hypothyroidism, further monitoring may be required for development of neonatal Graves' disease.

5. Children with large liver hemangiomas may develop hypothyroidism due to tumor overexpression of the enzyme type 3 deiodinase, which inactivates circulating thyroid hormone. These patients often require treatment with high doses of LT4, and in some cases with triiodothyronine (T3) as well.

Practice Option #5: Infants with Compensated Primary Hypothyroidism (Elevated TSH and Normal fT4)

Data on the benefit of treatment with LT4 are less clear in this population than in patients with overt hypothyroidism (low fT4).

1. Treatment is recommended for patients with serum TSH above 20 mIU/L. The starting dose of LT4 is 10–15 µg/kg daily, depending on the severity of TSH elevation.
2. If TSH is elevated but not above 20 mIU/L, management is controversial. Options include:
   a. Treatment with LT4.
   b. Close observation of TSH and fT4 levels every 1–2 weeks, with initiation of LT4 if fT4 falls below normal, if TSH increases above 20 mIU/L, or if the patient has clinical signs of hypothyroidism (Table 45.3).
   c. If TSH remains elevated but below 20 mIU/L for 3–4 weeks, LT4 treatment should be considered in discussion with the patient's family. While many practitioners recommend treatment in this situation, whether this improves medical or developmental outcomes is unclear.

Practice Option #6: Infants with Hypothyroxinemia (Normal or Low TSH and Low fT4)

1. In an otherwise healthy male infant, congenital deficiency of TBG should be considered. This X-linked condition is characterized by normal TSH, low total T4, and normal fT4; however, many widely available fT4 assays may be unreliable in the presence of abnormal TBG, so assay of fT4 by the gold standard method of equilibrium dialysis may be necessary. Diagnosis is confirmed by a low serum level of TBG. Because the HPT axis is intact and fT4 is normal, this condition is benign and requires no treatment.
2. Central hypothyroidism should be considered in any infant with normal or low TSH, low fT4, and signs of a possible hypothalamic or pituitary abnormality. These may include midline defects (e.g., cleft palate), central nervous system defects, hypoglycemia, conjugated hyperbilirubinemia, microphallus (in a male infant), or diabetes insipidus. Magnetic resonance imaging of the brain can be used to assess for a hypothalamic or pituitary abnormality. Confirmed central hypothyroidism should be treated with LT4 (10–15 µg/kg daily) with the goal of maintaining serum fT4 in the upper half of the normal range; monitoring of TSH is not indicated in central hypothyroidism. Assessment for additional pituitary hormone deficits is mandatory, as these are present in most cases.
3. Infants of mothers with Graves' disease may have central hypothyroidism due to suppression of the HPT axis induced by fetal thyrotoxicosis. This condition is usually transient but may persist in rare cases.
4. In preterm or LBW infants, the finding of low fT4 without TSH elevation is common and is often termed "transient hypothyroxinemia of prematurity" (THOP). Although the presence of THOP is correlated with poor outcomes, treatment of THOP has

not been proven to improve outcomes, and the risks of treatment remain unclear. Nevertheless, treatment with LT4 (8 µg/kg daily) may be considered in patients born under 27 weeks' gestational age or in infants with clinical signs suggestive of hypothyroidism (Table 45.3).

IMPLEMENTATION OF GUIDELINE

DESCRIPTION OF IMPLEMENTATION STRATEGY

Create written protocol for newborn screening of infants for hypothyroidism, including protocol for repeat screening in high-risk infants.

QUALITY METRICS

Proportion of at-risk infants receiving repeat newborn screening between 2 and 4 weeks of age; time to normalization of fT4 (goal 1 week) and TSH (goal 2 weeks) in infants with primary hypothyroidism.

SUMMARY

Neonatal hypothyroidism is common and is associated with poor neurodevelopmental outcomes. All newborns should be screened for hypothyroidism (following local newborn screening protocols where applicable), and treatment should be initiated promptly when hypothyroidism is confirmed. Close follow-up is necessary to ensure rapid restoration and consistent maintenance of euthyroidism, which can prevent most developmental sequelae of neonatal hypothyroidism.

BIBLIOGRAPHIC SOURCE(S)

Cao XY, Jiang XM, Dou ZH, et al. Timing of vulnerability of the brain to iodine deficiency in endemic cretinism. *N Engl J Med.* 1994;331(26):1739-44.

Connelly KJ, Boston BA, Pearce EN, et al. Congenital hypothyroidism caused by excess prenatal maternal iodine ingestion. *J Pediatr.* 2012;161(4):760-2.

Delahunty C, Falconer S, Hume R, et al. Levels of neonatal thyroid hormone in preterm infants and neurodevelopmental outcome at 5 1/2 years: millennium cohort study. *J Clin Endocrinol Metab.* 2010;95(11):4898-908.

Garber JR, Cobin RH, Gharib H, et al. Clinical practice guidelines for hypothyroidism in adults: cosponsored by the American Association of Clinical Endocrinologists and the American Thyroid Association. *Endocr Pract.* 2012;18(6):988-1028.

La Gamma EF, Paneth N. Clinical importance of hypothyroxinemia in the preterm infant and a discussion of treatment concerns. *Curr Opin Pediatr.* 2012;24(2):172-80.

Larson C, Hermos R, Delaney A, Daley D, Mitchell M. Risk factors associated with delayed thyrotropin elevations in congenital hypothyroidism. *J Pediatr.* 2003;143(5):587-91.

Leger J, Olivieri A, Donaldson M, et al. European Society for Paediatric Endocrinology consensus guidelines on screening, diagnosis, and management of congenital hypothyroidism. *Horm Res Paediatr.* 2014;81(2):80-103.

Rose SR, Brown RS, Foley T, et al. Update of newborn screening and therapy for congenital hypothyroidism. *Pediatrics.* 2006;117(6):2290-303.

van Wassenaer AG, Kok JH, de Vijlder JJ, et al. Effects of thyroxine supplementation on neurologic development in infants born at less than 30 weeks' gestation. *N Engl J Med.* 1997;336(1):21-6.

van Wassenaer AG, Westera J, Houtzager BA, Kok JH. Ten-year follow-up of children born at <30 weeks' gestational age supplemented with thyroxine in the neonatal period in a randomized, controlled trial. *Pediatrics.* 2005;116(5):e613-8.

Vigone MC, Caiulo S, Di Frenna M, et al. Evolution of thyroid function in preterm infants detected by screening for congenital hypothyroidism. *J Pediatr.* 2014;164(6):1296-302.

WHO/UNICEF/ICCIDD. Assessment of iodine deficiency disorders and monitoring their elimination: a guide for programme managers. 3rd ed. Geneva, Switzerland: World Health Organization; 2007.

Williams FL, Simpson J, Delahunty C, et al. Developmental trends in cord and postpartum serum thyroid hormones in preterm infants. *J Clin Endocrinol Metab.* 2004;89(11):5314-20.

Disorders of Calcium, Phosphorus, and Vitamin D

Sarah N. Taylor, MD, MSCR

SCOPE

DISEASE/CONDITION(S)

Neonatal hypocalcemia.

GUIDELINE OBJECTIVE(S)

Describe mechanisms, causes, and effects of neonatal hypocalcemia, and its management.

BRIEF BACKGROUND

In the normal transition to extrauterine life, circulating calcium levels reach a nadir at 24–48 hours post-birth. By 48 hours, parathyroid hormone (PTH) responds to this dip with a gradual increase in serum calcium levels. This occurs via a vitamin D–independent mechanism. This normal mechanism can be in disarray if hypomagnesemia leading to poor parathyroid function or, in a subset of infants, PTH does not respond to the calcium nadir in a timely manner, or if end-organ unresponsiveness to PTH occurs for a short time period. Infants who are most at risk for symptomatic early hypocalcemia include preterm infants (<32 weeks), infants of diabetic mothers, and asphyxiated infants. Other infants with risk factors for hypocalcemia include small for gestational age (SGA) infants with other morbidity, infants of pre-eclamptic mothers, and infants of hyperparathyroid mothers. Late hypocalcemia occurs at 7–8 days and historically was due to high phosphate loads with bovine milk and early formulas. Other causes of late hypocalcemia include hypoparathyroidism, vitamin D deficiency, maternal hyperparathyroidism, and renal insufficiency. It is difficult to provide adequate calcium through a peripheral intravenous route, and central venous access is required to avoid tissue necrosis from extravasation. Solubility of calcium and phosphorus limits the amounts that can be provided in parenteral infusions, and such intake is also limited by amino acid intake, volume, cysteine, pH, time, temperature, and lipids. Phosphate salts that improve solubility are available in Europe but not in the United States. Historically, studies to identify the calcium-to-phosphorus molar ratio optimal for retention of both minerals point to a ratio of 1.3:1. However, this research is limited, and a range of molar ratios from 0.8:1 to 1.5:1 may result in similar retention. In fact, studies with high parenteral protein infusion demonstrate optimal calcium and phosphorus retention at a molar ratio of 1:1 for at least the first postnatal days.

RECOMMENDATIONS

MAJOR RECOMMENDATIONS

Calcium infusion should be provided by 24 hours of life for preterm infants and "sick" infants of diabetic mothers, and asphyxiated infants. Calcium 60–80 mg/kg/day should be provided parenterally. Central access is required to provide this concentration of calcium infusion. Phosphorus 48–60 mg/kg/day should be provided. This amount of phosphorus is difficult to provide intravenously. Absolute minimum parenteral intake amounts to avoid bone demineralization and fracture risk are 52 mg/kg/day of calcium and 31 mg/kg/day of phosphorus. Symptoms of hypocalcemia which include neurological, cardiovascular, neuromuscular irritability (jittery, exaggerated startle), seizures, heart failure, and prolonged QT interval are clear indications for treatment with intravenous calcium.

PRACTICE OPTIONS

Practice Option #1

In early days, normal serum ionized is 1.1–1.3 mmol/L and hypocalcemia <1 mmol/L and <0.9 for preterm infants in early days. Normal serum total is 8.8–12 mg/dL, and hypocalcemia is defined as <7 mg/dL with normal albumin.

Practice Option #2

The World Health Organization recommends at least 40 mg/kg/day elemental calcium. To match in utero accretion, 90–120 mg/kg/day is required. With the limitations in current parenteral nutrition products, 60–80 mg/kg/day is a realistic goal and should provide adequate intravenous calcium intake. This amount of calcium requires central access for delivery.

Practice Option #3

Provide 1.3 mmol/kg/day (perhaps 1 mmol/kg/day) phosphorus to avoid bone mineralization deficit and fracture.

SCOPE

DISEASE/CONDITION(S)

Preterm infant receiving early parenteral protein delivery.

GUIDELINE OBJECTIVE(S)

Recognize mineral metabolism associated with sustaining preterm infant nutrition from placental to parenteral nutrition.

BRIEF BACKGROUND

Current nutritional practices for very preterm infants include protein delivery to at least match intrauterine support. Very low birth weight infant in-hospital growth is improved with parenteral protein delivery of 3–3.5 g/kg/day. Historically, preterm infants did not receive mineral delivery in the first postnatal days, and most received dextrose water after birth, perhaps supplemented with calcium. When protein was not delivered in the early days, cellular metabolism was in a dormant state and intracellular ions, such as potassium and phosphorus, were not needed. Now that protein is delivered immediately after birth, cellular metabolism is active, and therefore intracellular minerals such as potassium and phosphorus are transported into the cell for this activity. Without a nutritional source of phosphorus, cellular phosphorus supply is maintained by resorption of bone phosphorus stores. In this circumstance, calcium is removed from bone with the phosphorus and becomes elevated in the circulation. Therefore, early protein delivery is associated with hypophosphatemia and hypercalcemia when inadequate parenteral phosphorus is delivered. This phenomenon has been termed *placental incompletely restored feeding syndrome*. Two approaches to avoid these early mineral dyscrasias are published. One investigative group in Europe provided 1.3 mmol/kg in the first day and 1.76 mmol/kg/day through the first week phosphorus. A decrease in the incidence of hypophosphatemia was observed, but it still occurred in 37% of infants. Of note, the parenteral compound calcium glycerophosphate, which allowed these concentrations of phosphorus to be delivered without calcium/phosphorus precipitation, is not available in the United States. In a second quality improvement study, an institution in the United States initiated a practice change to provide early parenteral phosphorus after a high prevalence of hypercalcemia was appreciated in the first postnatal week. The change in practice included starter parenteral nutrition with calcium but with initiation of individualized parenteral nutrition containing 1.2–2 mmol/kg/day phosphorus at a ratio of 1:1, with calcium as soon as possible. With this practice change, first postnatal week mean serum phosphorus levels increased from 3.52 ng/mL to 4.3 ng/mL. In addition, the prevalence of hypercalcemia and severe hypercalcemia decreased from 77% and 50% to 52% and 21%, respectively.

RECOMMENDATIONS

MAJOR RECOMMENDATIONS

With early protein delivery, phosphorus should also be provided. The recommendation is to provide parenteral phosphorus in the first parenteral nutrition ordered after the "starter" fluid. Starter parenteral nutrition with phosphorus has not been studied and therefore is not recommended at this time. The calcium-to-phosphorus ratio should be at the lower limit of the recommended parenteral ratio in the first week of parenteral nutrition (0.8–1:1 calcium to phosphorus). Infants should be monitored for electrolyte dyscrasias and supplemented with phosphorus as needed to maintain a serum level of at least 4 mg/dL.

PRACTICE OPTIONS

Practice Option #1
Transition from starter parenteral nutrition to individualized parenteral nutrition containing phosphorus as soon as possible.

Practice Option #2
Give parenteral calcium and phosphorus at a 0.8–1:1 ratio at least in the first week. Ratio can be increased to 1.3–1.5:1 if infant remains on parenteral nutrition long-term and with normal serum phosphorus concentration.

Practice Option #3
Monitor for hypercalcemia and hypophosphatemia in the first week of parenteral protein. Treatment of both dyscrasias is to increase phosphorus delivery.

IMPLEMENTATION OF GUIDELINE

DESCRIPTION OF IMPLEMENTATION STRATEGY

If delivering parenteral protein, initiate parenteral phosphorus delivery as soon as possible at a concentration of 1.1–2 mmol/kg/day and at a ratio of 0.8–1:1 calcium to phosphorus. Follow serum phosphorus to ensure adequate supplementation.

QUALITY METRICS

Incidence of hypercalcemia; incidence of hypophosphatemia; parenteral delivery of phosphorus.

SUMMARY

With delivery of early parenteral protein, cellular metabolism is active, and therefore a phosphorus supply is needed to support these metabolic processes. In contrast to the historically high early serum phosphorus concentrations observed for preterm infants, with early parenteral protein delivery the prevalence of hypophosphatemia is high. Further research is needed, but early retrospective cohort studies support providing 1.2–2 mmol/kg/day phosphorus at a ratio of 1:1 calcium to phosphorus as soon as possible. In addition, serum phosphorus concentrations should be observed, as the incidence of hypophosphatemia continues to occur despite this higher phosphorus supplementation.

SCOPE

DISEASE/CONDITION(S)

Calcium and phosphorus fortification of feeds.

GUIDELINE OBJECTIVE(S)

Review roles of calcium and phosphorus in healthy bone mineralization; identify heightened risk for metabolic bone disease due to calcium and phosphorus dyscrasias; identify the best method to supply adequate calcium and phosphorus to avoid metabolic bone disease.

BRIEF BACKGROUND

The majority of calcium and phosphorus deposition into bone occurs from 24 weeks to term age. Eighty percent of fetal calcium and phosphorus is accrued in the third trimester, with peak accretion at 36–38 weeks' gestation. Studies investigating how to achieve fetal calcium and phosphorus accretion in the preterm infant receiving enteral nutrition indicate that delivery of 120–200 mg/kg/day calcium and 70–120 mg/kg/day phosphorus is sufficient. To attain this nutrition would take 300 mL/kg/day unfortified human milk and is therefore not realistic. Instead, preterm infants receive fortified human milk. Randomized controlled trials (RCTs) of only calcium and phosphorus supplementation have not been performed. Instead, multicomponent human milk fortifier is the product available to provide calcium and phosphorus for preterm infant bone mineralization. RCT studies of multicomponent human milk fortifier effect on bone mineralization show no difference in whole-body bone mineralization but show a significant improvement when evaluating specifically radial bone mineral content. Further studies comparing fortified and unfortified human milk intake are unlikely to be performed. Currently available commercial multicomponent human milk fortifiers provide adequate calcium and phosphorus with no specific product proven to be superior for bone mineralization. Randomized trials studying how early feed fortification can be initiated have shown tolerance to fortification with bovine-based fortifier at 20 mL/kg/day, with human-based fortifier at 40 mL/kg/day, and with high-protein bovine-based fortifiers at 80–100 mL/kg/day. If targeted fortification instead of multicomponent fortification is being practiced, steps should be taken to ensure adequate calcium and phosphorus delivery. Questions that remain include at what degree of prematurity routine calcium and phosphorus fortification is required, and when to discontinue human milk fortification. Dexamethasone and diuretics are two common therapies in preterm infant care, and both are associated with increased losses of calcium and phosphorus and deleterious effect on bone. These medications may counteract the benefit of calcium and phosphorus fortification. Diuretics, especially loop diuretics, and less so thiazides, induce urinary calcium loss and thereby diminish bone mineralization. Catch-up bone mineralization likely occurs with discontinuation of these medications. Dexamethasone alters bone formation and resorption and is associated with hypercalciuria and hyperphosphaturia. However, the long-term effect on bone and growth is not clear.

RECOMMENDATIONS

MAJOR RECOMMENDATIONS

Provide preterm infants with multicomponent human milk fortifier. Data are limited regarding the birth gestational age or birth weight at which a preterm infant bone mineralization is adequate without feed fortification. Dexamethasone and diuretics are two common therapies in preterm infant care whose use should be minimized.

PRACTICE OPTIONS

Practice Option #1

Initiation of fortification with a multicomponent human milk fortifier at least by 100 mL/kg/day of feed volume. Overlap with parenteral nutrition to promote steady delivery of nutrients.

Practice Option #2

Continue multicomponent fortification at least through hospitalization or term age. Calcium and phosphorus supplementation of feeds post-hospitalization has not been shown to add benefit for preterm infants. Multicomponent fortification may be required post-hospitalization for delivery of other nutrients.

Practice Option #3

Calcium and phosphorus fortification of feeds may be inadequate to overcome deleterious effects of medications such as dexamethasone and diuretics. In circumstances where indication for these medications is not clear, their effect on bone health should be taken into consideration.

CLINICAL ALGORITHM(S)

Use of a standard feeding protocol is associated with less necrotizing enterocolitis. Include fortification of feeds in a standardized feeding advancement protocol.

IMPLEMENTATION OF GUIDELINE

DESCRIPTION OF IMPLEMENTATION STRATEGY

A written protocol for every neonatal unit for standardization of human milk feed fortification is desirable. Human milk fortification should be continued until at least term age and/or hospital discharge to support infants' calcium and phosphorus needs. Fortification with calories and protein may be required longer to support adequate growth. Because of the potential harmful effects of dexamethasone and diuretic therapy on bone mineralization, these medications should be used only when essential.

QUALITY METRICS

Monitor compliance with feeding protocol, incidence of metabolic bone disease, and especially fractures, infant linear growth, and use of corticosteroids and diuretics.

SUMMARY

Fortification of human milk with a multicomponent human milk fortifier should be initiated at least by 100 mL/kg/day of feed volume. To match in utero calcium and phosphorus accretion, fortification should be continued until term age and/or hospital discharge. Limiting preterm infant exposure to dexamethasone and diuretics is beneficial for calcium and phosphorus mineralization of bone.

SCOPE

DISEASE/CONDITION(S)

Metabolic bone disease of prematurity.

GUIDELINE OBJECTIVE(S)

Describe causes and risk factors for metabolic bone disease of prematurity, its effects, and methods of prevention and mitigation.

BRIEF BACKGROUND

Metabolic bone disease (MBD) or osteopenia of prematurity is multifactorial and can include inadequate supply of phosphorus, calcium, and vitamin D to the preterm infant. In addition, the decreased and abnormal physical movement of the preterm infant compared to the fetus plays a role. Exposure to medications such as steroids and diuretics greatly increase the risk of developing MBD. Eighty percent of fetal calcium and phosphorus is accrued in the third trimester, with peak accretion at 36–38 weeks' gestation. Of total body levels, 98–99% of calcium and 85–88% of phosphorus resides in bone. The majority of deposition of calcium and phosphorus into bone occurs from 24 weeks to term age. Studies comparing enteral nutrition and bone outcomes have shown that unfortified mother's milk is not adequate for bone growth unless an intake of almost 300 mL/kg/day is provided. Studies of current fortifiers and formulas show that bone mineralization is improved at hospital discharge with intake of preterm formula through term age. Comparisons between preterm products show no consistent differences in bone mineralization or growth. To support bone mineralization, 120–200 mg/kg/day enteral calcium and 70–120 mg/kg/day enteral phosphorus supply is required to equal in utero accretion. Diuretics, especially loop and less so with thiazides, induce urinary calcium loss, and bone mineralization is compromised. Catch-up bone mineralization may be possible. Dexamethasone alters bone formation and resorption and is associated with hypercalciuria and hyperphosphaturia. However, the long-term effect on bone and growth is not clear.

RECOMMENDATIONS

MAJOR RECOMMENDATIONS

Enteral intake of 120–200 mg/kg/day calcium is adequate calcium supply for bone mineralization, unless calcium losses are increased as a side effect of respiratory care interventions.

PRACTICE OPTION

Practice Option #1

Preterm infants should receive human milk fortified with calcium and phosphorus to increase linear growth during hospitalization and improve bone mineralization.

BIBLIOGRAPHIC SOURCE(S)

Atkinson S, Tsang RC. Calcium and phosphorus. In: Tsang RC, Uay R, Koletzko B, Zlotkin SH, eds. *Nutrition of the Preterm Infant: Scientific Basis and Practice*. 2nd ed. Cincinnati, OH: Digital Educational Publishing, Inc; 2005:245-75.

Berseth CL, Van Aerde JE, Gross S, Stolz SI, Harris CL, Hansen JW. Growth, efficacy, and safety of feeding an iron-fortified human milk fortifier. *Pediatrics*. 2004;114(6):e699-706.

Bonsante F, Iacobelli S, Latorre G, et al. Initial amino acid intake influences phosphorus and calcium homeostasis in preterm infants–it is time to change the composition of the early parenteral nutrition. *PLoS One*. 2013;8(8):e72880.

Brown JV, Embleton, ND, Harding JE, McGuire, W. Multi-nutrient fortification of human milk for preterm infants. *Cochrane Database Syst Rev*. 2016;5:Cd000363.

Hair AB, Chetta KE, Bruno AM, Hawthorne KM, Abrams SA. Delayed introduction of parenteral phosphorus is associated with hypercalcemia in extremely preterm infants. *J Nutr.* 2016;146(6):1212-6.

Hillman LS, Salmons SJ, Slatopolsky E, McAlister WH. Serial serum 25-hydroxyvitamin D and mineral homeostasis in very premature infants fed preterm human milk. *J Pediatr Gastroenterol Nutr.* 1985;4(5):762-70.

Kim JH, Chan G, Schanler R, et al. Growth and tolerance of preterm infants fed a new extensively hydrolyzed liquid human milk fortifier. *J Pediatr Gastroenterol Nutr.* 2015;61(6):665-71.

Koo WW, Hockman EM. Physiologic predictors of lumbar spine bone mass in neonates. *Pediatr Res.* 2000;48(4):485-9.

Lapillonne A, Salle BL, Glorieux FH, Claris O. Bone mineralization and growth are enhanced in preterm infants fed an isocaloric, nutrient-enriched preterm formula through term. *Am J Clin Nutr.* 2004;80(6):1595-603.

Lucas A, Morley R, Cole TJ. Randomised trial of early diet in preterm babies and later intelligence quotient. *BMJ.* 1998;317(7171):1481-7.

Marinella MA. The refeeding syndrome and hypophosphatemia. *Nutr Rev.* 2003;61(9):320-3.

Moya F, Sisk PM, Walsh KR, Berseth CL. A new liquid human milk fortifier and linear growth in preterm infants. *Pediatrics.* 2012;130(4): e928-35.

Nicholl RM, Gamsu HR. Changes in growth and metabolism in very low birthweight infants fed with fortified breast milk. *Acta Paediatr.* 1999;88(10):1056-61.

Pelegano JF, Rowe JC, Carey DE, et al. Effect of calcium/phosphorus ratio on mineral retention in parenterally fed premature infants. *J Pediatr Gastroenterol Nutr.* 1991;12(3):351-5.

Porcelli P, Schanler R, Greer F, et al. Growth in human milk-fed very low birth weight infants receiving a new human milk fortifier. *Ann Nutr Metab.* 2000;44(1):2-10.

Prestridge LL, Schanler RJ, Shulman RJ, Burns PA, Laine LL. Effect of parenteral calcium and phosphorus therapy on mineral retention and bone mineral content in very low birth weight infants. *J Pediatr.* 1993;122(5 Pt 1):761-8.

Reis BB, Hall RT, Schanler RJ, et al. Enhanced growth of preterm infants fed a new powdered human milk fortifier: a randomized, controlled trial. *Pediatrics.* 2000;106(3):581-8.

Rigo J, De Curtis M, Pieltain C, Picaud JC, Salle BL, Senterre J. Bone mineral metabolism in the micropremie. *Clin Perinatol.* 2000;27(1):147-70.

Ryan S. Nutritional aspects of metabolic bone disease in the newborn. *Arch Dis Child Fetal Neonatal Ed.* 1996;74(2):F145-8.

Senterre T, Abu Zahirah I, Pieltain C, de Halleux V, Rigo J. Electrolyte and mineral homeostasis after optimizing early macronutrient intakes in VLBW infants on parenteral nutrition. *J Pediatr Gastroenterol Nutr.* 2015;61(4):491-8.

Shah SD, Dereddy N, Jones TL, Dhanireddy R, Talati AJ. Early versus delayed human milk fortification in very low birth weight infants-a randomized controlled trial. *J Pediatr.* 2016;174: 126-31.e1.

Sullivan S, Schanler RJ, Kim JH, et al. An exclusively human milk-based diet is associated with a lower rate of necrotizing enterocolitis than a diet of human milk and bovine milk-based products. *J Pediatr.* 2010;156(4):562-7.e1.

Warner JT, Linton HR, Dunstan FD, Cartlidge PH. Growth and metabolic responses in preterm infants fed fortified human milk or a preterm formula. *Int J Clin Pract.* 1998;52(4):236-40.

Wauben IP, Atkinson SA, Shah JK, Paes B. Growth and body composition of preterm infants: influence of nutrient fortification of mother's milk in hospital and breastfeeding post-hospital discharge. *Acta Paediatr.* 1998;87(7):780-5.

Hypoglycemia

Prem S. Shekhawat, MD • Gautham K. Suresh, MD, DM, MS, FAAP

SCOPE

DISEASE/CONDITION(S)

Hypoglycemia in the late preterm and full-term neonate.

GUIDELINE OBJECTIVE(S)

To describe the identification and management of neonatal hypoglycemia in the late preterm and full-term neonate, to delineate the debated aspects of the definition of hypoglycemia, and to emphasize the importance of identification and management of persistent hypoglycemia.

BRIEF BACKGROUND

Hypoglycemia is common in late preterm and term infants (with a prevalence as high as 15–20%) because of an increased number of infants born between 34 and 38 weeks' gestation over the past 20 years, increasing births of large for gestational age (LGA) infants (a consequence of increasing prevalence of maternal obesity with associated gestational diabetes), and a high prevalence of intrauterine growth restriction (IUGR) (with associated low glycogen and fat stores and hence higher incidence of hypoglycemia) as a consequence of poor prenatal care, smoking, and drug use among pregnant women. Hypoglycemia further complicates transitional conditions such as hypothermia, respiratory distress, and poor feeding.

Glucose is an essential fuel for cellular metabolism and is the primary fuel of choice for certain cells such as the neurons, and most other cells utilize glucose as their main source of energy in the form of adenosine triphosphate (ATP). Clinical signs of hypoglycemia occur relatively late when there is failure to generate enough ATP for adequate cellular function. This may be due to not only hypoglycemia but also deficiency of alternative fuels or inability to break down stored energy sources. Because it is difficult to measure available alternative fuels for ATP generation clinically, the availability of fuel source is estimated by the blood levels of glucose, a surrogate molecule.

During gestation, there is a reliable transfer of maternal glucose to the fetus, and the fetus utilizes the minimum amount of energy for its own metabolism and stores the transported glucose in the form of glycogen and fat. This in utero physiologic state is interrupted at birth, and the neonate's metabolic needs increase substantially after birth. Thus there is an initial drop in glucose, followed by a slow and steady rise in its blood glucose to the acceptable normal range. For these reasons, coming up with a definition of hypoglycemia in the neonate has been a challenge, since blood sugar fluctuations are common in the first several hours after birth. The American Academy of Pediatrics (AAP) and the Pediatric Endocrine Society (PES) have both tried to come to a consensus for a safe range of glucose in neonates. It is now accepted that plasma glucose values drop down to 30 mg/dL (1.67 mmol/L) in the first 2 hours of life and subsequently rise to a value of at least 45 mg/dL (2.5 mmol/L) before stabilizing at around 12–24 hours. The AAP defines hypoglycemia as a numerical plasma glucose value of less than 47 mg/dL (2.6 mmol/L) in all neonates, whether term or preterm.

Although in clinical practice a single value of plasma glucose is often used to identify and treat hypoglycemia, a specific plasma glucose level that consistently causes brain injury cannot be pinpointed, because brain injury can result at a variety of glucose levels. Adherence to AAP and PES guidelines of maintaining blood sugars >47 mg/dL in the first 48 hours of life and >60 mg/dL after 48 hours of life is thought to mitigate the occurrence of hypoglycemic brain injury.

Etiopathogenesis of Hypoglycemia

The majority of late preterm and term neonates diagnosed with hypoglycemia in the first 48 hours after birth have a transitional condition where they are unable to maintain serum glucose in the normal range due to either low tissue stores of glycogen and fat or inability to upregulate enzymes involved in gluconeogenesis. They usually are appropriate for gestational age (AGA), and in rare cases could be IUGR or LGA, or infants born to diabetic mothers (IDM) (Figure 47.1). When supported with feeds, these infants with transient hypoglycemia generally do well and are able to increase their blood sugars to the acceptable normal range within 24–48 hours when the AAP protocol is followed as outlined in Table 47.1 and Figure 47.2. These infants do not warrant further investigation and can be cared for in the normal newborn nursery or even stay with their mothers.

In contrast, infants with prolonged or persistent hypoglycemia require emergent and prolonged management. These infants have a severe condition where they are unable to raise their blood sugar due to decreased production from glycogen stores or excessive utilization of glucose, or fail to mount an adequate counterregulatory response through their adrenal glands. Newborns utilize their circulating glucose within 20–30 minutes after birth. After that, to avoid hypoglycemia they must break down glycogen and at the same time produce new glucose. During fetal life, there is a minimal amount of gluconeogenesis in the liver, and enzymes involved in this metabolic pathway are poorly expressed; thus the newborn must express and activate several enzymes to kick-start this process. The principal enzymes involved in this process are glucose-6-phosphatase, fructose-1,6-diphosphatase, pyruvate carboxylase, and phenol pyruvate carboxykinase (PEPCK), where PEPCK happens to be the rate-limiting enzyme.

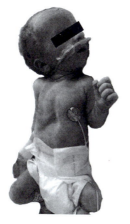
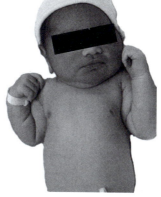

IUGR	LGA/IDM
↓ Glycogen stores	↑ Insulin production
↓ Fat stores	↑ Glycogen stores
↓ Muscle mass	↑ Fat stores
↓ Counterregulatory hormone secretion	↑ Glucose consumption
↓ Gluconeogenesis	↓ Gluconeogenesis
↑ Glucose consumption	↓ Glucagon production

FIGURE 47.1 • Salient metabolic differences between IUGR and LGA/IDM infants.

TABLE 47.1. Causes of Hypoglycemia in Late Preterm and Term Neonates

Transient Hypoglycemia	Persistent Hypoglycemia
1. Prematurity	1. Infant of diabetic mother
2. SGA	2. Hyperinsulinism due to sulfonylurea receptor mutations
3. Perinatal events such as asphyxia	3. Isolated growth hormone deficiency
4. IUGR	4. Congenital hypopituitarism
5. Sepsis	5. Congenital adrenal hypo/hyperplasia
6. Hypothermia	6. Beckwith-Wiedemann syndrome
7. Infant of a diabetic mother (mild)	7. Organic acidemias (MSUD, MMA, glutaric acidemia, tyrosinemia)
8. Gluconeogenesis disorders (mild PEPCK deficiency)	8. Fatty acid oxidation disorders (carnitine deficiency, CPT-1 and -2, CT, MCAD, SCHAD, LCHAD, VLCAD, HMG CoA synthase/lyase deficiency)
9. Tocolytic agents such as β-blockers	9. Glut-1 and -2 deficiency
10. High glucose infusion to mother before delivery	10. Sotos syndrome

CT, carnitine translocase; HMG CoA synthase, hydroxymethylglutaryl-CoA synthase; IUGR, intrauterine growth restriction; LCHAD, long-chain 3-hydroxy-acyl CoA dehydrogenase; MCAD, medium-chain acyl CoA dehydrogenase; MMA, methylmalonic acidemia; MSUD, maple syrup urine disease; PEPCK, phenol pyruvate carboxykinase; SCHAD, short-chain 3-hydroxy-acyl CoA; SGA, small for gestational age; VLCAD, very long-chain acyl CoA dehydrogenase.

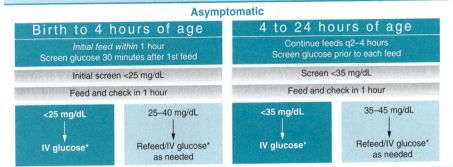

Screening and management of postnatal glucose homeostasis in late preterm and term SGA, IDM/LGA infants
(LPT infants 34–36 6/7 weeks and SGA [screen 0–24 h]; IDM and LGA [screen 0–12 h])

Symptomatic and <40 mg/dL ⟶ IV glucose

Asymptomatic

Birth to 4 hours of age	4 to 24 hours of age
Initial feed within 1 hour	Continue feeds q2–4 hours
Screen glucose 30 minutes after 1st feed	Screen glucose prior to each feed
Initial screen <25 mg/dL	Screen <35 mg/dL
Feed and check in 1 hour	Feed and check in 1 hour

<25 mg/dL	25–40 mg/dL	<35 mg/dL	35–45 mg/dL
IV glucose*	Refeed/IV glucose* as needed	IV glucose*	Refeed/IV glucose* as needed

Target glucose screen ≥45 mg/dL prior to routine feeds

*Glucose dose = 200 mg/kg (dextrose 10% at 2 mL/kg) and/or IV infusion at 5–8 mg/kg per min (80–100 mg/kg per d). Achieve plasma glucose level of 40–50 mg/dL.

Symptoms of hypoglycemia include: Irritability, tremors, jitteriness, exaggerated Moro reflex, high-pitched cry, seizures, lethargy, floppiness, cyanosis, apnea, poor feeding.

FIGURE 47.2 • Management of high-risk asymptomatic infants based on the AAP Guidelines. (From Committee on Fetus and Newborn, Adamkin DH. Postnatal glucose homeostasis in late-preterm and term infants. *Pediatrics* 2011;127;575-9.)

Prenatal glucocorticoids are known to upregulate expression of PEPCK and thus may help prevent hypoglycemia in some late preterm infants.

Glycogen stores are limited in IUGR infants, and even in AGA infants these stores can be depleted within 2–3 hours after birth. At this stage, the unfed newborn must rely on breakdown and metabolism of fatty acids to produce ATP. IUGR/SGA infants are at a great disadvantage due to their limited stores of fat—especially brown fat, which is found around the scapulae and retroperitoneal part of abdomen and generates heat and triglycerides when stimulated by the sympathetic nerve endings that innervate it. Triglycerides, a very basic form of fat, are utilized by the process of β-oxidation in the mitochondria. There are nearly 25 enzymes and transporters involved in transport and metabolism of fat to produce ATP. Thus, a defect in this pathway leads to failure to generate ATP during fasting and stressful situations, and certain organs such as the myocardium and liver, which must utilize fatty acids for their normal sustenance, begin to show signs of failure.

Excessive utilization of glucose by peripheral tissues occurs in some LGA and IDM infants and in those with overwhelming sepsis. Excess production of insulin leads to increased expression of Glut-4 in insulin-sensitive organs, excessive tissue uptake of glucose, subsequent conversion to glycogen, and ultimately reduced ability to generate ATP. Hypoglycemia in these infants is persistent and at times intractable. Hyperinsulinism has also been described in rare cases of short-chain 3-hydroxy-acyl CoA (SCHAD) deficiency and erythroblastosis fetalis. Other causes of persistent hypoglycemia include hypoxic–ischemic encephalopathy, polycythemia, hypothermia, and genetic causes such as Beckwith-Wiedemann syndrome and Sotos syndrome. Hypoglycemia is also observed in several hormone deficiency states such as hypofunctioning adrenal gland (cortex as well as medulla), growth hormone deficiency, and glucagon deficiency. The hypoglycemia in these infants is persistent and requires hormone replacement therapy usually for life, and extensive endocrine workup is needed before therapy can be initiated.

Prognosis

Mild asymptomatic late preterm and term infants with hypoglycemia usually have a normal outcome with no long-term sequelae, but infants with persistent hypoglycemia are at risk for brain injury on follow-up studies. Hypoglycemia, when persistent, leads to increased production of glutamate and increased blood flow initially, followed by neuronal swelling and death via apoptosis leading to the typical pattern of injury. The duration, severity, and the number of hypoglycemia events closely correlate with the outcome of hypoglycemia. Hypoglycemic brain injury does not necessarily follow the pattern of brain blood supply, so is a unique form of brain injury that can be visualized on MRI scanning, where hyperintense shadows are visualized mainly in the occipital cortex of brain. Hypoglycemia delays astrocyte proliferation and affects several parts of brain such as the sensorimotor cortex, thalamus, midbrain, brainstem, cerebellar vermis, and the occipital cortex. Hypoglycemic brain injury may cause a long-term effect on the developing nervous system and may cause developmental delay, cerebral palsy, and neuropsychiatric disorders. It is frequently associated with small head size and poor cognitive abilities, and neurodevelopmental follow-up of these infants is highly recommended.

RECOMMENDATIONS

MAJOR RECOMMENDATIONS

All neonates at risk of hypoglycemia should have screening blood glucose levels obtained, and neonates with symptoms attributable to hypoglycemia should undergo blood glucose testing. If the results of bedside glucose testing show low values, the result should be confirmed by laboratory assessment. The definition of hypoglycemia is debated, although action thresholds for blood glucose have been recommended based on available evidence and expert opinion. Blood glucose levels below the action thresholds can be treated with enteral feeds, intravenous dextrose, intramuscular glucagon, or buccal dextrose gel. Persistent hypoglycemia is a marker for endocrine, metabolic, or genetic disorders and requires endocrine consultation, specialized investigation, and treatment of the underlying disorder in addition to supplemental glucose.

PRACTICE OPTIONS

Practice Option #1: Diagnosis of Hypoglycemia

Most preterm and term neonates with hypoglycemia are asymptomatic, and hypoglycemia is diagnosed on routine bedside glucose monitoring. They may appear to be normal AGA infants or show signs of being IUGR or LGA (Figure 47.1). Infants at risk—late preterm and term neonates who are small for gestational age (SGA), IDM, and LGA babies—should all be routinely screened for low glucose levels, even if they are asymptomatic and feeding well (Figure 47.2).

Symptoms associated with hypoglycemia can be attributed to neuroglycopenia, or may be due to activation of the sympathetic nervous system. The symptoms in many

cases are vague and nonspecific, and may consist of sweating, pallor, temperature instability, irritability, hunger, tremulousness, tachycardia, and vomiting. Thus hypoglycemia should be suspected in any sick neonate. The neuroglycopenic manifestations occur
later, and are apnea, hypotonia, seizures, and coma. Death may result if the hypoglycemia is left untreated.

In infants with hypoglycemia, especially if prolonged and severe, a detailed feeding
history and detailed family history including any history of sudden infant deaths and
other genetic conditions should be obtained. Clues to the diagnosis may be found on a
thorough physical examination—hepatosplenomegaly, stigmata of Beckwith-Wiedemann
syndrome, midline defects associated with pituitary abnormalities (cleft lip/palate, central
incisor tooth, eye globe defects, micropenis), ambiguity of genitalia, and other phenotypic
features of specific genetic conditions.

Practice Option #2: Measurement of Glucose Levels

In clinical practice, blood glucose values are usually first obtained by point-of-care glu-
cometers. These devices often underestimate or overestimate the true glucose value,
and in the range of hypoglycemia, they may deviate from the true value by as much as
10–15 mg/dL in either direction. Therefore, all low glucose values on bedside testing
should be confirmed by a blood sample sent to the clinical laboratory for confirmatory testing. When such a sample is sent, delays in processing and assaying glucose
can reduce the glucose concentration by up to 6 mg/dL/hour. Whole blood glucose
values are around 15% lower than plasma glucose concentrations. Higher hematocrit
produces a reduction in the blood glucose value measured. Finally, accurate glucose
measurement requires adequate tissue perfusion.

When frequent blood sampling for glucose levels and ancillary tests is needed, obtaining arterial access may be prudent to avoid repeated needle pricks to the heels or toes
and the pain and tissue damage they cause.

Practice Option #3: Management of Asymptomatic and Mild Hypoglycemia

In clinical practice, all decisions to manage hypoglycemia are based on glucose levels,
the presence of clinical manifestations, and the likely underlying cause. The likelihood
of availability of alternate sources of metabolic fuel to the brain cells is not considered
in decision-making. Asymptomatic infants can be managed using the AAP guidelines
in most cases (Figure 47.2). There are four interventions that can be used to quickly
raise blood glucose levels: enteral feeds of milk, intravenous dextrose-containing fluid,
intramuscular injection of glucagon, and oral dextrose gel (a recent and increasingly
used intervention). All symptomatic infants must be treated emergently with intravenous glucose.

1. In hypoglycemic infants who are able to take oral feeds, enteral feeding with breast
   milk or formula is often a quick and effective way to raise the blood glucose. A glucose level should be checked 20–30 minutes after the feed ends to ensure that the it
   has increased to normal level.
2. Hypoglycemia can be treated by administration of parenteral dextrose, starting with the
   "mini-bolus" approach of 200 mg/kg of 10% dextrose in water (2 mL/kg D10W) followed by constant intravenous infusion and a recheck of blood sugar after 30 minutes
   later and then hourly. The goal is to immediately raise blood sugar with the bolus

and then provide a continuous glucose infusion rate (GIR) of 6–8 mg/kg/min. This is particularly important in preterm and low birth weight infants, since it is equivalent to the glucose that would have been provided by the liver via gluconeogenesis. A lower dextrose infusion rate of 3–5 mg/kg/min may be used for infants born to mothers with diabetes to provide minimal stimulation to their pancreas to secrete insulin. With these interventions, if an infant does not attain normoglycemia it is prudent to go up on the GIR to 8, 10, 12, and then 15 mg/kg/min over a period of 24 hours. A dextrose concentration of higher than 12.5% calls for central venous access. Dextrose-containing fluids are usually administered in a special care nursery or ICU. The dextrose solution is gradually weaned until glucose values are maintained in the desirable range.

3. In situations where intravenous access is difficult or impossible to obtain, intramuscular injection of glucagon in a dose of 0.5–1.0 mg/kg can help in raising serum glucose levels but requires the presence of adequate glycogen stores to be effective, and its effects can be blunted if the neonate's mother was on treatment with a beta blocker. The effect of glucagon lasts for 2–4 hours, giving the clinician enough time to arrange transport of such infants to a tertiary medical center.

4. Oral (buccal) administration of 40% dextrose gel is an emerging and promising treatment for hypoglycemia in relatively stable late-preterm and term infants who can feed orally. It has been shown to be effective and offers the advantages of improving serum glucose levels in infants who do not respond solely to enteral feeds of milk or formula. It may help avoid admission to the neonatal intensive care unit, avoid intravenous dextrose infusion, prevent separation of mothers and babies, and help promote breastfeeding and bonding.

Practice Option #4: Management and Diagnostic Workup of Persistent Hypoglycemia

When hypoglycemia is severe and persists beyond 48 hours of life, the neonate should be investigated for a persistent hypoglycemic disorder. Specifically, if the preprandial plasma glucose cannot be maintained above 50 mg/dL in the first 48 hours of life and above 60 mg/dL after 48 hours of age, a persistent hypoglycemic disorder should be suspected.

Conditions that lead to persistent or recurrent hypoglycemia include infant of diabetic mothers who are persistently hyperinsulinemic, infants with congenital hypopituitarism, congenital adrenal hyperplasia, and inborn errors of metabolism such as maple syrup urine disease, glycogen storage disorders, fructose intolerance, and fatty acid enzyme deficiencies, and those with rare conditions such as Beckwith-Wiedemann syndrome, Turner syndrome, Down syndrome, Costello syndrome, and Sotos syndrome. When such a disorder is suspected, endocrinology and metabolic specialist consultation should be required, and such infants must be transferred to a tertiary care center.

Treatment of persistent hypoglycemic disorders will depend on the cause. In neonates with a suspected persistent hypoglycemia disorder, the PES recommends maintaining a plasma glucose level above 70 mg/dL. In some forms of hyperinsulinism, diazoxide may be effective in stabilizing glucose levels and allow intravenous dextrose supplementation to be weaned. Diazoxide use can be associated with fluid retention and with the development of pulmonary hypertension, and therefore requires close monitoring for these disorders. A diuretic is sometimes used concurrently with diazoxide to prevent fluid retention.

Other medications that may be helpful in persistent hypoglycemic disorders are stress dose of hydrocortisone (4 mg/kg/day) (which enhances gluconeogenesis in the liver and reduces insulin sensitivity), nifedipine (which reduces glucose tolerance and insulin secretion), and octreotide (which decreases pancreatic insulin secretion, similar to diazoxide). Infants who have congenital neonatal hypoglycemia, depending on the cause, may require long-term treatment with cortisol, growth hormone, and special formulas or diets for those who have inborn errors of metabolism. Pancreatic resection is performed for infants with persistent hyperinsulinemic hypoglycemia of infancy who are resistant to medications.

To identify the cause of persistent hypoglycemia, sophisticated laboratory testing is required. Most such tests are not informative if performed when the glucose level is normal, therefore a blood sample should be obtained when the glucose level is low (as confirmed in the clinical laboratory, not just on point-of-care testing), and before treatment. Such a sample is known as a "critical sample," and should include levels of serum insulin, C-peptide, β-hydroxybutyrate, free fatty acids, cortisol, growth hormone, bicarbonate, and lactate. Extra plasma can be held in reserve for specific tests such as plasma total and free carnitine and acyl carnitine for suspected disorders of fatty acid oxidation. To diagnose adrenal insufficiency, the simultaneous measurement of adrenocorticotropic hormone (ACTH) and cortisol, and an ACTH stimulation test are required. The results of the state newborn metabolic screening test, if available, should be reviewed. A detectable insulin level in the face of blood sugar of less than 30 mg/dL is suggestive of hyperinsulinism.

If a critical sample cannot be obtained, a provocative fasting testing test for 6–8 hours (the exact duration should be tailored to the condition suspected) should be performed. When the plasma glucose decreases to 50 mg/dL, the critical sample described above should be obtained and the infant fed. During the fasting test, the neonate's vital signs, plasma glucose levels, and β-hydroxybutyrate levels should be monitored closely. If at any time during the test the infant's vital signs are unstable or if the β-hydroxybutyrate level exceeds 2.5 mmol/L, the fast should be terminated and the infant fed. When the fasting test is performed in infants with suspected hyperinsulinism, a dose of glucagon should be given intravenously, intramuscularly, or subcutaneously when the plasma glucose decreases to 50 mg/dL, and plasma glucose should be measured. An exaggerated "glycemic response" with an increase in plasma glucose of greater than 30 mg/dL is highly suggestive of hyperinsulinism.

Further investigation for persistent hypoglycemia disorder may include obtaining a detailed metabolic profile using mass spectrometric analysis of various metabolites, genetic studies, and imaging to look for pathology in the pancreas and the adrenal and pituitary glands.

CLINICAL ALGORITHM(S)

See Figure 47.2 for a suggested algorithm for screening and management of hypoglycemia.

IMPLEMENTATION OF GUIDELINE

QUALITY METRICS

Percentage of at-risk infants undergoing appropriate screening per unit protocol, time taken in hypoglycemic infants to restore blood glucose values to above the desired threshold, neonatal intensive care unit admissions due to hypoglycemia, and neurodevelopmental outcomes in hypoglycemic infants.

BIBLIOGRAPHIC SOURCE(S)

Adamkin DH, Polin RA. Imperfect advice: neonatal hypoglycemia. *J Pediatr.* 2016;176:195-6.

Committee on Fetus and Newborn, Adamkin DH. Clinical report. Postnatal glucose homeostasis in late-preterm and term infants. *Pediatrics.* 2011;127(3):575-9.

Güemes M, Rahman SA, Hussain K. What is a normal blood glucose? *Arch Dis Child.* 2016;101(6):569-74.

Rozance PJ, Hay WW Jr. New approaches to management of neonatal hypoglycemia. *Matern Health Neonatol Perinatol.* 2016;2:3.

Sharma A, Davis A, Shekhawat PS. Hypoglycemia in the preterm neonate: etiopathogenesis, diagnosis, management and long-term outcomes. *Transl Pediatr.* 2017;6(4):335-48.

Stanley CA, Rozance PJ, Thornton PS, et al. Re-evaluating "transitional neonatal hypoglycemia": mechanism and implications for management. *J Pediatr.* 2015;166(6):1520-5.

Thornton PS, Stanley CA, De Leon DD, et al; Pediatric Endocrine Society. Recommendations from the Pediatric Endocrine Society for evaluation and management of persistent hypoglycemia in neonates, infants, and children. *J Pediatr.* 2015;167(2):238-45.

Adrenal Insufficiency

Prem S. Shekhawat, MD • Gautham K. Suresh, MD, DM, MS, FAAP

SCOPE

DISEASE/CONDITION(S)

Insufficiency of the adrenal cortex in the neonate.

GUIDELINE OBJECTIVE(S)

Identification, management, and monitoring of adrenocortical insufficiency in the neonate.

BRIEF BACKGROUND

Normal Physiology: The Hypothalamic–Pituitary–Adrenal Axis

The cortex of the adrenal gland produces the hormone cortisol, which helps maintain blood pressure, electrolyte balance, and vascular permeability and helps mature the lungs, cardiovascular system, GI tract, and several metabolic pathways. It also facilitates renal free-water excretion, modulates central nervous system processing and behavior, and most importantly, during periods of stress, suppresses the body's inflammatory responses. Cortisol production is regulated by adrenocorticotrophin (ACTH) produced by the anterior pituitary, which is in turn regulated by corticotrophin-releasing hormone (CRH) secreted from the hypothalamus. Activation of this hypothalamic–pituitary–adrenal (HPA) axis and release of cortisol are critical in mounting a response to stress. Factors influencing the release of CRH and ACTH include neurological inputs from the normal diurnal rhythm, and acute physiological stressors, as well as negative feedback from circulating cortisol.

Fetal and Postnatal Physiology

The adrenal gland develops from the mesoderm and undergoes a remarkable transformation during fetal life to mature into a functioning gland to sustain extrauterine survival. The fetal adrenal cortex consists of a fetal zone (80%) and smaller definitive and transitional zones (20%). The fetal zone gradually involutes and gets replaced by the definitive and transitional zones near term and shortly after birth. The fetal zone expresses high levels of sulfotransferases and very low levels of 3β-hydroxysteroid dehydrogenase (3β-HSD) which leads to production of inactive glucocorticoids and low levels of cortisol exposure to the growing fetus while at the same time providing substrate to placenta for estrogen production. During fetal life, maternal cortisol, while crossing the placenta, is converted to its inactive form cortisone by the enzyme 11β-hydroxysteroid dehydrogenase 2 (11β-HSD2). Maternal stress leading to production of high levels of cortisol can escape inactivation by 11β-HSD2 and lead to fetal growth restriction and inhibition of fetal HPA axis. Human fetal cortisol levels tend to be as low as <5 μg/dL until about near-term gestation (Figure 48.1). Extremely preterm infants born during this phase of adrenal development are therefore likely to suffer from RAI and unable to mount a stress response.

As gestation progresses to near term, there is an increase in cortisol production by the fetal adrenal gland mediated by maternal stress of labor and increasing activity of the adrenal 3β-HSD leading to maturation of fetal organs like the lungs, cardiovascular system, and liver enzymes. Caesarean section without labor is associated with lack of the "cortisol surge" leading to higher incidence of respiratory distress and delayed lung fluid clearance in these infants. Infants born at extremely low birth weight are more likely to suffer from hypoglycemia, hypotension, delayed lung fluid clearance, severe grade of intraventricular hemorrhage, develop hemodynamically significant patent ductus arteriosus (PDA), and necrotizing enterocolitis. Thus, a normal functioning adrenal gland is critical to ensure a good neonatal outcome. Adrenal gland maturation is enhanced in infants born to mothers with chorioamnionitis and those with intrauterine fetal growth restriction. Maturation of adrenal gland is delayed in large for gestational age infants and infants of poorly controlled diabetic mothers. Some late preterm and near-term infants

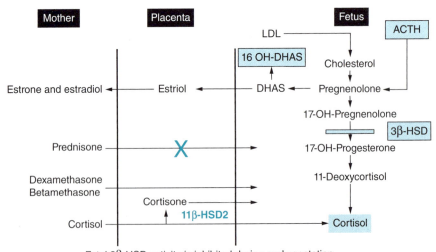

FIGURE 48.1 • Maternal–placental–fetal steroid interactions.

also demonstrate RAI and clinically develop conditions mentioned above leading to increased morbidity and mortality in this population.

Antenatal steroid therapy in the form of two doses of betamethasone given 12 hours apart is prescribed to mothers likely to deliver preterm infants at <34 weeks' gestation to help avoid these complications. Lately, antenatal steroids are being tried for late preterm pregnancies as well to avoid these morbidities and improve outcomes.

RECOMMENDATIONS

PRACTICE OPTIONS

Practice Option #1: Identification of Infants at Risk of, or With Existing Adrenal Insufficiency

A term neonate produces roughly 6–8 mg/m^2/day of cortisol. In comparison, a preterm neonate produces only 2–4 mg/m^2/day. Some preterm neonates such as those born between 22 and 24 weeks produce much less than 2–4 mg/m^2/day, and therefore their HPA axis produces insufficient cortisol for their physiological needs and for the degree of illness or stress they are experiencing. This leads to physiological instability, increase in severity of illness, and increased morbidity and mortality.

Table 48.1 lists conditions that result in a deficiency in the production of cortisol, ACTH, or CRH. In addition to the listed specific diseases, critically ill neonates and extremely preterm infants are likely to develop relative adrenal insufficiency (RAI), also known as transient adrenocortical insufficiency of prematurity (TAP). This is analogous to a condition known as "critical illness-related corticosteroid insufficiency" (CIRCI), sometimes seen in critically ill adults where there is inadequate cellular corticosteroid activity for the severity of the patient's illness.

TABLE 48.1. Causes of Adrenal Insufficiency

- Congenital adrenal hyperplasia (enzymatic defects such as 21-hydroxylase, 3β-hydroxysteroid dehydrogenase, and 11-hydroxylase deficiency leading to impaired biosynthesis of glucocorticoids, often accompanied by impaired biosynthesis of mineralocorticoid that leads to salt wasting)
- RAI due to late maturation of adrenal cortex commonly seen in the preterm neonates and infants born to poorly controlled diabetic mothers
- Adrenal hemorrhage
- Genetic conditions affecting the adrenal gland (e.g., neonatal adrenoleukodystrophy, Wolman disease, Smith-Lemli-Opitz syndrome; mitochondrial disorders such as Kearns-Sayre syndrome; and storage diseases such as Niemann-Pick disease)
- Adrenal suppression from exogenously administered medications— corticosteroids (including occasionally from topical and inhaled corticosteroids), ketoconazole, etomidate, lopinavir/ritonavir combination
- Adrenal infection (including meningococcemia, other bacterial infections, cytomegalovirus, HIV, and tuberculosis)
- Tissue resistance to glucocorticoids as a result of effects of cytokines, nitric oxide, and HIV infection is also reported
- Autoimmune process affecting the adrenal gland which usually occurs later in life

Asymptomatic neonates with one or more of the following conditions are at risk of adrenal insufficiency—ambiguous genitalia, midline defects (cleft palate, central incisor tooth, septo-optic dysplasia), adrenal hemorrhage, elevated 17-hydroxyprogesterone levels on routine newborn metabolic screening, treatment with the medications listed in Table 48.1, and extreme prematurity.

Adrenal insufficiency should be suspected in neonates with hypotension or shock, particularly if it is refractory to vasopressors, and in neonates with persistent hypoglycemia.

Low cortisol levels in neonates have been associated with hypotension, inflammation, and bronchopulmonary dysplasia.

Practice Option #2: Assessment and Diagnosis of Adrenal Insufficiency

There is a paucity of evidence to inform clinicians about which patients should be tested for adrenal insufficiency, the tests to use, and how to interpret the results of these tests. The currently available low-dose ACTH stimulation provides a "yes" or "no" answer to the question of whether a functioning adrenal gland is present or not. This test is unable to diagnose RAI commonly seen in preterm, late preterm, and some near-term infants.

Measurement of serum cortisol levels is not helpful in diagnosing adrenal insufficiency because it does not correlate with normal functioning of adrenal gland. Most neonates, especially extremely preterm neonates, have a low basal cortisol level and the only clinically useful level of cortisol is >20 µg/dL where adrenal insufficiency can be ruled out. This level is again unable to predict whether these infants are capable of handling a stressful event like surgery for PDA ligation or exploratory laparotomy since serum cortisol does not reflect the reserve capacity of adrenal gland. Also, elevated serum cortisol levels in critically ill patients may result from increased production, decreased metabolism, and decreased excretion, besides resistance to its actions at cellular level, and it is impossible to distinguish these three causes. The cortisol level must be interpreted in association with clinical features, postnatal age, antenatal corticosteroids usage, and the level of stress experienced by the infant. A 24-hour urinary excretion of cortisol metabolites, though cumbersome to measure, can be useful in assessing production capacity of neonatal adrenal gland.

The ability of the neonatal adrenal gland to increase the production of cortisol in response to synthetic ACTH (1-24) is tested, under the guidance of a pediatric endocrinologist, using an ACTH stimulation test, in which a single dose of ACTH (1 µg/kg, range 0.1–1.0 µg/kg) is injected intravenously and the serum cortisol level is measured immediately before, 30 minutes, and 60 minutes after the injection. Adrenal insufficiency is confirmed if the cortisol response is subnormal, especially in the setting of stress. Generally, an increase in cortisol level to >20 µg/dL rules out adrenal insufficiency or when there is doubling of cortisol level from the basal level at 30 minutes is considered an adequate response, although there is uncertainty about the exact levels for neonates, especially for preterm ones.

If a condition listed in Table 48.1 is suspected to exist, additional targeted laboratory and imaging tests should be performed to identify it.

Practice Option #3: Management of Adrenal Insufficiency

Only low-quality evidence is available to inform the treatment of adrenal insufficiency in neonates.

RAI with hemodynamic instability is treated with exogenously administered hydrocortisone (which is identical to native cortisol), intravenously initially, and enteral hydrocortisone sodium succinate (Solu-cortef), or prednisolone after the neonate is stable and if prolonged administration is required, as in patients with congenital adrenal hyperplasia. Supplemental dextrose infusion may be required to maintain euglycemia and volume expansion with crystalloid solution and inotropic support may be required to maintain blood pressure in the acute phase shortly after birth. Additional specific treatment is required based on the underlying conditions identified, such as aldosterone substitutes (fludrocortisone) and supplemental intake of sodium chloride in congenital adrenal hyperplasia and replacement of other deficient hormones in cases of panhypopituitarism.

In extremely preterm infants, hydrocortisone therapy given simultaneously with indomethacin or ibuprofen is associated with an increased risk of spontaneous gastrointestinal perforation. Therefore, use of hydrocortisone along with either of these medications should be avoided. When treating refractory neonatal hypotension with hydrocortisone, the use of high or "stress" doses (4 mg/kg divided every 6 hours) is recommended for short periods of time, usually not more than 3–4 days. Stress dose of hydrocortisone has been used in late preterm and near-term neonates to treat persistent pulmonary hypertension of newborn, to avoid the need for extra-corporeal membrane oxygenation, although the quality of evidence for this practice is low. This stress dose can be followed by a dose of 0.5–1.0 mg/kg divided every 12 hours while the response in terms of normalization of blood pressure is closely monitored. The clinical response to hydrocortisone therapy is commonly witnessed after 12 hours of starting the medication since its effects are mediated through up-regulation of α-receptors and several other proteins which mediate cellular steroid action. Long-term and high-dose steroid use, especially fluorinated steroids such as dexamethasone, should be avoided since these have been shown to be associated with neurodevelopmental delays, cerebral palsy, poor postnatal growth, and long-term complications like hypertension, cardiovascular disease, and chronic kidney disease. Using lower, less frequent, short-duration doses should decrease the chances of suppression of HPA axis, and if clinical situation warrants long term use of >2–3 weeks, then steroids should be gradually weaned.

RAI in extremely preterm neonates is usually transient but may last till close to term post-menstrual age, so low-dose supplementation may be considered based on clinical needs like oxygen or ventilator dependency. Term and late preterm neonates are more likely to be successfully weaned off hydrocortisone in a few days. Postnatal hydrocortisone helps mature 3β-HSD enzyme in the adrenal gland and thus helps endogenous production of cortisol.

BIBLIOGRAPHIC SOURCE(S)

Aucott SW, Watterberg KL, Shaffer ML, Donohue PK; PROPHET Study Group. Do cortisol concentrations predict short-term outcomes in extremely low birth weight infants? *Pediatrics.* 2008;122(4):775-81.

Auron M, Raissouni N. Adrenal insufficiency. *Pediatr Rev.* 2015;36(3):92-102.

Chung HR. Adrenal and thyroid function in the fetus and preterm infant. *Korean J Pediatr.* 2014;57(10):425-33.

Fernandez EF, Watterberg KL. Relative adrenal insufficiency in the preterm and term infant. *J Perinatol.* 2009;29(Suppl 2):S44-9.

Finken MJ, van der Voorn B, Heijboer AC, de Waard M, van Goudoever JB, Rotteveel J. Glucocorticoid programming in very preterm birth. *Horm Res Paediatr.* 2016;85(4):221-31.

Gyamfi-Bannerman C, Thom EA, Blackwell SC, et al; NICHD Maternal–Fetal Medicine Units Network. Antenatal betamethasone for women at risk for late preterm delivery. *N Engl J Med.* 2016;374(14):1311-20.

Gyurkovits Z, Maróti Á, Rénes L, Németh G, Pál A, Orvos H. Adrenal haemorrhage in term neonates: a retrospective study from the period 2001-2013. *J Matern Fetal Neonatal Med.* 2015;28(17):2062-5.

Higgins S, Friedlich P, Seri I. Hydrocortisone for hypotension and vasopressor dependence in preterm neonates: a meta-analysis. *J Perinatol.* 2010;30(6):373-8.

Johnson PJ. Hydrocortisone for treatment of hypotension in the newborn. *Neonatal Network.* 2015;34(1):46-51.

Ng PC. Is there a "normal" range of serum cortisol concentration for preterm infants? *Pediatrics.* 2008;122(4):873-5.

Quintos JB, Boney CM. Transient adrenal insufficiency in the premature newborn. *Curr Opin Endocrinol Diabetes Obes.* 2010;17(1):8-12.

Shaffer ML, Baud O, Lacaze-Masmonteil T, Peltoniemi OM, Bonsante F, Watterberg KL. Effect of rophylaxis for early adrenal insufficiency using low-dose hydrocortisone in very preterm infants: an individual patient data meta-analysis. *J Pediatr.* 2018;pii:S0022-3476(18)31416-1.

Watterberg KL, Hintz SR, Do B, et al; SUPPORT Study Group of the Eunice Kennedy Shriver National Institute of Child Health and Human Development Neonatal Research Network. Adrenal function links to early postnatal growth and blood pressure at age 6 in children born extremely preterm. *Pediatric Research.* 2018. doi: 10.1038/s41390-018-0243-1.

Zadik Z. Adrenal insufficiency in very low birth weight infants. *J Pediatr Endocrinol Metab.* 2010;23(1-2):1-2.

Congenital Adrenal Hyperplasia

Yunru Shao, MMSc, LCGC • Oluyemisi A. Adeyemi-Fowode, MD, FACOG • Duong D. Tu, MD • Sheila K. Gunn, MD • Marni Elyse Axelrad, PhD, ABPP • Vernon R. Sutton, MD • Lefkothea Karaviti, MD, PhD

SCOPE

DISEASE/CONDITION(S)

Congenital adrenal hyperplasia in the neonate.

GUIDELINE OBJECTIVE(S)

Describe the etiology, pathophysiology, and management of congenital adrenal hyperplasia in the neonate.

BRIEF BACKGROUND

Congenital adrenal hyperplasia (CAH) comprises a group of autosomal recessive disorders in which impaired cortisol biosynthesis by the adrenal glands leads to overproduction of hypothalamic corticotrophin-releasing hormone (CRH) and the secretion of pituitary adrenocorticotrophic hormone (ACTH), with consequent hyperplasia of adrenal tissue. In addition, diversion of precursor products into alternate pathways causes elevated levels of other classes of corticosteroid, particularly gonadal steroid hormones.

Cortisol is produced by the adrenal cortex under the regulation of ACTH from the anterior pituitary, which in turn is regulated by CRH from the hypothalamus—the hypothalamic–pituitary–adrenal (HPA) axis. Cortisol concentration in the serum

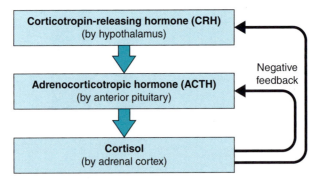

FIGURE 49.1 • The hypothalamic–pituitary–adrenal (HPA) axis.

modulates the resting activity of the HPA axis via negative feedback on ACTH and CRH secretion (Figure 49.1).

Steroid hormone biosynthesis commences with cholesterol translocation from the cytoplasm to the inner membrane of the mitochondrion, a rate-limiting step mediated by the steroidogenic acute regulatory (StAR) protein. Catalyzed by side-chain cleavage (P450scc), cholesterol is converted into pregnenolone, the common precursor for all other steroids. Glucocorticoid (cortisol), mineralocorticoid (aldosterone), and adrenal androgen are all synthesized from pregnenolone, after sequential processing by the appropriate steroidogenic enzymes.

Deficiency in one of the critical steroidogenic enzymes leads to impaired production of cortisol, which leads to increased secretion of both CRH and ACTH. Excessive ACTH causes hyperplasia of the adrenal cortex and also stimulates melanocytes, with an excess of ACTH potentially leading to hyperpigmentation.

With the block in the biosynthesis of cortisol, common precursors at supraphysiologic concentrations are shunted into an alternative pathway, which can lead to either increased or decreased androgen production. As a result, the target organ is subject to either undesired, long-term exposure or deprivation of the sex steroid hormones. Overvirilization in females (such as in 21-hydroxylase deficiency [21-OHD]), and undervirilization in males (from 3β-hydroxysteroid dehydrogenase deficiency [3B-HSD]), can be seen during gestation or at birth, presenting as atypical genitalia, or occasionally diagnosed at a later time.

The regulation of aldosterone secretion is via plasma renin. Depending on where the enzyme blockage is, mineralocorticoid levels may be low (due to enzyme block) or high (due to excessive synthesis through alternative pathways). The neonate might present with features of mineralocorticoid disturbances and manifest hyponatremia and shock in the context of 21-OHD, or with hypertension when 11β-hydroxylase is deficient.

There are several different forms of CAH depending on the defective enzyme involved (Table 49.1 and Figure 49.2). These include StAR protein deficiency, 21-OHD, 3B-HSD, 17α-hydroxylase deficiency, and 11β-hydroxylase deficiency. Though this group of disorders shares similar pathophysiologic mechanisms and overlapping features, their clinical manifestations and biochemical profiles are distinguishable and reflect the consequences of specific blocks at different steps of the steroidogenic pathway.

Infants with CAH are at increased risk of mortality from hypovolemic shock, electrolyte disturbances, and hypoglycemia.

TABLE 49.1. Clinical Presentation and Biochemical Characteristics of CAH due to Different Enzyme Deficiency in Neonates

	Girls	Boys	Androgen	Mineralocorticoid
21-Hydroxylase deficiency	Virilization, adrenal crisis	Adrenal crisis	Excess	Deficiency
11β-Hydroxylase deficiency	Virilization, later hypertension	Isosexual virilization Later hypertension	Excess	Excess
17α-Hydroxylase deficiency	Hypertension	Hypertension, lack of virilization	Deficiency	Excess
3β-Hydroxysteroid dehydrogenase deficiency	Mild virilization, adrenal crisis	Undervirilization, adrenal crisis	Deficiency	Deficiency
Steroidogenic acute regulatory protein (StAR) deficiency	Adrenal crisis	Adrenal crisis, undervirilization to complete feminization	Deficiency	Deficiency

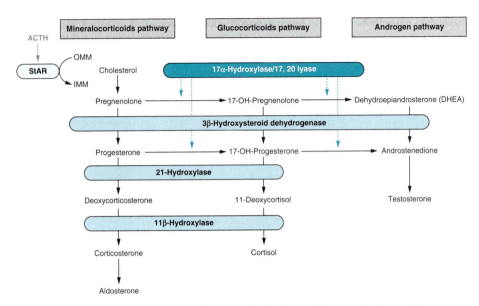

FIGURE 49.2 • Five main types of congenital adrenal hyperplasia and the corresponding enzymes are shown in the steroidogenic pathway in adrenal gland.

RECOMMENDATIONS

MAJOR RECOMMENDATIONS

CAH is a group of autosomal recessive disorders that are characterized by defects in cortisol biosynthesis and hyperplasia of the adrenal cortex. Depending on where the enzyme block is in the steroidogenic pathway, patients may also exhibit symptoms of mineralocorticoid and sex steroid synthesis abnormalities. Using genetic data, we now have a better understanding of these conditions, and using evidence-based medicine, can better differentiate and treat CAH cases. 21-OHD is responsible for over 90% of cases and is by far the most common cause of CAH. Appropriate and immediate medical management effectively is of the utmost importance, although challenges still exist that necessitate careful evaluation and additional monitoring. Prenatal treatment, despite being controversial, has been made available and can prevent fetal virilization during pregnancy. In general, managing newborns is extremely challenging to the medical team. An interdisciplinary approach and psychological support are essential in providing the appropriate care for the affected families and individuals, and to assure both short-term and long-term clinical benefits. Figure 49.3 depicts the initial approach to management of an infant with suspected CAH identified in the unit.

PRACTICE OPTIONS

Practice Option #1: When to Suspect CAH in a Neonate

Initial suspicion of CAH usually arises in the neonatal period with one of the following scenarios:

1. *Atypical external genitalia or external genitalia that are discordant from the sex chromosome constitution.* Depending on the steroidogenic enzyme involved and the severity of its disruption, both boys and girls can present with discordance between their genetic sex and external genitalia owing to intra-utero exposure to abnormal

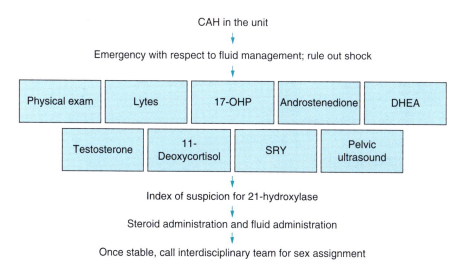

FIGURE 49.3 • Action flowchart for suspected congenital adrenal hyperplasia identified in the neonatal unit.

levels of androgens. The severity of the genital abnormality can vary widely from mild overvirilization/undervirilization to sex reversal (Table 49.1). In contrast to many other disorders of sex development, in CAH the internal reproductive organs are normal. The initial evaluation of a neonate with atypical genitalia is described in Chapter 50.

2. *The newborn screen is suggestive of CAH.* Currently, all US newborn screening programs, and those of many other countries, screen for CAH, usually employing a radioimmunoassay for 17-hydroxyprogesterone. This screening is valuable given that 21-OHD deficiency can be lethal if left untreated, as shock, hyponatremia, and hyperkalemia can occur. Furthermore, cost-effective universal screening can efficiently identify infants, especially at-risk males, with no distinguishable physical features at birth, and expedite the diagnosis of females with atypical genitalia. Abnormal newborn screening results should always lead to a follow-up with further evaluations or, if necessary, immediate treatment based on regional protocols to prevent adrenal crises. A substantial number of non-classical cases can also be identified through newborn screening, which allows monitoring and early treatment for prepubertal growth acceleration and other problems in childhood.

3. *A neonate who initially appears healthy experiences a salt-wasting crisis in the first or second week of life.* This event is seen in the most severe cases and should immediately prompt an evaluation for CAH. Neonates with CAH-induced aldosterone deficiency will typically present at 7–14 days of life with adrenal crisis, characterized by vomiting, weight loss, lethargy, dehydration, hyponatremia, and hyperkalemia, and can present in shock, leading to serious illness and even death. Early recognition and treatment can prevent morbidity and mortality. Such salt-losing crises happen more frequently in undetected and untreated male infants because of the lack of external visible sexual ambiguity and delays in the results of newborn screening tests.

Practice Option #2: Management of Electrolyte and Glucocorticoid Imbalance

For classic CAH, the management is as follows (Figure 49.4). The priority is to focus on the adrenal crisis in salt-losing cases. A secondary goal is to reduce excessive androgen

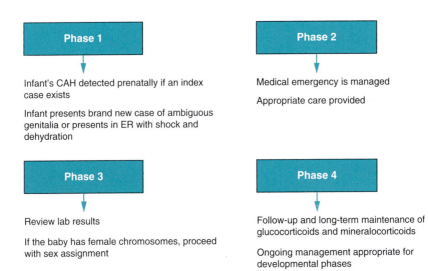

FIGURE 49.4 • Phases of recommended perinatal management of congenital adrenal hyperplasia.

secretion by replacing deficient hormones. Appropriate treatment with glucocorticoids can prevent adrenal crisis and virilization, allowing normal growth and development. In practice, the clinical management of classic CAH is a difficult balance between hyperandrogenism and hypercortisolism.

Immediate Intervention Regarding Stress Management. In the neonatal period, after samples are obtained to measure stat electrolytes, blood sugar, 17-hydroxyprogesterone, plasma renin, androstenedione, and testosterone concentrations, the patient with a suspicion of adrenal insufficiency should be immediately treated with glucocorticoids. Treatment should not be withheld while awaiting confirmatory results, as this condition is life-threatening. In patients who are sick and have signs of adrenal insufficiency, therapy should consist of stress doses of hydrocortisone (100 mg/m^2 administered as an initial dose), followed by $100 \text{ mg/m}^2/\text{d}$ IV, divisible into 6-hourly doses, with progressive dose tapering as the patient gets stabilized and the management is converted to maintenance therapy.

Maintenance Therapy. Adequate glucocorticoid replacement should prevent excessive concentrations of ACTH from stimulating the adrenal glands to produce extra adrenal androgens that provoke further virilization. In growing patients with classic CAH, long-term maintenance therapy with hydrocortisone is recommended. The dose should be tailored to each individual patient, but the average is $10–15 \text{ mg/m}^2/\text{day}$, administered as three doses (i.e., every 8 hours).

Salt Replacement. Patients with dehydration, hyponatremia, or hyperkalemia, and a possible salt-wasting form of adrenal hyperplasia with shock, should receive an intravenous (IV) bolus of isotonic sodium chloride solution (20 mL/kg or 450 mL/m^2) over 30 minutes as needed to restore their intravascular volume and blood pressure. Following the fluid bolus, replacement should be commenced with normal saline supplemented with 5% dextrose for children, and 10% for infants. Fludrocortisone and sodium chloride supplements for newborns and those in early infancy are recommended for all patients diagnosed with classic CAH. A dose of 2.5 g/day (6–8 meq/kg/day) is appropriate after the initial hyponatremia hyperkalemia has been corrected.

Practice Option #3: Management of Genitalia at Birth

The assessment of atypical genitalia and the importance of management by a coordinated multidisciplinary specialist team is described in Chapter 50.

In most cases, girls with classic 21-OHD CAH manifest with atypical genitalia or complete male-appearing external genitalia. Affected male infants are usually normally developed, but the phallus is almost invariably enlarged and the scrotum hyperpigmented in virilizing and salt-wasting forms. In other forms of CAH, undervirilized male patients typically present with a chordee, with perineal hypospadia. Rarely does the urethra extend to the tip of the phallus.

The surgical management of children born with atypical genitalia is complex and controversial due to the clinical presentation of the genitalia as well as concern for future psychological well-being of the patient. Currently, the practice guideline consensus by the Endocrine Society suggest consideration of clitoral and perineal reconstruction surgery in infancy, however, this surgery should not proceed without extensive counseling about timing and alternatives.

Practice Option #4: Clinical Options and Controversies

Prenatal Diagnosis and Prenatal Therapy. For couples with one child affected by CAH, an autosomal recessive condition, the risk of recurrence in a subsequent child is one in four. In a pregnancy at risk for CAH, dexamethasone treatment administered to the mother may suppress fetal androgen production and reduce female genital virilization, which in turn may diminish the need for postnatal reconstructive surgery and the parental emotional distress associated with the birth of a child with atypical genitalia. However, the risk-versus-benefit ratio of prenatal dexamethasone therapy and the optimum treatment regimen are uncertain, and this therapy should be used only when the parents fully understand the risks and benefits, and the therapy is monitored by an Institutional Review Board-approved clinical trial. Since virilization of the external genitalia begins by 8 weeks of gestation, prenatal dexamethasone therapy must be started as soon as pregnancy is confirmed. Since only affected females (1 in 8 fetuses) will benefit from this prenatal treatment, DNA and chromosome testing to confirm the diagnosis and chromosomal sex should be undertaken as early in the pregnancy as is possible, generally by 10 weeks of gestation. Unnecessary prenatal treatment should be discontinued after obtaining the genetic diagnosis and fetal sex. Prenatal treatment does not change the need for lifelong adrenocortical hormonal replacement therapy.

Sex of Rearing and Sex Assignment. This is described in detail Chapter 50. In terms of congenital adrenal hyperplasia, particularly 21-OHD, and based on existing evidence, sex assignment is generally recommended in accordance with the chromosomal sex if no other defects are involved. This recommendation is based on preservation of reproductive potential and evidence showing that gender identity is generally consistent with genetic sex.

In some genetically female infants with completely male-appearing genitalia, particularly those who have been raised as a male for several months, a male sex assignment could be discussed as an alternative but is associated with long-term consequences of management of the sex organs and the lack of reproductive potential, and possible gender dysphoria.

Surgical Procedures. Surgical management is intended to achieve a near-normal appearance of the genitalia while striving to assure functionality, and is associated with extensive debate in the literature (see Practice Option #3). Feminizing genital surgery can be extensive, depending on the degree of virilization. It comprises some or all of the following: neurovascular-sparing clitoroplasty to address clitoromegaly, if present; mobilization of the urogenital sinus to separate the urethra and vaginal opening; vaginoplasty or neovaginoplasty; and labial fashioning to create a more feminine appearance. Only surgeons with specific training in disorders of sexual differentiation should perform these procedures, with an emphasis placed on functional outcome (preserving sensation and preventing urologic sequelae) over aesthetics.

The timing of genital reconstructive surgery in patients with CAH is controversial. Specifically, the risks and benefits of the traditional "one-step" surgery compared to multi-stage repair are unknown.

BIBLIOGRAPHIC SOURCE(S)

Araújo VG, Oliveira RS, Gameleira KP, Cruz CB, Lofrano-Porto A. 3β-hydroxysteroid dehydrogenase type II deficiency on newborn screening test. *Arq Bras Endocrinol Metabol.* 2014;58:650-5.

Auchus RJ. The genetics, pathophysiology, and management of human deficiencies of P450c17. *Endocrinol Metab Clin North Am.* 2001;30:101-19, vii.

Axelrad ME, Berg JS, Coker LA, et al. The gender medicine team: 'it takes a village'. *Adv Pediatr.* 2009;56:145-64.

Baker BY, Lin L, Kim CJ, et al. Nonclassic congenital lipoid adrenal hyperplasia: a new disorder of the steroidogenic acute regulatory protein with very late presentation and normal male genitalia. *J Clin Endocrinol Metab.* 2006;91:4781-5.

Baskin LS. Anatomical studies of the female genitalia: surgical reconstructive implications. *J Pediatr Endocrinol Metab.* 2004;17:581-7.

Bose HS, Sato S, Aisenberg J, Shalev SA, Matsuo N, Miller WL. Mutations in the steroidogenic acute regulatory protein (StAR) in six patients with congenital lipoid adrenal hyperplasia. *J Clin Endocrinol Metab.* 2000;85:3636-9.

Carroll MC, Campbell RD, Porter RR. Mapping of steroid 21-hydroxylase genes adjacent to complement component C4 genes in HLA, the major histocompatibility complex in man. *Proc Natl Acad Sci U S A.* 1985;82:521-5.

Chang YT, Kulin HE, Garibaldi L, Suriano MJ, Bracki K, Pang S. Hypothalamic-pituitary-gonadal axis function in pubertal male and female siblings with glucocorticoid-treated nonsalt-wasting 3 beta-hydroxysteroid dehydrogenase deficiency congenital adrenal hyperplasia. *J Clin Endocrinol Metab.* 1993;77:1251-7.

Clayton PE, Miller WL, Oberfield SE, Ritzén EM, Sippell WG, Speiser PW; ESPE/ LWPES CAH Working Group. Consensus statement on 21-hydroxylase deficiency from the European Society for Paediatric Endocrinology and the Lawson Wilkins Pediatric Endocrine Society. *Horm Res.* 2002;58:188-95.

Crouch NS, Creighton SM. Long-term functional outcomes of female genital reconstruction in childhood. *BJU Int.* 2007;100:403-7.

Dessens AB, Slijper FME, Drop SLS. Gender dysphoria and gender change in chromosomal females with congenital adrenal hyperplasia. *Arch Sex Behav.* 2005;34:389-97.

Furtado PS, Moraes F, Lago R, Barros LO, Toralles MB, Barroso U Jr. Gender dysphoria associated with disorders of sex development. *Nat Rev Urol.* 2012;9:620-7.

Geller DH, Auchus RJ, Mendonca BB, Miller WL. The genetic and functional basis of isolated 17,20-lyase deficiency. *Nat Genet.* 1997;17:201-5.

Joehrer K, Geley S, Strasser-Wozak EM et al. CYP11B1 mutations causing non-classic adrenal hyperplasia due to 11 beta-hydroxylase deficiency. *Hum Mol Genet.* 1997;6:1829-34.

Khattab A, Yuen T, Sun L, et al. Noninvasive prenatal diagnosis of congenital adrenal hyperplasia. *Endocr Dev.* 2016;30:37-41.

Kim CJ. Congenital lipoid adrenal hyperplasia. *Ann Pediatr Endocrinol Metab.* 2014;19:179-83.

Krone N, Arlt W. Genetics of congenital adrenal hyperplasia. *Best Pract Res Clin Endocrinol Metab.* 2009;23:181-92.

Lachance Y, Luu-The V, Labrie C, et al. Characterization of human 3 beta-hydroxysteroid dehydrogenase/delta 5-delta. *J Biol Chem.* 1990;265:20469-75.

Lee PA, Houk CP, Ahmed SF, Hughes IA. Consensus statement on management of intersex disorders. International Consensus Conference on Intersex. *Pediatrics.* 2006;118:e488-500.

Lee P, Schober J, Nordenström A, et al. Review of recent outcome data of disorders of sex development (DSD): emphasis on surgical and sexual outcomes. *J Pediatr Urol.* 2012;8:611-5.

Lutfallah C, Wang W, Mason JI, et al. Newly proposed hormonal criteria via genotypic proof for type II 3beta-hydroxysteroid dehydrogenase deficiency. *J Clin Endocrinol Metab.* 2002;87:2611-22.

McCann-Crosby B, Chen MJ, Lyons SK, et al. Nonclassical congenital adrenal hyperplasia: targets of treatment and transition. *Pediatr Endocrinol Rev.* 2014;12:224-38.

Mermejo LM, Elias LL, Marui S, Moreira AC, Mendonca BB, de Castro M. Refining hormonal diagnosis of type II 3beta-hydroxysteroid dehydrogenase deficiency in patients with premature pubarche and hirsutism based on HSD3B2 genotyping. *J Clin Endocrinol Metab.* 2005;90:1287-93.

Mieszczak J, Houk CP, Lee PA. Assignment of the sex of rearing in the neonate with a disorder of sex development. *Curr Opin Pediatr.* 2009;21:541-7.

Miller WL, Auchus RJ. The molecular biology, biochemistry, and physiology of human steroidogenesis and its disorders. *Endocr Rev.* 2011;32:81-151.

Mouriquand PDE, Gorduza DB, Gay CL, et al. Surgery in disorders of sex development (DSD) with a gender issue: If (why), when, and how? *J Pediatr Urol.* 2016;12:139-49.

Nakae J, Tajima T, Sugawara T, et al. Analysis of the steroidogenic acute regulatory protein (StAR) gene in Japanese patients with congenital lipoid adrenal hyperplasia. *Hum Mol Genet.* 1997;6:571-6.

New M, Karavit L, Crawford C. Congenital adrenal hyperplasia. In: *Current Pediatric Therapy.* Philadelphia: WB Saunders; 1993;14:292-6.

New MI. Extensive clinical experience: nonclassical 21-hydroxylase deficiency. *J Clin Endocrinol Metab.* 2006;91: 4205-14.

Nimkarn S, New MI. Steroid 11beta- hydroxylase deficiency congenital adrenal hyperplasia. *Trends Endocrinol Metab.* 2008;19:96-9.

Olgemoller B, Roscher AA, Liebl B, Fingerhut R. Screening for congenital adrenal hyperplasia: adjustment of 17-hydroxyprogesterone cut-off values to both age and birth weight markedly improves the predictive value. *J Clin Endocrinol Metab.* 2003;88:5790-4.

Pang S. Newborn screening for congenital adrenal hyperplasia. *Pediatr Ann.* 2003;32:516-23.

Reisch N, Högler W, Parajes S, et al. A diagnosis not to be missed: nonclassic steroid 11beta-hydroxylase deficiency presenting with premature adrenarche and hirsutism. *J Clin Endocrinol Metab.* 2013;98:E1620-5.

Rosler A, Leiberman E, Cohen T. High frequency of congenital adrenal hyperplasia (classic 11 beta-hydroxylase deficiency) among Jews from Morocco. *Am J Med Genet.* 1992;42:827-34.

Sahakitrungruang T, Tee MK, Speise, PW, Miller WL. Novel P450c17 mutation H373D causing combined 17alpha-hydroxylase/17,20-lyase deficiency. *J Clin Endocrinol Metab.* 2009;94:3089-92.

Simard J, Ricketts ML, Gingras S, Soucy P, Feltus FA, Melner MH. Molecular biology of the 3beta-hydroxysteroid dehydrogenase/delta5-delta4 isomerase gene family. *Endocr Rev.* 2005;26:525-82.

Speiser PW, Azziz R, Baskin LS, et al. Congenital adrenal hyperplasia due to steroid 21-hydroxylase deficiency: an Endocrine Society clinical practice guideline. *J Clin Endocrinol Metab.* 2010;95: 4133-60.

Speiser PW, Dupont B, Rubinstein P, Piazza A, Kastelan A, New MI. High frequency of nonclassical steroid 21-hydroxylase deficiency. *Am J Hum Genet.* 1985;37:650-67.

Therrell BL. Newborn screening for congenital adrenal hyperplasia. *Endocrinol Metab Clin North Am.* 2001;30:15-30.

Therrell BL Jr, Berenbaum SA, Manter-Kapanke V, et al. Results of screening 1.9 million Texas newborns for 21-hydroxylase-deficient congenital adrenal hyperplasia. *Pediatrics.* 1998;101:583-90.

Warne GL. Long-term outcome of disorders of sex development. *Sex Dev Genet Mol Biol Evol Endocrinol Embryol Pathol Sex Determ Differ.* 2008;2:268-77.

White PC. Neonatal screening for congenital adrenal hyperplasia. *Nat Rev Endocrinol.* 2009;5:490-8.

White PC, Curnow KM, Pascoe L. Disorders of steroid 11 beta-hydroxylase isozymes. *Endocr Rev.* 1994;15:421-38.

Yanase T, Simpson ER, Waterman MR. 17 alpha-hydroxylase/17,20-lyase deficiency: from clinical investigation to molecular definition. *Endocr Rev.* 1991;12:91-108.

Yoo HW, Kim GH. Molecular and clinical characterization of Korean patients with congenital lipoid adrenal hyperplasia. *J Pediatr Endocrinol Metab.* 1998;11:707-11.

Zhu Y-S, Cordero JJ, Can S, et al. Mutations in CYP11B1 gene: phenotype-genotype correlations. *Am J Med Genet A.* 2003;122A:193-200.

Atypical Genitalia

Paraskevi Georgiadis, MD, FAAP • Johanna Viau Colindres, MD
• Yunru Shao, MMSc, LCGC • Marni Elyse Axelrad, PhD, ABPP
• Vernon R. Sutton, MD • Duong D. Tu, MD
• Sridevi Devaraj, PhD, DABCC, FAACC, FRSC, CCRP
• Lefkothea Karaviti, MD, PhD • Sheila K. Gunn, MD

SCOPE

DISEASE/CONDITION(S)

The neonate with atypical genitalia at birth.

GUIDELINE OBJECTIVE(S)

Define the terminology and language used to describe neonates with atypical genitalia, the causes and mechanisms of this condition, and the management of infants with atypical genitalia.

BRIEF BACKGROUND

The preferred term for neonates with atypical genitalia is "disorders of sex development" (DSD), defined as any congenital condition in which the development of chromosomal, gonadal, and/or anatomic sex is atypical. Terms such as "intersex," "sex reversal," "hermaphroditism," and "pseudo-hermaphroditism" should be avoided.

NORMAL SEXUAL DEVELOPMENT

Major Genes Involved in Sexual Development

Multiple genes are involved in normal gonadal development, the most important being the *SRY* gene. Others include the *SOX9* gene, the steroidogenic factor 1 gene *(SF1* or *NR5A1)*, the desert hedgehog gene *(DHH)*, the *DAX1 (NR0B1)* gene, the Wilms tumor gene, the *WT-1, WnT-4,* and *Wnt-7a* genes, the fibroblast factor receptor 2 gene, and the *ATRX* gene. Defects of any of these can lead to DSD.

Early Fetal Life

In early fetal development, both 46,XX and 46,XY fetuses have similar reproductive tissue. The Wolffian (mesonephric) and Müllerian (paramesonephric) ducts start developing in both sexes. The bipotential internal genital structures can further differentiate into male or female depending on gene expression. Around the fourth or fifth week of gestation, germ cells migrate from the yolk sac, and paired gonadal ridges develop from the urogenital ridge. The germs cells intermingle with pre-Sertoli and pre-granulosa cells. A summary of the process of sex development is depicted in Figure 50.1.

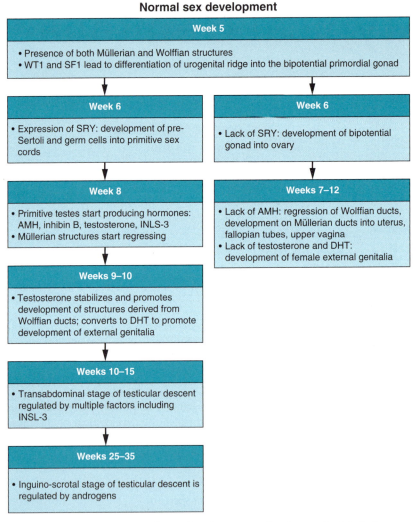

Normal sex development

Week 5
- Presence of both Müllerian and Wolffian structures
- WT1 and SF1 lead to differentiation of urogenital ridge into the bipotential primordial gonad

Week 6
- Expression of SRY: development of pre-Sertoli and germ cells into primitive sex cords

Week 6
- Lack of SRY: development of bipotential gonad into ovary

Week 8
- Primitive testes start producing hormones: AMH, inhibin B, testosterone, INLS-3
- Müllerian structures start regressing

Weeks 7–12
- Lack of AMH: regression of Wolffian ducts, development on Müllerian ducts into uterus, fallopian tubes, upper vagina
- Lack of testosterone and DHT: development of female external genitalia

Weeks 9–10
- Testosterone stabilizes and promotes development of structures derived from Wolffian ducts; converts to DHT to promote development of external genitalia

Weeks 10–15
- Transabdominal stage of testicular descent regulated by multiple factors including INSL-3

Weeks 25–35
- Inguino-scrotal stage of testicular descent is regulated by androgens

FIGURE 50.1 • The process of sex development. In the early fetal stage, both 46,XX and 46,XY fetuses have similar reproductive tissue with Wolffian (mesonephric) and Müllerian (paramesonephric) ducts. These bipotential internal genital structures further differentiate or regress into male or female depending on the gene expression and hormonal milieu.

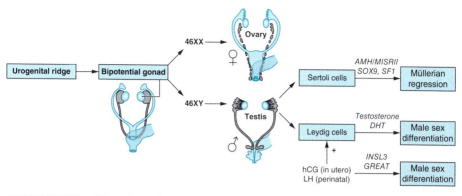

FIGURE 50.1 • (*Continued*)

Normal Female Development

In XX fetuses, in the absence of *SRY* expression, the bipotential gonad develops into an ovary. In the absence of anti-Müllerian hormone (AMH), the Wolffian ducts regress and the Müllerian structures develop into the upper vagina, uterus, and fallopian tubes. In the absence of testosterone, dihydrotestosterone (DHT), or normal androgen receptors, the genital tubercle becomes a clitoris, the urogenital folds become the labia minora, and the labioscrotal swelling develops to the labia majora. The separation of the vagina and the urethra is complete by 12 weeks of gestation.

Normal Male Development

In XY fetuses, around the 6th week of gestation, the pre-Sertoli cells and germ cells develop into primitive sex cords under the influence of the expression of the sex-determining region of the Y chromosome gene, *SRY*. At approximately 8 weeks of gestation, the primitive testes begin to produce hormones. The Sertoli cells produce AMH and inhibin B, and the Leydig cells produce insulin-like factor 3 (INSL3) and testosterone. AMH leads to the regression of the Müllerian (female) ducts. INLS3 is important for the testicular descent.

Testosterone production in the testis is initially stimulated by placental human chorionic gonadotropin (hCG) and subsequently by fetal pituitary luteinizing hormone (LH). Testosterone stabilizes the Wolffian duct and promotes the development of the epididymis, vas deferens, and seminiferous tubules. The enzyme 5α-reductase catalyzes the conversion of testosterone to DHT, a more potent androgen necessary for the virilization of the external genitalia. DHT induces the posterior fusion of the genital folds to form the urethra, the fusion of the labioscrotal folds to form the scrotum, and the growth of the genital tubercle into a phallic structure. The genitalia become sexually distinct at about 9 weeks of gestation. The external genital development is complete by 17 weeks of gestation.

DISORDERS OF SEXUAL DEVELOPMENT

A defect at any stage or level of sexual development may result in a DSD. Major DSDs occur in approximately 1 out of 4500 to 5500 children, and when all congenital abnormalities of the genitalia are considered, including cryptorchidism and hypospadias, the rate is as high as 1 in 200 to 300 children. There are three categories of DSDs (Table 50.1).

TABLE 50.1. Classification of Disorders of Sexual Differentiation

46,XX DSD	46,XY DSD	Sex Chromosome DSD
Disorders of ovarian development • Gonadal dysgenesis • Ovotesticular DSD • Testicular DSD **Androgen excess** • Fetal: 21OH deficiency, 3β-HSD deficiency, 11β hydroxylase deficiency • Fetoplacental: aromatase deficiency • Maternal: virilizing drugs and tumors **Other** • Syndromic associations: cloacal malformations • Müllerian agenesis and uterine abnormalities	**Disorders of testicular development** • Gonadal dysgenesis • Ovotesticular DSD • Testis regression **Disorders of androgen synthesis** • LH receptor mutations • Smith-Lemli-Opitz • Steroidogenic regulatory protein mutations • 3β-HSD deficiency, 17α-hydroxylase deficiency, 17β-HSD deficiency, 5α- reductase deficiency **Disorders of androgen action** • Androgen insensitivity syndrome **Other** • Congenital hypogonadotropic hypogonadism • Syndromic associations: cloacal malformation, Robinow, Aarskog, etc. • Persistent Müllerian duct syndrome • Vanishing testis syndrome • Isolated hypospadias • Cryptorchidism	• Turner syndrome (45,XO) and variants • Klinefelter syndrome (47,XXY) and variants • Mixed gonadal dysgenesis (45,X/46,XY) and variants • Sex chromosome mosaicism and chimerism (46,XX/46,XY)

46,XX Disorders of Sex Development

46,XX DSDs are subdivided into disorders of gonadal (ovarian) development and disorders associated with androgen excess.

Disorders of Ovarian Gonadal Development

1. **Ovotesticular disorders.** These are characterized by the presence of both testicular and ovarian tissue, which requires histological confirmation for diagnosis. Patients can present with ambiguous genitalia as well as a mixture of ovarian and testicular structures. Most cases are associated with a 46,XX karyotype.
2. **Testicular disorders.** These are characterized by the presence of testes alone in the absence of ovarian tissue or Müllerian structures in a 46,XX individual. Patients may present in the neonatal period with atypical appearing genitalia or later in life with infertility.

3. **Gonadal dysgenesis.** This DSD is characterized by abnormal ovarian development in a 46,XX individual. Most patients have a normal female phenotype and are diagnosed in adolescence due to a lack of secondary sexual characteristics.

Disorders of Androgen Excess

1. **Congenital adrenal hyperplasia.** This condition is described in Chapter 49.
2. **Aromatase deficiency.** In this rare disorder, the placenta cannot convert androgen precursors produced by the fetal adrenal glands to endogenous estrogen. Instead, dehydroepiandrosterone is converted to androstenedione and testosterone, leading to the virilization of both the mother and the female fetus.
3. **Maternal exposures and hyperandrogenemia.** Rarely, progestin or androgen ingestion or other causes of maternal hyperandrogenemia (e.g., maternal congenital adrenal hyperplasia (CAH), virilizing adrenocortical tumors, ovarian tumors, or luteomas) can cause the virilization of a 46,XX fetus.

46,XY Disorders of Sex Development

46,XY DSDs are subdivided into disorders of gonadal development and disorders of androgen synthesis and action.

Congenital Hypogonadotropic Hypogonadism. This is a group of conditions caused by deficient production, secretion, or action of gonadotropin-releasing hormone (GnRH) or the gonadotropins luteinizing hormone (LH) and follicle-stimulating hormone (FSH). In male infants, the initial testosterone production and genital development are regulated by maternal hCG. In the latter part of pregnancy, fetal gonadotropins are required for androgen production and subsequent testicular descent and penile growth. Therefore, male neonates with congenital hypogonadotropic hypogonadism may present with micropenis and cryptorchidism. There may be associated deficiencies of other pituitary hormones (which may lead to hypoglycemia and adrenal crisis), and clinical findings such as midline defects, anosmia, and features of different syndromes. When associated with anosmia, the condition is termed *Kallmann syndrome.*

Disorders of Testicular Gonadal Development

1. **Ovotesticular disorders (see above).** Approximately 10% of cases have a 46,XY karyotype. Patients often present with atypical genitalia, and many have a genetic defect involving the *SRY* gene.
2. **Complete 46,XY gonadal dysgenesis (Swyer syndrome).** In this condition there is absence of testicular development and the presence of female external genitalia, intact Müllerian ducts, and streak gonads. Most patients are diagnosed at adolescence.
3. **XY partial gonadal dysgenesis.** This is a heterogeneous group of disorders in which the degree of testicular development leads to varying degrees of virilization and various stages of Müllerian duct persistence. Hormonal evaluation typically reveals decreased levels of AMH and testosterone as well as a poor response to an hCG stimulation test.
4. **Gonadal regression (Vanishing testes syndrome).** In this DSD there is absence of testes, thought to be the result of perinatal thrombosis, testicular torsion, or endocrinopathy. The degree of virilization is related to the timing of testicular regression in utero.

Disorders of Androgen Synthesis and Action

1. **Persistent Müllerian duct syndrome.** This DSD, caused by a mutation in either the *AMH* gene or in the *AMH* receptor gene, leads to normal external male genitalia in

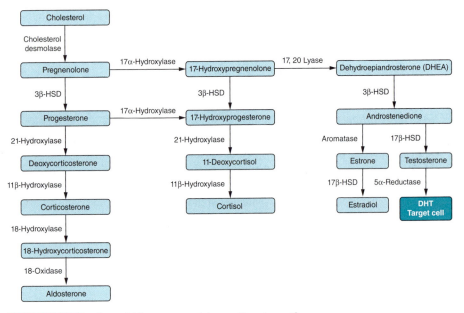

FIGURE 50.2 • Steroid hormones biosynthesis pathway.

the presence of Müllerian derivatives (e.g., the uterus and fallopian tubes) and variable testicular descent.

2. **Testosterone biosynthesis enzyme defect.** Testosterone is derived from cholesterol (Figure 50.2). A defect in any of the enzymatic steps required to synthesize cholesterol or testosterone can lead to the undervirilization of a 46,XY individual (Figure 50.3). Conditions in this category are:
   a. Smith-Lemli-Opitz syndrome
   b. Lipoid congenital adrenal hyperplasia
   c. P450 side-chain cleavage (P450scc) enzyme deficiency
   d. 3β-HSD type II deficiency
   e. 17α-Hydroxylase deficiency
   f. 17,20-Lyase deficiency
   g. Testicular 17β-hydroxysteroid dehydrogenase type 3 deficiency
3. **5α-Reductase deficiency.** 46,XY neonates present with varying degrees of genital ambiguity, but normal testes, normal internal (Wolffian) structures, and normal testosterone production. At puberty, virilization may occur, given increased testosterone levels. This condition is inherited in an autosomal recessive pattern. Biochemically, it is characterized by an elevated testosterone-to-DHT ratio.
4. **Leydig cell aplasia or hypoplasia.** Testosterone levels are low, the hCG stimulation test is nonresponsive (because it acts through LH receptors which are defective in this condition), and there are normal levels of testosterone precursors (from the adrenal glands).
5. **Androgen action defects and androgen insensitivity syndrome (AIS).** In this condition (with 70% of cases inherited in an X-linked recessive pattern) mutations in the androgen receptor gene lead to a lack of response to androgens. Patients with the complete form are phenotypic females with testes (bilateral inguinal or labial swellings) who typically present in the adolescent period with secondary amenorrhea. The partial form (PAIS) usually presents earlier, with ambiguous genitalia.

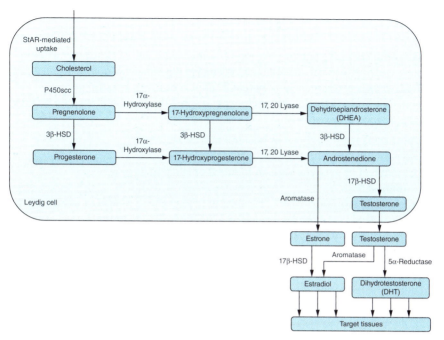

FIGURE 50.3 • Testicular androgen biosynthesis.

6. **Gestational endocrine disruptors.** In utero exposure to phenytoin, phenobarbital, or endocrine-disrupting chemicals (through environmental exposure) may result in hypospadias or atypical genitalia in male fetuses.

Sex Chromosome Disorders of Sex Development

Sex chromosome DSD is a heterogeneous group that includes abnormalities in a number of sex chromosomes as well as mosaicism, with two different cell lines. Infants with 45,X/46,XY mixed gonadal dysgenesis (MGD) and 46,XX/46,XY MGD often have genital ambiguity and are at higher risk of gonadoblastoma.

RECOMMENDATIONS

MAJOR RECOMMENDATIONS

The evaluation and management of neonates with atypical genitalia is challenging for both the clinician and the family. Best practices include having a multidisciplinary team composed of experts in neonatology, endocrinology, genetics, urology, gynecology, laboratory medicine, psychology, ethics, and social work. The neonatologist is a key member of this team and should prioritize efforts to

1. Recognize cases of atypical genitalia in a timely manner.
2. Rule out or treat medical emergencies that could be associated with atypical genitalia, such as CAH and hypopituitarism.
3. Coordinate all members of the team to provide optimal care, including psychosocial support, a thorough diagnostic workup, and sex assignment.

PRACTICE OPTIONS

Practice Option #1: Evaluation of Patients with Suspected DSDs

Neonates with atypical genitalia pose multiple challenges for the clinician, including ruling out or treating medical emergencies, a complex diagnostic workup, a broad differential diagnosis, sex assignment, and parental support during a stressful period.

Neonates who have the following clinical features should be evaluated for a DSD:

1. Micropenis
2. Hypospadias with unilateral or bilateral nonpalpable testes
3. Bilateral nonpalpable testes
4. Apparent female genitalia with an inguinal or labial mass
5. Clitoromegaly
6. Posterior labial fusion
7. Discrepancy between prenatal karyotype and postnatal phenotype
8. Elevated 17-hydroxyprogesterone in newborn screening

History. A thorough maternal and prenatal history should be elicited. Medications like progestins (used for amenorrhea and menstrual cycle regulation), finasteride (a 5α-reductase inhibitor used to treat alopecia), and phenytoin can interfere with normal fetal genital development. Severe IUGR can lead to hypospadias and undervirilization of a 46,XY fetus. Signs of maternal virilization could indicate excessive androgen production by androgen-secreting tumors in the adrenal gland or ovary. A detailed family history of consanguinity, genital ambiguity in siblings or the family, neonatal deaths, and infertility or amenorrhea can be of great diagnostic value.

Physical Examination

General. A complete newborn examination is essential to identify features that may be associated with certain syndromes or diseases that could lead to DSDs. Some important findings include:

1. Dysmorphic features suggesting genetic syndromes (e.g., Smith-Lemli-Opitz syndrome and Denys-Drash syndrome). Some syndromes associated with DSDs are described in Table 50.2.
2. Midline defects suggesting hypothalamic-pituitary causes for hypogonadism.
3. State of hydration and blood pressure abnormalities suggestive of CAH. Most patients with severe forms of CAH develop salt-wasting crises between the 4th and 15th day of life. Depending on the enzymatic defect, some patients with CAH may be hypertensive.
4. Hyperbilirubinemia may be secondary to concomitant thyroid or cortisol deficiency.

External Genitalia. The external genitalia exam should focus on the following:

1. **Genital tubercle (penis/clitoris).** The genital tubercle is the structure that develops into a penis in the male and a clitoris in the female. This structure should be measured on its dorsal surface from pubic ramus to the tip, and its width should be measured in the middle. A penile length <2.5 cm in a term male neonate is considered a micropenis. Different standards are available for premature neonates, or the formula PL = 2.27 + 0.16 GA, where PL is the penile length in centimeter and GA is gestational age in weeks, can be used for premature infants. A normal clitoris size in a term female neonate is less than 9 mm in length with a width varying between 2 mm and 6 mm. Standards for preterm infants are also available.

TABLE 50.2. Syndromes Associated with Disorders of Sexual Development

Syndrome	Pathophysiology	Description of DSD	Associated Features
Campomelic dysplasia	SOX9 gene sequence variant or structural rearrangement	Undervirilized 46,XY	Bowed lower extremities Skeletal malformations Large head
Smith-Lemli-Opitz syndrome	Deficiency of 7-dihydrocholesterol reductase resulting in decreased steroid hormone synthesis	Undervirilized 46,XY	Microcephaly Micrognathia Low-set and posterior rotated ears Cleft palate Syndactyly of 2nd and 3rd toes Developmental delay
X-linked adrenal hypoplasia, congenital	NR0B1 sequence variant leading to deficiency of DAX1 protein	Undervirilized 46,XY	Adrenal insufficiency
WAGR syndrome	Continuous gene deletion including WT1 and PAX6	Undervirilized 46,XY	Wilms tumor Aniridia Developmental delay
Denys-Drash syndrome and Fraser syndrome	Mutations in WT1	Undervirilized 46,XY	Wilms tumor Diffuse glomerulosclerosis
IMAGe syndrome	Mutations in CDKN1C gene	Undervirilized 46,XY	Adrenal hypoplasia Intrauterine growth restriction Metaphyseal dysplasia

2. **Urethral opening.** The penile urethra forms as a result of the fusion of the medial edges of the endodermal urethral folds. The specific mechanisms involved in this process are not well understood. However, exposure to testosterone seems to play a role in the fusion of the folds as well as the elongation of the urethra. Therefore, hypospadias is common in infants with early undervirilization. There are many classifications of hypospadias, especially since its characterization is often complicated by other penile abnormalities such as chordae. At a minimum, the anatomical location of the urethral opening should be documented (Figure 50.4).
3. **Genital folds (labia/scrotum) and anogenital ratio.** The genital folds develop into the scrotum and labia in males and females, respectively. The anogenital distance (distance between the center of the anus and the junction of the posterior convergence of the fourchette in females or the junction of the smooth perineal skin and rugated scrotal skin in males) is a sexually dysmorphic characteristic, being 2–2.5 times longer in males. It has been used as a marker of in utero exposure to androgens. The anogenital ratio, which is calculated by dividing the anogenital

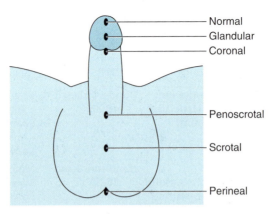

FIGURE 50.4 • Basic classification of hypospadias.

distance (AG) by the distance from the anus to the tip of the genital tubercle (AT; Figure 50.5), has a normal distribution and does not vary by gestational age or weight. In the normal female infant, this ratio is less than 0.3; a ratio of more than 0.5 exceeds the 95% confidence interval and reflects significant virilization. Finally, hyperpigmentation of the genital skin should be noticed, as it is associated with increased androgens and with increased ACTH secretion in the setting of a primary cortisol deficiency.

4. **Gonads.** Testicular descent occurs in two prenatal phases: transabdominal and inguinoscrotal. The transabdominal phase occurs between the 10th and the 15th week of gestation and is mediated by the INSL3, a growth factor produced by the Leydig cells. In this phase, the testicle remains close to the inguinal canal; by contrast, the ovary moves further away from the inguinal canal. During the inguinoscrotal phase (25–35 weeks of gestation) the intraperitoneal testes leave the abdomen. Based on models of AIS, this process seems to be androgen dependent. Therefore, cryptorchidism can be a sign of hypogonadism and/or abnormal Leydig cell function.

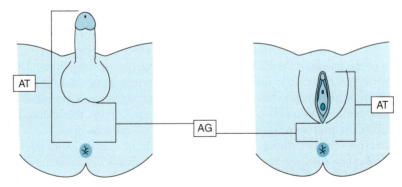

FIGURE 50.5 • Anogenital distance and anogenital ratio. The anogenital ratio is calculated by dividing the anogenital distance (AG) by the distance from the tip of the tubercle and the anus (AT). A ratio of more than 0.5 is associated with significant virilization.

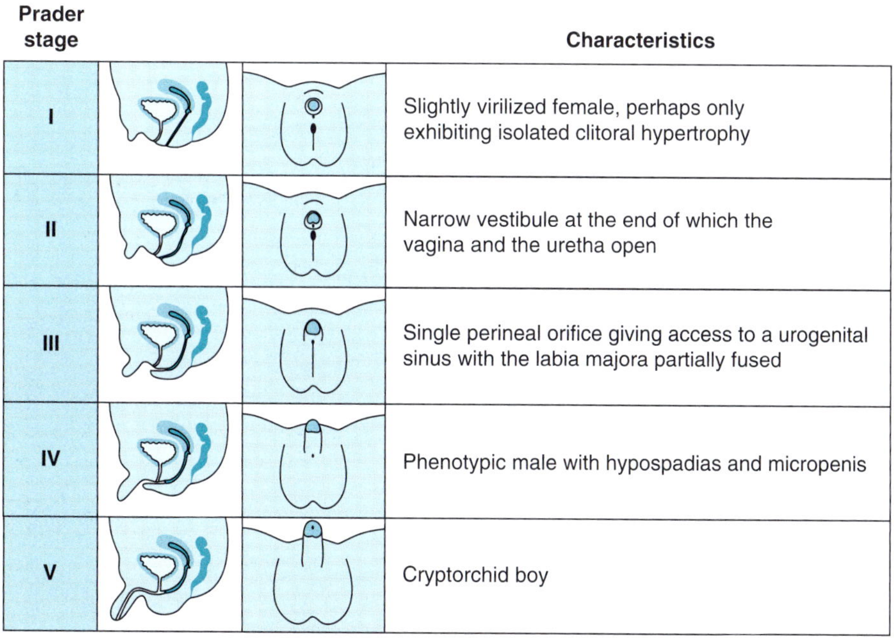

Prader stage			Characteristics
I			Slightly virilized female, perhaps only exhibiting isolated clitoral hypertrophy
II			Narrow vestibule at the end of which the vagina and the uretha open
III			Single perineal orifice giving access to a urogenital sinus with the labia majora partially fused
IV			Phenotypic male with hypospadias and micropenis
V			Cryptorchid boy

FIGURE 50.6 • Prader classification.

Conversely, gonads located in the inguinal canal of a phenotypical female usually contain a component of testicular tissue and therefore need to be evaluated.

5. **Virilization score.** Based on the above findings on a physical exam, neonates can be described using the standards by Prader (Figure 50.6). Virilization is a continuum, and Prader staging is limited in that it only describes the genital tubercle and urethral position.

Practice Option #2: Laboratory Evaluation

Evaluation of infants with a DSD should be individualized based on the physical examination findings. A suggested algorithm is provided in Figure 50.7. The potential studies are described below.

Genetic Analysis

1. **High-resolution chromosomal analysis (karyotype).** This test identifies aneuploidies (sex chromosome DSDs) and the presence or absence of a Y chromosome as well as large structural rearrangements. This test, in addition to assessment of the *SRY* gene by FISH (see below) is the first-line testing.

2. **FISH studies.** Specific probes are used for a targeted chromosomal region. X chromosome centromere and *SRY* gene FISH analyses are the most frequently used first-tiered testing.

3. **Single-gene analysis.** This method detects sequence variants and small deletions and duplications in a single gene of interest. It is useful once the differential diagnosis has been narrowed based on clinical presentation and hormonal analysis. Some of the genes that can be analyzed include *CYP21A2* (21-hydroxylase gene), *SRY, NR5A1, SRD5A3, DHH, AR, NR0B1,* and *AMH.* Gene panels that simultaneously analyze

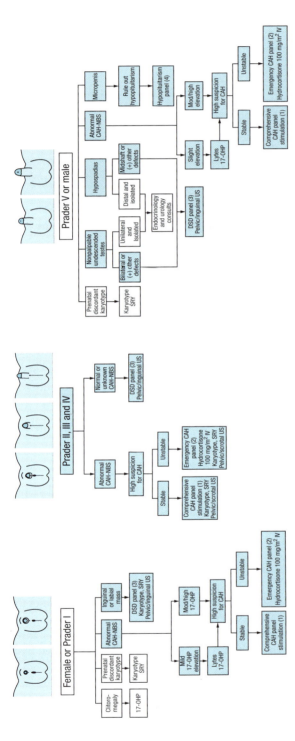

FIGURE 50.7 • Evaluation of neonates with suspected DSD. Evaluation of infants with a suspected DSD should be tailored based on the physical examination and reason for concern. For example, when CAH is suspected, the evaluation should focus on evaluating the adrenal biosynthetic pathway, keeping in mind that if the patient is unstable, steroids should be started immediately after baseline labs are obtained. (1) Comprehensive CAH panel/stimulation: includes baseline and 60 minutes post ACTH stimulation measurements of the following sex steroids: progesterone, pregnenolone, 17-OH pregnenolone, 17-OH progesterone, 11-deoxycortisol, aldosterone, plasma renin, DHEA, testosterone, androstenedione, and cortisol. Should identify the majority of patients with CAH, including the less common forms. (2) Emergency CAH panel: includes a baseline measurement of 17-OH progesterone, androstenedione, testosterone, cortisol, and plasma renin activity. Should identify the majority of patients with 21-hydroxylase deficiency. (3) DSD panel: includes a baseline measurement of 17-OH progesterone, gonadotropins, testosterone, and AMH, as well as karyotype and FISH SRY. (4) Hypopituitarism panel: includes baseline electrolytes, glucose, thyroid function studies (TSH, free T4), and gonadotropins as well as a low-dose ACTH stimulation test to evaluate for adrenal insufficiency.

multiple genes are now commercially available and have become widely adopted for a higher diagnostic yield.

4. **Chromosomal microarray analysis (CMA).** This methodology detects genome-wide microdeletions and microduplications of chromosome segments that include or interrupt genes associated with DSDs. CMA is an effective tool in determining the genetic causes of DSD. Apart from SRY region rearrangement, CMA was reported to have a detection rate of 25–28% for DSD cases with syndromic features and a variable rate of 5–21.5% for atypical genitalia in general.

5. **Whole-exome sequencing (WES).** The exons or coding regions of thousands of genes are analyzed simultaneously using next-generation sequencing techniques. Due to its cost as well as the complexity of its result, it should be reserved for difficult-to-diagnose patients, and counseling should be offered before and after the test by genetic specialists.

Hormonal Tests

1. **17-Hydroxyprogesterone (17-OHP).** Since CAH is the most common cause of DSD and missing the diagnosis is life-threatening (given adrenal insufficiency), all patients with DSDs need to have 17-OHP levels evaluated. In many cases, CAH is suspected by an elevated 17-OHP level in newborn screen. However, when the newborn screen is pending and there is a high suspicion for CAH, 17-OHP levels and electrolytes should be obtained promptly, as an emergency screen. An elevated 17-OHP is highly suggestive of CAH. However, this value may be unreliable in infants <36 hours old. A more comprehensive analysis involves the adrenal steroid synthesis pathway (including **dehydroepiandrosterone** [DHEA], **17-hydroxypregnenolone**, **11-deoxycortisol**, and **plasma renin activity**) should be obtained in patients with an elevated 17-OHP, patients with high suspicion for CAH, even in the absence of an elevated 17-OHP (higher blocks such as 3-beta-hydroxysteroid dehydrogenase [3β-HSD] or StAR protein deficiency have low or normal 17-OHP) or in patients in whom steroids are going to be started due to their clinical condition (Figure 50.7). A high-dose cosyntropin stimulation test (125 μg in infants less than 3 kg or 250 μg in infants more than 3 kg) with a comprehensive assessment of the steroid synthesis pathway at 0 and 60 minutes may be needed in cases where the baseline tests are nondiagnostic.

2. **LH and FSH.** Gonadotropins are useful to evaluate for hypogonadotropic hypogonadism as well as primary gonadal failure. In hypogonadotropic hypogonadism, LH and FSH are typically low, while in primary gonadal failure, these are elevated due to a lack of negative feedback. Reference values based on gestational age and day of life are available.

3. **Testosterone and AMH.** Testosterone and AMH are useful markers of Leydig and Sertoli masses as well as testosterone synthesis mechanisms, and may help narrow the differential diagnosis. Since testosterone levels start rising at 7 to 14 days of life, repeated measurements may be needed.

4. **Testosterone and DHT.** The relationship between testosterone and DHT after hCG stimulation is used to test the activity of the 5α-reductase enzyme.

Imaging

1. **Pelvic and labioscrotal ultrasound.** Pelvic and labioscrotal ultrasound is the first-line imaging study to evaluate anatomy including the presence of Müllerian structures (e.g., uterus, uterine remnants) and the location of gonads. Depending on the size

and the location, gonadal characteristics such as the presence of follicles or testicular-like structures can point toward the characterization of the gonads. Frequently, in small infants or prior to surgical interventions, other imaging modalities such as abdominal magnetic resonance imaging and urethrocystoscopy/vaginoscopy may be required. In some complicated cases, laparoscopic visualization with gonadal biopsy may be required.

Practice Option #3: Management of Patients with DSDs

Infants with DSDs should be managed by a multidisciplinary team of experts including neonatology, endocrinology, genetics, laboratory medicine, psychology, urology, gynecology, and ethics. The neonatologist should coordinate diagnostic and treatment efforts, and serve as the primary source of communication, support, and education for parents. Gender-specific terms (boy/girl, he/she, penis/clitoris, testes/ovaries, etc.) that may form or accentuate preconceptions should not be used before the diagnostic workup and sex assignment are completed.

Sex Assignment with Atypical Genitalia. Sex assignment should be performed only after the patient is completely evaluated by the multidisciplinary team and the diagnosis is confirmed. The two main factors influencing sex assignment are gender satisfaction and family preferences.

The most important long-term outcome for sex assignment in DSDs is gender satisfaction. Although most patients with DSDs are satisfied with their assigned gender, this population has higher rates of gender dysphoria than the general population. This reflects the fluid rather than dichotomous character of sex as well as our suboptimal understanding of the development of gender identity and the early interaction between the brain and androgens.

The DSD Consensus Group has suggested the following recommendations: female sex assignment for 46,XX with CAH, 46,XY with CAIS, and 46,XY with LH-receptor deficiency given that 90–100% of individuals with these traits develop a female gender identity; male sex assignment is recommended for individuals with 5α-reductase deficiency given that 60% of those individuals identify as male, and >50% of those with a 17-βHSD deficiency assigned females reassign to male later in life.

The ultimate decision about sex assignment should incorporate family preferences, including cultural and religious beliefs. Therefore, the family should be educated about the genetic, chromosomal, anatomic, functional, and reproductive aspects of sex, the major factors that are relevant to sex assignment, and long-term outcomes. Sex assignment is a social and legal procedure and does not imply intervention measures. Many families opt for hormonal and surgical interventions, although this is a separate process. Decisions about the timing and character of the irreversible interventions (e.g., surgeries, gonadectomy, and testosterone therapy, among others) include consideration of social norms as well as patient autonomy.

BIBLIOGRAPHIC SOURCE(S)

Baskin LS, Erol A, Jegatheesan P, Li Y, Liu W, Cunha GR. Urethral seam formation and hypospadias. *Cell Tissue Res.* 2001;305:379-87.

Bianco SD, Kaiser UB. The genetic and molecular basis of idiopathic hypogonadotropic hypogonadism. *Nat Rev Endocrinol.* 2009;5:569-76.

Boehm U, Bouloux PM, Dattani MT, et al. Expert consensus document: European Consensus Statement on congenital hypogonadotropic hypogonadism–pathogenesis, diagnosis and treatment. *Nat Rev Endocrinol.* 2015;11:547-64.

Brennan J, Capel B. One tissue, two fates: molecular genetic events that underlie testis versus ovary development. *Nat Rev Genet.* 2004;5:509-21.

Callegari C, Everett S, Ross M, Brasel JA. Anogenital ratio: measure of fetal virilization in premature and full-term newborn infants. *J Pediatr.* 1987;111:240-3.

Cohen-Kettenis PT. Psychosocial and psychosexual aspects of disorders of sex development. *Best Pract Res Clin Endocrinol Metab.* 2010;24:325-34.

Feldman KW, Smith DW. Fetal phallic growth and penile standards for newborn male infants. *J Pediatr.* 1975;86:395-8.

Ferlin A, Foresta C. Insulin-like factor 3: a novel circulating hormone of testicular origin in humans. *Ann N Y Acad Sci.* 2005;1041:497-505.

Fisher AD, Ristori J, Fanni E, Castellini G, Forti G, Maggi M. Gender identity, gender assignment and reassignment in individuals with disorders of sex development: a major of dilemma. *J Endocrinol Invest.* 2016;39(11):1207-24.

Furtado PS, Moraes F, Lago R, Barros LO, Toralles MB, Barroso U Jr. Gender dysphoria associated with disorders of sex development. *Nat Rev Urol.* 2012;9:620-7.

Gibbons RJ, Wada T, Fisher CA, et al. Mutations in the chromatin-associated protein ATRX. *Hum Mutat.* 2008;29:796-802.

Hutson JM, Li R, Southwell BR, Newgreen D, Cousinery M. Regulation of testicular descent. *Pediatr Surg Int.* 2015;31:317-25.

Jones ME, Boon WC, McInnes K, Maffei L, Carani C, Simpson ER. Recognizing rare disorders: aromatase deficiency. *Nat Clin Pract Endocrinol Metab.* 2007;3:414-21.

Josso N, De Grouchy J, Auvert J, et al. True hermaphroditism with Xx-Xy mosaicism, probably due to double fertilization of the ovum. *J Clin Endocrinol Metab.* 1965;25:114-26.

Kousta E, Papathanasiou A, Skordis N. Sex determination and disorders of sex development according to the revised nomenclature and classification in 46,XX individuals. *Hormones (Athens).* 2010;9:218-131.

Larson A, Nokoff NJ, Travers S. Disorders of sex development: clinically relevant genes involved in gonadal differentiation. *Discov Med.* 2012;14:301-9.

Lee PA, Nordenstrom A, Houk CP, et al. Global disorders of sex development update since 2006: perceptions, approach and care. *Horm Res Paediatr.* 2016;85:158-80.

Levitt SB, Reda EF. Hypospadias. *Pediatr Ann.* 1988;17:48-9, 53-4, 7.

Litwin A, Aitkin I, Merlob P. Clitoral length assessment in newborn infants of 30 to 41 weeks gestational age. *Eur J Obstet Gynecol Reprod Biol.* 1991;38:209-12.

McCann-Crosby B, Sutton VR. Disorders of sexual development. *Clin Perinatol.* 2015;42: 395-412, ix-x.

Mendonca BB, Costa EM, Belgorosky A, Rivarola MA, Domenice S. 46,XY DSD due to impaired androgen production. *Best Pract Res Clin Endocrinol Metab.* 2010;24:243-62.

Merriman LS, Arlen AM, Broecker BH, Smith EA, Kirsch AJ, Elmore JM. The GMS hypospadias score: assessment of inter-observer reliability and correlation with post-operative complications. *J Pediatr Urol.* 2013;9:707-12.

Nordenvall AS, Frisen L, Nordenstrom A, Lichtenstein P, Nordenskjold A. Population based nationwide study of hypospadias in Sweden, 1973 to 2009: incidence and risk factors. *J Urol.* 2014;191:783-9.

Oberfield SE, Mondok A, Shahrivar F, Klein JF, Levine LS. Clitoral size in full-term infants. *Am J Perinatol.* 1989;6:453-4.

Okeigwe I, Kuohung W. 5-Alpha reductase deficiency: a 40-year retrospective review. *Curr Opin Endocrinol Diabetes Obes.* 2014;21:483-7.

Ortenberg J, Oddoux C, Craver R, et al. SRY gene expression in the ovotestes of XX true hermaphrodites. *J Urol.* 2002;167:1828-31.

Phillip M, De Boer C, Pilpel D, Karplus M, Sofer S. Clitoral and penile sizes of full term newborns in two different ethnic groups. *J Pediatr Endocrinol Metab.* 1996;9:175-9.

Prader A. Genital findings in the female pseudo-hermaphroditism of the congenital adrenogenital syndrome; morphology, frequency, development and heredity of the different genital forms. *Helv Paediatr Acta.* 1954;9:231-48.

Salehi P, Koh CJ, Pitukcheewanont P, Trinh L, Daniels M, Geffner M. Persistent Mullerian duct syndrome: 8 new cases in Southern California and a review of the literature. *Pediatr Endocrinol Rev.* 2012;10:227-33.

Sathyanarayana S, Grady R, Redmon JB, et al. Anogenital distance and penile width measurements in The Infant Development and the Environment Study (TIDES): methods and predictors. *J Pediatr Urol.* 2015;11:76 e1-6.

Sax L. How common is intersex? A response to Anne Fausto-Sterling. *J Sex Res.* 2002;39:174-8.

Schaefer AA, Erbes J. Hypospadias. *Am J Surg.* 1950;80:183-91.

Thankamony A, Pasterski V, Ong KK, Acerini CL, Hughes IA. Anogenital distance as a marker of androgen exposure in humans. *Andrology.* 2016;4:616-25.

Tuladhar R, Davis PG, Batch J, Doyle LW. Establishment of a normal range of penile length in preterm infants. *J Paediatr Child Health.* 1998;34:471-3.

Unger S, Scherer G, Superti-Furga A. Campomelic dysplasia. In: Pagon RA, Adam MP, Ardinger HH, et al, eds. GeneReviews®. Seattle, WA; 1993.

Yu T, Wang J, Yu Y, et al. X-linked adrenal hypoplasia congenita and hypogonadotropic hypogonadism: identification and in vitro study of a novel small indel in the NR0B1 gene. *Mol Med Rep.* 2016;13:4039-45.

Yucel S, Cavalcanti AG, Desouza A, Wang Z, Baskin LS. The effect of oestrogen and testosterone on the urethral seam of the developing male mouse genital tubercle. *BJU Int.* 2003;92:1016-21.

Neurological Issues

Hypoxic Ischemic Encephalopathy

Hallie Morris, MD • Amit M. Mathur, MBBS, MD, MRCP(UK)

SCOPE

DISEASE/CONDITION(S)

Evaluation and initial treatment of encephalopathy in newborns following acute perinatal event.

GUIDELINE OBJECTIVE(S)

Review common mechanisms of injury; identify encephalopathy on physical examination; recommendations for initiation of hypothermia therapy; early management of the infant undergoing hypothermia.

BRIEF BACKGROUND

Hypoxic ischemic encephalopathy (HIE) will occur in 1–6/1000 births, or approximately 9000–12,000 newborns in the United States each year. Given the high rate of mortality and morbidity attributed to the condition, it is imperative for pediatricians to have a high index of suspicion and feel comfortable examining a newborn soon after birth, especially in the setting of an acute perinatal event, concerning history or abnormal cord blood gases. The Sarnat physical examination is a reliable scoring system to differentiate mild, moderate, and severe encephalopathy. For patients with moderate or severe encephalopathy, whole-body cooling is now the standard of care in neonatal intensive care units to decrease brain metabolism and help prevent secondary neuronal injury. Neonatal cooling has been found to decrease the composite primary outcome of death or major neurodevelopmental disability at 18 months from 63% to 48%, and was statistically significant for newborns with both moderate and severe HIE. These patients often require sedation and continuous EEG monitoring, and may require further cardiovascular and respiratory support depending on the extent of their illness. All cooled patients should have MRI imaging following cooling to help physicians and family anticipate long-term prognosis. Further research continues on the potential neuroprotective effects of erythropoietin, melatonin, and xenon as well as the free radical scavenging abilities of N-acetylcysteine and allopurinol to determine if any of these agents may further decrease long-term disease burden in this population.

RECOMMENDATIONS

MAJOR RECOMMENDATIONS

When evaluated and treated promptly, randomized trials show that neonatal cooling of infants with moderate or severe encephalopathy leads to improved morbidity and mortality in approximately 1/7 cooled infants. Although treatment will require care in a neonatal intensive care unit, initial evaluation and initiation of cooling can be considered in any facility with a physician comfortable in Sarnat examination scoring, and with minimal equipment investment.

PRACTICE OPTIONS

Practice Option #1: Evaluation of Whether a Patient is Demonstrating Moderate or Severe Encephalopathy

A neonatal encephalopathy assessment tool allows a physician to systematically determine the severity of a patient's encephalopathy, and should be printed or easily accessible in the electronic medical record for hourly scoring. The infant should be scored on level of consciousness (normal, hyperalert, lethargic, or coma), spontaneous activity (normal, decreased, or absent), muscle tone (normal, hypotonic, or flaccid), posture (normal, mild distal flexion, strong distal flexion, or decerebrate), primitive reflexes (suck and moro: normal, weak, or exaggerated, respectively, intermittently absent, or incomplete, absent), and autonomic function (pupils dilated, constricted or fixed and dilated, heart rate normal, tachycardic, bradycardic, or variable, and respirations normal, periodic breathing, or apnea). In infants who meet the perinatal criteria, the presence of three or more moderate or severe scores, or the occurrence of seizures, constitute criteria for initiation of therapeutic hypothermia. If the infant does not meet these criteria, they should continue to be scored hourly for 6 hours after birth to determine if their status is improving or worsening.

Practice Option #2: Determine Whether the Patient Meets Criteria for Cooling

At minimum, the infant should be >36 weeks' gestational age and <6 hours old, exhibiting moderate to severe encephalopathy on clinical examination, with any one of the following perinatal factors: 1) pH <7.0 or base deficit >16 mmol/L in either umbilical cord blood or blood obtained within 60 minutes of life; 2) chest compression, intubation, or mask ventilation ongoing at 10 minutes of life; or 3) APGAR score ≤5 at 10 minutes of life. Some institutions may widen those criteria to capture more infants with potential HIE who may benefit from cooling, such as by including infants >34 or 35 weeks' gestation, considering blood pH <7.1 or base deficit >12 as sufficient, or including seizures or concern for seizure activity as predictive of HIE regardless of encephalopathy.

Practice Option #3: Initiation of Therapeutic Hypothermia

Infants who satisfy eligibility criteria should begin passive cooling prior to transfer to the neonatal intensive care unit. Preferably before cooling, vascular access should be obtained, as cooling will induce vasoconstriction. Pediatricians should be in touch with accepting neonatal intensive care unit to discuss laboratory studies to send simultaneously. Once these are complete, passive cooling will require a rectal thermometer able to read low temperatures. Document temperature every 15 minutes, with target temperature of 33.5°C. The infant should be draped with a light blanket with the radiant warmer off; however, should infant's temperature drop below 33.5°C, the warmer should be turned on to the lowest servo-control setting. Once the infant is again >34°C, the team can turn the warmer back off. Be sure to maintain adequate sedation so that infant does not shiver; morphine is the drug of choice.

IMPLEMENTATION OF GUIDELINE

DESCRIPTION OF IMPLEMENTATION STRATEGY

1) Randomized trials and meta-analysis support the use of neonatal hypothermia as the standard of care in the setting of neonatal encephalopathy, and cooling should be initiated within 6 hours of birth. 2) For those who do not qualify for neonatal cooling, such as those less than 35 weeks' gestation or outside the 6-hour window, it is reasonable to monitor temperature closely to at least avoid hyperthermia, although the evidence is not as strong for this practice. 3) Patients undergoing cooling should be cared for in a neonatal intensive care unit setting; however, the implementation of passive cooling is reasonable following the use of Sarnat examination scoring and with the use of close rectal temperature monitoring.

Recommend written guidelines for Sarnat encephalopathy scoring at all delivering hospitals; pediatricians, pediatric hospitalists, and nurse practitioners should be comfortable at least discussing scoring with the neonatology team to determine if passive cooling should be initiated. Sarnat guidelines should have easy to fill-in-the-blank documentation that can be followed over a 6-hour time period. Score sheet can be accompanied by neonatal encephalopathy assessment tool definitions, describing the examination features to look for. Consider automatic alerts to the pediatrician on call whenever there is an umbilical cord pH <7.1 or base deficit >12. Delivering hospitals and transport teams should be equipped with rectal thermometers sensitive to low temperatures. Infants should be started on continuous video EEG monitoring as soon as possible. Fluid intake should be restricted to 60 mL/kg/d and titrated based on urine output and electrolytes. Close monitoring of coagulation studies, blood glucose, gases, and electrolytes is warranted. Maintaining a normal metabolic milieu is important during recovery. Total parenteral nutrition should be considered once laboratory parameters have normalized.

SUMMARY

HIE is a relatively common newborn complication and has the potential to lead to significant lifetime morbidity and mortality. Neonatal cooling is currently the only evidence-based treatment for this disease process and should be available to all newborns who qualify, even when treatment requires transfer to a neonatal intensive care unit. All delivering facilities and pediatric transport teams should educate themselves to evaluate a newborn for encephalopathy using a Sarnat scoring tool and equip their teams to potentially begin passive cooling after discussion with the accepting neonatal intensive care unit. Each NICU should develop a guideline to standardize neurological examination, EEG monitoring, timing and type of neuroimaging, and frequency of laboratory investigation in this population.

BIBLIOGRAPHIC SOURCE(S)

Higgins RD, Raju T, Edwards AD, et al. Hypothermia and other treatment options for neonatal encephalopathy: an executive summary of the Eunice Kennedy Shriver NICHD workshop. *J Pediatr*. 2011;159(5):851-8.e1.

Jacobs SE, Berg M, Hunt R, et al. Cooling for newborns with hypoxic ischaemic encephalopathy. *Cochrane Database Syst Rev*. 2013;CD003311.

Martin RJ, Fanaroff AA, Walsh MC. *Fanaroff and Martin's Neonatal-Perinatal Medicine: Diseases of the Fetus and Infant*. Philadelphia, PA: Elsevier/Saunders; 2015.

Shankaran S, Laptook AR, Ehrenkranz RA, et al. Whole-body hypothermia for neonates with hypoxic-ischemic encephalopathy. *N Engl J Med*. 2005;353:1574.

St. Louis Children's Hospital. SLCH Neonatal ICU Therapeutic Hypothermia Guidelines for Outborn Infants. 2016.

Tagin MA, Woolcott CG, Vincer MJ, et al. Hypothermia for neonatal hypoxic ischemic encephalopathy: an updated systematic review and meta-analysis. *Arch Pediatr Adolesc Med*. 2012;166:558.

Perinatal Stroke

Sudeepta K. Basu, MD • Gautham K. Suresh, MD, DM, MS, FAAP

SCOPE

DISEASE/CONDITION(S)

Arterial and venous stroke in neonates.

GUIDELINE OBJECTIVE(S)

Review frequency, types, impact, and causes of perinatal stroke. Describe the preferred methods to investigate and acutely treat patients with stroke.

BRIEF BACKGROUND

Perinatal stroke is a focal or multifocal ischemic or hemorrhagic infarction of the neonatal brain due to cerebrovascular injury during the immediate prenatal, intranatal, or postnatal period. It is defined as "a group of heterogeneous conditions with a focal disruption of cerebral flow secondary to an arterial or a venous thrombosis or embolization between the 20 week of fetal life through the 28 post-natal day, and confirmed by neuroimaging or neuropathological studies." Perinatal arterial ischemic stroke (PAIS), cerebral sinovenous thrombosis (CSVT), and other entities such as hemorrhagic infarct, periventricular hemorrhagic infarction (PVHI), and presumed perinatal stroke with considerable overlap are included under the umbrella term *perinatal stroke*.

Epidemiology and Pathogenesis

PAIS is reported in 1 in 2300–5000 live births and is caused by an embolus arising from the placenta or the heart passing through the patent foramen ovale (or rarely from a blood vessel or other causes). A large cerebral artery, most commonly the left middle cerebral artery, is occluded, leading to infarction of the region of arterial supply.

Sometimes small vessels are involved, and this leads to multifocal involvement in the regions of the thalamus or the basal ganglia.

CSVT is less common, affecting 1–2 in 100,000 deliveries and results from a thrombus partially or completely occluding a cranial venous sinus, a large deep vein, or a smaller cortical or deep vein. A CSVT commonly occurs in the superior sagittal system, the internal cerebral veins, and the straight sinus leading to hemorrhagic infarction secondary to impaired venous drainage. Neonatal CSVT might be associated with mechanical factors such as occipital bone compression of the superior sagittal sinus in the supine posture. A hemorrhagic stroke can result from bleeding into the brain as a result of rupture of an arteriovenous malformation, trauma, inherited or acquired coagulopathy (including that caused by maternal ingestion of phenobarbital, phenytoin, or warfarin), or thrombocytopenia.

Risk factors associated with perinatal stroke include maternal and placental disorders (e.g., chorioamnionitis, maternal pre-eclampsia, intrauterine growth restriction, emergency cesarean section), low Apgar scores at 1 and 5 minutes, need for resuscitation at birth, perinatal asphyxia, assisted ventilation at birth, cardiac disorders, coagulation disorders, polycythemia, infection, trauma, and drugs. The risk factors and clinical presentation can overlap with those of global hypoxic ischemic encephalopathy and can occur concurrently. Prothrombotic disorders involving protein C, protein S, antithrombin III, Factor V Leiden mutation, prothrombin mutation, phospholipid antibody, or a homocysteine defect are common (40–70%) and may be contributory among neonates with PAIS.

Clinical Presentation

A neonatal ischemic stroke most commonly presents as seizures or apneas, hypotonia, hemiparesis, and poor feeding during the first few days of life. A CSVT can have variable, subtle, and nonspecific manifestations such as increased intracranial pressure, subdural effusion/hematomas, hydrocephalus, and seizures. In some cases the perinatal stroke is undetected during the neonatal period and manifests in later infancy with delayed milestones, neurological deficit, seizures, or early handedness.

Prognosis

Long-term prognosis depends on the extent and location of infarction. Magnetic resonance imaging (MRI) plays an important role in predicting motor outcome. Concomitant involvement of cerebral hemisphere, basal ganglia, and posterior limb of internal capsule is highly predictive of contralateral spastic cerebral palsy. Most survivors have lifelong neurodevelopmental impairment, primarily hemiparetic cerebral palsy. Cognitive or behavioral disorders and epilepsy are also common.

RECOMMENDATIONS

MAJOR RECOMMENDATIONS

The possibility of a perinatal stroke should be considered in all neonates who present with acute neurologic manifestations and in those who have neurologic deficits, particularly asymmetric ones, following NICU discharge. The goals of acute management are to ensure clinical stability, identify and treat life-threatening conditions, prevent further brain injury, and identify the causal conditions so that specific treatment may be initiated.

PRACTICE OPTIONS

Practice Option #1: Neuroimaging and Laboratory Investigation

The diagnosis is confirmed by cranial imaging, with head ultrasound often being the first imaging modality, although it may be normal within the first few days of onset of symptoms. MRI is the gold standard. Within the first few days and up to the first week of PAIS, T2-weighted images (T2WI) show high signal intensity in affected cortex leading to loss of contrast between cortex and white matter, also known as the "missing-cortex sign." On T1-weighted images (T1WI), the signal intensity is lower in the cortex and white matter. By end of the first week, T2WI shows a lower signal intensity, whereas T1WI shows a high signal intensity known as "cortical highlighting."

Supplemental techniques such as diffusion-weighted imaging (DWI) and spectroscopy may provide additional information. DWI has high sensitivity in detecting ischemic lesions in the early acute phase, with high signal intensity on DWI or low signal intensity on the apparent diffusion coefficient (ADC) map within first 24–72 hours even before conventional T1WI or T2WI changes are detected. After the first week, diffusion changes appear to be normalized, known as "pseudonormalization." In selected cases, a magnetic resonance angiography and magnetic resonance venography may be done to delineate vessel patency and vascular anatomy. CT scans should be avoided because of the adverse effects of radiation exposure. Findings of a CSVT are often subtle and can be missed. An intraventricular hemorrhage in a term infant is often a marker of a deep system CSVT, especially if there is associated thalamic infarction or bleeding. In infants who cannot be transported out of the unit for MRI, bedside cranial ultrasonography, although limited, may help identify parenchymal hemorrhage and allow gross anatomic evaluation of the supratentorial structures.

Investigations for coagulation disorders are often performed in neonates with a stroke, but the role of such testing is debated because 1) it is difficult to reliably diagnose some of these conditions in the neonatal period, particularly in the aftermath of a stroke, and repeat testing in later infancy and testing of the parents and other family members is often required; 2) immediate management is usually not altered by identifying these conditions; and 3) a large volume of blood is required for testing.

Practice Option #2: Supportive Treatment

Treatment consists of supportive care that may include intubation and mechanical ventilation in infants with respiratory failure from encephalopathy, maintenance of blood gases within the normal range, maintenance of adequate blood pressure to ensure cerebral perfusion, maintenance of adequate levels of hemoglobin and coagulation factors (including antithrombin and protein C where they are deficient), platelets, electrolytes, and glucose. Seizures should be controlled with anticonvulsant medications and should be monitored with continuous electroencephalographic monitoring. Hyperthermia should be avoided, but the role of therapeutic hypothermia, erythropoietin, or stem cells is yet to be proven.

Practice Option #3: Management of the Thrombus

Anticoagulation is controversial; but heparin is sometimes used in PAIS with ongoing cardioembolic source and in CSVT to prevent extension and recurrence of thrombosis. Anticoagulation carries the risk of causing or extending intracranial hemorrhage. The American College of Chest Physicians recommends unfractionated heparin followed by low molecular weight heparin for 6–12 weeks in infants with CSVT without intracranial hemorrhage. In neonates with an MTHFR mutation, supplementation with folate and B vitamins is used to normalize homocysteine levels. Long-term anticoagulation may be required for patients with prothrombotic disorders. There is no evidence to support thrombolytic therapy, and it is generally not used. Contraindications for thrombolytic therapy are active bleeding and recent surgery.

Practice Option #4: Surgical Options

In general there is no role for thrombolysis, embolectomy, or surgical procedures to restore vessel patency. In selected patients with a stroke, there may be a role for surgical evacuation of a hematoma that is exerting pressure, or for ventricular drainage of hydrocephalus.

IMPLEMENTATION OF GUIDELINE

DESCRIPTION OF IMPLEMENTATION STRATEGY

Infants with suspected perinatal stroke should be managed in institutions where subspecialist consultation from neurology and advanced diagnostic imaging are available. If such resources are not available, the patient should be transferred to an institution with such resources. These infants should be managed collaboratively by the neonatology and neurology teams. If anticoagulation is initiated, specialists from hematology should be involved and should guide the use of heparin or coagulation factors. To ensure consistency of care, clinicians should follow a unit guideline that is developed on the basis of best available evidence and consensus among local experts, and that specifies the assessment, evaluation, and management of infants with perinatal stroke.

BIBLIOGRAPHIC SOURCE(S)

Benders MJ, Groenendaal F, Uiterwaal CS, et al. Maternal and infant characteristics associated with perinatal arterial stroke in the preterm infant. *Stroke.* 2007;38(6):1759-65.

Cole L, Dewey D, Letourneau N, et al. Clinical characteristics, risk factors, and outcomes associated with neonatal hemorrhagic stroke: a population-based case-control study. *JAMA Pediatr.* 2017;171(3):230-8.

Lee S, Mirsky DM, Beslow LA, et al. Pathways for neuroimaging of neonatal stroke. *Pediatr Neurol.* 2017;69:37-48.

Monagle P, Chan AKC, Goldenberg NA, et al. Antithrombotic therapy in neonates and children: antithrombotic therapy and prevention of thrombosis. 9th ed. American College of Chest Physicians Evidence-Based Clinical Practice Guidelines. *Chest.* 2012;141(2 Suppl):e737S-e801S.

Raju TN, Nelson KB, Ferriero D, Lynch JK, NICHD-NINDS Perinatal Stroke Workshop Participants. Ischemic perinatal stroke: summary of a workshop sponsored by the national institute of child health and human development and the national institute of neurological disorders and stroke. *Pediatrics.* 2007;120(3):609-16.

Ramenghi LA, Govaert P, Fumagalli M, Bassi L, Mosca F. Neonatal cerebral sinovenous thrombosis. *Semin Fetal Neonatal Med.* 2009;14(5):278-83.

Ricci D, Mercuri E, Barnett A, et al. Cognitive outcome at early school age in term-born children with perinatally acquired middle cerebral artery territory infarction. *Stroke.* 2008;39(2):403-10.

van der Aa NE, Benders MJ, Groenendaal F, de Vries LS. Neonatal stroke: a review of the current evidence on epidemiology, pathogenesis, diagnostics and therapeutic options. *Acta Paediatr.* 2014;103(4):356-64.

Neonatal Seizures

Stephanie Si-Tang Lee, MD • Amit M. Mathur, MBBS, MD, MRCP(UK)

SCOPE

DISEASE/CONDITION(S)

Neonatal seizures; neonatal epilepsy syndromes.

GUIDELINE OBJECTIVE(S)

Recommendations for diagnosis, treatment, and monitoring of seizures in neonates.

BRIEF BACKGROUND

Seizures in neonates are often multifactorial, ranging from acute brain injury from hypoxic-ischemic events to epilepsy syndromes from structural, metabolic, or genetic etiologies. While broad, diagnosis of seizures, whether clinical or subclinical, acute or refractory, can help direct management and improve morbidity or mortality for the neonate, keeping in mind that outcomes may still largely depend on the underlying disease process and degree of brain injury. While no national guidelines are established for acute treatment of neonatal seizures and institutional practices may differ, treatment options have been published in the literature as described below.

RECOMMENDATIONS

MAJOR RECOMMENDATIONS

The overall goal of management is to quickly identify and stop electrographic seizures, determine underlying etiology, and prevent secondary brain injury. The priorities for managing seizures are ensuring clinical stability, stopping the seizures, treating easily treatable conditions, and rapidly identifying life-threatening conditions and initiating immediate treatment for them. This should be followed by more detailed attempts to identify the cause of the seizures and underlying conditions. Neonatal seizures are difficult to identify clinically as they are often subclinical. Seizures should be identified and monitored using clinical assessment, bedside cardiorespiratory monitoring, and electroencephalographic monitoring, with close collaboration between neurology, neonatology, and other subspecialists as required. When seizures are refractory to treatment, clinicians often have to weigh the benefits of extinguishing every single seizure against the adverse effects of anticonvulsants. Choice of antiepileptic medications currently used for acute symptomatic seizure treatment is challenging because of a lack of evidence about them. Vitamin-responsive epilepsy should be considered early in those infants that are refractory to treatment.

PRACTICE OPTIONS

Practice Option #1: Seizure Monitoring and Detection

Clinical manifestations suggestive of seizures, such as eye deviations, generalized myoclonic jerks, clonic jerking of the extremities associated with autonomic features, etc., are only approximately 30–50% accurate for seizure detection. Neonates often have subclinical seizures in the setting of severe brain injury or receiving anti-epileptic medications. Thus management based on clinical diagnosis alone is not recommended. Neonates at high risk for or with clinical suspicion for seizures can undergo monitoring using the following methods either alone or together:

1. **Conventional video-EEG (cEEG)** is the gold standard for seizure detection. Electrode placement is based on the International 10–20 system modified for neonates. Electrographic seizures are defined as a sudden abnormal EEG event characterized by a repetitive evolving pattern with a minimum 2uV amplitude and duration of at least 10 seconds. Status epilepticus is defined as the summed duration of seizures to be ≥50% of an arbitrarily defined 1-hour epoch.

2. **Amplitude-integrated EEG (aEEG)** is a simplified bedside tool that utilizes heavily processed limited channel EEG signal recording for seizure detection. Seizures on aEEG present as an increase in both the minimum and maximum amplitudes with confirmation of electrographic seizure on raw EEG trace. Although it has a lower sensitivity and specificity than cEEG, its ease of use by the bedside clinician can allow for more rapid real-time recognition and management of seizures.

Duration of monitoring is dependent on the indication for EEG evaluation. Based on American Clinical Neurophysiology Society guidelines, EEG monitoring should be maintained until patient is seizure-free for at least 24 hours, after seizures were ruled out after three to four events were captured, or at the discretion of the neurology team.

Practice Option #2: Diagnosis of Etiology

1. **Acute symptomatic seizures:** Obtain the following:
   a. Blood glucose, electrolytes, calcium, magnesium, phosphorus, complete blood count, culture
   b. Urine culture
   c. CSF culture, glucose, protein, cell count, HSV PCR
   d. Head ultrasound/MRI.
2. **Chronic/refractory seizures:** Obtain the following:
   a. Blood lactate/pyruvate, amino acids, ammonia, creatine kinase, carnitine, acylcarnitine, biotinidase, uric acid, cholesterol, fatty acids, pipecolic acid, copper/ceruloplasmin

TABLE 53.1. **Etiology Based on Time of Onset**

Day 1	Day 2	Day 3	Day 4	Day 5	Day 6+
Structural, developmental brain abnormalities Congenital infections Pyridoxine dependent/pyridoxal phosphate responsive epilepsy					
HIE, sepsis, hypoglycemia, perinatal stroke, perinatal trauma, periventricular hemorrhage, neonatal abstinence syndrome					
	Hypoglycemia, hypocalcemia, benign familial neonatal convulsions				
		Aminoacidopathies, galactosemia, ketotic and nonketotic hyperglycinemia, folinic acid–responsive seizures, glucose transporter type 1 deficiency, Ohtahara syndrome, early myoclonic epilepsy			
			Benign neonatal seizures, migrate partial seizures of infancy		

   b. Urine organic acids, sulfites, uric acid, acylglycines, xanthine, hypoxanthine, pipecolic acid, guanidinoacetate

   c. CSF lactate/pyruvate, amino acids, neurotransmitter metabolites

   d. Congenital infection screen

   e. Head ultrasound/MRI if not already obtained

3. Etiology can be based on time of onset, as shown in Table 53.1.

Practice Option #3: Treatment

There is scant evidence to guide the choice of antiepileptic medications in neonates and the optimal treatment regimens. Controversy exists regarding who to treat, when to treat, which drug to use, and for how long to treat, yet the evidence for recurrent seizures to have a potentially adverse effect on immature brain development argues that treatment may be beneficial. Neurology consultation is recommended. If the decision is made to treat, Table 53.2 provides a list of frequently used anticonvulsant drugs to consider for acute treatment of seizures without underlying correctable metabolic abnormality.

For seizures that are refractory to acute treatment above, it is important to consider a therapeutic trial of vitamins in the event that the underlying etiology is a vitamin-responsive epilepsy due to inborn errors of metabolism. Vitamins to consider are listed in Table 53.3.

CLINICAL ALGORITHM(S)

Figure 53.1 is an example of a possible algorithm for treatment of neonatal seizures.

IMPLEMENTATION OF GUIDELINE

DESCRIPTION OF IMPLEMENTATION STRATEGY

Every unit should have written guidelines for seizure detection, evaluation, and management. These guidelines should specify the timing of diagnostic testing and imaging in relationship to treatment, the choice of the antiepileptic medications to be used for acute management of seizures, and the sequence of use of the various medications.

TABLE 53.2. Anticonvulsants for Acute Treatment of Seizures

Drug	Loading Dose	Maintenance Dose	Discontinue	Side Effects	Monitoring
Phenobarbital	20 mg/kg IV; can repeat if needed up to maximum total of 40 mg/kg	3–5 mg/kg/d IV or PO Target level 40–60 μg/mL	Irritability, altered sleep, tremors	Respiratory depression, depressed level of consciousness, hypotension, hypotonia, skin rash, hepatotoxicity, blood dyscrasia	Blood pressure, EEG
Phenytoin/ Fosphenytoin	15–20 mg/kg IV	3–5 mg/kg/d IV Target level 10–20 μg/mL	At removal of IV lines	Dysrhythmia, infusion site reaction, skin rash, hepatotoxicity, blood dyscrasia	EEG
Levetiracetam	20–40 mg/kg IV	20–60 mg/kg/d divided into 2–3 doses	Consult neurology	Mild sedation/drowsiness and irritability Limited data in neonates	EEG

Drug	Dose			Adverse effects	Monitoring
Midazolam	0.05–0.2 mg/kg IV followed by continuous infusion at 0.05–0.3 mg/kg/h	May adjust infusion by 0.05–0.1 mg/kg increments up to 1.0 mg/kg/h	If seizure free for 24 h	Temporary reduction of blood pressure and cerebral blood flow, respiratory depression, depressed level of consciousness	Blood pressure
Lidocaine (not to be used if treated with phenytoin/ fosphenytoin or with congenital heart disease)	2 mg/kg IV over 10 min	Continuous infusion at 6 mg/kg/h for 12–24 h	After 12–24 h of treatment: 4 mg/kg/h After 24–36 h: 2 mg/kg/h After 36–48 h: stop	Arrhythmia, seizures, hypotension	ECG, EEG, blood pressure
Lorazepam	0.05–0.1 mg/kg IV			Respiratory depression, depressed level of consciousness, hypotension	EEG
Clonazepam	0.15 mg/kg IV repeat once or twice	0.1 mg/kg/d	If seizure free for 24 h		

TABLE 53.3. **Treatment for Vitamin-Responsive Epilepsy**

Drug	Loading Dose	Maintenance Dose	Discontinue	Monitoring
Pyridoxine	50–200 mg IV followed by 100 mg every 10 minutes until a maximum of 500 mg or 30 mg/kg given	15–18 mg/kg/d in divided doses to a maximum of 500 mg daily	If no effect: stop	EEG
Pyridoxal phosphate	30–50 mg/kg/d PO divided in 3–4 doses or 3–5 days	30–50 mg/kg/d in divided in 4–6 doses	If no effect: stop	EEG
Folinic acid	3–5 mg/kg/d PO for 3–5 days	3–5 mg/kg/d PO	If no effect: stop	EEG
Biotin	5–10 mg IV or PO BID	5–10 mg IV or PO BID	If no effect: stop	EEG

They should also address initiation of maintenance medications and criteria for discontinuation to minimize long-term side effects from antiepileptic medications. Because the evidence for diagnosis and management of neonatal seizures is scant and of very low quality, these guidelines should be based on available literature and local consensus between neonatologists and neurologists in the institution. The response of the patient to each attempted intervention should be closely monitored and adjusted as required. Every institution should ensure that there are mechanisms to rapidly obtain a neurology consultation, electroencephalography, diagnostic imaging, and testing for genetic and metabolic disorders, as well as urgent neurosurgical intervention when required. In the absence of such resources, unless the seizures are brief and a benign reversible condition is found, the neonate should be transferred to a higher-level institution where such resources are available.

QUALITY METRICS

Monitor time to treatment of seizures after recognition, duration of seizures/seizure burden, time to diagnosis of etiology, length of treatment.

SUMMARY

Neonates are at a higher risk for seizures than other age groups, and those who do have seizures are at a higher risk for increased mortality, epilepsy, and other neurodevelopmental delays. Improved recognition and detection of seizures using cEEG and/or aEEG can help facilitate prompt treatment in the hope of decreasing seizure burden and improving long-term outcomes. While evidence is lacking for optimal strategies for seizure management with antiepileptic medications, establishing institutional treatment guidelines can improve outcomes by preventing unnecessary delays in treatment.

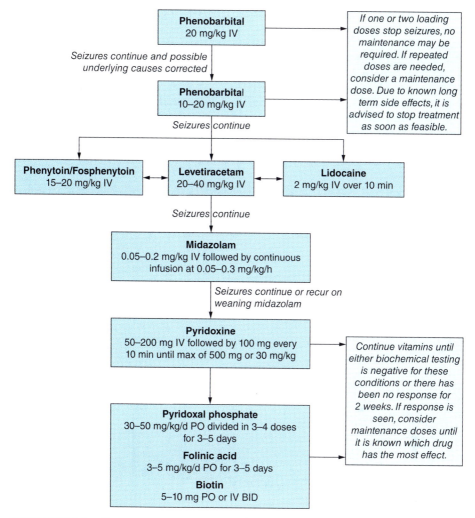

FIGURE 53.1 • Suggested algorithm for treatment of neonatal seizures.

BIBLIOGRAPHIC SOURCE(S)

Booth D, Evans DJ. Anticonvulsants for neonates with seizures. *Cochrane Database Syst Rev.* 2004;(4):Cd004218.

Glass HC. Neonatal seizures: advances in mechanisms and management. *Clin Perinatol.* 2014;41(1):177-90.

Glass HC, Kan J, Bonifacio SL, Ferriero DM. Neonatal seizures: treatment practices among term and preterm infants. *Pediatr Neurol.* 2012;46(2):111-5.

Gospe SM Jr. Neonatal vitamin-responsive epileptic encephalopathies. *Chang Gung Med J.* 2010;33(1):1-12.

Hart AR, Pilling EL, Alix JJ. Neonatal seizures. Part 2: Aetiology of acute symptomatic seizures, treatments and the neonatal epilepsy syndromes. *Arch Dis Child Educ Pract Ed.* 2015;100(5):226-32.

Hellstrom-Westas L, Boylan G, Agren J. Systematic review of neonatal seizure management strategies provides guidance on anti-epileptic treatment. *Acta Paediatr.* 2015;104(2):123-9.

Hellström-Westas L, Rosén I, de Vries LS, Greisen G. Amplitude-integrated EEG classification and interpretation in preterm and term infants. *NeoReviews*. 2006;7(2):e76-e87.

Holmes GL, The long-term effects of neonatal seizures. *Clin Perinatol*. 2009;36(4):901-14, vii-viii.

Murray DM, Boylan GB, Ali I, Ryan CA, Murphy BP, Connolly S. Defining the gap between electrographic seizure burden, clinical expression and staff recognition of neonatal seizures. *Arch Dis Child Fetal Neonatal Ed*. 2008;93(3):F187-91.

Shah DK, Mackay MT, Lavery S, et al. Accuracy of bedside electroencephalographic monitoring in comparison with simultaneous continuous conventional electroencephalography for seizure detection in term infants. *Pediatrics*. 2008;121(6):1146-54.

Shellhaas RA, Chang T, Tsuchida T, et al. The American Clinical Neurophysiology Society's Guideline on Continuous Electroencephalography Monitoring in Neonates. *J Clin Neurophysiol*. 2011;28(6):611-7.

Scher MS. Seizures in neonates. In: Martin RJ, Walsh MC, eds. *Fanaroff and Martin's Neonatal-Perinatal Medicine*. A.A.F. Philadelphia, PA: Elsevier Saunders; 2015:927-49.

Scher MS, Alvin J, Gaus L, Minnigh B, Painter MJ. Uncoupling of EEG-clinical neonatal seizures after antiepileptic drug use. *Pediatr Neurol*. 2003;28(4):277-80.

The Hypotonic Infant

Monica Hsiung Wojcik, MD • Sarah U. Morton, MD, PhD
• Pankaj B. Agrawal, MD, MMSc

SCOPE

DISEASE/CONDITION(S)

Neonatal hypotonia.

GUIDELINE OBJECTIVE(S)

Review possible etiologies of neonatal hypotonia, an approach to the diagnostic evaluation, and options for clinical management.

BRIEF BACKGROUND

Neonatal hypotonia can result from a variety of underlying disease conditions. In contrast to weakness, which is a reduction in maximum voluntary power of the muscles, hypotonia is defined by decreased resistance to passive range of motion or loss of postural control against gravity. Here we consider conditions characterized by hypotonia, which may or may not be accompanied by weakness.

Conditions Causing Hypotonia

Hypotonia in infants may result from central or peripheral causes (Figure 54.1). Central nervous system disorders represent the underlying etiology for primary hypotonia in 60–80% cases, whereas neuromuscular disorders (involving either peripheral nerve, neuromuscular junction, or muscle) are present in 15–30% (Figure 54.1).

Central Nervous System Disorders. These conditions affect the structure or function of the brain or spinal cord. They are often associated with axial hypotonia, normal or exaggerated deep tendon reflexes (DTRs), and relative preservation of strength with or without altered consciousness, seizures, feeding difficulties, abnormal

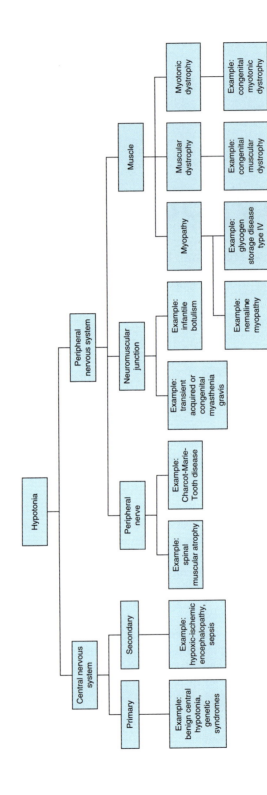

FIGURE 54.1 • Causes of hypotonia.

brainstem reflexes, and abnormal extraocular movements. Included in this category would be encephalopathy, such as hypoxic-ischemic encephalopathy or acute infectious encephalopathy, intracranial hemorrhage, cerebral malformations (such as schizencephaly, lissencephaly, or holoprosencephaly), trauma, and malformations including the spinal cord, such as a Chiari malformation or syringomyelia. Systemic conditions causing secondary hypotonia, such as sepsis or certain inborn errors of metabolism, often present with central hypotonia. Also in this category are infants with delayed myelination of the brain seen on MRI, and those with no abnormalities found on imaging or other evaluation (benign congenital hypotonia). These infants often normalize over time and may become indistinguishable from their peers, particularly if only gross motor delays are present.

Neuromuscular Disorders

Peripheral Nerve Disorders. These are characterized by normal alertness, absent DTRs, and profound weakness. This includes anterior horn cell disease such as spinal muscular atrophy (SMA), caused by a loss of motor neurons in the spinal cord and characterized by proximal weakness, absent DTRs, facial sparing, paradoxical breathing, and tongue fasciculation. Peripheral neuropathies, characterized by predominantly distal symptoms, absent DTRs, and pes cavus, such as congenital motor sensory neuropathy (Charcot-Marie-Tooth disease) and hereditary sensory and autonomic neuropathy, would also be included in this category.

Neuromuscular Junction Disorders. These may present with preserved DTRs and include transient acquired neonatal myasthenia (placental transfer of maternal antibodies against acetylcholine receptor), congenital myasthenia gravis (notable for including bulbar weakness, can be rapidly progressive), magnesium or aminoglycoside toxicity, or infantile botulism.

Muscle Disorders. These are characterized by the presence of both hypotonia and weakness. Specific conditions in this category include congenital myopathies (such as nemaline, central core, multiminicore, centronuclear, and congenital fiber type disproportion), congenital muscular dystrophy, and congenital myotonic dystrophy, in addition to inborn errors of metabolism primarily affecting muscle, such as certain glycogen storage diseases.

RECOMMENDATIONS

MAJOR RECOMMENDATIONS

Immediate concerns when faced with a hypotonic infant involve stabilization and treatment of possible life-threatening conditions, after which a workup to determine the precise etiology can proceed. Once the infant is medically stable, the diagnostic evaluation may proceed, targeted to the salient features of the presenting case. After an underlying explanation is discovered, specific treatments may be available. In the event that no disease-targeted therapies exist, palliative care is often considered for infants with a poor long-term prognosis. Pediatric subspecialists in neurology or medical genetics may often be of assistance in the evaluation and management of these infants.

PRACTICE OPTIONS

The items to pursue in the evaluation of a hypotonic infant are listed sequentially next.

Practice Option #1: Immediate Stabilization

Prior to embarking upon a diagnostic investigation, it is important to ensure medical stability in the hypotonic infant. Respiratory status is an immediate concern, and evaluation for the possible need for intubation and mechanical ventilation, or the provision of continuous positive airway pressure (CPAP) can be aided by arterial, venous, or capillary blood gas measurement. As some conditions resulting in hypotonia can also manifest with cardiac disease, assessment for signs of cardiac dysfunction or failure, including physical examination, chest x-ray, and laboratory values such as an arterial blood gas and lactate is also important. Even an infant with a stable cardiorespiratory status may decompensate upon oral feeding, as hypotonia is often accompanied by a poor sucking and swallowing ability, so prohibiting attempts at oral feeding and providing intravenous dextrose and hydration may be warranted.

Practice Option #2: History and Physical Examination

For the initial evaluation of all hypotonic infants, a careful history and physical examination must be performed, including the maternal and obstetric history. This may uncover important features directing further diagnostic evaluation.

The history should include the obstetric history and family history, tailored to the presenting features of the case. Infants with hypotonia can present with reduced fetal movements in utero, and this is an important item to determine from the obstetric history. A history regarding prenatal screening is important to obtain, as many women are now screened for carrier status for SMA, or have cell-free DNA testing to evaluate for risk of aneuploidy—both conditions that can present with infantile hypotonia. The birth history may also contribute, though poor Apgar scores at birth may be reflective of either a perinatal event causing hypoxic-ischemic encephalopathy and secondary hypotonia, or of an underlying neurologic disorder. For infants who present later in the neonatal period or infancy, careful questioning for possible toxic exposures is necessary.

On physical examination, it is important to recognize that many factors can influence tone, including gestational age, infant state (level of alertness), and ligamentous laxity, in addition to medications. These must be considered when determining whether or not an infant is truly hypotonic. Many hypotonic infants exhibit a particular resting position, with the legs abducted and externally rotated and the arms extended. Common maneuvers to assess tone in infants include pulling the infant to a seated position from supine to assess for head lag (which should be nearly absent by 2 months of age), holding an infant upright with the examiner's hands beneath the shoulders to assess if the infant slips through the examiner's hands, or holding the infant in ventral suspension (prone, over the examiner's hand) to assess for the ability to lift the head. As previously mentioned, hypotonia and weakness may or may not be present concurrently. Assessment of DTRs is helpful in distinguishing central from non-central etiologies of hypotonia, and assessment of muscle bulk may point toward a neuromuscular disorder.

Aside from the neurologic examination, the remainder of the physical examination can point to systemic conditions causing secondary hypotonia. Dysmorphic features may suggest a genetic etiology, such as Prader-Willi syndrome or trisomy 21, and the presence of hepatosplenomegaly or petechiae may suggest a systemic infection such as a TORCH (toxoplasmosis, rubella, cytomegalovirus, or herpesvirus) infection.

Practice Option #3: Diagnostic Evaluation

Once the examiner has determined whether the hypotonia is most likely central or peripheral, a targeted diagnostic evaluation can be undertaken (see Clinical Algorithm later).

First, an evaluation for systemic conditions leading to secondary hypotonia should be undertaken, particularly for cases of central hypotonia. This may include a blood gas with lactate, electrolyte panel, thyroid function tests, and a sepsis evaluation including blood count, blood culture, and urine and cerebrospinal fluid studies. Umbilical cord blood gases may help to diagnose cases of hypoxic-ischemic encephalopathy, in combination with the history, physical examination, and amplitude-integrated EEG (aEEG). If hypotonia is accompanied by other multisystem manifestations, particularly after an initial period of stability and normal tone in a newborn, certain inborn errors of metabolism should be considered, such as Pompe disease or a glycogen storage disease. Many of these conditions can be detected by a newborn state screen, or can be found by a basic evaluation for inborn errors of metabolism consisting of ammonia, total and free carnitine, plasma amino acids, blood acylcarnitine profile, urine organic acids, and urine acylglycines. Very long chain fatty acids and blood plasmalogens can also be sent to evaluate for peroxisomal disorders, which often present with characteristic facial features or brain or other organ system abnormalities. Congenital disorders of glycosylation can be found by serum transferrin isoelectric focusing or by measurement of N- and O-linked glycans; genetic testing is also available for many of these conditions. With the exception of these rare inborn errors of metabolism, systemic diseases such as sepsis and perinatal depression represent the majority of conditions leading to central hypotonia and are important to exclude prior to pursuing further diagnostic evaluations for primary neurologic conditions.

If systemic conditions are thought to be less likely, brain imaging with magnetic resonance imaging (potentially accompanied by magnetic resonance spectroscopy) can identify brain malformations causing central hypotonia. Electroencephalography (EEG) can also be considered to evaluate for epileptic encephalopathy, which can cause hypotonia in addition to altered mental status. In addition, genetic or metabolic conditions are responsible for over 50% of infantile hypotonia cases. Infants with dysmorphic features should have a comprehensive genetic evaluation, ideally involving a medical geneticist, including karyotype (to detect aneuploidies such as trisomy 21, 18, or 13), chromosomal microarray (to detect microdeletion and microduplication disorders such as 22q11 deletion syndrome or cri-du-chat syndrome), and possible targeted testing for specific conditions depending on the presenting features of the infant. Smith-Lemli-Opitz syndrome can present with hypotonia and dysmorphic features, including midline defects such as cleft palate, abnormal genitalia, and 2-3 syndactyly of the toes. Testing for this condition consists of a 7-dehydrocholesterol level and sequencing of the gene *DHCR* to look for biallelic pathogenic variants. Prader-Willi syndrome presents with hypotonia in the newborn period (this disorder has been seen in up to 10% of infants who present with hypotonia) and poor feeding (hyperphagia does not appear until school age) and is best diagnosed by methylation analysis to evaluate for abnormal imprinting leading to this condition. It can on occasion be detected by chromosomal microarray, as a microdeletion of the paternal allele on chromosome 15 can be responsible. Depending on the microarray technology, maternal uniparental disomy (inheriting both copies of the chromosomal region from the mother) can also be detected. Finally, many additional

Mendelian syndromic disorders can also present with infantile hypotonia, often accompanied by congenital anomalies or characteristic dysmorphic features. These may be exceedingly difficult to diagnose clinically in the newborn period, and often require gene sequencing panels to examine multiple genes at once, or exome sequencing, consisting of sequencing all the coding regions of the genome.

For cases of suspected peripheral nervous system disease (neuromuscular disorders), there may be particular presenting features suggesting a specific diagnosis that warrant genetic testing as a first-line test, bypassing the typical tiered evaluation. For example, a family history of Charcot-Marie-Tooth disease or myotonic dystrophy or of known parental carrier status for SMA may direct toward a molecular genetic test to evaluate for that particular condition. Otherwise, the initial evaluation typically consists of measuring serum creatine kinase (highly elevated in the dystrophinopathies or other myopathies) in addition to obtaining nerve conduction studies and electromyography. Muscle biopsy is being performed less frequently in favor of molecular genetic techniques, but can be helpful in identifying classic features of certain muscle disorders.

As mentioned earlier, the hallmark disorder of the anterior horn cell is SMA, caused by biallelic pathogenic variants in the *SMN* gene—typically a deletion of exon 7, detectable by deletion/duplication analysis. Currently, direct testing of this gene is the typical diagnostic approach before performing other invasive tests such as muscle biopsy. Peripheral nerve disease is rare in the infant period, but conditions such as Charcot-Marie-Tooth disease can present in this age group and are detectable by genetic testing. Nerve conduction studies can suggest a diagnosis in this category, although the particular disorder may require a more specific test, such as gene sequencing.

Disorders of the neuromuscular junction, including congenital myasthenic syndromes, can be diagnosed by genetic testing. A diagnosis of transient acquired neonatal myasthenia gravis (transmission of maternal antibodies) is typically made based on a known maternal history of myasthenia gravis; another potential sign in the maternal history would be difficult labor due to fatigue. Serum antibodies to the acetylcholine receptor (anti-AChR, anti-MuSK) can also be measured, and repetitive nerve stimulation studies can also be performed. Congenital myasthenia gravis, which can be rapidly progressive and involve the bulbar muscles, can be suspected by IV pyridostigmine administration, with affected infants improving after this medication is given, and repetitive nerve stimulation studies, with the exact etiology found by genetic testing. Infantile botulism is another important disorder of the neuromuscular junction to recognize, typically by presentation of acquired, progressive paralysis and a history of ingestion to a substance that may contain *Clostridium botulinum* spores, such as honey.

Muscle disorders were historically diagnosed by muscle biopsy and are therefore named by the histopathologic features—for example, central core disease, nemaline myopathy, multiminicore, congenital fiber type disproportion, and myotubular myopathy. As noted earlier, these conditions are now more typically diagnosed by genetic testing. Congenital muscular dystrophies are also marked by abnormal muscle biopsy and can also have involvement of other tissues such as the brain. Congenital myotonic dystrophies are often maternally inherited, and a feature suggestive of this disorder in adults is grip myotonia, where a slow release after a tight hand grip is seen. Clinical suspicion for congenital myotonic dystrophy is important to direct genetic testing for this disorder, as it typically involves a triplet repeat expansion that may not be easily detected by standard sequencing techniques.

TABLE 54.1. Treatments Available for Selected Specific Causes of Infant Hypotonia

Category of Disease	Condition	Treatment
Inborn errors of metabolism	Pompe disease	Enzyme replacement
Neuromuscular disorder	Spinal muscular atrophy Congenital myasthenic syndrome Infantile botulism	Intrathecal nusinersen Intravenous pyridostigmine Intravenous human botulism immune globulin

Practice Option #4: Selected Treatments

In addition to the treatment of underlying conditions that can lead to secondary neonatal- or infantile-onset hypotonia, such as the treatment of systemic bacterial infections with antibiotics, specific treatment options are available for a limited number of rare diseases (Table 54.1). These include enzyme replacement treatments for certain metabolic disorders such as Pompe disease, and newer therapies such as nusinersen for SMA. As many disorders causing both central or peripheral hypotonia have an underlying genetic component, it is possible that additional, gene-directed therapies will be developed in the next several years. For disorders for which there is no treatment, supportive therapies such as home ventilation services and home enteral feeding supplies may be indicated, and some families may choose to provide palliative or hospice care only after the diagnosis of a severe congenital disorder presenting with neonatal hypotonia. Early diagnosis is therefore important where possible for these infants, to allow families to consider the full range of management options.

CLINICAL ALGORITHM(S)

General steps in evaluation after initial stabilization are summarized in Figure 54.2.

IMPLEMENTATION OF GUIDELINE

DESCRIPTION OF IMPLEMENTATION STRATEGY

All providers caring for newborns should receive training and education in the medical assessment and stabilization of hypotonic infants and should have a basic understanding of the possible categories of disease. Specific diagnostic investigations, however, may be best conducted under the guidance of specialists in neurology or medical genetics to best assist in the choice of test and interpretation of results. Once a diagnosis is made, a multidisciplinary care team is often required to provide medical treatment and/or support to the infant and family.

SUMMARY

A diverse array of conditions, some congenital and some acquired, can present in the infant period with hypotonia. Providers caring for the hypotonic infant should first ensure clinical stability and then pursue a targeted diagnostic evaluation. Central

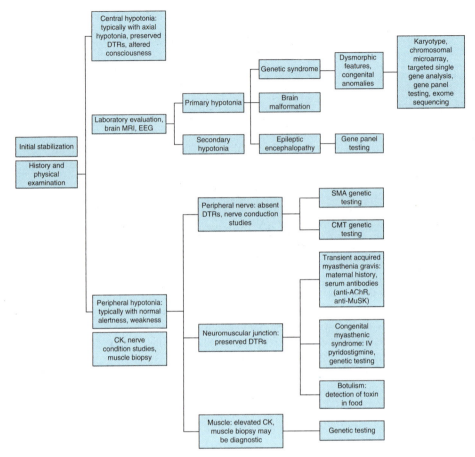

FIGURE 54.2 • Approach to the evaluation of the hypotonic infant. CMT, Charcot-Marie-Tooth disease; SMA, spinal muscular atrophy.

hypotonia should be distinguished from peripheral causes; if the hypotonia is determined to be central, an evaluation for systemic conditions should be undertaken. If peripheral, a variety of neuromuscular diseases should be considered, many of which have underlying genetic etiologies. Treatment of hypotonia in infancy, aside from initial medical stabilization, is highly dependent upon the underlying etiology. In some cases, no treatment or cure is presently available and palliative care is often pursued.

BIBLIOGRAPHIC SOURCE(S)

Bertini E, D'Amico A, Gualandi F, Petrini S. Congenital muscular dystrophies: a brief review. *Semin Pediatr Neurol*. 2011;18(4):277-88.

Birdi K, Prasad AN, Prasad C, Chodirker B, Chudley E. The floppy infant: retrospective analysis of clinical experience (1990–2000) in a tertiary care facility. *J Child Neurol*. 2005;20(10):803-8.

Bodensteiner JB. The evaluation of the hypotonic infant. *Semin Pediatr Neurol*. 2008;15(1):10-20.

Bönnemann CG, Wang CH, Quijano-Roy S, et al. Diagnostic approach to the congenital muscular dystrophies. *Neuromuscul Disord*. 2014;24(4):289-311.

Das AS, Agamanolis DP, Cohen BH. Use of next-generation sequencing as a diagnostic tool for congenital myasthenic syndrome. *Pediatr Neurol.* 2014;51(5):717-20.

Driscoll DJ, Miller JL, Schwartz S, et al. Prader-Willi Syndrome. 1998 [Updated 2017]. In: Adam MP, Ardinger HH, Pagon RA, et al, eds. GeneReviews® [Internet]. Seattle, WA: University of Washington, Seattle; 1993-2018. Available from https://www.ncbi.nlm.nih.gov/books/NBK1330/.

Engel AG. Current status of the congenital myasthenic syndromes. *Neuromuscul Disord.* 2012;22(2):99-111.

Hart AR, Sharma R, Rittey CD, Mordekar SR. Neonatal hypertonia - a diagnostic challenge. *Dev Med Child Neurol.* 2014;1-11.

Lorenzoni PJ, Scola RH, Kay CSK, Werneck LC. Congenital myasthenic syndrome: a brief review. *Pediatr Neurol.* 2012;46(3):141-8.

North KN. Clinical approach to the diagnosis of congenital myopathies. *Semin Pediatr Neurol.* 2011;18(4):216-20.

North KN, Wang CH, Clarke N, et al. Approach to the diagnosis of congenital myopathies. *Neuromuscul Disord.* 2014;24(2):97-116.

Peredo DE, Hannibal MC. The floppy infant: evaluation of hypotonia. *Pediatr Rev.* 2015;30(9):e66-76.

Prasad AN, Prasad C. Genetic evaluation of the floppy infant. *Semin Fetal Neonatal Med.* 2011;16(2):99-108.

Prior TW, Finanger E. Spinal muscular atrophy. 2000 [Updated 2016]. In: Adam MP, Ardinger HH, Pagon RA, et al, eds. GeneReviews® [Internet]. Seattle, WA: University of Washington, Seattle; 1993-2018. Available from https://www.ncbi.nlm.nih.gov/books/NBK1352/.

Tuysuz B, Kartal N, Erener-Ercan T, et al. Prevalence of Prader-Willi syndrome among infants with hypotonia. *J Pediatr.* 2014;164(5):1064-7.

Meningitis

Sourabh Dutta, MBBS, MD, PhD • Rajendra Prasad Anne, MBBS, MD, DM

SCOPE

DISEASE/CONDITION(S)

Neonatal bacterial meningitis.

GUIDELINE OBJECTIVE(S)

To address the following aspects of diagnosis and management of neonatal bacterial meningitis:

1. When should neonatal bacterial meningitis be suspected and a lumbar puncture performed in neonates?
2. How to interpret cerebrospinal fluid (CSF) findings.
3. Role of rapid diagnostic tests (including C-reactive protein [CRP]) in diagnosis.
4. Optimal duration and choice of antibiotics.
5. Role of adjunctive therapies in management.

BRIEF BACKGROUND

The highest incidence of meningitis across all age groups is in the neonatal period. Neonatal bacterial meningitis is a potentially devastating disease. Not only does it increase the risk of mortality, it can also have disastrous long-term neurodevelopmental consequences. The risk of mortality in neonates with meningitis has been reported to be 16–58% in various studies throughout the world. The risk of moderate to severe neurodevelopmental disability following meningitis depends upon the etiologic organism, and is markedly increased compared to controls without meningitis, with 11–56% of neonates surviving meningitis suffering from such impairment. Two specific neurologic sequelae of meningitis are sensorineural hearing loss, which occurs in around 4% of cases, and hydrocephalus, reported in 3% of cases. The above data suggest that neonatal meningitis is a serious disease, and one cannot afford to miss the diagnosis. Neonates with bacterial meningitis may demonstrate encephalopathy, seizures, a bulging anterior fontanel, signs of raised intracranial pressure, or other neurologic findings. However, the manifestations of neonatal meningitis are usually nonspecific or absent. Therefore, unlike in older children and adults, one cannot rely on clinical signs to decide whether to perform a lumbar puncture (LP). The currently acceptable reference standard for the diagnosis of neonatal meningitis is a positive CSF culture or Gram stain. Because CSF culture positivity rates are low in routine clinical practice and it takes about 48–72 hours to get a culture report, clinicians tend to rely on rapid diagnostic tests performed on CSF to arrive at a diagnosis. These include the total CSF white blood cell count, glucose level, and protein level. However, the diagnosis of neonatal meningitis based on rapid diagnostic tests is beset with controversy; because the levels of these parameters change with postnatal age, abnormal levels are not clearly defined, the sensitivity and specificity of these tests is uncertain, and CSF samples are often contaminated with blood from a traumatic lumbar puncture.

RECOMMENDATIONS

MAJOR RECOMMENDATIONS

LP should be performed in neonates based on the probability of their having meningitis, and not based purely on the presence or absence of clinical manifestations.

In attempting to identify meningitis, CSF examination, culture, and Gram stain results represent the reference standard. Several parameters (CSF white blood cell count, glucose level, and protein level) are commonly used for rapid diagnosis. However, no single parameter or combination of these commonly used parameters is diagnostic.

As with suspected sepsis, antibiotic therapy for meningitis should be initiated with antibiotics that provide broad coverage and adequate CSF penetration. Both epidemiologic and local microbiologic data should be used when choosing antibiotics for such broad coverage. Antibiotic therapy should be narrowed after culture results are obtained.

Based on current evidence, adjunctive therapies such as dexamethasone and therapies for increased intracranial pressure cannot be routinely recommended in the management of neonatal meningitis.

Cranial imaging with ultrasonography or magnetic resonance imaging should be performed in all neonates with meningitis after the completion of therapy, or with the development of any clinical complications during the course of therapy.

PRACTICE OPTIONS

Practice Option #1: Neonates with Suspected Early-Onset Sepsis and Respiratory Distress Syndrome

The incidence of meningitis is so low among neonates with suspected early-onset sepsis or asymptomatic neonates with only risk factors of early-onset sepsis that performing LP in such patients is not justified. Irrespective of the severity of the risk factors, as long as the neonate is asymptomatic, LP must not be performed. However, patients with early-onset sepsis who are symptomatic and have a positive blood culture have a high incidence of meningitis, and these patients must be subjected to a CSF examination.

The incidence of meningitis is so low among neonates with respiratory distress syndrome who were started on antibiotics to "cover the possibility" of pneumonia that performing LP among such patients is not justified.

Practice Option #2: Neonates with Suspected Late-Onset Sepsis

An LP must be performed in all patients with late-onset sepsis (LOS) because the incidence of meningitis is reasonably high in mixed populations of neonates who have both blood culture–positive as well as blood culture–negative LOS. At the time of onset of LOS, it is not possible to predict which patients will turn out to have a positive blood culture, therefore an LP should be performed in all patients with clinically suspected LOS. Clinicians should not wait for the blood culture report before deciding on an LP, because antibiotic treatment in the interim is likely to lead to false negative results on the CSF examination.

Practice Option #3: Diagnosis of Neonatal Meningitis

A diagnosis of meningitis should not be based on a single abnormal rapid diagnostic CSF test. The analysis should include CSF WBC count, glucose level, and protein level, in addition to Gram stain and culture. The presently available CSF parameters and the standard cutoffs suggested in the literature do not clearly confirm or rule out the diagnosis of meningitis. Clinicians should not rely on a single cutoff value of CSF WBC count and CSF protein at all postnatal ages. Unfortunately, there are no cutoff values that help identify the presence or absence of meningitis at different weeks of postnatal age.

Among preterm infants, the areas under the receiver operating curve for WBC count, protein, and glucose are 0.8 (95% CI 0.73, 0.86), 0.72 (0.64, 0.8), and 0.63 (0.54, 0.73), respectively. Among the three, the WBC count is the most preferable. Using likelihood ratios of these diagnostic tests, the pretest probability of meningitis in a given infant can be used to derive the post-test probability. Based on one study, if the presence of any one or more of the three is taken as indicative of meningitis, the likelihood ratio of a positive test (LR+) is 2.2 and the likelihood ratio of a negative test (LR−) is 0.3. If the presence of all three is required to make a diagnosis of meningitis, the LR+ is 8.7 and LR− is 0.8. If all the parameters are negative, the presence of meningitis is highly unlikely. In term infants, based on one study, a WBC range of 22 to 100 had an LR+ of 4.2, glucose <20 mg/dL had an LR+ of 22 and protein >120 had an LR+ of 2.0. However, none of the ranges described in the study had an LR less than 1.

When interpreting CSF parameters, it is also important to remember that CSF WBC count and protein (but not glucose levels) decrease with postnatal age. Traumatic LPs are common in neonates. In such cases, methods to "adjust" or correct the CSF WBC count based on the CSF RBC count should not be used. Instead, according to Greenberg et al., the "unadjusted" WBC count should be used to estimate the probability of meningitis. This method will result in a higher false-positive rate of diagnosis of meningitis and excess use of antibiotics, but it will miss less cases of meningitis compared to an approach that uses "adjustment."

The incidence of meningitis is higher among patients with positive blood cultures. This may have an implication for the interpretation of the CSF results, as the pretest probability of meningitis is higher in such patients. A few days of antibiotic exposure does not significantly alter the CSF WBC, protein, and glucose level. Prior exposure to antibiotics is therefore not a good enough reason to avoid doing an LP. CSF lactate does not have a diagnostic role. There are scant and conflicting reports regarding the utility of CRP in the diagnosis of neonatal meningitis.

Practice Option #4: Antibiotic Therapy for Neonatal Meningitis

The evidence for the optimal duration of antibiotics for neonatal meningitis is of very low quality. The conventional practice has been to give 14 days of therapy for gram-positive infections, and 21 days for gram-negative infections. When there are complications of meningitis such as brain abscess, empyema, or ventriculitis, antibiotic duration is extended to 4–6 weeks or longer. The duration of antibiotics for culture-negative meningitis (diagnosis based solely on abnormal CSF cytology and/or biochemistry) is unclear. The choice of antibiotics depends on organisms prevalent in the community and the neonatal unit. For meningitis suspected as a part of early-onset sepsis, in communities where Group B Streptococcus colonization is common, ampicillin should be included in the empiric management of neonatal meningitis. An aminoglycoside should be added to cover gram-negative organisms. In late-onset meningitis, an empiric antibiotic regimen to cover for *Staphylococci* and gram-negative organisms is usually chosen.

IMPLEMENTATION OF GUIDELINE

Consensus-based unit guidelines should be developed for investigation and management of neonates with suspected sepsis and meningitis. Some clinicians may feel reluctant to perform LP in neonates with suspected LOS, or feel that they are unnecessary—this may cause infants with meningitis to be undertreated and to suffer from relapse of meningitis and from complications of meningitis. After a CSF sample is obtained, the WBC level and glucose levels decrease steadily over time, and a delayed analysis can lead to a missed diagnosis of meningitis. Therefore a CSF sample is ideally analyzed within 30 minutes of collection. Central venous access is usually necessary for prolonged antibiotic administration for meningitis. Consultations from neurology and neurosurgery are required if complications of meningitis develop. Infants surviving meningitis should have their hearing assessed at discharge and subsequently, and also have close long-term follow-up to identify and manage neurodevelopmental impairment.

BIBLIOGRAPHIC SOURCE(S)

Bedford H, de LJ, Halket S, Peckham C, Hurley R, Harvey D. Meningitis in infancy in England and Wales: follow up at age 5 years. *BMJ.* 2001;323(7312):533-6.

BenGershom E, Briggeman-Mol GJ, de Zegher F. Cerebrospinal fluid C-reactive protein in meningitis: diagnostic value and pathophysiology. *Eur J Pediatr.* 1986;145(4):246-9.

Chadwick SL, Wilson JW, Levin JE, Martin JM. Cerebrospinal fluid characteristics of infants who present to the emergency department with fever: establishing normal values by week of age. *Pediatr Infect Dis J.* 2011;30(4):e63-7.

Furyk JS, Swann O, Molyneux E. Systematic review: neonatal meningitis in the developing world. *Trop Med Int Health.* 2011;16(6):672-9.

Greenberg RO, et al. Traumatic lumbar punctures in neonates: test performance of the cerebrospinal fluid white blood cell count. *Pediatr Infect Dis J.* 2008;27:1047-51.

Hendricks-Munoz KD, Shapiro DL. The role of the lumbar puncture in the admission sepsis evaluation of the premature infant. *J Perinatol.* 1990;10(1):60-4.

Hoque MM, Ahmed AS, Chowdhury MA, Darmstadt GL, Saha SK. Septicemic neonates without lumbar puncture: what are we missing? *J Trop Pediatr.* 2006;52(1):63-5.

Hristeva L, Bowler I, Booy R, King A, Wilkinson AR. Value of cerebrospinal fluid examination in the diagnosis of meningitis in the newborn. *Arch Dis Child*. 1993;69(5 Spec No):514-7.

Johnson CE, Whitwell JK, Pethe K, Saxena K, Super DM. Term newborns who are at risk for sepsis: are lumbar punctures necessary? *Pediatrics*. 1997;99(4):E10.

Kumar P, Sarkar S, Narang A. Role of routine lumbar puncture in neonatal sepsis. *J Paediatr Child Health*. 1995;31(1):8-10.

Mathur NB, Garg A, Mishra TK. Role of dexamethasone in neonatal meningitis: a randomized controlled trial. *Indian J Pediatr*. 2013;80(2):102-7.

Mathur NB, Kharod P, Kumar S. Evaluation of duration of antibiotic therapy in neonatal bacterial meningitis: a randomized controlled trial. *J Trop Pediatr*. 2015;61(2):119-25.

Ogunlesi TA, Odigwe CC, Oladapo OT. Adjuvant corticosteroids for reducing death in neonatal bacterial meningitis. *Cochrane Database Syst Rev*. 2015(11):CD010435.

Philip AG, Baker CJ. Cerebrospinal fluid C-reactive protein in neonatal meningitis. *J Pediatr*. 1983;102(5):715-7.

Rajesh NT, Dutta S, Prasad R, Narang A. Effect of delay in analysis on neonatal cerebrospinal fluid parameters. *Arch Dis Child Fetal Neonatal Ed*. 2010;95(1):F25-9.

Shah SS, Ebberson J, Kestenbaum LA, Hodinka RL, Zorc JJ. Age-specific reference values for cerebrospinal fluid protein concentration in neonates and young infants. *J Hosp Med*. 2011;6(1):22-7.

Sivanandan S, Soraisham AS, Swarnam K. Choice and duration of antimicrobial therapy for neonatal sepsis and meningitis. *Int J Pediatr*. 2011;2011:712150.

Smith PB, Garges HP, Cotton CM, Walsh TJ, Clark RH, Benjamin DK Jr. Meningitis in preterm neonates: importance of cerebrospinal fluid parameters. *Am J Perinatol*. 2008;25(7):421-6.

Srinivasan L, Shah SS, Padula MA, Abbasi S, McGowan KL, Harris MC. Cerebrospinal fluid reference ranges in term and preterm infants in the neonatal intensive care unit. *J Pediatr*. 2012;161(4):729-34.

Stevens JP, Eames M, Kent A, Halket S, Holt D, Harvey D. Long term outcome of neonatal meningitis. *Arch Dis Child Fetal Neonatal Ed*. 2003;88(3):F179-84.

Stoll BJ, Hansen N, Fanaroff AA, et al. To tap or not to tap: high likelihood of meningitis without sepsis among very low birth weight infants. *Pediatrics*. 2004;113(5):1181-6.

Weiss MG, Ionides SP, Anderson CL. Meningitis in premature infants with respiratory distress: role of admission lumbar puncture. *J Pediatr*. 1991;119(6):973-5.

Germinal Matrix Hemorrhage

Ashley M. Lucke, MD, FAAP • Amy R. Mehollin-Ray, MD

SCOPE

DISEASE/CONDITION(S)

Periventricular-intraventricular hemorrhage (PIVH) in preterm infants.

GUIDELINE OBJECTIVE(S)

Review the frequency, classification, pathogenesis, and sequelae of germinal matrix hemorrhage in preterm infants. List methods of prevention and management, including screening.

BRIEF BACKGROUND

PIVH remains a significant cause of morbidity among premature neonates. While the incidence of intraventricular hemorrhage (IVH) has declined since the 1970s, the total number of cases has not changed over the past few decades due to increased survival of neonates at progressively earlier gestational ages. IVH occurs in approximately 20% of neonates born <1500 g.

PIVH originates from the subependymal germinal matrix, a highly vascular structure surrounding the entire lateral ventricle but most apparent in the sagittal plane near the caudate nucleus. Proliferating neuronal and glial cells migrate outward from the germinal matrix toward the cortex; thus disruption of these structures from PIVH can lead to neurodevelopmental impairment.

TABLE 56.1. Grading Classification of Intraventricular Hemorrhage

Grade	Description
1	Hemorrhage confined within the germinal matrix
2	Germinal matrix hemorrhage with extension into the ventricle
3	Germinal matrix hemorrhage with extension into the ventricle *with hemorrhage filling and distending the ventricle*
4/PVHI	Germinal matrix and intraventricular hemorrhage plus parenchymal hemorrhage

Predisposition for PIVH: Review of Germinal Matrix Structure

Multiple critical protective structural elements are reduced in the germinal matrix vessels as compared to normal capillaries elsewhere in the body due to the high rate of angiogenesis and endothelial cell turnover. Protective pericytes which strengthen the vessels and produce extracellular matrix are reduced. The germinal matrix basal lamina in neonates is deficient in fibronectin compared to white and grey matter areas. Studies of fibronectin knockout animal models have shown propensity for cerebral hemorrhage, and it is hypothesized that a similar connection exists in human neonates. Astrocyte processes (end-feet) also comprise a proportion of the blood-brain barrier by wrapping around the blood vessels. In premature neonates these end-feet are deficient in glial fibrillary acidic protein (GFAP), a key component of the supportive cytoskeleton. The combination of reduced pericytes, basal lamina fibronectin, and astrocyte GFAP render the germinal matrix endothelium highly susceptible to hemorrhage.

Classification

PIVH is classified into four categories (Table 56.1). If ventricular dilation is noted on cranial ultrasound it must be carefully reviewed to determine if dilation is secondary to an acute filling and distention by blood products (grade 3) or due to post-hemorrhagic hydrocephalus. In addition, in the past, grade 4 PIVH was incorrectly thought to be an extension of hemorrhage from the lateral ventricles into surrounding periventricular white matter. As blood accumulates in the ventricles, there is progressive compression of the surrounding venous drainage, resulting in obstruction and secondary venous infarction. Therefore, grade 4 PIVH has been more appropriately renamed periventricular hemorrhagic infarction (PVHI).

Pathogenesis

Cerebral blood flow is pressure-passive in premature neonates, and significant alterations in arterial or venous flow cause PIVH. Clinical causes of PIVH are listed in Table 56.2.

Prognosis and Counseling of Families

Traditionally, the severity of neurodevelopmental impairment has been predicted based on PIVH classification (grade 1 to PVHI), with the worst outcomes expected for PVHI with PHH and mild or possibly no impairment in grade 1 PIVH. Many reviews and meta-analyses group grades 1 and 2 together for comparison against grades 3 and 4 with similar results; however, many studies do not account for confounding factors and report unadjusted data. Families should be counseled that risk for long-term

TABLE 56.2. Clinical Causes of Intraventricular Hemorrhage

Respiratory	Fluid/Electrolytes
Respiratory distress syndrome	Hyperosmolarity
Pneumothorax	Hypoglycemia
Hypercarbia/CO_2 fluctuations	Sodium bicarbonate infusions
Multiple intubation attempts	Rapid volume expansion (fluid bolus)
High peak inspiratory pressures	**Hematologic**
Asphyxia	Anemia
Tracheal suctioning	Platelet dysfunction/coagulopathy
Cardiac	**Other**
Hypotension	Hypothermia
Hypertension	Excessive handling/stimulation
Myocardial failure	Labor and vaginal delivery
Patent ductus arteriosus	Postnatal transport

neurodevelopmental impairment increases in continuum with severity of PIVH; however, individual studies have reported a proportion of patients with normal neurodevelopmental outcomes in infants with grade 1–3 PIVH and less frequently in PVHI.

RECOMMENDATIONS

MAJOR RECOMMENDATIONS

All preterm infants should be considered at risk for PIVH and should be managed with practices that minimize perturbations of cerebral blood follow. Conditions that impair hemostasis should be quickly identified and corrected. Infants at higher risk for PIVH should undergo routine screening with cranial ultrasonography. Infants with severe PIVH are at significant risk of long-term neurodevelopmental impairment, and counseling of families of such patients often involves discussions about redirection of care to provide comfort measures only. Such discussions should be guided by accurate data on long-term outcomes in infants who received maximal intensive care.

PRACTICE OPTIONS

Practice Option #1: Preventive Practices

Antenatal corticosteroids given to pregnant women at risk of delivering preterm at least 24 hours prior to delivery, maternal transportation prior to delivery, delayed cord clamping, and volume mode ventilation are associated with decreased rates of PIVH. While prophylactic indomethacin has been shown to reduce incidence of severe IVH, follow-up studies have not shown significant differences in neurodevelopmental outcomes. The role of cesarean delivery in preventing PIVH is uncertain.

Practice Option #2: Screening with Cranial Ultrasonography

The American Academy of Neurology practice parameter on neuroimaging in the neonate (2002) recommends all infants <30 weeks' gestational age receive a screening cranial ultrasound at 7–14 days of life. There are insufficient data at this time to recommend repeat cranial ultrasound or MRI at term, as it is unclear if these studies provide additional information to inform clinical care which justifies the cost, resource utilization, and parental anxiety.

Practice Option #3: Treatment

Treatment of PIVH is supportive with the goal of minimizing derangements known to cause extension of PIVH (Table 56.2). Immediate clinical signs of PIVH can include changes in muscle tone and altered mental status, bulging anterior fontanel, a precipitous drop in hematocrit, hyperglycemia, metabolic acidosis, seizures, apnea, and bradycardia events. Acid-base balance, glucose, blood pressure, and respiratory status should be carefully monitored and maintained in the optimal ranges in the acute phase.

Practice Option #4: Post-Hemorrhagic Hydrocephalus

Post-hemorrhagic hydrocephalus (PHH) affects 25–50% of all premature neonates with PIVH (any grade) and can present in an acute or chronic manner. In the acute presentation, clotted blood products inside the ventricles may obstruct cerebrospinal fluid (CSF) flow and lead to a rapid onset of hydrocephalus within days. In the chronic presentation, CSF flow may be impeded by ependymal inflammatory changes and gliosis which occurs over the course of weeks.

After diagnosis of PIVH, a cranial ultrasound should be repeated to assess progression and development of PHH. Of neonates who develop PHH, 60% will have spontaneous cessation of progression and 40% will require neurosurgical intervention (external ventricular drain, ventriculosubgaleal shunt, endoscopic third ventriculostomy). The American Association of Neurological Surgeons (AANS) 2014 guidelines do not recommend serial lumbar punctures, intraventricular thrombolytic agents, acetazolamide, or furosemide to prevent progression of PHH. Frequent examination of the anterior fontanel and daily head circumference measurements should be used to monitor the status of infants with PHH in the intervals between ultrasounds. There is no standardized age or weight requirement for neurosurgical intervention; however, the benefits of waiting several weeks for growth and optimal peritoneal absorptive surface area must be weighed against ongoing injury from inflammation and ischemia.

IMPLEMENTATION OF GUIDELINE

DESCRIPTION OF IMPLEMENTATION STRATEGY

Perinatal programs should routinely review their rate of antenatal steroid usage and improve it if there are gaps in performance. Regional systems of care should ensure the birth of preterm infants in regional referral centers instead of being born elsewhere and transported postnatally. Images from routine cranial ultrasonographic screening should be interpreted by radiologists with expertise in neonatal ultrasonography. Ideally, images should be obtained through supplemental acoustic (lambdoid, mastoid, and lateral fontanels) windows as well. If severe PIVH is discovered on cranial imaging, clinicians should counsel the families about the high risk of long-term neurodevelopmental impairment and depending on the overall condition of the baby and family preferences, guide the family in decision-making about provision of comfort measures only, and withdrawal of life-sustaining intensive care.

QUALITY METRICS

Every neonatal unit should monitor the rate of PIVH in admitted patients and compare these rates with other similar units. Such data are available in databases such as the Vermont Oxford Network, Canadian Neonatal Network, and Pediatrix databases.

Data should be analyzed separately for inborn and outborn neonates. A comparatively high rate of PIVH or an increase in this rate compared to previous rates should lead to review of the care provided to affected infants, and of the overall process of care, particularly in the first 2 days of life, to identify opportunities for improvement.

SUMMARY

Risk and incidence of PIVH is inversely related to gestational age in weeks. Screening cranial ultrasounds should be performed on neonates less than 30 weeks' gestational age.

BIBLIOGRAPHIC SOURCE(S)

Bassan H. Intracranial hemorrhage in the preterm infant: understanding it, preventing it. *Clin Perinatol.* 2009;36(4):737-62.

Christian EA, Melamed BA, Peck E, et al. Surgical management of hydrocephalus secondary to intraventricular hemorrhage in the preterm infant. *J Neurosurg Pediatr.* 2016;17:278-84.

Fowlie PW, Davis PG, McGuire W. Prophylactic intravenous indomethacin for preventing mortality and morbidity in preterm infants. *Cochrane Database Syst Rev.* 2010;7:000174.

Mazzola CA, Choudhri AF, Auguste KI, et al. Pediatric hydrocephalus: systematic literature review and evidence-based guidelines. Part 2: Management of posthemorrhagic hydrocephalus in premature infants. *J Neurosurg Pediatr.* 2014;14(Suppl):8-23.

McDonald SJ, Middleton P, Dowswell T, et al. Effect of timing of umbilical cord clamping of term infants on maternal and neonatal outcomes. *Evid Based Child Health.* 2014;9(2):303-97.

Ment LR, Bada HS, Barnes PD, et al. Practice parameter: neuroimaging of the neonate. *Neurology.* 2002;58:1726-38.

Mukerji A, Shah V, Shah PS. Periventricular/intraventricular hemorrhage and neurodevelopment outcomes: a meta-analysis. *Pediatrics.* 2015;136(6):1132-43.

Murphy BP, Inder TE, Rooks V, et al. Posthaemorrhagic ventricular dilatation in the premature infant: natural history and predictors of outcome. *Arch Dis Child Fetal Neonatal Ed.* 2002;87(1):F37-41.

Papile LA, Burstein J, Burstein R, et al. Incidence and evolution of subependymal and intraventricular hemorrhage: a study of infants with birth weights less than 1,500 gm. *J Pediatr.* 1978;92(4):529-34.

Stoll BJ, Hansen NI, Bell EF, et al; Eunice Kennedy Shriver National Institute of Child Health and Human Development Neonatal Research Network. Neonatal outcomes of extremely preterm infants from the NICHD Neonatal Research Network. *Pediatrics.* 2010;126(3):443-56.

Volpe JJ. *Neurology of the Newborn.* Philadelphia: WB Saunders; 2008.

Developmental Care

Joan R. Smith, PhD, RN, NNP-BC • Mary R. Raney, MSN, NNP-BC, WCC • Roberta Pineda, PhD, OTR/L

SCOPE

DISEASE/CONDITION(S)

An extended stay in the newborn intensive care unit (NICU) places newborns, preterm and term, at an increased risk for alterations in neurodevelopment.

GUIDELINE OBJECTIVE(S)

Review essential components of developmentally supportive care; recommend strategies to protect neurodevelopment in the NICU.

BRIEF BACKGROUND

Premature infants admitted to the NICU lose the protection of the intrauterine environment, placing them at risk for alterations in neurodevelopment. It is vital for neonatal healthcare professionals and families to adapt and optimize the NICU environment in order to protect the preterm brain during critical and sensitive periods of development. All care delivered to hospitalized newborns has the potential to positively or negatively impact neurodevelopment. Developmentally supportive care is a holistic, family-centered philosophy of care that promotes neurodevelopment of preterm infants, decreases discordance between the womb and NICU environments, and alters the micro- and macro-environments to match the infant capabilities. Critical to this philosophy of care is the development of a positive parent-infant relationship that is life-long and essential for long-term development. Parents are recognized as partners of the healthcare team. The following recommendations are aligned with the developmental care core measures published by the National Association of Neonatal Nurses (NANN).

RECOMMENDATIONS

MAJOR RECOMMENDATIONS: PROMOTE A HEALING ENVIRONMENT

A healing environment of care includes not only the physical environment but also the culture of an organization that recognizes patients as human beings with physical, social, psychological, and spiritual needs. A healing environment reduces stress and anxiety and promotes harmony of mind, body, and spirit, which positively affects health. The working environment defines the NICU culture; therefore, healthcare workers should strive to create a positive environment/culture so that safe, effective, and evidenced-based care can be delivered. Professionals in the NICU are challenged to provide a healing environment to infants and families during one of the most vulnerable and frightening periods of their lives. Compassionate professionals should guide parents through their shock, fear, and grief experiences by providing physical, emotional, and psychological support. This will empower families to parent, advocate, and partner with medical professionals to care for their babies. The physical surroundings of the NICU should be welcoming, aesthetically pleasing, and provide space and privacy for parents to engage with their infants. Specific design recommendations are set forth by the Committee to Establish Recommended Standards for Newborn ICU Design. The healing environment for the infant includes care that minimizes pain and stress, promotes uninterrupted sleep, supports the developing sensory system, encourages parental attachment, optimizes nutrition, provides a neutral thermal environment, and meets the infant's medical needs to restore health. Such an environment allows medical professionals to deliver individualized, age appropriate, and neuroprotective care for every infant in their care.

PRACTICE OPTIONS

Practice Option #1: Provide Appropriate Sensory Exposure

Preterm birth removes the fetus from the protective gravity-free fluid uterine environment, with sensory experiences modulated by the physical barrier of the womb and maternal activity. These early sensory experiences are critical for optimal growth and health. Fetal sensory development occurs in the following sequence: 1) tactile, 2) vestibular, 3) olfactory/gustatory, 4) auditory, and 5) visual. A preterm neonate experiences an interruption of this normal progression, and is exposed in the NICU to unexpected, intense, poorly timed sensory stimuli. Such exposure may be harmful to the developing sensory system and impair long-term neurological and behavioral outcomes.

Professionals caring for preterm infants in the NICU should ensure that such infants are exposed to properly timed sensory experiences that match the post-menstrual age (PMA), and that are guided by infant cues. Care should consist of positive tactile experiences, modulated auditory exposure, avoidance of excessive noise, and protection from inappropriate visual stimuli. Care should also include boundaries and containment that encourage proprioception, supported changes in position (including holding) that provide positive vestibular stimulation, and exposure to mother's scent with protection from noxious odors.

Recommended interventions include:

- Educate parents/families to provide age-appropriate tactile and auditory interventions; promote skin-to-skin care (SSC) early and often; introduce other tactile stimulation, including massage, holding, and gentle human touch; encourage parents to read, talk, or sing to the infant; play recorded or live music after 32 weeks PMA.

- Monitor infant behavioral and physiologic stability prior to and during all care activities. Adapt sensory exposure based on responses. All movement should be deliberate and supported to maintain alignment, safety, and security.
- Care professionals should quietly and respectfully introduce themselves to the infant prior to hands-on activity.
- Provide gentle rocking, movement, and infant engagement out of the bed when medically stable to promote vestibular and kinesthetic development.
- Expose the infant to positive olfactory input: maternal scent, nuzzling at the breast, SSC.
- Avoid opening noxious odors (e.g., alcohol, betadine, etc.) inside the incubator or near the infant; use non-scented products within the infant's microsystem environment (e.g., diaper creams, detergents, fabric softeners, etc.); avoid exposure to secondhand cigarette smoke.
- Limit potentially noxious environmental noise (e.g., answer alarms quickly, gently close incubator portholes and doors) and direct light (e.g., shield eyes).
- Limit noise to 50 decibels (dB) for sleep; transient noise should not exceed 65 dB; infants prior to term gestation should only be exposed to indirect lighting; focused procedure light and task lighting should be provided for caregivers.
- Promote circadian rhythm by using cycled lighting starting at 32 weeks PMA.
- Involve age-appropriate therapy services when medically stable to enhance neurobehavioral/sensory progression, to train parents on appropriate therapeutic interventions, and to evaluate the need for therapy services at discharge.

Practice Option #2: Optimize Positioning

Flexion has developmental importance, as it is the basis of early movement. The intrauterine environment provides a confined and protected space for fetal flexion with the ability for the infant to move into extension with proprioceptive feedback for return to midline flexion. This occurs during a critical period of brain development in which the formation of synaptic connections and pathways are formed. Flexion is important because it is developmentally regulated, promotes self-regulation, and fosters optimal reflex development and fine and gross motor skills. Critically ill and preterm infants who are removed from the intrauterine environment have inadequate tone and strength to maintain midline flexion and positioning, putting them at risk for extended posture, hip and shoulder abduction, neck rotation, and movement asymmetries. The goals of neonatal positioning are to ensure good joint alignment, promote physiological stability, encourage sleep, and optimize development. Positioning aids or boundaries are important components of neonatal positioning. This can include swaddling with a blanket, providing boundaries with a nest, or using commercial positioning aids. It is also important to consider pressure points when positioning neonates and distribute contact with the surface evenly, and to change positioning frequently to prevent abnormal head shaping, tightness, and posturing.

While nesting in supine may achieve positioning goals in many infants, some infants may benefit from prone positioning, which can improve ventilation, oxygen saturation, and chest wall synchrony, decrease incidence of apnea, decrease symptoms of gastroesophageal reflux, and promote better sleep. However, transitioning infants to their backs for sleep prior to NICU discharge is critical to reduce the risk of sudden infant death. Recommended interventions include:

- Promote midline flexion with the use of positioning aids to facilitate: 1) neutral alignment of the neck; 2) flexion of the trunk, elbows, hips, and knees; and 3) midline orientation of hips and upper extremities with hands close to face.
- Prevent pressure ulcers, mechanical pain and contractures, and promote optimal head shaping by changing positions with care as tolerated and initiate the use of pressure redistribution surfaces (e.g., gel mattress, pillows/cushions).
- Consult therapy services to assist with optimal positioning and alignment.

Practice Option #3: Protect Sleep

The intrauterine environment promotes optimal sleep and wake patterns, but this is lost following preterm birth. Sleep is essential to brain growth and maturation, including the formation of new neural pathways that provide permanent brain circuits and connections that impact future memory, learning, long-term brain connectivity, and the preservation of brain plasticity. However, procedures, care, evaluations, and noise from other healthcare professionals and infants can frequently disrupt sleep in the NICU, and disruption of normal sleep cycles may be detrimental to health. Promoting an environment to support sleep requires healthcare professionals and families to be able to recognize infant sleep states and to alter their caregiving/interaction based on infant sleep states. Recommended interventions include:

- Avoid multiple sleep disturbances; coordinate nonemergent caregiving/examinations to preserve normal sleep cycles; in the event that a sleep cycle must be interrupted, take the time afterward to help the infant return to a resting sleep state.
- Promote sleep by delivering calming activities into daily routine care (e.g., comforting touch, massage, SSC care, swaddled bathing, audible parental voice, cycled lighting, etc.) based on infant readiness.
- Implement the use of cycled lighting to promote nocturnal sleep and support infant growth and development.
- Educate parents on the importance of sleep and support family involvement in care practices that promote sleep (e.g., SSC care—infants have better sleep cycles during SSC care when provided greater than 1 hour in duration).

Practice Option #4: Mitigate Pain and Stress

Neonatal care necessitates many painful/stressful interventions to enhance the survival of infants born prematurely and term infants with life-threatening conditions. The perception of pain is active at 20 weeks' gestation, but the descending inhibitory pathways are not completely mature and active until approximately 48 weeks' gestation. The immaturity of the integrated pain circuitry may make the pain experience more diffuse and potentially more intense for a premature infant. In addition, the ability to discriminate between touch and nociception does not emerge until approximately 35–37 weeks' gestation. Therefore, premature infants may respond to routine care interventions with pain-like behaviors and physiologic changes. The cumulative effect of repetitive pain and unrelieved stress is linked to epigenetic changes that affect brain maturation, somatosensory processing, pain signaling, and hypothalamic–pituitary–adrenal axis programming. Frequent and prolonged exposures to undermanaged pain and chronic stressors have been linked to changes in brain structure and function and to poorer cognitive outcomes in premature infants. Neonatal healthcare providers need to be acutely aware of the potential adverse consequences of unmanaged and undermanaged pain in infants.

Neonatal pain assessment tools rely on behavioral and physiologic parameters, facial expressions, and the clinical experience of the caregiver. Selected validated neonatal pain scales include the Premature Infant Pain Profile (PIPP), Neonatal Postoperative Pain Assessment Score (CRIES), Neonatal Infant Pain Scale (NIPS), and the Neonatal Pain Agitation and Sedation Scale (N-Pass). These tools are meant to assist, not replace, the expert assessment of the care provider. The lack of response to an intervention by a preterm infant may represent an exhaustion of their response capability and not a lack of pain perception. In the instance of prolonged unmanaged or undermanaged pain, the infant may become unresponsive and energy-depleted as well as may demonstrate dangerous drops in heart rate, respiratory rate, and oxygen consumption.

Preemptive analgesia should be provided for any painful/stressful procedure or medical intervention. Nonpharmacologic interventions ameliorate the physical symptoms of infant pain during mild to moderate painful interventions and can serve as an adjunct to pharmacologic therapies for moderate to severe painful interventions. Nonpharmacologic interventions assist the infant in maintaining homeostasis, and include facilitated tuck, nonnutritive suck, sucrose, SSC care, and breastfeeding. These interventions may be more effective when used in combination, rather than alone, and should be employed during mild-moderate painful procedures (e.g., heel lance, feeding tube placement, peripheral IV start, endotracheal suctioning, etc.) and routine care.

Pharmacologic interventions include the use of opioids, acetaminophen, sedatives, and local anesthetics. Opioids are the most effective for moderate to severe pain, providing both analgesia and sedation. Morphine and fentanyl are the most commonly used opioids in the NICU. High-dose opioids in preterm infants, especially the extremely premature infant, may be associated with increased adverse events, and chronic use should be managed conservatively and with caution. The addition of acetaminophen may minimize the need for opioids for adequate pain control intraoperatively and in the postoperative period. It is also effective for mild pain control in conjunction with nonpharmacologic interventions. Midazolam is a short-acting benzodiazepine that provides sedation and anxiolysis, possibly decreasing stress related to NICU care. It provides no analgesia. Due to adverse events and poor neurologic outcomes in preterm infants who received midazolam, its routine use is not recommended in preterm infants. Dexmedetomidine use in the NICU requires further study to establish its safety and efficacy but holds promise. It provides potent sedative effects and provides some analgesia.

Local anesthetics, eutectic mixture of local anesthetics (EMLA), and lidocaine can reduce pain in some acute procedures in infants. However, they are not effective for heel lance, the most frequent painful procedure in the NICU.

Recommended interventions include:

- Utilize valid pain assessment tool to routinely assess for pain/stress.
- Document and assess the efficacy of intervention used to relieve pain/stress.
- Minimize laboratory testing; use noninvasive monitoring when appropriate; consider arterial access for frequent laboratory studies to limit repeated heel lances or venipunctures; limit unsuccessful attempts of painful procedures.
- Provide pharmacologic pain control for all moderate to severe painful procedures and provide nonpharmacologic support as an adjunct therapy.

- Prevent pain/stress during daily care by providing nonpharmacologic support (e.g., use two-person technique for suctioning [one person to maintain facilitated tuck and the other to suction] when available).
- Educate parents about infant pain and stress cues; encourage parents to provide comfort and use nonpharmacologic interventions to control stress/pain.

Practice Option #5: Promote Family-Centered Care

Family-centered care (FCC) incorporates parents as partners in the care of their infant in the NICU to foster the development of the parent-infant relationship, preserve the integrity of the family, and promote parents' competence and confidence. Early separation between parents and their infant admitted to the NICU strains the parent-infant relationship, disrupts attachment, results in high levels of distress (e.g., increased anxiety, depression, and trauma symptoms) and alters the parenting role (e.g., helplessness, loss of control, inadequacy, poor confidence, and fear). Such effects on the early parent-child relationship can have long-term implications. A positive parent-infant relationship is essential and provides infants with early life experiences that lay the foundation for neural and synaptic connections that ultimately promote cognitive development, infant self-confidence, security, emotional stability, readiness to learn, and social competence. Four tenets are vital for FCC: dignity and respect, information sharing, participation, and collaboration.

Recommended interventions include:

- Develop a supportive FCC culture—develop an interdisciplinary FCC committee that includes parents; educate physicians, nurses, therapists, and all members of the care team to adopt FCC approaches.
- Integrate FCC into neonatal transport by assessing parents' emotional needs, offering clear, concise, honest, accurate, and compassionate communication; provide opportunities for the parents to see and touch their infant; provide photographs for parents and/or opportunities for parents to view their infant on transport or upon arrival to the NICU via iPads, smartphones, telemedicine, etc.; minimize separation and reunite families with their infants at the earliest opportunity; encourage and collect colostrum before the transport team departs.
- Assess parent experiences and their readiness to assimilate information; exercise cultural sensitivity; adapt and optimize communication, which may include but is not limited to availability of translation specialists and materials that are available in both English and other languages/dialects.
- Encourage parental presence and participation with supportive unit policies and resources; provide parents 24-hour/365-day access to the NICU; include parents in medical rounds; encourage presence during invasive and resuscitative procedures; integrate families into daily caregiving and provide a welcoming and unrestricted environment for parents, grandparents, siblings, and other individuals identified by the parents (e.g., inpatient rooms with comfortable furniture and family space; NICU waiting area with toys, furniture, and books for siblings and children; a private and quiet space for respite for families).
- Educate parents on their child's cues and behaviors, empowering them to actively participate in daily activities including feeding, changing diapers, bathing, and reading to their child, SSC care, and/or massage to enhance parental competence and confidence.
- Provide peer-to-peer social support (e.g., parent education hours [offered by former NICU parents who are properly screened, prepared, trained, and supported

themselves]), parent scrapbooking, mothers' milk club, monthly milestone calendars, journaling, and special holiday activities.

- Provide access to resources to support parenting skills, decision-making, and overall psychological, emotional, and physical well-being, including access to written or online educational materials or websites (e.g., family resource library); provide access to designated family support personnel (e.g., March of Dimes NICU specialist), a lactation consultant, discharge coordinator, neonatal therapists, financial support personnel, mental health experts, social workers, and chaplains.
- Provide access to palliative care and bereavement support—provide opportunities to create family memories while the infant is alive (e.g., SSC care, cuddling, breastfeeding, dressing, diapering, bathing, etc.) and support ethnic or cultural differences surrounding end-of-life traditions.
- Provide transition-to-home support starting at admission, including hands-on caregiving practices, parent education classes and workshops, and opportunities for parents to spend the night(s) with their infant prior to going home in order to help individualize the content of discharge planning for their specific family needs.

IMPLEMENTATION OF GUIDELINE

DESCRIPTION OF IMPLEMENTATION STRATEGY

Parent and staff education; facilitators, experts, and champions to develop and implement clinical practice guidelines related to developmentally supportive care.

QUALITY METRICS

Parental satisfaction, maternal mental health, pain/stress scores, behavioral and sleep/wake states, physiologic stability, neurobehavioral assessment, and post-discharge neurodevelopmental assessment.

SUMMARY

Converging evidence supports the importance of providing developmentally supportive care within the NICU environment, since neurodevelopment continues outside the natural protective intrauterine environment. In an effort to protect the brain and positively influence short- and long-term neurological and behavioral outcomes in preterm and term newborns, caregivers are encouraged to partner with families to optimize the NICU environment in an effort to provide neuroprotective care. Through this partnership, neurodevelopment can be optimized through a healing environment that provides appropriate sensory exposures, optimizes positioning, reduces pain, improves sleep quality, and promotes the early parent-child relationship.

BIBLIOGRAPHIC SOURCE(S)

Aden U. Maternal singing for preterm infants during kangaroo care comforts both the mother and baby. *Acta Paediatr.* 2014;103(10):995-6.

Allen MC, Capute AJ. Tone and reflex development before term. *Pediatrics.* 1990;85(3 Pt 2):393-9.

Als H. Program Guide Newborn Individualized Developmental Care and Assessment Program (NIDCAP). NIDCAP Federation International Voice of the Newborn; 2000.

Altimier L, Phillips RM. The neonatal integrative developmental care model: seven neuroprotective core measures for family-centered developmental care. *Newborn Infant Nurs Rev*. 2013;13(1):9-22.

American Academy of Pediatrics. *Guidelines for Perinatal Care*. Elk Grove Village, IL: American Academy of Pediatrics; 2012.

American Academy of Pediatrics, Committee on Fetus and Newborn, et al. Prevention and management of pain in the neonate: an update. *Pediatrics*. 2006;118(5):2231-41.

Anand K. Prevention and treatment of neonatal pain. UpToDate.com. 2015. Available from http://www.uptodate.com/contents/prevention-and-treatment-of-neonatal-pain?source=search_result&search=prevention+and+treatment+of+neonatal+pain&selectedTitle=1~6.

Anderson P, Doyle LW; Victorian Infant Collaborative Study G. Neurobehavioral outcomes of school-age children born extremely low birth weight or very preterm in the 1990s. *JAMA*. 2003;289(24):3264-72.

Ariagno RL, van Liempt S, Mirmiran M. Fewer spontaneous arousals during prone sleep in preterm infants at 1 and 3 months corrected age. *J Perinatol*. 2006;26(5):306-12.

Artley K, Miller, C, Gephart, S. Facilitated tucking to reduce pain in neonates, evidence for best practice. *Adv Neonatal Care*. 2015;15(3):201-8.

Bahman Bijari B, Iranmanesh S, Eshghi F, Baneshi MR. Gentle Human Touch and Yakson: The Effect on Preterm's Behavioral Reactions. *ISRN Nurs*. 2012;2012:750363.

Blomqvist YT, Rubertsson C, Kylberg E, Joreskog K, Nyqvist KH. Kangaroo mother care helps fathers of preterm infants gain confidence in the paternal role. *J Adv Nurs*. 2012;68(9):1988-96.

Brandon DH, Holditch-Davis D, Belyea M. Preterm infants born at less than 31 weeks' gestation have improved growth in cycled light compared with continuous near darkness. *J Pediatr*. 2002;140(2):192-9.

Brummelte S, Grunau RE, Chau V, et al. Procedural pain and brain development in premature newborns. *Ann Neurol*. 2012;71(3):385-96.

Caskey M, Stephens B, Tucker R, Vohr B. Adult talk in the NICU with preterm infants and developmental outcomes. *Pediatrics*. 2014;133(3):e578-84.

Cleveland LM. Parenting in the neonatal intensive care unit. *J Obstet Gynecol Neonatal Nurs*. 2008;37(6):666-91.

Cooper L, Morrill A, Russell RB, Gooding JS, Miller L, Berns SD. Close to me: enhancing kangaroo care practice for NICU staff and parents. *Adv Neonatal Care*. 2014;14(6):410-23.

Coughlin M. *Transformative Nursing in the NICU: Trauma-Informed Age-Appropriate Care*. New York, NY: Springer; 2014.

Coughlin M, Gibbins S, Hoath S. Core measures for developmentally supportive care in neonatal intensive care units: theory, precedence and practice. *J Adv Nurs*. 2009;65(10):2239-48.

Doesburg SM, Chau CM, Cheung TPL, et al. Neonatal pain-related stress, functional cortical activity and visual-perceptual abilities in school-age children born at extremely low gestational age. *Pain*. 2013;154(10):1946-52.

Fabrizi L, Slater R, Worley A, et al. A shift in sensory processing that enables the developing human brain to discriminate touch from pain. *Curr Biol*. 2011;21(18):1552-8.

Fern D. *A Neurodevelopmental Care Guide to Positioning and Handling the Premature, Fragile or Sick Infant*. New York, New York: DF Publishing 2011.

Ferrari F, Bertoncelli N, Gallo C, et al. Posture and movement in healthy preterm infants in supine position in and outside the nest. *Arch Dis Child Fetal Neonat Ed*. 2007;92(5):F386-90.

Fitzgerald M, Walker SM. Infant pain management: a developmental neurobiological approach. *Nat Clin Pract Neuro*. 2009;5(1):35-50.

Franck LS, Oulton K, Bruce E. Parental involvement in neonatal pain management: an empirical and conceptual update. *J Nurs Scholarsh*. 2012;44(1):45-54.

Gelfer P, Cameron R, Masters K, Kennedy KA. Integrating "back to sleep" recommendations into neonatal ICU practice. *Pediatrics*. 2013;131(4):e1264-70.

Goddard S. *Reflexes, Learning and Behavior: A Window Into the Child's Mind*. Eugene, OR: Fern Ridge Press; 2005.

Gooding JS, Cooper LG, Blaine AI, Franck LS, Howse JL, Berns SD. Family support and family-centered care in the neonatal intensive care unit: origins, advances, impact. *Semina Perinatol.* 2011;35(1):20-8.

Goto K, Mirmiran M, Adams MM, et al. More awakenings and heart rate variability during supine sleep in preterm infants. *Pediatrics.* 1999;103(3):603-9.

Graven S. Sleep and brain development. *Clin Perinatol.* 2006;33(3):693-706, vii.

Graven S, Browne, J. Sensory development in the fetus, neonate, and infant: introduction and overview. *Newborn Infant Nurs Rev.* 2008;8(4):169-72.

Grunau RE. Neonatal pain in very preterm infants: long-term effects on brain, neurodevelopment and pain reactivity. *Rambam Maimonides Med J.* 2013;4(4):e0025.

Guyer C, Huber R, Fontijn J, et al. Cycled light exposure reduces fussing and crying in very preterm infants. *Pediatrics.* 2012;130(1):e145-51.

Hall RW. Anesthesia and analgesia in the NICU. *Clin Perinatol.* 2012;39(1):239-54.

Hall RW, Anand KJ. Pain management in newborns. *Clin Perinatol.* 2014;41(4):895-924.

Institute for Patient and Family Centered Care. Advancing the practice of patient- and family-centered care in hospitals: how to get started. Available at http://www.ipfcc.org/pdf/getting_started.pdf.

Johnston C, Campbell-Yeo M, Fernandes A, Inglis D, Streiner D, Zee R. Skin-to-skin care for procedural pain in neonates. *Cochrane Database Syst Rev.* 2014;1:CD008435.

Kanagasabai PS, Mohan D, Lewis LE, Kamath A, Rao BK. Effect of multisensory stimulation on neuromotor development in preterm infants. *Indian J Pediatr.* 2013;80(6):460-4.

Kenner C, McGrath J. *Developmenatal Care of Newborns and Infants.* Glenview: National Association of Neonatal Therapists; 2010.

Korja R, Maunu J, Kirjavainen J, et al. Mother-infant interaction is influenced by the amount of holding in preterm infants. *Early Hum Devel.* 2008;84(4):257-67.

Krueger C. Exposure to maternal voice in preterm infants: a review. *Adv Neonatal Care.* 2010;10(1):13-8; quiz 9-20.

Lacina L, Casper T, Dixon M, et al. Behavioral observation differentiates the effects of an intervention to promote sleep in premature infants: a pilot study. *Adv Neonatal Care.* 2015;15(1):70-6.

Lickliter R. The integrated development of sensory organization. *Clin Perinatol.* 2011;38(4):591-603.

Liu WF, Laudert S, Perkins B, et al. The development of potentially better practices to support the neurodevelopment of infants in the NICU. *J Perinatol.* 2007;27(Suppl 2):S48-74.

Madlinger-Lewis L, Reynolds L, Zarem C, Crapnell T, Inder T, Pineda R. The effects of alternative positioning on preterm infants in the neonatal intensive care unit: a randomized clinical trial. *Res Devel Disabili.* 2014;35(2):490-7.

Malkin J. The business argument for creating a healing environment 2003. Available from http://www.capch.org/wp-content/uploads/2012/10/hosp031_r_malkin1.pdf.

McPherson C, Grunau RE. Neonatal pain control and neurologic effects of anesthetics and sedatives in preterm infants. *Clin Perinatol.* 2014;41(1):209-27.

Milgrom J, Newnham C, Anderson PJ, et al. Early sensitivity training for parents of preterm infants: impact on the developing brain. *Pediatr Res.* 2010;67(3):330-5.

Monterosso L, Kristjanson LJ, Cole J, Evans SF. Effect of postural supports on neuromotor function in very preterm infants to term equivalent age. *J Paediatr Child Health.* 2003;39(3):197-205.

Montirosso R, Del Prete A, Bellu R, Tronick E, Borgatti R; Neonatal Adequate Care for Quality of Life Study Group. Level of NICU quality of developmental care and neurobehavioral performance in very preterm infants. *Pediatrics.* 2012;129(5):e1129-37.

Morag I, Ohlsson A. Cycled light in the intensive care unit for preterm and low birth weight infants. *Cochrane Database Syst Rev.* 2013;8:Cd006982.

Mullaney DM, Edwards WH, DeGrazia M. Family-centered care during acute neonatal transport. *Adv Neonatal Care.* 2014;14(Suppl 5):S16-23.

Neu M, Robinson J, Schmiege SJ. Influence of holding practice on preterm infant development. *MCN Am J Matern Child Nurs.* 2013;38(3):136-43.

Pepino VC, Mezzacappa MA. Application of tactile/kinesthetic stimulation in preterm infants: a systematic review. *J Pediatr.* 2015;91(3):213-33.

Picheansathian W, Woragidpoonpol P, Baosoung C. Positioning of preterm infants for optimal physiological development: a systematic review. *JBI Libr Syst Rev.* 2009;7(7):224-59.

Pillai Riddell R, Racine N, Turcotte K, et al. Nonpharmacological management of procedural pain in infants and young children: an abridged Cochrane review. *Pain Res Manage.* 2011;16(5):321-30.

Ranger M, Grunau RE. Early repetitive pain in preterm infants in relation to the developing brain. *Pain Manag.* 2014;4(1):57-67.

Rattaz C, Goubet N, Bullinger A. The calming effect of a familiar odor on full-term newborns. *J Dev Behav Pediatr.* 2005;26(2):86-92.

Reynolds LC, Duncan MM, Smith GC, et al. Parental presence and holding in the neonatal intensive care unit and associations with early neurobehavior. *J Perinatol.* 2013;33(8):636-41.

Seifert P, Hickman DS. Enhancing patient safety in a healing environment. *Topics in Advanced Practice Nursing eJournal.* 2005;5(1). Available from http://www.medscape.com/viewarticle/499690.

Short MA, Brooks-Brunn JA, Reeves DS, Yeager J, Thorpe JA. The effects of swaddling versus standard positioning on neuromuscular development in very low birth weight infants. *Neonatal Netw.* 1996;15(4):25-31.

Smith GC, Gutovich J, Smyser C, et al. Neonatal intensive care unit stress is associated with brain development in preterm infants. *Ann Neurol.* 2011;70(4):541-9.

Standley J. Music therapy research in the NICU: an updated meta-analysis. *Neonatal Netw.* 2012;31(5):311-6.

Stevens B, Yamada J, Lee GY, Ohlsson A. Sucrose for analgesia in newborn infants undergoing painful procedures. *Cochrane Database Syst Rev.* 2013;1:CD001069.

Sweeney JK, Gutierrez T. Musculoskeletal implications of preterm infant positioning in the NICU. *J Perinat Neonatal Nurs.* 2002;16(1):58-70.

Task Force on Sudden Infant Death Syndrome. SIDS and other sleep-related infant deaths: expansion of recommendations for a safe infant sleeping environment. *Pediatrics.* 2011;128(5):1030-9.

Treyvaud K, Lee KJ, Doyle LW, Anderson PJ. Very preterm birth influences parental mental health and family outcomes seven years after birth. *J Pediatr.* 2014;164(3):515-21.

Turnage-Carrier C, McLane KM, Gregurich MA. Interface pressure comparison of healthy premature infants with various neonatal bed surfaces. *Adv Neonatal Care.* 2008;8(3):176-84.

Vaivre-Douret L, Ennouri K, Jrad I, Garrec C, Papiernik E. Effect of positioning on the incidence of abnormalities of muscle tone in low-risk, preterm infants. *Eur J Paediatr Neurol.* 2004;8(1):21-34.

Vergara E, Bigsby R, eds. *Developmental and Therapeutic Interventions in the NICU.* Baltimore: Paul H. Brooks; 2004.

Visscher MO, Lacina L, Casper T, et al. Conformational positioning improves sleep in premature infants with feeding difficulties. *J Pediatr.* 2015;166(1):44-8.

Voos KC, Miller L, Park N, Olsen S. Promoting family-centered care in the NICU through a parent-to-parent manager position. *Adv Neonatal Care.* 2015;15(2):119-24.

Walden M, Gibbins S. *Practice Guideline for Newborn Pain Assessment and Management.* 3rd ed. Glenview, IL: National Association of Neonatal Nurses; 2012.

Walden M, Jorgensen K. Pain assessment and nonpharmacologic management. In: Kenner C, McGrath J, eds. *Developmental Care of Newborns and Infants.* Glenview, IL: National Association of Neonatal Nurses; 2010.

Webb AR, Heller HT, Benson CB, Lahav A. Mother's voice and heartbeat sounds elicit auditory plasticity in the human brain before full gestation. *Proc Nat Acad Sci USA.* 2015;112(10):3152-7.

White RD, Smith JA, Shepley MM. Recommended standards for newborn ICU design, eighth edition. *J Perinatol.* 2013;33(Suppl 1):S2-16.

White-Traut RC, Nelson MN, Silvestri JM, et al. Effect of auditory, tactile, visual, and vestibular intervention on length of stay, alertness, and feeding progression in preterm infants. *Devel Med Child Neurol.* 2002;44(2):91-7.

Long-Term Neurodevelopmental Impairment

Shannon N. Liang, MD • Cynthia E. Rogers, MD
• Christopher D. Smyser, MD, MSCI

SCOPE

DISEASE/CONDITION(S)

Neurodevelopmental impairment in infants born preterm.

GUIDELINE OBJECTIVE(S)

To review the frequency and impact (medical, social, and economic) of and contributors to long-term neurodevelopmental impairment in preterm infants. To discuss methods to predict and improve neurodevelopmental outcomes in these infants. Outcomes in term infants are not addressed in this chapter.

BRIEF BACKGROUND

Prevalence of Neurodevelopmental Impairment

The improved survival rates for preterm infants over the past several decades have not translated into improvements in long-term neurodevelopmental outcomes. Preterm birth remains a leading cause of neurological and neurodevelopmental disabilities worldwide. In the United States alone, the medical costs associated with preterm birth amount to $17 billion per year, with combined costs of medical and social services amounting to more than $26 billion.

Very Preterm Infants (Born <32 Weeks' Gestation)

Infants born at the earliest gestational ages experience the greatest rates of adverse neurodevelopmental sequelae. Impairments include cognitive, language, motor, social, and behavioral disability, with 30–50% of very preterm (VPT) children experiencing impairments across multiple developmental domains. Approximately 10% of VPT infants experience severe deficits associated with functional disability, including cerebral palsy (CP), intellectual disability (IQ <70), and/or severe visual or hearing impairments. Many deficits are identifiable by 2 years of age. Mild to moderate deficits are seen in an additional 30–50% of VPT infants, with some impairments not evident until school age. Table 58.1 provides a summary of the literature regarding the prevalence of neurodevelopmental challenges for VPT infants.

TABLE 58.1. Neurodevelopmental Impairment in Very Preterm Children

Type of Neurodevelopmental or Functional Impairment	Patient Category and Prevalence
Cognitive impairment or intellectual disability	Severe in 10% of VPT infants Mild to moderate in 30–50% of VPT infants >50% of VLBW young adults have an IQ >1 SD below the mean
Cerebral palsy	Severe in 5–15% of VPT infants* Mild to moderate in 30–50% of VPT infants
Visual impairment	Unilateral or bilateral blindness in 1–10% of extremely-low-birthweight infants Mild to moderate in 30–50% of VPT infants
Hearing impairment	Up to 14% in VPT infants (10% require amplification)
Language impairment	20–35% in VPT infants
Impaired school performance	More likely to leave school at an earlier age Less likely to graduate from high school† Less likely to attend college and graduate from 4-year universities
Behavioral and psychiatric problems	Behavioral problems in 25–28% of VPT children Higher rates of subclinical psychiatric symptoms‡ Autism spectrum disorder in 8% of extremely preterm infants ADHD§ in 15–27% of VLBW children Increased risk-taking behaviors (e.g., smoking, drinking alcohol, and drug use) Less likely to establish an independent adult life¶

*The most common form of cerebral palsy is spastic diplegia (40–50%), followed by spastic quadriplegia and hemiplegia.

†56–74% graduated from high school in one study.

‡Social withdrawal, introversion, neuroticism, anxiety, inattention, autistic traits, psychosis, schizophrenia, and mood disorders.

§Mainly symptoms of inattention.

¶Including leaving their parental home, cohabiting with partners, and having children.

ADHD, attention deficit hyperactivity disorder; VLBW, very low birthweight; VPT, very preterm.

TABLE 58.2. Neurodevelopmental Impairment in Moderate-to-Late Preterm Children

Type of Neurodevelopmental or Functional Impairment	Risk in Moderate-to-Late Preterm Infants
Cognitive, language, and social impairments	Up to 2 × risk
Cerebral palsy and/or motor delays	2–3 × risk
Impaired school performance	Worse school performance, commonly with reading and writing 71% of moderate-preterm achieve below expected grade level 36% of late-preterm achieve below expected grade level
Behavioral and psychiatric problems	Mixed evidence—some reports of increased rates of psychiatric disorders (particularly anxiety) during childhood, while other reports find this risk is not present by adulthood

Moderate and Late Preterm Infants (Born at 32–36 Weeks' Gestation)

Approximately 75% of preterm births include infants born between 32 and 36 weeks' gestation, accounting for ~8% of all live births. It is estimated that late preterm infants account for 20–25% of neonatal intensive care unit (NICU) admissions, but many are observed in special care or normal newborn nursery settings. Compared to full-term infants, moderate-to-late preterm infants have higher morbidity, including temperature instability, hypoglycemia, hyperbilirubinemia, respiratory distress, apnea, infection, poor feeding, and inadequate nutrition. While a majority of the literature focuses on neurodevelopmental outcomes of VPT infants, there is also growing evidence regarding the increased risk for adverse neurodevelopmental outcomes among moderate and late preterm infants. There seems to be a gradient of risk, with a greater proportion of preterm infants born at later gestational ages within this group facing milder and/or more subtle symptoms, as summarized in Table 58.2.

Common Causes of Impaired Neurodevelopmental Outcomes

Brain Injury

Intraventricular Hemorrhage and Post-Hemorrhagic Hydrocephalus. It is estimated that the lifetime cost of care for those with intraventricular hemorrhage (IVH) in the United States is $4 billion. IVH increases the risk for developmental delay, intellectual disability, CP, post-hemorrhagic hydrocephalus (PHH), and seizures, with the nature and prevalence of these morbidities related to hemorrhage location and severity (Figure 58.1). About 10–15% of very low birthweight (VLBW) infants develop severe IVH (grades III/IV with ventricular dilation), and of these, >75% have CP and/or intellectual disability. The risk of CP increases two- to sixfold in the setting of grade III/IV IVH. In addition, ~10% of all premature infants with IVH develop epilepsy. However, for low-grade IVH (grades I and II without ventricular dilation), the data are mixed as to whether the IVH is an independent risk factor for long-term neurodevelopmental sequelae.

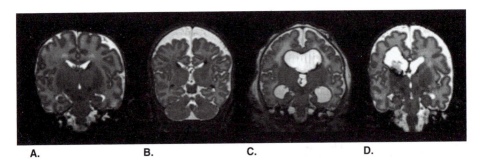

A.   B.   C.   D.

FIGURE 58.1. • Intraventricular hemorrhage. High-resolution coronal T2-weighted MR images demonstrating progressively severe forms of intraventricular hemorrhage using criteria defined according to Papile. **A.** Grade I, defined as germinal matrix hemorrhage. **B.** Grade II, defined as intraventricular hemorrhage without ventricular dilatation. **C.** Grade III, defined as intraventricular hemorrhage with ventricular dilatation. **D.** Grade IV, defined as intraventricular hemorrhage with extension into the surrounding brain parenchyma.

PHH is associated with increased rates of seizures, as well as motor, cognitive, and visual disabilities, correlating with the severity of associated parenchymal injury. While shunt surgery may be associated with reduced risk of mortality, morbidity is not affected by shunt placement.

White Matter Injury. White matter injury (WMI) (Figure 58.2) is more predictive of later neurodevelopmental impairments than gestational age or other perinatal risk factors. About 25–50% of VLBW infants suffer WMI. The most common form

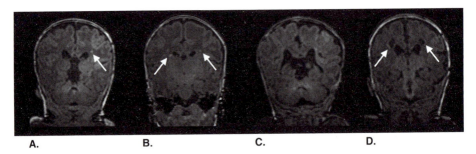

A.   B.   C.   D.

FIGURE 58.2. • White matter injury. High-resolution coronal T1-weighted MR images demonstrating progressively severe forms of white matter injury. **A.** Grade I white matter injury was defined by the presence of punctate lesions ≤3 mm in size in the periventricular white matter on either or both of the T1/T2-weighted images. **B.** Grade II PVL was distinguished from grade I by the presence of lesions in bilateral corticospinal tracts or, more extensively, with ≥3 lesions per hemisphere. **C.** Grade III PVL was defined as the presence of extensive lesions along the wall of the lateral ventricles with high signal on T1-weighted images. **D.** Grade IV PVL was defined as the presence of cystic lesions in periventricular white matter. Arrows denote focal areas of injury.

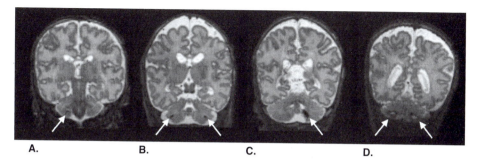

A. **B.** **C.** **D.**

FIGURE 58.3. • Cerebellar hemorrhage. High-resolution coronal T2-weighted MR images demonstrating progressively severe forms of cerebellar injury. **A.** Grade I is defined as unilateral punctate lesions ≤3 mm in size. **B.** Grade II is classified by the presence of bilateral punctate lesions (≤3 mm in size). **C.** Grade III is distinguished by the presence of a unilateral lesion >3 mm in size. **D.** Grade IV is identified by bilateral lesions >3 mm in size. Arrows denote focal areas of injury.

of WMI is noncystic periventricular leukomalacia (PVL), which has been shown to affect cognitive more than motor outcomes. In one recent study, the risk of intellectual disability at school age was 28% with mild PVL and 77% with severe PVL. A rare (~5%), but severe form of WMI is cystic PVL, which is strongly associated with motor disability. Cystic PVL typically presents with spastic diplegia, as the pattern of injury incorporates the corticospinal tracts, which control lower extremity movements. The risk for CP increases three- to tenfold with cystic PVL; 90% with severe PVL develop CP, while 50% with mild PVL develop CP. In addition, behavioral problems are seen in one-third of children with PVL. WMI is also associated with increased rates of visual and cognitive impairments at school age, including intelligence, language, and executive functioning.

Cerebellar Injury. Cerebellar injury (Figure 58.3) can arise from destructive lesions such as infarction and hemorrhage, or from primary underdevelopment. It most commonly occurs in the inferior cerebellar artery distribution, affecting the ventral posterior lobes and inferior vermis. In VPT infants, the rate of cerebellar hemorrhage is reported to be between 7% and 19%. Cerebellar lesions are often associated with supratentorial injury, such as IVH or PVL, so determining neurodevelopmental impairments attributable to cerebellar injury is often confounded. About two-thirds of infants with cerebellar injury have neurologic abnormalities, including cognitive, language, behavioral, socialization, and motor impairments. Rates of cognitive impairment are as high as 40–45% in isolated cerebellar injury, possibly related to subsequent cerebral atrophy, and is associated with attention and learning problems. Language impairments (receptive and expressive) occur in ~40% of former preterm infants with isolated cerebellar injury. Also, motor delays are seen in about half of former VPT infants with cerebellar injury. However, rates of CP are not as high (5–10%), with affected children manifesting a mixed pattern including spasticity, dystonia, and ataxia. In addition, one-third of those with cerebellar injury show autism spectrum disorder symptoms.

Other Factors Contributing to Neurodevelopmental Impairment. In addition to brain injury, there are many other clinical variables which can influence brain development and contribute to adverse neurodevelopmental outcomes. Preterm infants have been shown to be susceptible to the effects of noxious exposures (e.g., pharmacology, stress, pain), the physical environment, other environmental exposures, and nutrition status.

RECOMMENDATIONS

Care of preterm infants managed in the NICU should include meticulous evidence-based clinical practices (described elsewhere in this textbook) to prevent the common forms of brain injury described above and mitigate the resulting deleterious neurodevelopmental effects. Serial, detailed medical and neurological examinations will prove valuable in identification of infants at risk for adverse neurodevelopmental outcomes. Motor, language, social, and cognitive development are interrelated and hinge upon the basic senses of vision, hearing, and touch—thus hearing and vision must be evaluated early. Neuroimaging, including head ultrasound (HUS) and brain magnetic resonance imaging (MRI) studies, provides valuable prognostic information regarding the presence and severity of brain injury that increases risk for adverse neurological outcomes. In addition, general interventions targeted toward improving neurodevelopmental outcomes, such as developmental care and therapy services, should be implemented. Further, throughout the hospitalization, parents of high-risk infants should receive education regarding typical developmental progress and risks for neurodevelopmental challenges according to the clinical picture. Finally, particularly toward discharge, infants at risk for impaired neurodevelopmental outcome should be identified so that indicated supportive services and early intervention programs can be initiated and caregivers can receive appropriate education.

PRACTICE OPTIONS: INTERVENTIONS TO IMPROVE OUTCOMES

Practice Option #1: Developmental Care

As detailed, infants in the NICU are at risk for various neurodevelopmental delays, and developmental care interventions starting in the hospital may improve outcomes. The goal should be to reduce stress (limiting pain), control external stimuli (noise), cluster care, promote flexion positioning, and involve parents in care, as these interventions may benefit cognitive and psychomotor development. Encouraging an emotional connection and calming cycle routine between the parent and infant includes interventions such as skin-to-skin contact, sustained eye contact, and vocalizations. Generally, developmental care including nurturing interactions and stress minimization may positively impact neurodevelopment, though long-term evidence is not available.

Practice Option #2: Early Initiation of Therapies

Understanding the neurodevelopmental risks faced by preterm children, as detailed above, is important in initiating appropriate therapies to minimize potential sequelae. When medically stable, infants in the NICU should receive physical, occupational, and speech therapies. Physical and occupational therapies can address tone abnormalities, range of motion, and positioning. Critically ill neonates may develop a head turn preference, usually to the right due to convention of bedside care, and increased severity of the head turn may be a marker for poor developmental outcome. Proper positioning can also promote flexion of extremities and minimize plagiocephaly. Speech therapy can promote oral-motor and feeding skills, frequently critical for graduating from the NICU. There is evidence that sensory–motor–oral stimulation with nonnutritive sucking in VPT infants can shorten the time to independent oral feeding and also shorten the length of hospitalization. Finally, given the higher risks for neurosensory impairment, hearing and vision screens should be universally performed prior to discharge.

Practice Option #3: Optimal Nutrition

In order to leverage the plasticity of the developing neonatal brain, ensuring optimal nutrition to provide necessary substrates is critical. Weight gain, linear growth, and head circumference are markers of nutritional status, and have been associated with long-term neurodevelopment. Thus, growth parameters should be followed, and nutrition optimized (including fortification of formula or breast milk) for appropriate weight and head circumference growth. Essential fatty acids, particularly the long-chain polyunsaturated fatty acids, are important for the developing fetal and postnatal brain. Also, docosahexaenoic acid (DHA), an omega 3 fatty acid, may be beneficial for visual or cognitive development.

Practice Option #4: Neurodevelopmental Follow-Up

All preterm infants should be followed after nursery discharge by medical providers who can evaluate their developmental progress at regular intervals. This could include newborn medicine, developmental pediatrics, neurology, physiatry, child psychiatry/psychology, and/or therapists based upon available local resources. In the first years of life, developmental follow-up should occur every 3–6 months at minimum. Hearing and vision should also be regularly evaluated, more frequently if there are concerns. Subsequent visits may occur at wider-spaced intervals pending the individual developmental needs of the child, which may evolve over time. In this way, mild and/or emerging developmental challenges may be identified early, and appropriate interventions can be initiated proactively.

Practice Option #5: Early Intervention/Therapy Services

All preterm infants are at risk for neurodevelopmental challenges and should be evaluated for and receive appropriate early intervention services following nursery discharge. These services can be provided through state early intervention programs, local hospitals, and/or private therapy companies. Services may include physical, occupational, speech, vision, and feeding therapies, as well as hearing aids if impaired.

PRACTICE OPTIONS: CLASSIFICATION OF RISK AND NEURODEVELOPMENTAL OUTCOME PREDICTION

Practice Option #6: Neurological Examination

A detailed neurological examination in the NICU may assist in identifying infants at risk for neurodevelopmental delays. First described in 1990, the Prechtl General Movement Assessment has been evaluated as a tool to identify infants at risk for motor and cognitive impairments. Using this tool, preterm infants are typically more hyperexcitable and have less flexor tone than age-matched term infants. Abnormalities in the quality of spontaneous movements have been associated with later motor impairments. For example, persistent cramped, synchronized movements which lack fluidity may predict CP. Asymmetry of limb movements or reflexes may be associated with brain injury, such as neonatal stroke, intracranial hemorrhage, or WMI. However, in the neonatal period, infants with focal CNS injuries often have symmetric examinations. A disorganized sucking pattern and/or swallowing problems occur in about 35–50% of neonates with brain injuries and can predict poor neurodevelopmental outcomes.

Practice Option #7: Cranial Imaging: Ultrasonography and Magnetic Resonance Imaging

HUS is a low-cost screening tool to evaluate for brain injury in neonates at the bedside. HUS can elucidate ventriculomegaly, IVH, hemorrhage, and sometimes ischemic stroke, with most institutions having guidelines detailing the frequency at which HUS studies should be performed (detailed elsewhere in this textbook). However, there are inherent limitations in the type and level of detail of information that can be obtained. In contrast, MRI provides greater ability to assess brain development, including key variables such as cortical folding and early myelination, while providing increased sensitivity and specificity for detecting brain injury. Unlike HUS, MRI typically requires transportation to a scanner outside the NICU, which adds additional risk for critically ill infants. However, clinical practice and research demonstrate these studies can be performed safely and effectively in non-sedated infants with limited specialized equipment.

Brain MRIs at term-equivalence may help to predict neurodevelopmental outcomes in childhood although the utility of routine MRI imaging of VPT infants is questionable. CP is strongly associated with white matter volume loss, cystic lesions, delayed myelination, and parenchymal lesions. In addition, white matter abnormalities are associated with cognitive delay, language delay, and significant motor impairment. In contrast, larger total brain tissue, white matter, and cerebellar volumes on brain MRI at term-equivalence are associated with better cognitive and language development. With respect to gray matter development, delayed cortical folding and enlarged extra-axial spaces are seen in one-third to one-half of brain MRIs of VPT infants. Infants with cortical gray matter abnormalities demonstrate lower cognitive and motor development, with increased rates of CP at 24 months. Deep gray matter injury, involving reduced basal ganglia and thalamic size, may be associated with impaired learning, attention, and memory. Decreased cerebellar size is seen in more than 50% of VPT infants at term-equivalence, with cerebellar lesions in 20% of these infants. Cerebellar lesions are usually unilateral, hemispheric, and coincident with supratentorial lesions including IVH. Injury confined to the cerebellar hemispheres is associated with cognitive disability, while injury to the cerebellar vermis is associated with motor delays as well as global developmental deficits. Interestingly, isolated small punctate cerebellar lesions have not been associated with cognitive impairment.

CLINICAL ALGORITHM(S)

With any preterm child, the goal is to maximize their neurodevelopmental outcome and minimize morbidity. During the nursery course, perform regular medical and neurological examinations and neuroimaging studies (e.g., HUS and brain MRI) per institutional guidelines to identify high-risk infants. Developmental care, therapy services, and optimized nutrition should be initiated early in the nursery course for all infants, followed by regular evaluation of the evolving needs of each child in coordination with the multidisciplinary team caring for each infant. Following discharge, ensure that each child undergoes interval developmental assessments, receives early intervention services if indicated, and follows with appropriate specialty services, including neurology, psychiatry/psychology, physiatry, audiology, and/or ophthalmology.

IMPLEMENTATION OF GUIDELINE

DESCRIPTION OF IMPLEMENTATION STRATEGY

Gather community resources and create a multidisciplinary team of medical providers and therapists who understand the psychosocial and medical complexities of caring for preterm children. Empower caretakers to promote developmental growth and advocate for their child.

SUMMARY

Despite improving survival rates, VPT infants continue to demonstrate increased rates of neurodevelopmental disability across domains, including cognitive, motor, language, hearing, vision, behavioral, and psychiatric deficits. More recently, moderate-to-late preterm infants have also been increasingly recognized to face neurodevelopmental challenges, most notably with cognitive impairments and poor school performance. Our understanding of the scope and scale of these deficits continues to grow and evolve. Increasing numbers of tools such as MRI are now available to better identify children at risk for adverse outcomes. Similarly, attention is focused on interventions designed to optimize developmental outcomes in this population, including minimizing infant stress through family-based interventions and developmental care strategies, early initiation of therapies, and optimal nutrition. All considered, while preterm infants remain at risk for adverse neurodevelopmental outcomes, a multidisciplinary approach which recognizes these challenges and successfully utilizes appropriate tools and interventions remains fundamental to allowing each infant to realize their neurodevelopmental potential.

BIBLIOGRAPHIC SOURCE(S)

Allen MC. Neurodevelopmental outcomes of preterm infants. *Curr Opin Neurol.* 2008;21:123-6.

Anderson PJ, Cheong JLY, Thompson DK. The predictive validity of neonatal MRI for neurodevelopmental outcome in very preterm children. *Sem Perinatol.* 2015;39:147-58.

Arpino C, Compagnone E, Montanaro ML. Preterm birth and neurodevelopmental outcome: a review. *Childs Nerv Syst.* 2010;26:1139-49.

Aylward GP. Cognitive and neuropsychological outcomes: more than IQ scores. *Ment Retard Dev Disabil Res Rev.* 2002;8:234-40.

Bhutta AT, Cleves MA, Casey PH, et al. Cognitive and behavioral outcomes of school-aged children who were born preterm: a meta-analysis. *JAMA.* 2002;288:728-37.

Brossard-Racine M, du Plessis AJ, Limperopoulos C. Developmental cerebellar cognitive affective syndrome in ex-preterm survivors following cerebellar injury. *Cerebellum.* 2015;14:151-64.

Chan E, Quigley MA. School performance at age 7 years in late preterm and early term birth: a cohort study. *Arch Dis Child Fetal Neonatal Ed.* 2014;99:F451-7.

Cheong JL, Thompson DK, Spittle AJ, et al. Brain volumes at term-equivalent age are associated with 2-year neurodevelopment in moderate and late preterm children. *J Pediatr.* 2016;174:91-7.

Choi JY, Rha DW, Park ES. The effects of the severity of periventricular leukomalacia on the neuropsychological outcomes of preterm children. *J Child Neurol.* 2016;31:603-12.

De Schuymer L, De Groote I, Beyers W, et al. Preverbal skills as mediators for language outcome in preterm and full term children. *Early Hum Devel.* 2011;87:265-72.

Dunsirn S, Smyser C, Liao S, et al. Defining the nature and implications of head turn preference in the preterm infant. *Early Hum Dev.* 2016;96:53-8.

Einspieler C, Prechtl HF. Prechtl's assessment of general movements: a diagnostic tool for the functional assessment of the young nervous system. *Ment Retard Dev Disabil Res Rev.* 2005;11:61-7.

Fazzi E, Bova S, Giovenzana A, et al. Cognitive visual dysfunctions in preterm children with periventricular leukomalacia. *Dev Med Child Neurol.* 2009;51:974-81.

Ferrari F, Cioni G, Einspieler C, et al. Cramped synchronized general movements in preterm infants as an early marker for cerebral palsy. *Arch Pediatr Adolesc Med.* 2002;156:460-7.

Fucile S, Gisel E, Lau C. Oral stimulation accelerates the transition from tube to oral feeding in preterm infants. *J Pediatr.* 2002;141:230-6.

Futagi Y, Toribe Y, Ogawa K, et al. Neurodevelopmental outcome in children with intraventricular hemorrhage. *Pediatr Neurol.* 2006;34:219-24.

Guarini A, Sansavini A, Fabbri C, et al. Reconsidering the impact of preterm birth on language outcome. *Early Hum Devel.* 2009;85:639-45.

Hack M. Adult outcomes of preterm children. *J Dev Behav Pediatr.* 2009;30:460-70.

Hane AA, Myers MM, Hofer MA, et al. Family nurture intervention improves the quality of maternal caregiving in the neonatal intensive care unit: evidence from a randomized controlled trial. *J Dev Behav Pediatr.* 2015;36:188-96.

Heinonen K, Kajantie E, Pesonen A-K, et al. Common mental disorders in young adults born late-preterm. *Psychol Med.* 2016;46:2227-38.

Himpens E, van den Broeck C, Ocastra A, et al. Prevalence, type, distribution and severity of cerebral palsy in relation to gestational age: a meta-analytic review. *Dev Med Child Neurol.* 2008;50:334-40.

Hutchinson EA, De Luca CR, Doyle LW, et al. School-age outcomes of extremely preterm or extremely low birth weight children. *Pediatrics.* 2013;131:e1053-61.

Institute of Medicine of the National Academies. Preterm birth: causes, consequences, and prevention. 2007. Available at http://www.nap.edu/catalog/11622.html.

Johnson S, Evans TA, Draper ES, et al. Neurodevelopmental outcomes following late and moderate prematurity: a population-based cohort study. *Arch Dis Child Fetal Neonatal Ed.* 2015;100:F301-8.

Johnson S, Hollis C, Kochhar P, et al. Psychiatric disorders in extremely preterm children: longitudinal finding at age 11 years in the EPICure study. *J Am Acad Child Adolesc Psych.* 2010;49:453-63.

Kajantie E, Hovi P, Räikkönen K, et al. Young adults with very low birth weight: leaving the parental home and sexual relationships—Helsinki study of very low birth weight adults. *Pediatrics.* 2008;122:e62-72.

Kerstjens JM, de Winter AF, Bocca-Tjeertes IF, et al. Developmental delay in moderately preterm-born children at school entry. *J Pediatr.* 2011;159:92-8.

Kidokoro H, Neil JJ, Inder TE. New MR imaging assessment tool to define brain abnormalities in very preterm infants at term. *Am J Neuroradiol.* 2013;34:2208-14.

Latal B. Prediction of neurodevelopmental outcome after preterm birth. *Pediatr Neurol.* 2009;40:413-9.

Limperopoulos C, Bassan H, Gauvreau K, et al. Does cerebellar injury in premature infants contribute to the high prevalence of long-term cognitive, learning, and behavioral disability in survivors? *Pediatrics.* 2007;120:584-93.

Lohaugen GC, Gramstad A, Evensen KA. Cognitive profile in young adults born preterm at very low birthweight. *Dev Med Child Neurol.* 2010;52:1133-8.

Lund LK, Vik T, Lydersen S, et al. Mental health, quality of life and social relations in young adults born with low birth weight. *Health Qual Life Outcomes.* 2012;10:146-55.

Lund LK, Vik T, Skranes J, et al. Low birth weight and psychiatric morbidity; stability and change between adolescence and young adulthood. *Early Hum Devel.* 2012;88:623-9.

Luu TM, Ment LR, Schneider KC, et al. Lasting effects of preterm birth and neonatal brain hemorrhage at 12 years of age. *Pediatrics.* 2009;123:1037-44.

Mathur AM, Neil JJ, McKinstry RC, et al. Transport, monitoring, and successful brain MR imaging in unsedated neonates. *Pediatr Radiol.* 2008;38:260-4.

McCrea HJ, Ment LR. The diagnosis, management, and postnatal prevention of intraventricular hemorrhage in the preterm neonate. *Clin Perinatol.* 2008;35:777–92.

McGowan JE, Alderdice FA, Holmes VA, et al. Early childhood development in late-preterm infants: a systematic review. *Pediatrics.* 2011;127:1111-24.

Miller SP, Ferriero DM, Leonard C, et al. Early brain injury in premature newborns detected with magnetic resonance imaging is associated with adverse early neurodevelopmental outcome. *J Pediatr.* 2005;147:609-16.

Mirmiran M, Barnes PD, Keller K, et al. Neonatal brain magnetic resonance imaging before discharge is better than serial cranial ultrasound in predicting cerebral palsy in very low birth weight preterm infants. *Pediatrics.* 2004;114:992-8.

Montirosso R, Del Prete A, Bellù R, et al. Level of NICU quality of developmental care and neurobehavioral performance in very preterm infants. *Pediatrics.* 2012;129:e1129-37.

Moster D, Terje Lie R, Markestad T. Longterm medical and social consequences of preterm birth. *N Engl J Med.* 2008;359(3):262–73.

Murray AL, Scratch SE, Thompson DK, et al. Neonatal brain pathology predicts adverse attention and processing speed outcomes in very preterm and/or very low birth weight children. *Neuropsychology.* 2014;28:552-62.

Ohlsson A, Jacobs SE. NIDCAP: a systematic review and meta-analyses of randomized controlled trials. *Pediatrics.* 2013;131:e881-93.

Omizzolo C, Scratch SE, Stargatt R, et al. Neonatal brain abnormalities and memory and learning outcomes at 7 years in children born very preterm. *Memory.* 2014;22:605-15.

Patra K, Wilson-Costello D, Taylor G, et al. Grades I-II intraventricular hemorrhage in extremely low birth weight infants: effects on neurodevelopment. *J Pediatr.* 2006;149:169-73.

Pavlova MA, Krägeloh-Mann I. Limitations on the developing preterm brain: impact of periventricular white matter lesions on brain connectivity and cognition. *Brain.* 2013;136:998-1011.

Petrini JR, Dias T, McCormick MC, et al. Increased risk of adverse neurological development for late preterm infants. *J Pediatr.* 2009;154:169-76.

Radic JAE, Vincer M, McNeely PD. Outcomes of intraventricular hemorrhage and posthemorrhagic hydrocephalus in a population-based cohort of very preterm infants born to residents of Nova Scotia from 1993 to 2010. *J Neurosurg Pediatr.* 2015;15:580-8.

Raju TNK, Pemberton VL, Saigal S, et al. Long-term health outcomes of preterm birth: an executive summary of a conference sponsored by the National Institutes of Health. *J Pediatr.* 2017;181:309-18.

Rocha AD, Lopes Moreira ME, Pimenta HP, et al. A randomized study of the efficacy of sensory-motor-oral stimulation and non-nutritive sucking in very low birthweight infant. *Early Hum Dev.* 2007;83:385-8.

Rogers CE, Lenze SN, Luby JL. Late preterm birth, maternal depression, and risk of preschool psychiatric disorders. *J Am Acad Child Adolesc Psych.* 2013;52:309-18.

Saidkasimova S, Bennett DM, Butler S, et al. Cognitive visual impairment with good visual acuity in children with posterior periventricular white matter injury: a series of 7 cases. *J AAPOS.* 2007;11:426-30.

Sansavini A, Guarini A, Justice LM, et al. Does preterm birth increase a child's risk for language impairment? *Early Hum Devel.* 2010;86:765-72.

Sansavini A, Guarini A, Savini S, et al. Longitudinal trajectories of gestural and linguistic abilities in very preterm infants in the second year of life. *Neuropsychology.* 2011;49:3677-88.

Seitz J, Jenni OG, Molinari L, et al. Correlations between motor performance and cognitive functions in children born <1250 g at school age. *Neuropediatrics.* 2006;37:6-12.

Sherlock RL, Anderson PJ, Doyle LW, et al. Neurodevelopmental sequelae of intraventricular haemorrhage at 8 years of age in a regional cohort of ELBW/very preterm infants. *Early Hum Devel.* 2005;81:909-16.

Slattery J, Morgan A, Douglas J. Early sucking and swallowing problems as predictors of neuro-developmental outcome in children with neonatal brain injury: a systematic review. *Dev Med Child Neurol.* 2012;54(9):796-806.

Spittle AJ, Cheong J, Doyle LW, et al. Neonatal white matter abnormality predicts childhood motor impairment in very preterm children. *Dev Med Child Neurol.* 2011;53:1000-6.

Stephens BE, Vohr. Neurodevelopmental outcome of the premature infant. *Pediatr Clin North Am.* 2009;56:631-46.

Thompson DK, Thai D, Kelly CE, et al. Alterations in the optic radiations of very preterm children-perinatal predictors and relationships with visual outcomes. *Neuroimage Clin.* 2013;4:145-53.

Valkama AM, Paakko ELE, Vainionppa LK, et al. Magnetic resonance imaging at term and neuro-motor outcome in preterm infants. *Acta Paediatr.* 2000;89:348-55.

Vohr BR. Neurodevelopmental outcomes of extremely preterm infants. *Clin Perinatol.* 2014;41:241-55.

Volpe JJ. Cerebellum of the premature infant: rapidly developing, vulnerable, clinically important. *J. Child Neurol.* 2009;24(9):1085-104.

Wallin L, Eriksson M. Newborn individual development care and assessment program (NIDCAP): a systematic review of the literature. *Worldviews Evid Based Nurs.* 2009;6:54-69.

Woodward LJ, Anderson PJ, Austin NC, Howard K, Inder TE. Neonatal MRI to predict neurode-velopmental outcomes in preterm infants. *N Engl J Med.* 2006;355:685-94.

Woodward LJ, Clark CAC, Bora S, Inder TE. Neonatal white matter abnormalities an important predictor of neurocognitive outcome for very preterm children. *PLoS One.* 2012;7(12):9.

Woodward LJ, Moor S, Hood KM, et al. Very preterm children show impairments across multiple neurodevelopmental domains by age 4 years. *Arch Dis Child Fetal Neonatal Ed.* 2009;94:F339-44.

Wy PA, Rettiganti M, Li J, et al. Impact of intraventricular hemorrhage on cognitive and behavioral outcomes at 18 years of age in low birth weight preterm infants. *J Perinatol.* 2015;35:511-5.

Zayek MM, Benjamin JT, Maertens P. Cerebellar hemorrhage: a major morbidity in extremely preterm infants. *J Perinatol.* 2012;32:699-704.

Renal Issues

Acute Renal Failure

Grant J. Shafer, MD, MA, FAAP • Poyyapakkam R. Srivaths, MD, MS, FAAP
• Gautham K. Suresh, MD, DM, MS, FAAP

SCOPE

DISEASE/CONDITION(S)

Acute kidney injury (AKI) in neonates.

GUIDELINE OBJECTIVE(S)

Review the definition, risk factors, pathogenesis, clinical symptoms, diagnosis, outcomes, and clinical management of neonatal AKI.

BRIEF BACKGROUND

AKI is a challenging and frequent condition in the neonatal intensive care unit (NICU).

While the definition of AKI in the neonate is controversial, one or more of the following indicate the presence of AKI: an elevated serum creatinine (SCr) for gestational age, an increase in SCr to 1.5 times the baseline value or higher, an increase in SCr by 0.3 mg/dL over 48 hours, or decrease in urine output (UOP). It should be noted that SCr has limitations as a biomarker for AKI including a 48- to 72-hour lag in rise after injury to the kidneys, presence of maternal creatinine at birth, and varying degrees of reabsorption in the proximal renal tubules. Research to identify other biomarkers for AKI is ongoing, but SCr remains the best accepted criterion at present. Table 59.1 lists the complete criteria for diagnosis of neonatal AKI.

The incidence of AKI varies depending on the definition applied as well as the characteristics of the study population, but ranges from 18% to 48% in recent studies.

AKI can be classified as prerenal due to inadequate renal perfusion, intrinsic due to intrarenal pathology, and postrenal due to obstructed urinary flow. Prerenal AKI

TABLE 59.1. Proposed Neonatal AKI Definition Modifications from KDIGO Pediatric AKI Definition Using Scr and Urine Output Criteria

Stage	Serum Creatinine Criteria (in mg/dL)			Urine Output Criteria (in mL/kg/h)*		
	Pediatric Definition	Neonatal Modification 2012	Neonatal Modification 2015–2016	Pediatric Definition	Neonatal Modification 2013	Neonatal Modification 2016
1	≥0.3 rise within 48 h or ≥1.5–1.9 × rise from baseline[†] within 7 days	≥0.3 rise or ≥1.5–1.9 × rise from baseline (defined as previous lowest/trough value)	>0.3 rise within 48 h or >1.5–1.9 × rise from baseline (previous lowest value) within 7 days	<0.5 for 8 h	<1.5 for 24 h	<1 for 24 h
2	≥2–2.9 × rise from baseline	Unchanged	Unchanged	<0.5 for ≥16 h	<1 for 24 h	≤0.5 for 24 h
3	≥3 × rise from baseline or eGFR <35 mL/min per 1.73 m² or RRT initiation	≥3 × rise from baseline or ≥2.5 or RRT initiation	≥3 × rise from baseline or ≥2.5 or RRT initiation	<0.3 for ≥24 h or anuria for ≥12 h	<0.7 for 24 h or anuria for 12 h	≤0.3 for 24 h

*The published Kidney Diseases: Improving Global Outcomes (KDIGO) definition proposes timing cutoffs for low urine output to be ≥6 h for stage 1 (instead of >8 h) and >12 h for stage 2 (instead of 16 h). The pediatric literature to date has consistently utilized urine output decrease timing cutoffs as displayed in the table.

†Baseline SCr: no clear guideline on how to define pediatric baseline SCr. In the literature, baseline SCr has most commonly been defined as the lowest SCr measure in the previous 3 months.

Reprinted from Zappitelli M, Ambalavanan N, Askenazi DJ, et al. Developing a neonatal acute kidney injury research definition: a report from the KIDDK neonatal AKI workshop. Retrieved from https://www.nature.com/articles/pr2017136/tables/1. Copyright 2017 by Springer Nature.

accounts for 75–80% of cases, while intrinsic and postrenal categories comprise 10–15% and 3–5%, respectively.

The neonatal kidney is particularly vulnerable to AKI due to perinatal changes in renal blood flow, reduced glomerular filtration rate (GFR), functional renal tubular immaturity (inability to concentrate urine as well as suboptimal regulation of electrolytes, metabolic waste, and acid–base balance), and large insensible water losses in the neonatal period. Preterm infants are at even higher risk than term infants, as preterm kidneys have incomplete nephronogenesis—a process that is completed around 34–36 weeks' gestation—and the renal tubules are even more functionally immature. This underlying susceptibility along with certain risk factors can lead to AKI. Known risk factors include maternal exposure to angiotensin-converting enzyme (ACE) inhibitors or nonsteroidal anti-inflammatory drugs (NSAIDs), birthweight less than 1500 g, perinatal asphyxia, sepsis, exposure to nephrotoxic medications, treatment with extracorporeal membrane oxygenation (ECMO), and cardiac surgery in the neonatal period. The risk of neonatal AKI increases with decreasing gestation age and birthweight as well as increasing severity of illness.

Neonatal AKI leads to derangements in fluid balance, electrolytes, acid–base status, and to accumulation of metabolic waste products. The clinical presentation is variable. Some neonates have abnormally high SCr in the absence of any clinical manifestations. These asymptomatic infants are often identified due to routine surveillance of at-risk populations. In symptomatic patients, the clinical manifestations are wide-ranging, and can provide important clues to the underlying etiology of the AKI.

Even with prompt recognition and treatment, neonatal AKI is associated with increased mortality as well as longer length of hospital stay. The presence of oliguria or anuria portends a worse outcome, with mortality ranging from 25% to 78%. Patients who survive an episode of neonatal AKI are at higher risk of developing chronic kidney disease (CKD) with progression to renal failure. Therefore, neonates with AKI should be monitored long-term for abnormalities in renal function status and blood pressure.

RECOMMENDATIONS

MAJOR RECOMMENDATIONS

Identification of neonatal AKI depends on recognition of at-risk neonates, evaluation of SCr, and UOP.

Management of neonatal AKI includes treatment of the underlying etiology, and supportive care while waiting for renal function recovery. Treatment of the etiology might include ablation of posterior urethral valves, performance of a nephrostomy to establish an alternate pathway for urinary drainage, fluid repletion, treatment of sepsis, discontinuation of nephrotoxic medication, or strategies to improve cardiac output such as initiation of prostaglandin E1 for ductal-dependent cardiac lesions. Supportive care includes correction of the ensuing fluid imbalance as well as the electrolyte and metabolic derangements, close monitoring, and treatment of complications. In a minority of patients, renal replacement therapy (RRT) might have to be used, despite the technical challenges associated with its application in neonates, and lack of high-quality evidence for it in this age group.

Preventing AKI remains challenging in the neonate; however, there are several strategies to decrease the risk of kidney injury. One is avoiding nephrotoxic medications such as aminoglycosides, vancomycin, amphotericin, and indomethacin whenever possible. If their use is required, then they should be used for the shortest duration required, at the lowest possible dose, and with modification of the treatment regimen based on renal function. Maintaining adequate renal blood flow is also important to help prevent AKI. This includes avoidance of hypovolemia using close monitoring of intake and output with regular adjustments to volume administration as needed. Use of vasoactive medications to maintain adequate blood pressure for renal perfusion in volume-replete patients is important as well.

PRACTICE OPTIONS

Practice Option #1: Diagnosis of AKI and Evaluation for the Underlying Etiology

For neonates at high risk to develop AKI, routine surveillance using SCr is indicated. This includes patients with the following conditions: prenatal diagnosis of hydrops fetalis, hydronephrosis, or other forms of obstructive uropathy, gestational age less than 32 weeks, birth weight less than 1500 g, perinatal asphyxia, treatment with ECMO, congenital heart disease, sepsis, and receipt of total parenteral nutrition. For neonates without risk factors, lack of UOP by 48 hours of life, a sustained decrease in urine volume, or development of edema or hypertension should prompt investigation for AKI. After confirming the presence of AKI, the clinician should undertake a stepwise, comprehensive evaluation to ascertain the underlying etiology.

History. History of maternal exposure to ACE inhibitors (e.g., enalapril) or NSAIDs (e.g., indomethacin), which decrease the GFR in utero increases the likelihood of neonatal AKI. Additionally, polyhydramnios, oligohydramnios, hydronephrosis, or hydrops in utero may be a sign of underlying renal abnormalities. Antenatal imaging and family history should also be examined for abnormalities or familial syndromes which may be the cause of AKI in the neonatal period.

Perinatal asphyxia is an important risk factor for kidney injury, and these patients should be monitored closely for the development of AKI. Postnatal exposure to nephrotoxic medications (aminoglycosides, prostaglandin synthesis inhibitors, amphotericin B, and vancomycin being the most common ones used in the NICU) is another important clue in the history.

A micturition history can be helpful, although it should be noted that normal UOP (>1 mL/kg/h) is present in 13–33% of neonates with AKI. Also, up to 7% of normal newborns will not void in the first 24 hours. For patients with intrinsic AKI, there may be an initial oliguric or anuric phase, followed by a high-output, post-AKI diuresis as the damaged kidneys are unable to appropriately concentrate urine.

The clinician should also evaluate the patient's history for evidence of hypovolemia, including bleeding, diarrhea, increased evaporative losses (e.g., phototherapy, skin compromise, increased skin thinness in extremely premature infants) or a clinical course suggesting impaired cardiac output (e.g., congenital heart disease, myocardial injury, complete heart block) or increased third spacing (e.g., shock or sepsis).

Physical Examination and Vital Signs. Assessment of volume status is important, as either hypovolemia or hypervolemia may be present. Hypotension, tachycardia, weak peripheral pulses or poor perfusion indicates intravascular depletion and a prerenal AKI. Edema indicates fluid overload, generally from intrinsic AKI. Body weight is another important clue for either volume depletion or overload, and should be followed closely. Hypertension (persistent systolic and/or diastolic blood pressure greater than the 95th percentile for gestational age) can be due to either fluid overload or intrinsic renal causes such as renal vasculature disease (thrombosis or stenosis of the renal vasculature).

It is important to assess for other abnormalities on examination that can offer clues to the nature of the AKI. Palpable kidneys should raise suspicion for renal vein thrombosis or severe hydronephrosis. A suprapubic mass indicates a palpable bladder and possible post-renal obstruction to urinary flow. If possible, the urinary stream in males should be observed, as a thin stream, dribbling, or large post-void residual suggests a postrenal obstruction. The presence of dysmorphic features may indicate a syndromic etiology.

Laboratory Investigations. In addition to SCr, other laboratory studies play an important role in AKI. Urinary indices are helpful in differentiating between prerenal and intrinsic AKI. Of the available tests, fractional excretion of sodium (FENa) is the most accepted. It is important to note that the urine sample to calculate a FENa must be obtained prior to fluid or diuretic challenge. FENa is calculated according to the following formula:

$$FENa = \frac{\text{Urine sodium (mEq/L)} \times \text{serum creatinine (mg/dL)}}{\text{Serum sodium (mEq/L)} \times \text{urine creatinine (mg/dL)}} \times 100$$

Cutoffs vary by gestational age as preterm neonates lose more sodium in the urine, but a FENa greater than 3% in term neonates and greater than 6% in preterm neonates indicates intrinsic AKI.

A urinalysis (UA) should also be obtained, as the presence of granular or hyaline casts, red blood cells, protein or tubular cells suggests an intrinsic renal etiology. Of note, the UA for patients who experience perinatal asphyxia will show a transient microscopic hematuria with leukocytes, increased epithelial cells, and low-molecular-weight proteins (such as beta-2 glycoprotein).

Imaging. A renal ultrasound (RUS) should be obtained for all patients with neonatal AKI to evaluate for the presence of kidneys as well as potential structural abnormalities. Concomitant Doppler studies can evaluate for occlusion of the renal vasculature. If the RUS demonstrates bilateral severe hydronephrosis or severe unilateral hydronephrosis in a solitary kidney, the clinician should suspect an obstructive postrenal AKI, which warrants consultation with a pediatric urologist, who may recommend a voiding cystourethrogram.

Practice Option #2: Management of Fluid Balance, Hypertension, and Metabolic Derangements

Fluid Balance. Restoring neutral fluid balance is crucial to successfully treating neonatal AKI. As hypovolemia-induced prerenal AKI is the most common etiology, a fluid challenge can be diagnostic as well as therapeutic. A fluid challenge of 10–20 mL/kg of intravenous isotonic saline should be administered to all neonates with AKI and oliguria except those with clinical evidence of fluid overload such as edema or hypertension. Normal saline is the superior choice compared to colloid administration (e.g., albumin or fresh frozen plasma), which risks protein leakage into the lungs and pulmonary edema.

A positive response to fluid challenge is any UOP in an anuric patient, increase in UOP to greater than 1 mL/kg/h in an oliguric patient, or improvement in the SCr. For patients who respond, the next steps are correction of the fluid deficit followed by replacement of ongoing fluid losses. If the patient does not respond to an initial fluid challenge, it should be repeated as long as the infant does not have clinical signs of volume overload. Persistent lack of response indicates intrinsic AKI.

On the other end of the spectrum, there may be fluid overload in patients with neonatal AKI. Management is with restriction of the patient's fluid intake to insensible losses plus UOP. Daily insensible losses in the neonate vary by birthweight from 15–25 mL/kg/d for neonates greater than 2500 g to 30–60 mL/kg/d for neonates less than 1500 g. In addition, radiant warmers increase insensible losses by 25–100%, and treatment with phototherapy by approximately 20 mL/kg. Continuous monitoring of UOP with appropriate adjustments to the volume of fluid administration is also necessary.

Treatment with loop diuretic therapy (diuretics) is controversial. Studies indicate that diuretics do not alter the natural course of neonatal AKI. The increased UOP seen following diuretic administration reflects enhanced UOP from the remaining functional nephrons without an overall impact on renal status or shortened time to recovery. Treatment with diuretic therapy also increases the risk of ototoxicity. However, patients with fluid overload may benefit from treatment with diuretics to improve fluid status—particularly if decreasing volume overload allows for administration of adequate nutrition. Thus, a trial of diuretic therapy (typically furosemide at a 1- to 2-mg/kg dose) is reasonable to induce diuresis in patients with fluid overload secondary to AKI.

Hypertension. Patients with neonatal AKI have a 10–20% risk of developing hypertension—usually due to fluid overload but can be due to intrinsic renal injury as well. Treatment is with fluid restriction and diuresis, then additional pharmacologic therapy as indicated for persistent hypertension not responsive to the first two measures.

Metabolic Derangements. Electrolyte disturbances are common in patients with neonatal AKI. Two of the most common abnormalities are hyponatremia and hyperkalemia.

Hyponatremia is dilutional from water retention in the setting of diminished UOP. Initial treatment is with free water restriction, which should lead to a gradual normalization of sodium values. Extreme hyponatremia (<120 mEq/L) or the development of neurologic sequelae such as seizure are indications for active replacement of sodium with hypertonic saline using the formula:

$$\text{Sodium required (mEq)} = [\text{sodium desired (mEq/L)} - \text{sodium actual (mEq/L)}] \times \text{body weight (kg)} \times 0.8 \text{ (to account for higher body water in neonates)}$$

In general, the clinician should take care to not increase serum sodium values by more than 0.5 mEq/L/h.

Hyperkalemia is one of the most dangerous complications of neonatal AKI. It is the result of a reduction in GFR and urinary potassium secretion as well as acidosis and immature renal tubular response to aldosterone and cellular breakdown. High serum potassium levels can lead to life-threatening disturbances in cardiac conduction. Electrocardiographic (ECG) abnormalities associated with hyperkalemia include peaked T waves, flattened P waves, increased PR interval, and widening of the QRS complex. A serum potassium value above 7 mEq/L or the presence of ECG changes constitutes a medical emergency and warrants immediate intervention.

The first step is to discontinue all potassium-containing fluids as well as drugs which can worsen hyperkalemia (e.g., indomethacin, ACE-inhibitors and potassium-sparing diuretics). If ECG abnormalities are present, then calcium gluconate should be given. This will help stabilize myocardial excitability, but does not affect serum potassium levels. Therapeutic options to correct hyperkalemia include administration of the following: insulin bolus or drip (accompanied by a glucose bolus or infusion to prevent hypoglycemia), beta-agonist, or cation exchange resin (e.g., Kayexalate). Persistent hyperkalemia despite medical management is an indication for RRT, which is covered in further detail in Practice Option #3.

Unproven Therapies. Two unproven but utilized therapies for neonatal AKI should be addressed. There is currently no evidence to support the use of low-dose dopamine (1–5 µg/kg/min) for renal protective effect in critically ill neonates based on a recent meta-analysis, although its use for hypotension in the neonate remains a supported practice. Also, while recommended by the Kidney Diseases: Improving Global Outcomes (KDIGO) guidelines for neonates who experience perinatal asphyxia, prophylactic administration of theophylline is not supported for patients undergoing therapeutic hypothermia for hypoxic ischemic encephalopathy (HIE).

Practice Option #3: Use of Renal Replacement Therapy

For select groups of neonates with AKI, RRT should be considered. Indications for RRT include severe fluid overload with heart failure or pulmonary edema, inability to provide adequate nutrition due to fluid restriction, or metabolic derangements (e.g., hyponatremia, hypernatremia, hyperkalemia, or acidosis) not responsive to medical management. The purpose of RRT is to provide ultrafiltration (removal of water) as well as clearance (removal of solutes). Options for RRT in the neonate include peritoneal dialysis (PD), hemodialysis (HD), or continuous renal replacement therapy (CRRT), also known as continuous venovenous hemofiltration/dialysis (CVVH/CVVHD).

PD is currently the most common modality for RRT in the neonate. Peritonitis is a common complication. In certain cases, PD may be technically limited by abdominal wall defects, skin infections, or high ultrafiltration requirements. In these cases, CRRT or HD may be used. These modalities pose unique challenges in the neonatal population, as most equipment is designed for larger patients, although systems specifically designed for neonates are currently awaiting trials in the United States. Current CRRT machines in the United States are only approved for patients greater than 20 kg, but have been used off-label in neonates less than 5 kg.

The decision to initiate RRT in a neonate with AKI and minimal expectation for recovery of renal function or severe multisystem organ failure raises a number of ethical considerations. Discussions by a multidisciplinary team including neonatologists, pediatric nephrologists, and other specialists as indicated should occur prior to the initiation of therapy. For patients in whom RRT is being considered, prompt referral to a center with expertise in the management of its various forms is indicated.

CLINICAL ALGORITHM(S)

While not specific to neonates, the KDIGO guidelines offer guidance to the diagnosis and management of AKI with some special considerations noted in regard to neonatal AKI. The KDIGO definitions has been modified for neonates and is available online (https://www.nature.com/articles/pr2017136/tables/1).

Several other international societies have published recommendations on AKI, but these are pediatric based and not specific to the neonate.

IMPLEMENTATION OF GUIDELINE

DESCRIPTION OF IMPLEMENTATION STRATEGY

It is recommended that institutions develop clinical guidelines for the evaluation and management of neonatal AKI. This includes consensus on diagnostic and management strategies as well as guidelines for the use of RRT.

When feasible, neonates with suspected AKI should have a urinary catheter placed to enable accurate measurement of UOP. Fluid intake and output should be closely monitored. The infant should be weighed at least twice a day if stable enough. If the patient's status does not improve with initial supportive measures, or if RRT is likely to be required, consultation from a nephrologist should be obtained. If there is obstructive uropathy or bladder dysfunction (e.g., due to a neural tube defect) consultation from a urologist should be obtained.

QUALITY METRICS

There are currently no published quality metrics regarding neonatal AKI. NICUs should continue to monitor their incidence of neonatal AKI—especially in at-risk populations—as well as morbidity and mortality.

SUMMARY

AKI remains a common clinical problem in the NICU. It increases morbidity, mortality, and risk of long-term renal impairment in neonates. Prompt recognition, targeted therapy toward underlying etiologies, and thoughtful management of the resultant fluid balance, and metabolic derangements are essential.

BIBLIOGRAPHIC SOURCE(S)

Abrahamson DR. Glomerulogenesis in the developing kidney. *Semin Nephrol.* 1991;11(4):375-89.

Agarwal R. Acute renal failure. *AIIMS Protocols in Neonatology.* Delhi, India: CBS Publishers. 2014. http://www.newbornwhocc.org/clinicalproto.html. Accessed August 31, 2018.

Alparslan C, Yavascan O, Bal A, et al. The performance of acute peritoneal dialysis treatment in neonatal period. *Ren Fail.* 2012;34(8):1015-20.

Askenazi DJ, Griffin R, McGwin G, Carlo W, Ambalavanan N. Acute kidney injury is independently associated with mortality in very low birthweight infants: a matched case-control analysis. *Pediatr Nephrol.* 2009;24(5):991-7.

Askenazi DJ, Koralkar R, Hundley HE, Montesanti A, Patil N, Ambalavanan N. Fluid overload and mortality are associated with acute kidney injury in sick near-term/term neonate. *Pediatr Nephrol.* 2013;28(4):661-6.

Auron A, Mhanna MJ. Serum creatinine in very low birth weight infants during their first days of life. *J Perinatol.* 2006;26(12):755-60.

Blinder JJ, Goldstein SL, Lee VV, et al. Congenital heart surgery in infants: effects of acute kidney injury on outcomes. *J Thorac Cardiovasc Surg.* 2012;143(2):368-74.

Coca SG, Singanamala S, Parikh CR. Chronic kidney disease after acute kidney injury: a systematic review and metaanalysis. *Kidney Int.* 2012;81(5):442-8.

Hothi DK. Designing technology to meet the therapeutic demands of acute renal injury in neonates and small infants. *Pediatr Nephrol.* 2014;29(10):1869-71.

Jenik AG, Ceriani Cernadas JM, Gorenstein A, et al. A randomized, double-blind, placebo-controlled trial of the effects of prophylactic theophylline on renal function in term neonates with perinatal asphyxia. *Pediatrics.* 2000;105(4):E45.

Jetton J, Boohaker L, Sethi S, et al. Incidence and outcomes of neonatal acute kidney injury (AWAKEN): a multicentre, multinational, observational cohort study. *Lancet Child Adolesc Health.* 2017;1(3):184-94.

Kaddourah A, Goldstein SL. Renal replacement therapy in neonates. *Clin Perinatol.* 2014;41(3):517-27.

Kellum JA, M Decker J. Use of dopamine in acute renal failure: a meta-analysis. *Crit Care Med.* 2001;29(8):1526-31.

Kidney Diseases: Improving Global Outcomes (KDIGO) Acute Kidney Injury Work Group. KDIGO clinical practice guideline for acute kidney injury. *Kidney Int Suppl.* 2012;2(1):1-138.

Koralkar R, Ambalavanan N, Levitan EB, McGwin G, Goldstein S, Askenazi D. Acute kidney injury reduces survival in very low birth weight infants. *Pediatr Res.* 2011;69(4):354-8.

Mattoo T. Neonatal acute kidney injury: evaluation, management and prognosis. In: Post TW, ed. Waltham, MA: UpToDate; 2017.

Mattoo T. Neonatal acute kidney injury: pathogenesis, etiology, clinical presentation and diagnosis. In: Post TW, ed. Waltham, MA: UpToDate; 2017.

Miall LS, Henderson MJ, Turner AJ, et al. Plasma creatinine rises dramatically in the first 48 hours of life in preterm infants. *Pediatrics.* 1999;104(6):e76.

Moghal N, Embleton N. Management of acute renal failure in the newborn. *Semin Fetal Neonat Med.* 2006;11:207-13.

Momtaz HE, Sabzehei MK, Rasuli B, Torabian S. The main etiologies of acute kidney injury in the newborns hospitalized in the neonatal intensive care unit. *J Clin Neonatol.* 2014;3(2):99-102.

Oliveros M, Pham JT, John E, Resheidat A, Bhat R. The use of bumetanide for oliguric acute renal failure in preterm infants. *Pediatr Crit Care Med.* 2011;12(2):210-4.

Rhone ET, Carmody JB, Swanson JR, Charlton JR. Nephrotoxic medication exposure in very low birth weight infants. *J Matern Fetal Neonatal Med.* 2014;27(14):1485-90.

Selewski D, Charlton J, Jetton J, et al. Neonatal acute kidney injury. *Pediatrics.* 2015;136(2):e463-73.

Unal S, Bilgin L, Gunduz M, Uncu N, Azili MN, Tiryaki T. The implementation of neonatal peritoneal dialysis in a clinical setting. *J Matern Fetal Neonatal Med.* 2012;25(10):2111-4.

Viswanathan S, Manyam B, Azhibekov T, Mhanna MJ. Risk factors associated with acute kidney injury in extremely low birth weight (ELBW) infants. *Pediatr Nephrol.* 2012;27(2):303-11.

Yao LP, Jose PA. Developmental renal hemodynamics. *Pediatr Nephrol.* 1995;9(5):632-7.

Zappitelli M, Ambalavanan N, Askenazi DJ, et al. Developing a neonatal acute kidney injury research definition: a report from the NIDDK neonatal AKI workshop. *Pediatr Res.* 2017;82:569.

Index

Page numbers followed by *f* or *t* indicate figures or tables, respectively.